MECHANISMS
OF MEMORY

ELSEVIER
science & technology books

ELSEVIER

 Companion Web Site:

http://books.elsevier.com/companions/9780123749512

Mechanisms of Memory, Second Edition

Resources

- **All figures from the book available as PowerPoint slides.**
- **A collection of useful student and teacher support materials.**

Related Titles:
From Molecules to Networks, Second Edition, edited by John H. Byrne and James L. Roberts, 2009, ISBN: 978-0-12-374132-5
Concise Learning and Memory: The Editor's Selection, edited by John H. Byrne, 2009, ISBN: 978-0-12-374627-6

ELSEVIER

TOOLS FOR ALL YOUR TEACHING NEEDS
textbooks.elsevier.com

ACADEMIC PRESS

MECHANISMS OF MEMORY

Second Edition

J. David Sweatt
*Department of Neurobiology
and Evelyn F. McKnight Brain Institute
University of Alabama at
Birmingham*

AMSTERDAM • BOSTON • HEIDELBERG • LONDON • NEW YORK • OXFORD
PARIS • SAN DIEGO • SAN FRANCISCO • SINGAPORE • SYDNEY • TOKYO

Academic Press is an imprint of Elsevier

Academic Press is an imprint of Elsevier
32 Jamestown Road, London NW1 7BY, UK
30 Corporate Drive, Suite 400, Burlington, MA 01803, USA
525 B Street, Suite 1900, San Diego, CA 92101-4495, USA

First edition 2003
Second edition 2010

Notice
No responsibility is assumed by the publisher for any injury and/or damage to persons
or property as a matter of products liability, negligence or otherwise, or from any use or
operation of any methods, products, instructions or ideas contained in the material herein.
Because of rapid advances in the medical sciences, in particular, independent verification
of diagnoses and drug dosages should be made

British Library Cataloguing-in-Publication Data
A catalogue record for this book is available from the British Library

Library of Congress Cataloging-in-Publication Data
A catalog record for this book is available from the Library of Congress

ISBN : 978-0-12-374951-2

For information on all Academic Press publications
visit our website at www.elsevierdirect.com

Typeset by Macmillan Publishing Solutions
www.macmillansolutions.com

Printed and bound by CPI Group (UK) Ltd, Croydon, CR0 4YY
Transferred to digital print 2013

*How small the cosmos (a kangaroo's pouch
would hold it), how paltry and puny in comparison
to human consciousness, to a single individual
recollection, and its expression in words!*

Vladimir Nabokov—from *Speak, Memory*

This book is dedicated to the memory of my mother, Evelyn Ruth Sweatt. Through some miracle, despite spending the last years of her life suffering the ravages of Alzheimer's disease, she always maintained her cheerful outlook and sweet disposition.

Contents

Foreword to the First Edition

In 1967, the neuroscientist E. Roy John published *Mechanisms of Memory,* a substantial 468-page survey of how the brain learns and remembers. Now, in 2003, the neuroscientist J. David Sweatt has written a book about memory under the same title. A consideration of the differences between the two books provides a dramatic picture of the progress that has been made in recent years. Indeed, it is striking how dissimilar the two books are, beyond the title. Building from the techniques and tools available at the time, Roy John emphasized work at a global, structural level of analysis: for example, the problem of localization of function, representation of information in assemblies of neurons, and electrophysiological correlates of learning and memory. One chapter discussed how macromolecules might be important for memory storage, but the first studies of protein synthesis inhibition and memory had been done only a few years earlier, and molecular techniques were not available to take the problem further.

David Sweatt's comprehensive book shows not only that much has happened since the 1960s, but that the field has been revolutionized. Consider the range of discoveries, tools, and ideas that are part of contemporary memory research, but which were absent altogether in the 1960s: the development of *Drosophila* and *Aplysia* as model systems for studying the genetics and the synaptic changes underlying behavioral memory, the discovery of LTP, the concept of multiple memory systems, and an entire new discipline that is delineating the biochemistry and molecular biology of short-term and long-term neural plasticity. As one of the very few books available that surveys learning and memory from molecules to behavior, *Mechanisms of Memory* (vintage 2003) provides a welcome and readable treatment of these extraordinary developments. Progress in the neuroscience of behavior follows a slower, more gradual course than molecular biology or biochemistry, but across the time spanned by these two books about the mechanisms of memory, the progress is breathtaking.

Larry R. Squire
March, 2003

Preface to the First Edition

This book is primarily intended for advanced undergraduates, graduate students, and researchers interested in learning and memory. After a brief introduction to the basics of learning and memory at the psychological level, the book will describe current understanding of memory at the molecular and cellular level. Particular emphasis will be on the hippocampus and its role in declarative and spatial learning, although examples from other anatomical and behavioral systems will also be used. As the book overall progresses from chapter to chapter, I will deliberately move from well-established facts and background, to a description of current work and thinking in the area, to at last what should be clearly labeled speculation.

In my opinion, this book is appropriate for use in advanced undergraduate and graduate-level learning and memory courses, courses that typically are based in Psychology, Biology, and Neuroscience Departments at the University and Medical School levels. I hope that it provides a nice foundation for thinking about the molecular underpinnings of synaptic plasticity and information storage. However, the book is primarily targeted to active researchers (at all stages of their career development) in the learning and memory fields.

One goal of the book is to begin to embrace the complexity of mechanisms of learning and memory at the molecular level. Some who work on the cellular processes of learning and memory seem to want to ignore this complexity, deny its existence, or throw up their hands in frustration and imply that the problem is insoluble. I share none of these viewpoints. My hope in this book is to begin to organize a framework of thinking about synaptic plasticity and memory at the molecular level—one which recognizes and begins to incorporate this extreme biochemical complexity

into our thinking about memory. I note that building these models is at a relatively early stage, but one thing the reader hopefully will take from the book is some perspective on where we stand at present and where the future may lie.

Most of us have seen the large and complex schematic diagrams summarizing intermediary metabolism. Hundreds of discrete and highly regulated enzymatic steps are necessary for the relatively basic function of converting glucose into ATP. How can memory be any less complex than that at the molecular level? Human learning and memory is likely the most highly evolved and sophisticated biological process in existence. In my view, the ultimate molecular understanding of learning and memory will make processes such as intermediary metabolism seem simple in comparison. This book represents one first step at beginning to put together the complex puzzle of the molecular basis of memory.

While a strong case can be made that the molecular basis of memory will of necessity be quite complex at the biochemical level, a more difficult argument arises as to whether understanding these processes is even really important. Is it molecular stamp collecting? If all the nervous system really cares about is the firing of action potentials, isn't the underlying biochemistry really just housekeeping? A second point that I want to try to make with this book is that understanding the underlying molecular basis *is* important. Where possible, I will try to utilize examples illustrating that various molecular processes are being used for information processing; information processing that occurs at a level independent of patterns of action potential firing. Also, I want to highlight that action potentials and neurons *per se* are incapable of *storing* information. That is because all biological processes are subserved by biochemical phenomena. This book is written from the perspective that, in the limit, neurons are bags of chemicals and the fundamental unit of information storage is the molecule.

This book seeks to take the reader from a basic background of learning theory and synaptic physiology, to a detailed discussion of the biochemical mechanisms of long-term changes in synaptic function and information storage, to a discussion of the molecular basis of learning and memory disorders. Themes that are highlighted include:

- Genes and gene regulation in memory formation.
- The role of long-term changes in synaptic function in memory.
- Does Long Term Potentiation = Memory?
- Multimodal signal integration at the molecular level and its role in cognition as related to memory.
- Learning disorders with a focus on mental retardation syndromes.
- Memory disorders with a focus on Alzheimer's Disease.
- The biochemical basis of cellular information processing.
- Biochemical mechanisms for information storage.

A few comments concerning references are in order. There have been many thousands of publications in the fields that are covered by this book. The chapters covering LTP biochemistry, which is the area that the book covers in the greatest detail, are drawn from about 900 primary publications. Some single paragraphs in these sections summarize work from about 50 different research papers. In writing the book, I had to make a decision—I could write sentences like "Postsynaptic calcium is known to be involved in LTP induction: blocking a rise in postsynaptic calcium blocks LTP induction, elevating postsynaptic calcium elicits synaptic potentiation, and a rise in postsynaptic calcium has been shown to occur with LTP-inducing stimulation." Or I could write sentences like "X et al, Y et al, and Z et al. showed that injecting calcium chelators postsynaptically blocked LTP induction, P et al., Q et al, and Z et al. showed that...." The latter type of sentence, the historical narrative, obviously has

a more scholarly tone and gives appropriate credit to X et al., etc. However, it rapidly leads to bloated verbiage that is much more difficult to read. Taking all this into consideration, I decided to handle the citations in the following way. At the end of each chapter is a section titled "References" which is a little different from the typical list of references in terms of its content. It is not exhaustive. "References" is the short list of papers that were the principal papers I used in preparing the chapter, and there is a distinct bias toward citing reviews that I feel are particularly lucid and informative. In a real sense, the references are my list of recommended readings for further information. The cited reviews are a place where readers looking for more detailed references can find citations to the extensive list of primary literature. I apologize in advance to the many researchers whose primary papers I have not cited directly.

I strongly encourage anyone with any complaint, correction, criticism or suggested addition to e-mail me (david@cns. neusc.bcm.tmc.edu). Constructive criticism is the only means by which the content of the book may be improved in the future. So, when John Lisman wants to fire off a scathing critique of my inadequate representation of his work, I encourage him to send me an e-mail so that I can take his comments into consideration in future writing efforts. I want to emphasize that I encourage everyone to do this. I want the post-doc who spent two years optimizing assays for measuring protein kinase activation, so that they could measure an LTP-associated increase in CaMKII, to be able to e-mail me and get at least some recognition for their effort. In cases like this it is likely to be helpful to send me the relevant citation and a few sentences describing its significance and relevance. The overall goal of encouraging this sort of interaction is to allow a means for dynamically correcting and updating the book content.

Finally, I am more than happy to share Powerpoint files containing the figures from the book with anyone who would like to use them for teaching purposes, etc. An e-mail to the above address will suffice to get that particular ball rolling.

David Sweatt

Preface to the
Second Edition

In the six years since the publication of the first edition of *Mechanisms of Memory*, I have had many students tell me how much they appreciated the easy readability and relatively informal writing style that I used in writing the first edition of the book. For the second edition, I have striven to maintain that approach to the writing. I also have maintained a narrative approach to writing the second edition, trying to tell stories about the overall development of the field of memory research, and providing various anecdotal descriptions of specific seminal experiments in this area. These two aspects of the first edition, the story-telling approach and the informal writing style, were likely the most appealing aspects of the book from the "student perspective," based on the feedback I received. As with the first edition, I apologize in advance to all the many memory scientists whose specific work is not cited in detail, citations sacrificed on the altar of readability.

I have also tried to make this edition more student-friendly in new ways. For one thing, there is greater breadth to this edition, including new sections on human memory and cognition, working memory, neuroimaging, and "simple" invertebrate model systems. I feel these additions make the text more useful as an introductory volume. I have also included an appendix on hypothesis testing and experimental design that I hope will be very useful to aspiring young scientists, to help give them a framework for thinking about designing research projects. Finally, based on feedback that I have had from other instructors, I have diminished the level of detail of the multitudinous molecular mechanisms that contribute to memory formation, so that the text is at least somewhat more tractable for students not as well-versed in molecular biology and biochemistry.

I have also kept the teachers in mind in preparing the second edition, and this has manifested itself in several ways. As has always been the case, all the figures (plus some) for the book are available on my book website (http://www.neurobiology.uab.edu/sweatt_lab) freely available for download. (If anyone has any problems accessing them, just send me an e-mail at: dsweatt@uab.edu.) I have also added some new types of references. First, there is now a list of further reading at the end of each chapter that provides good sources of basic background information and additional specific topic-related information. I also have added recommended "Journal Club" articles that students can be assigned for outside reading. These articles are chosen to be representative of classic papers in the field, as examples of modern approaches to studying memory, or as representing particularly hot topics in the memory area. All of these papers will serve as good case studies for further detailed reading for students participating in any class based on this textbook.

Finally, I know that in many cases specific individual instructors will want to address particular topics in more detail than is presented in this book. Fortunately, there is now a comprehensive series of books available, comprising up-to-date chapters written by leading experts in specific areas of the memory field. The series is published by Elsevier and is titled *Learning and Memory, a Comprehensive Reference* (Jack Byrne, Series Editor, specific volumes edited by Howard Eichenbaum, Roddy Roediger, Randolph Menzel, and David Sweatt). The recent reviews published in this series are excellent, detailed reviews on specific topics that are touched on in the chapters in this book. I feel that many instructors (or advanced students) may wish to delve more deeply into the details of particular areas of memory research, or instructors may wish to assign advanced topics for term papers, etc. For this reason at the end of each chapter I have cross-referenced specific chapters from the *Learning and Memory, a Comprehensive Reference* series that relate to topics covered in the chapter. I feel that the combination of *Mechanisms of Memory* as a launching point for further reading, coupled with the detailed up-to-date information available in the *Learning and Memory, a Comprehensive Reference* series, provides an unparalleled resource for instruction in the area of memory mechanisms. Additional information for accessing reviews in the *Learning and Memory, a Comprehensive Reference* series is also available on my book website.

One overall goal of the book is to begin to embrace the complexity of mechanisms of learning and memory at the molecular level. My hope in this book is to begin to organize a framework of thinking about synaptic plasticity and memory at the molecular level—one which recognizes and begins to incorporate the known biochemical complexity into our thinking about memory. I note that building these models is at a relatively early stage, but one thing the reader will hopefully take from the book is some perspective on where we stand at present, and where the future may lie.

Most of us have seen the large and complex schematic diagrams summarizing intermediary metabolism. Hundreds of discrete and highly regulated enzymatic steps are necessary for the relatively basic function of converting glucose into ATP. How can memory be any less complex than that at the molecular level? Human learning and memory is likely the most highly evolved and sophisticated biological process in existence. In my view, the ultimate molecular understanding of learning and memory will make processes such as intermediary metabolism seem simple in comparison. This book represents one first step at

beginning to put together the complex puzzle of the molecular basis of memory.

This book seeks to take the reader from a basic background of learning theory and basic studies of human memory, to the level of synaptic physiology, and thence to a more detailed discussion of the biochemical mechanisms of long-term changes in synaptic function and information storage. The book finishes with a discussion of the molecular basis of learning and memory disorders, discussing clinical syndromes that are associated with human memory malfunction.

Themes that are highlighted include:

- Multiple memory systems in human cognition.
- Genes and epigenetic regulation in memory formation.
- The role of long-term changes in synaptic function in memory.
- The NMDA receptor as an information processing nexus.
- Multimodal signal integration at the cellular and molecular level and its role in cognition as related to memory.
- Learning disorders with a focus on mental retardation syndromes.
- Memory disorders with a focus on Alzheimer's disease.
- Invertebrate model systems for studying memory mechanisms.
- Biochemical mechanisms for perpetual information storage.

Finally, I strongly encourage anyone with any complaint, correction, criticism or suggested addition to e-mail me at: dsweatt@uab.edu.

David Sweatt
Memory Lane
Trussville Alabama

Acknowledgements

I want to begin by profusely thanking Felecia Hester for all the great work she did in putting together the second edition of *Mechanisms of Memory*. Felecia was my collaborator in all aspects of preparing the book for publication, she read every sentence with an editorial eye, and prepared many of the figures in the book. Preparing the book literally would not have been possible without her, and I thank her deeply and sincerely.

I also wish to thank my wife, Kim Strifert, to whom the first edition was dedicated. I am fortunate beyond belief to be married to such an interesting, encouraging, deep-thinking, and beautiful woman.

I have received tremendous support from the University of Alabama at Birmingham, and I thank my many colleagues here for their support, encouragement, and helpful discussions. I also thank the Evelyn F. McKnight Brain Research Foundation for their strong support in making so many great things possible here at the Evelyn F. McKnight Brain Institute. I gratefully acknowledge the research support I have received over the years from the NIH, in particular from the NIMH, NIA, and NINDS.

I thank my many colleagues and collaborators, from whom I have learned much over the years. I especially thank my former and current students and post-docs, from whom I have learned much more than I ever taught.

I also would like to thank my editor, Johannes Menzel, for his infectious enthusiasm for the book project and numerous suggestions to help improve the book, as well as his associate Clare Caruana for her help and input on many aspects of the book. The anonymous reviewers of the book proposal and the anonymous readers of the first edition who provided feedback also deserve recognition for their contributions in making the book better—they made many useful suggestions that I incorporated into the text.

Finally, I would like to specifically thank the many scientists who allowed me to use figures illustrating their research results and important concepts.

MECHANISMS
OF MEMORY

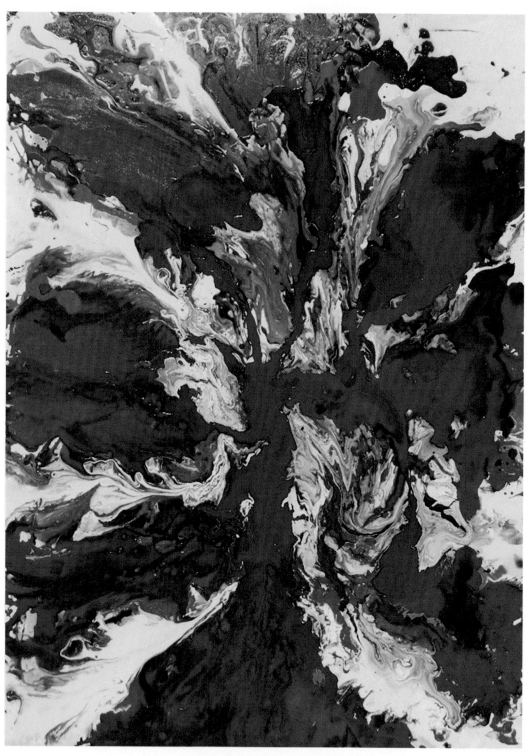

Multiple Memory Systems
J. David Sweatt, acrylic on canvas, 2008–2009

1

Introduction

*The Basics of Psychological Learning
and Memory Theory*

I. INTRODUCTION

Knowledge is power and learning is the tool we use to get it. For that reason humans have evolved extremely sophisticated mechanisms for learning new information and storing it for subsequent recall. This book will be a description of recent laboratory discoveries that have begun to scratch the surface of the amazingly complex phenomenon of learning and memory, focusing on their cellular and molecular bases.

An understanding of the cellular and molecular basis of learning and memory of course requires a firm foundation in understanding the behavioral processes these mechanisms subserve. This first chapter serves as an introduction to the basics of learning and memory, its theory and terminology. This will provide you with the fundamental terms most psychologists use to describe the types and forms of learning and memory that we will be discussing throughout the book.

What is learning? Before we can begin to effectively discuss categorizing types of learning and memory, it is useful to define both of the terms we will be using extensively throughout this book: "learning" and "memory." Both of these terms are so widely used and implicitly understood that there is a great temptation to say "learning is when you learn something and memory is when you remember it." This type of definition obviously is not going to take us very far.

Upon serious reflection it becomes clear that neither "learning" nor "memory" is easy to define, and indeed learning and memory psychologists continue to debate these definitions to this day. In this book we will define learning as: the acquisition of an *altered* behavioral response due to an environmental stimulus. In other words, learning is when an animal changes its behavior pattern in response to an experience. Note that what is defined is a change in a behavior from a pre-existing baseline. Don't get confused: learning is not a response to an environmental stimulus, but rather is an alteration in that response due to an environmental stimulus. An animal has a baseline response, experiences an environmental signal, and then has an altered response different from its previous response. This is learning (see Figure 1).

Memory is defined as the storage of the learned item, which of course must be subject to recall by some mechanism.

These definitions are functional definitions that lend themselves to experimental application. An experimentalist has to be able to observe something (and ideally measure it) in order to be able to test a hypothesis. The definitions of learning and memory that are used in this book derive directly from the experimentalist mindset. This practical orientation is both a strength and a weakness for the definitions— their ready application in practice leads to limitations for their use in theory.

For example, one criticism of this definition of learning is that it is too narrow. If someone learns my name and stores it as a perfectly legitimate memory, that learned item may never be manifest as an altered behavioral output on their part. This is a completely valid theoretical criticism and a limitation to the definition. The rebuttal to this argument is that in order for one to ever prove that such a memory exists, one would have to demonstrate an altered behavioral

output on the part of the person involved. For example, an experimenter would have to have them respond with "David" instead of "I don't know" when they showed them my picture. Nevertheless, it is important to remember that this definition is based in experimentation, not theory.

At the other end of the spectrum is the criticism that the definition is too broad. It certainly covers many types of alterations in behavior, such as simple sensitization and habituation, which most people would not consider as "real" learning (this is illustrated in Box 1, for example). Nevertheless, a considerable body of literature is available indicating that many simple forms of behavioral modification qualify as learned responses, and most researchers in the field agree with this. These forms of simple, non-associative learning are described in Section III of this chapter, and in more detail in Chapter 3 of this book.

A. Categories of Learning and Memory

This broad, umbrella-like definition of learning covers so many different types of behavioral modifications that some sort of organizing principle and attendant nomenclature are called for. We will use an organizational framework developed and promulgated by Larry Squire and Eric Kandel (1–3). As a starting point we will use their system, and I would be remiss if I did not credit their many significant and influential contributions in this area.

In this scheme human memory is typically divided into declarative and non-declarative types, also known respectively as explicit and implicit memory (see Figure 2). This type of system, subdividing memory into several separately identified components, distills the modern concept of multiple memory systems. It is now clear that different anatomical structures in the brain are involved in different types of memory formation. Moreover, the different systems can operate as parallel processors, operating independently. This allows multi-tasking, with conscious and unconscious memory systems operating simultaneously and increasing the overall "memory throughput" of the CNS. Figure 2 briefly summarizes the major subdivisions of human memory, along with the associated known areas of the CNS that are involved in those specific types of memory. We will discuss most of the major subdivisions listed in Figure 2 in greater detail later in this chapter, and in Chapter 3 of this book.

The multiple memory systems concept is important and soundly based on functional neuroanatomy. However, a different, cognitively based framework is also useful to consider. This additional system is based on whether different types of learning and memory are

Learning:	The acquisition of an altered behavioral response due to an environmental stimulus.
Memory:	The processes through which learned information is stored.
Recall:	The conscious or unconscious retrieval process through which this altered behavior is manifest.

FIGURE 1   Definitions of learning, memory, and recall.

BOX 1

LEARNING IN A PLANT? "SENSITIZATION" IN THE VENUS' FLYTRAP

Our functional definition of learning is: a change in an animal's behavioral responses as a result of a unique environmental stimulus. This broad definition is useful in that it encompasses various non-associative forms of learning such as sensitization and habituation, but the breadth of the definition can be criticized. This can be illustrated by consideration of "sensitization" in the Venus' flytrap plant.

Although plants are not thought of expressing behavior in the same sense as animals, plants can and do respond to environmental stimuli. We are all familiar with the phototactic responses of plants as they turn to follow the sun, foliage changes in response to cooling weather, and the nocturnal closing of certain flowers, just to name a few simple examples. However, these types of responses are really more akin to reflexive, non-learned behaviors in animals.

One intriguingly complex, multi-component response of a plant to an environmental stimulus is exhibited by *Dionaea muscipula*, commonly known as the Venus' flytrap. This carnivorous plant, indigenous to the peat bogs of the Carolinas in the southeastern United States, supplements its nutrition by capturing and digesting insects. Insects are trapped by *Dionaea* when they land in one of the plant's V-shaped leaves, which closes on the hapless victim like a miniature steel bear trap.

It is the triggering mechanism for closure of the trap that warrants our attention. Each half of the V-shaped trap has on its inward facing surface three trigger hairs. Mechanical stimulation of these hairs is what elicits closure of the trap. To eliminate "false alarms," *Dionaea*

has evolved a mechanism whereby stimulation of a single trigger hair is insufficient to cause closure of the trap. Two hairs must be stimulated in succession (or simultaneously) to trigger a trapping response. Thus, in one circumstance stimulating a particular trigger hair will give no response, whereas depending on recent history stimulating the same trigger hair will in another instance give trap closure. This is clearly an example of an altered response that depends on a prior environmental stimulus. In a sense, the mechanical stimulation of the first trigger hair could be viewed as analogous to "sensitizing" the plant, in order that it respond to the mechanical stimulation of the second hair. Venus' flytrap photograph by Muriel Weinerman.

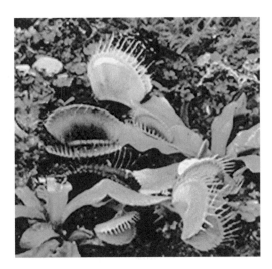

---

consciously or unconsciously processed. Thus, using this system one can divide learning into two broad classes—unconscious learning and conscious learning. For the purposes of this framework we also introduce a "recall" term (see Figure 3), and apply conscious and unconscious to it as well. Thus, any type of memory (with one exception, see below) falls into one of four categories: unconscious learning with unconscious recall; unconscious learning subject to conscious recall; conscious learning subject to unconscious recall; and conscious learning subject to conscious recall. Specific examples of each category are listed in Figure 3 for

illustrative purposes, and for the rest of this chapter and in Chapters 2 through 6 we will cover many specific examples in each category.

The nomenclature summarized in Figure 3 emphasizes that any given memory event is comprised of three components: learning; storage; and recall. An item or event is learned, stored for some period of time, and recalled. Highlighting these three components is necessary, because each corresponds to a distinct molecular and cellular set of events.

It is also important to note that the category for the learning, memory, and recall of a specific bit of

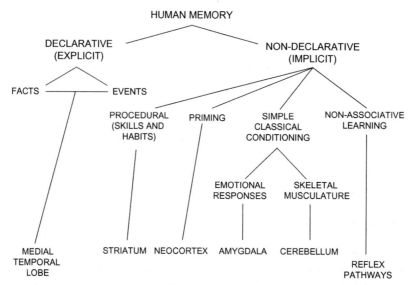

FIGURE 2 Subdivisions of human memory and associated brain regions. Human memory is typically divided into declarative and non-declarative types, also known as explicit and implicit memory, respectively. In addition to various types of memory described in the text, priming is also listed. Priming is unconscious memory formation. An example of priming is if one hears or reads a word, for a period of time afterward one is more likely to use that word in conversation or in a word completion task. This occurs even if no conscious memory for having heard the word is formed. Chart adapted from Milner, Squire, and Kandel (13).

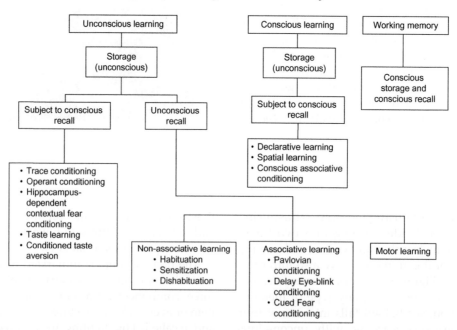

FIGURE 3 Hierarchical organization of memory. Short-term and long-term memory is subject to being learned by either conscious or unconscious processes. Similarly, memory can be recalled either consciously or unconsciously. Many forms of simple learning such as motor learning, simple associative conditioning, and non-associative learning can be learned and recalled unconsciously. More complex forms of learning typically involve conscious processes. Short-term working memory is listed as a separate category because it is essentially entirely conscious and not stored for more than a few seconds.

information is not static over time, but subject to change. This can be illustrated by considering the learning and recollection of a phone number that becomes familiar with repetition. One first looks up the number and consciously stores and recalls the number. Over time one repetitively punches in the number and it is subject to being learned unconsciously as a motor pattern, and recalled unconsciously in the same way. This is one example of how the same bit of information, over time, can be subject to conscious learning, unconscious learning, conscious recall, and unconscious recall.

Finally, note that storage is unconscious in this model. This emphasizes the underlying nature of the storage mechanisms—they do not require ongoing conscious rehearsal. This has critically important implications concerning the cellular and molecular processes that underlie memory storage. They must be stable and capable of self-perpetuation in the absence of ongoing conscious input.

This is not to say that all forms of memory are stored unconsciously—clearly several forms of short-term "working" memory are conscious. A good example of this is short-term storage of a phone number, where one can store information over time essentially by conscious repetition over a given time span. However, this form of memory is in a separate category from longer-term forms of memory from a cellular and molecular perspective (see Figure 3). Working memory can be stored as a short-term change in firing pattern in cortical neurons, for example in a reverberating circuit. As such, it does not require any persisting biochemical modification for its maintenance. Indeed, at the molecular level this seems likely to be the distinguishing characteristic of working memory. It is memory that cannot sustain itself in the absence of continuing neuronal firing.

These categories of learning and memory roughly correspond to the typically used "non-declarative memory" and "declarative memory" nomenclature popularized by Squire and Kandel (Figure 2), and widely accepted and utilized. I also emphasize the conscious/unconscious terminology because it highlights the cognitive differences between the two forms. Most importantly, this terminology semantically separates the learning from the memory storage from the recall—an important mindset to adapt as we seek to understand learning and memory events in molecular terms.

B. Memory Exhibits Long-Term and Short-Term Forms

Emphasized by Eric Kandel, Jim McGaugh, and many others (4), almost all forms of memory can be either short-lasting or long-lasting. With only a few exceptions (see Box 2), the duration of the memory for a learned event depends on the number of times an animal experiences a behavior-modifying stimulus. For example, a single repetition (or "training trial") may elicit a memory that lasts only a few minutes, whereas repeated stimulations will likely result in memory lasting hours to days. Repeated presentations of multiple training trials can elicit memory lasting for even more prolonged periods, up to the lifetime of the animal. Thus, the acquisition of memory is a *graded* phenomenon (see Figure 4).

One exciting area of contemporary learning research is to try to understand the basis for this attribute. It is intriguing to wonder how repeated presentations of the identical environmental stimulus can uniquely elicit a long-lasting behavioral alteration, especially when one considers that the behavioral output (e.g., enhanced responsiveness) is identical in the short- and long-lasting forms. This is still fairly mysterious at present for the various mammalian systems that we will be discussing; however, significant progress has been made addressing this issue in the *Aplysia* invertebrate model system that will be discussed in Chapter 3.

Long-term memory also has the general attribute that it undergoes a period of consolidation. Decades ago it was discovered that, for a period of time after the training period, generally on the order of hours, memories that were normally destined to become long-term memories were susceptible to disruption. Disruption of nascent long-term memories can be brought about by trauma, for example, or in a more refined manipulation application of inhibitors of protein synthesis can block memory consolidation (Figure 5). Thus it is clear that some set of molecular processes is occurring for some period of time after the training trial, which are necessary for memory to be established as truly long-lasting. Once the critical time window has passed, the same disruptive manipulations have no effect on memory storage. Studies of the cellular and molecular mechanisms contributing to the consolidation of long-term memory will be an area of emphasis in Chapters 2, 3, 6, and 10 of this book.

There has been a resurgence of interest in the consolidation phenomenon lately because several groups have reported that previously stored memories are subject to disruption in certain circumstances. Specifically, for some types of memory an event already learned and stored in long-term memory is selectively subject to disruption when it is recalled. The basic experimental observation is that while protein synthesis inhibitors do not wipe out stored memory, the same protein synthesis inhibitor treatment will disrupt memory if the subject is simultaneously

BOX 2

NON-GRADED ACQUISITION OF MEMORY—FOOD AVERSION AND IMPRINTING

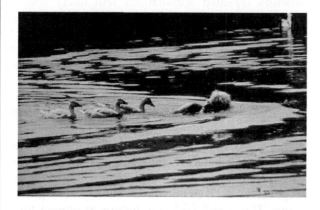

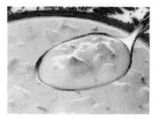

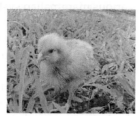

While most forms of long-term memory exhibit graded acquisition, some types of learning are so critical to an animal's survival that extremely robust learning mechanisms have evolved to subserve them. One striking example of this is *conditioned food avoidance*.

Generally, if an animal consumes a novel foodstuff that subsequently causes sickness, even after a single such experience the animal will exhibit a life-long aversion to that particular food. While for animals in the wild the survival value of this type of learning is obvious, the phenomenon can have unintended consequences. For example, I once got food poisoning after eating a bowl of New England clam chowder; to this day even the sight of a can of New England clam chowder on the grocery store shelf is enough to send me scurrying to the next aisle. This is a textbook case of conditioned food avoidance—being from Alabama, I had never had clam anything until that day. I certainly will fastidiously avoid future clam encounters of any kind.

While I have not personally experienced it, hatchling chicks exhibit a robust form of learning termed *imprinting*. A newborn bird will develop a strong, long-lasting affinity for whatever it sees in the first hour after hatching. In one famous example, a group of young geese imprinted on the experimental ethologist Konrad Lorenz. In experimental situations chicks will even imprint on inanimate objects, such as red boxes or dolls. Of course, in the wild this type of learning serves a useful purpose, as hatchlings will almost always first see their mother and imprint upon her. The chicks will then stick close by the mother as she guides and protects them through the perilous fledgling period.

required to recall the information (5–6). Thus, pairing protein synthesis inhibitors with a behavioral task requiring information recall can lead to a selective loss of a previously stored memory from long-term stores. This intriguing process is referred to as reconsolidation of memory. The necessity for a process of memory reconsolidation highlights the fact that previously formed, apparently stable, memories are labile after recall, and must be restabilized for continued storage.

The process of memory reconsolidation also illustrates that recall is its own unique process; recall is not simply a passive process that does not impact the underlying memory storage mechanism. Rather, recall, in at least some instances, directly impacts the molecular and cellular processes underlying memory storage

(the *engram*), changing them at least transiently and triggering a new process of memory reconsolidation.

Finally, to round out our terminology we need to introduce three terms related to the loss or suppression of memories: extinction; forgetting; and latent inhibition. Forgetting is woefully familiar to most of us, and its basis is essentially unexplored. At a minimum it can be defined as a failure over time of the storage or recall processes.

Extinction is the specific erasure of a previous memory in response to a new environmental stimulus. Extinction has largely been studied in the context of reversal of learning. For example, if your cafeteria serves hamburgers every Monday you will learn over time that the cafeteria always serves hamburgers on Monday. If at some later point they stop serving

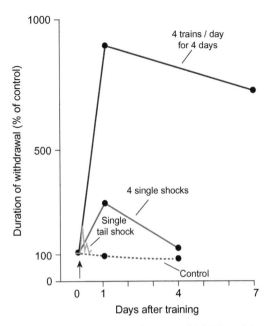

FIGURE 4 Graded acquisition of memory. Multiple training trials typically result in more robust and long-lasting memory formation. In this case sensitization of the gill-withdrawal reflex in *Aplysia californica* was measured by quantitating the duration of gill withdrawal in response to a slight touch (duration of withdrawal, Y-axis). Delivery of a tail shock to the animal elicits sensitization, and an increase in the magnitude of the protective gill withdrawal reflex (see Box 3 and text). Increasing numbers of training trials (tail shocks) increases both the duration of the memory (days of duration) and the magnitude of the learned response. Adapted from Kandel (14).

A few words about the particulars of the *Aplysia* model system are appropriate at this point, although we will discuss this system in much greater detail in later parts of the book. Much (but by no means all) of the work in *Aplysia* has been geared toward understanding the basis of sensitization in this animal. *Aplysia* has on its dorsum a respiratory gill-and-siphon complex, which is normally extended when the animal is in the resting state. If the gill or siphon is lightly touched (or experimentally, squirted with a Water-Pic), this elicits a defensive withdrawal reflex in order to protect the gill from potential damage. This defensive withdrawal reflex can undergo both habituation (by repeated light stimuli) and sensitization. Sensitization occurs when the animal receives an aversive stimulus, for example a modest tail-shock experimentally or a predatory nip in the wild (see Box 3). After sensitizing stimulation, the animal exhibits a more robust, longer-lasting gill-withdrawal in response to the identical light touch or water squirt. Acquisition of this sensitization response is graded; repetitive sensitizing stimuli can give sensitization lasting minutes to hours (one to a few shocks), or weeks (repeated training trials over a few days). We will return to the *Aplysia* system in later chapters of the book, where we will discuss several of the biochemical mechanisms underlying the short- and long-term modification of this behavioral response.

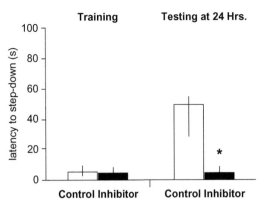

FIGURE 5 Protein synthesis inhibitors block consolidation of long-term memory. Inhibitors of protein synthesis typically block the ability of learned information to be consolidated into a long-lasting form. In this experiment rats were trained in a step-down avoidance paradigm (see Chapter 4). Animals are placed on an elevated platform in the middle of an electric grid and receive a mild foot shock when they step down from the platform. On the training day animals that received a saline infusion (CONTROL) or the protein synthesis inhibitor anisomycin (INHIBITOR) both quickly step down from the platform (latency to step-down, Y-axis). Twenty-four hours later the control animals exhibit a much longer latency to step down, indicating that they have learned to avoid the electrified floor. Animals treated with protein synthesis inhibitor have not consolidated their memory for the step-down training, and exhibit a short latency to step down just as they did on the first day. Additional experiments (not shown) have demonstrated that anisomycin treatment immediately after training is also effective at blocking memory consolidation, indicating that consolidation is a post-training phenomenon (5).

hamburgers on Monday it will take a while to relearn that contingency. Over time, you will no longer assume that if it's Monday that means hamburgers, and similarly will no longer infer that if they are serving hamburgers then it is Monday. This disassociation is an example of extinguishing a previously learned response. This is an extinction of a memory that Monday means hamburgers. Similar to forgetting, the unique mechanisms underlying extinction have not been extensively studied. One intriguing speculation is that the reconsolidation mechanism may be involved in some cases, the thinking being that perhaps reconsolidation is the process that has evolved to allow specific erasure of previously learned material, by opening up a period of susceptibility on recall (5–6).

Latent inhibition is the mirror image of extinction. Latent inhibition refers to the capacity of prior experience to suppress ("inhibit") new learning. The "latent" in latent inhibition refers to the attribute that the process is passive and not generally recognizable until one observes a failure of learning. Latent inhibition can be illustrated by the following example. Over a lifetime of food consumption you passively and unconsciously learn a wide variety of tastes. Familiar tastes from foods that you have repeatedly consumed are not subject to conditioned food avoidance (see Box 2) if they are paired with a nausea-inducing agent. The prior experience with the familiar taste leads to latent inhibition of subsequent aversive conditioning; having a latent memory that the taste has not been previously associated with malaise leads to an inhibition of the formation of a new, different association.

II. SHORT-TERM MEMORY

The quickest, earliest stages of memory of necessity deal with processing transient sensory and perceptual stimuli. The buffers for holding onto sensory information for seconds or a few minutes after their termination in the environment are referred to as *short-term memory*. The short-term memory system is divided into three basic components: sensory memory; short-term storage; and working memory, each with different functions.

It is important to realize that short-term memory is bidirectional. It is clear that short-term memory deals with sensory perceptions as already mentioned, but short-term memory also handles information that is recently recalled from long-term stores. Thus, short-term memory is both an input device and an output device. It not only handles new information freshly perceived, it also handles old information freshly recalled. Old information must be brought forward into a short-term memory store for utilization, and this is also a component of short-term memory.

A. Sensory Memory and Short-Term Storage

The first component of the short-term memory system deals exclusively with freshly perceived information, for example the face of someone you have just met. The sensory input (visual in this example) begins its journey into memory by passing into the first stage of the short-term memory system. This initial, transient stage of sensory information storage is referred to as sensory memory, or the sensory register (Figure 6A). While it is difficult to define exactly when perception ceases and short-term memory takes over, it is clear that sensory input, be it touch, taste, smell, sight or sound, must pass into a short-term store in order to be further processed as part of a lasting memory.

The sensory register is the first stage of processing new information into a memory. Presumably, each different sensory system has dedicated components of the sensory register that contribute to passing its unique information along to memory. However, two sensory registers have been widely studied, and have been poetically named. *Echoic memory* refers to the auditory sensory store, while *iconic memory* refers to the visual store.

Short-term storage refers to retention of information in the short-term system after the information has been processed and has reached consciousness. The "processing" may have been either the processing of new sensory input, or processing in the sense of recalling a previously stored memory, hence short-term storage operates on both new and old information (Figure 6A). In the case of handling new information, short-term storage may operate as a step in the sequence of events leading to long-term storage of that information.

If a person is distracted, information is rapidly lost from short-term storage. One commonly-used technique to counteract this fact (in humans at least) is ongoing repetition or rehearsal of the information held in short-term storage (Figure 6A). As a first approximation, the information in your short-term storage is the information of which you are consciously aware.

B. Working Memory

It is possible to hold a fact in short-term storage without doing anything with it. However, if the information is manipulated and further processed in any way, it is referred to as being held in working memory. Thus, the term working memory refers specifically to the type of memory system used to hold information for short periods of time while it is being utilized. A simple example is doing arithmetic calculations using remembered numbers (what is 4×56?). Mentally multiplying 4×56 is clearly a different memory task than simply remembering the number 224 for a few seconds.

Alan Baddeley has presented a refined model of the working memory component of short-term memory that is a significant addition to the simpler multi-store model presented in the previous section and in Figure 6A. In the Baddeley model, the passive sensory registers and short-term stores (Figure 6A) are also augmented by a working memory module (Figure 6B).

In the Baddeley module, three different storage systems contribute to the working memory component of short-term memory. The phonological loop is responsible for short-term storage of auditory and spoken language information. Limitations to the capacity of the phonological loop are responsible for the familiar limits on digit-span memory capacity, for example. The visuospatial sketchpad is conceptually similar to the phonological loop, except that it deals with visual and spatial information. The episodic buffer is the component that deals with holding and manipulating information recently recalled from long-term storage. These three components are regulated by a central executive system that coordinates and integrates their functions.

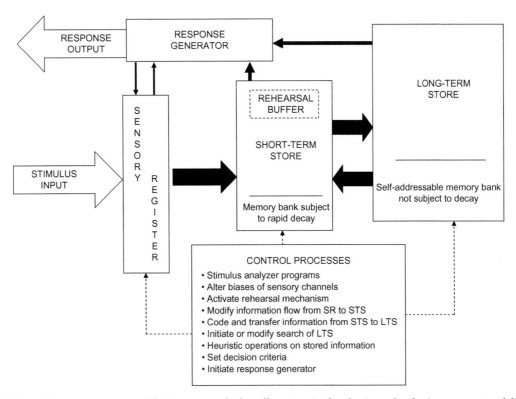

FIGURE 6A The multi-store memory model. Memory can be broadly categorized as having a few basic components, delineated by the timing of their participation. Sensory input impinges upon sensory organs (eyes, ears, etc.) and is held very briefly as a perception in a sensory register. Information then traverses to a short-term store where it is held (and potentially rehearsed and processed) for seconds to minutes. From the short-term store the information may be passed on for long-term storage for minutes to years. Higher-order control mechanism and processes such as attention-related systems orchestrate the overall process. (SR = sensory register; STS = short-term store; LTS = long-term store). Adapted, with permission, from the work of Shiffrin and Atkinson (1969). "Storage and retrieval processes in long-term memory." *Psychological Review* 76:179–193. Copyright 1969 by the American Psychological Association.

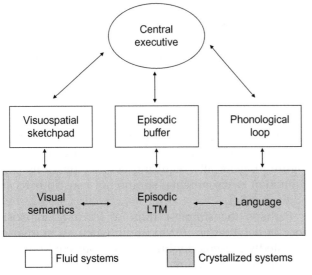

FIGURE 6B Baddeley's working memory module. An executive control system regulates the integration of three basic components of the working memory system. The system overall coordinates the processing of visual sensory information, verbal language, and information recalled from long-term episodic memory stores. (LTM = long-term memory). Adapted with permission from Baddeley (2001). "Is working memory still working?" *Am. Psychol.* 56:849–864. Copyright 2001 by the American Psychological Association.

C. The Prefrontal Cortex and Working Memory

What brain region does the work in working memory? There is very strong experimental support that the prefrontal cortex (PFC) is one anatomical site subserving working memory. The PFC in humans is large, is located in the rostral part of the frontal lobes, and occupies about one-third of the cerebral cortex. The PFC is immediately rostral to the premotor and motor cortices, and is extensively interconnected with other parts of the cerebral cortex and the hippocampus.

The laboratory of the late Patricia Goldman-Rakic pioneered studies in non-human primates that demonstrated a role for the PFC in working memory. These elegant studies combined discrete anatomical lesioning approaches, pharmacologic studies, and direct recordings *in vivo* from the PFC during working memory tasks. More recently, these studies have been reinforced by studies in humans using functional magnetic resonance imaging (fMRI).

Altogether, a convincing case has been made that the PFC contributes to working memory, and indeed Goldman-Rakic and colleagues have proposed that different PFC subregions contribute to different

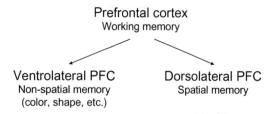

FIGURE 7 Anatomical subdomains of working memory. This model is based on work by Goldman-Rakic and co-workers.

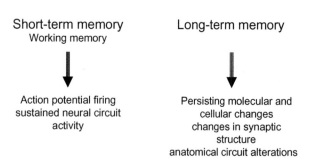

FIGURE 8 Mechanisms for storing short-term memory are distinct from those underlying long-term memory.

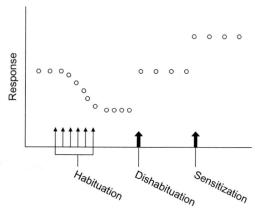

FIGURE 9 Some simple non-associative forms of learning. Habituation, dishabituation and sensitization are illustrated. Each circle represents a hypothetical response to an environmental stimulus. Habituation is a decrease in response (arbitrarily defined in this schematic example) with repeated presentation of the stimulus. Dishabituation is a recovery to normal baseline response when the animal receives a different environmental stimulus. Sensitization is an increase in the magnitude of the response above the original baseline.

III. UNCONSCIOUS LEARNING

A. Simple Forms of Learning

In this section we will explore several "simple," i.e., non-associative, forms of learning. Keep in mind that even those forms of learning that exhibit themselves in a fairly straightforward manner at the behavioral level involve elaborate underlying cellular and molecular machinery. In this section we will emphasize that several forms of *non-associative* learning are exhibited by animals, including: habituation; dishabituation; and sensitization (see Figure 9). These forms of learning involve altered responses to a single stimulus, and do not necessitate the animal forming any association between one environmental stimulus and another—that is, these forms of learning are non-associative. They also can occur unconsciously (see Figure 3), generally requiring neither conscious perception of environmental stimuli nor conscious recall of information.

Perhaps the simplest form of learning in existence is habituation; for example when an animal is repeatedly presented with an innocuous environmental stimulus, the animal's response to that stimulus decreases over time. For example, if someone moves from a small, quiet town to a street-level apartment in Manhattan, typically at first the street noises in the city are disturbing. However, over time, the newcomer becomes accustomed to the new environment, and the street noise is no longer so bothersome. This type of phenomenon is referred to as habituation. The

components of the working memory system. Specifically, they have proposed that persisting neuronal activity in the ventrolateral PFC contributes to non-spatial short-term memory (the color and shape of an object, for example) while the dorsolateral PFC contributes to spatial short-term memory (see Figure 7).

D. Reverberating Circuit Mechanisms Contrast with Molecular Storage Mechanisms for Long-Term Memory

The mechanisms underlying short-term memory and working memory involve persistent firing of neurons within the PFC and elsewhere in the CNS. Thus, the memory trace for short-term memory is based in a repetitively firing neural circuit actively encoding and holding information. It is important to emphasize that this mechanism contrasts with the mechanisms underlying long-term memory, which do not rely on persistent or reverberating neuronal action potential firing for their persistence (see Figure 8). Thus, short-term memory storage and long-term memory storage manifest a fundamental mechanistic difference. Moreover, the fact that long-term memories can be maintained in the absence of ongoing action potential firing (at least for long periods of time) means that the fundamental unit of information storage, the *engram*, must reside wholly or in part at the molecular and cell structural level in the case of long-term memory.

BOX 3

APLYSIA IN ITS NATURAL HABITAT

Given the popularity of *Aplysia* as an experimental system, one might be tempted to think of *Aplysia* as being indigenous to the aquaria of neurobiology laboratories. However, the most widely studied *Aplysia* species, *californica*, lives in the cool Pacific waters off the California coast. *Aplysia* spends its time in the tidal and near-coastal zones, where it feeds on a diet of seaweed. Except for the buffeting of the ocean waves and currents (and, one must assume, the occasional curious scuba diver), *Aplysia* lead a fairly peaceful existence. They are unsavory to fish and have very few natural predators; however, *Aplysia* can serve as prey to certain types of sea anemones. When an *Aplysia* is seriously perturbed, it exhibits its most dramatic behavioral response; inking. *Aplysia* possess an ink gland and can release a cloud of viscous purple ink, similar to the well known octopus. Although the precise function of the inking is unknown, two popular ideas are that the ink may contain noxious compounds to help ward off predators, or may serve to camouflage the animal from potential attackers. A strong aversive stimulus such as one that elicits inking by *Aplysia* also results in sensitization of the animal. For some period of time after inking an animal will exhibit enhancement of its baseline defensive withdrawal responses. This ethologically relevant form of behavior modification is the basis for laboratory study of sensitization in *Aplysia*.

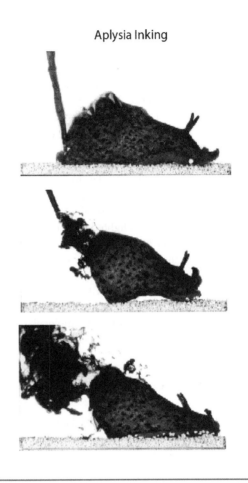

Aplysia Inking

teleologic explanation for habituation is that over time animals learn to ignore environmental stimuli that carry no unique informational content.

Habituation is a very robust behavioral phenomenon that exhibits itself in many forms—essentially all baseline behavioral responses more complex than the purest reflex responses habituate. Some of the more well studied habituation phenomena experimentally are habituation of the *Aplysia californica* gill-and-siphon defensive withdrawal response and habituation of reflexive leg-lifting in *Drosophila*. Habituation is also frequently encountered outside the laboratory setting; in particular it is frequently observed by teachers in the classroom lecture environment.

After a response is habituated, if you present another, unique, stimulus, dishabituation can occur. For example, even after becoming habituated to street noises, if one is expecting a visitor to be dropped off at their doorstep, street noises may once again become noticeable. It is worth noting that dishabituation is a useful tool to distinguish habituation from fatigue. A habituated response can be overcome by a dishabituating stimulus; however, a decreased response due to fatigue cannot.

Animals can also learn to become hyper-responsive to an environmental stimulus, a phenomenon known as sensitization. Sensitization is defined as an increased response over and above the normal baseline response which occurs in response to an environmental signal. Sensitizing stimuli typically can elicit an augmentation in response from either a non-habituated or a habituated starting point. In the second scenario a component of the increased responsiveness must, by definition, then be described as dishabituation (see Figure 9).

Keep in mind that in some ways the definitions of habituation, dishabituation, and sensitization are

BOX 4

HERMISSENDA—THE GOOD-LOOKING ONE IN THE FAMILY

While even a dedicated neurobiologist would be hard-pressed to describe *Aplysia* as aesthetically attractive, another popular invertebrate species used in studies of learning and memory is a clear winner in any molluscan beauty contest. With its bright coloration and striking profile, *Hermissenda* is the closest thing to a poster child available among the invertebrate species commonly studied by neurobiologists. *Hermissenda* is not just all looks and no brains, however. This system has been used to study the cellular and molecular basis of a particular form of associative learning exhibited by the animal. *Hermissenda* are normally phototactic; that is, they will move toward a lighted area. However, if the animal is trained that light predicts an upcoming aversive stimulus, in this case turbulence in the water surrounding the animal, the normal phototactic response is suppressed. The laboratories of Dan Alkon and Terry Crow have been instrumental in discovering the neuronal circuitry, cellular physiology, and molecular mechanisms underlying this form of associative conditioning.

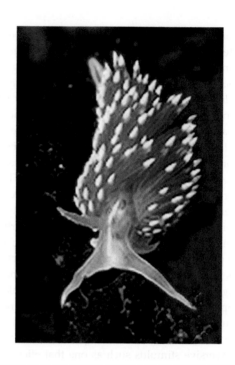

arbitrary. In the natural setting animals are constantly modifying their behaviors in response to the ongoing barrage of environmental signals. Thus, it is difficult to determine what a "baseline" response is outside of a stringently controlled experimental setting.

All of these non-associative forms of learning can exhibit themselves in either short-term or long-term forms. The duration of the memory for a learned event depends on the number of times an animal experiences a behavior-modifying stimulus. For example, a single sensitizing stimulation may elicit sensitization that lasts only a few minutes, whereas repeated stimulations will likely result in sensitization lasting hours to days (see Figure 4, for example). Repeated presentations of multiple training trials can elicit sensitization lasting for weeks.

One exciting area of contemporary neurobiological research is to try to understand the basis for short-term and long-term non-associative learning. Starting in the 1960s the mechanisms underlying habituation and sensitization began to be worked out at the cellular and biochemical level. Part of this watershed of new understanding of the basis of learning and memory came about as a result of the insight to capitalize on easily studied, simple forms of learning in special preparations that lent themselves to experimental investigation at the cellular level. In particular, the work of Eric Kandel (Figure 10) and his colleagues allowed enormous progress in our understanding of the cellular basis of behavior in general, and learning and memory specifically. Kandel and his colleagues Tom Carew, Jack Byrne, and Bob Hawkins, along with many others, have used the simple marine mollusk *Aplysia californica* (Figure 11) to great effect to study the behavioral attributes and cellular and molecular mechanisms of learning and memory.

B. Unconscious Learning and Unconscious Recall

Motor Learning

Motor learning, skills, and habits are the classic examples of unconsciously learned and unconsciously recalled memories. Walking is a good example. Walking is an extremely complex task involving intricate motor movements, which we generally perform automatically and with great facility. We learned to walk unconsciously as small children and, if anything, trying to exert conscious

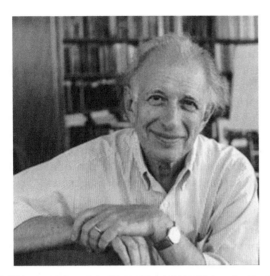

FIGURE 10 Dr Eric Kandel. Dr Kandel is a University Professor at Columbia University and Nobel Prize-winner who led pioneering studies on the cellular basis of learning and memory.

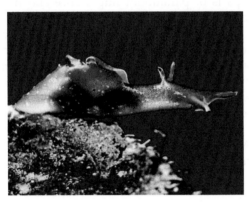

FIGURE 11 *Aplysia Californica. Aplysia*, a nudibranch mollusk found in the cool waters off the coast of California, popularized for its use in studies of simple forms of learning and memory.

control over our walking as adults likely leads to an awkward gait.

Another example of unconscious learning is learning to play an instrument such as the guitar or piano, at least as concerns the motor components. Repetition allows the development of finely tuned motor patterns that can be recalled without conscious thought. Learning of the motor components also occurs without much conscious control, although certainly there is conscious involvement when the initial motor patterns are beginning to be laid down. Even in this case, though, one does not consciously work out the pattern of firing of individual muscles—indeed we by-and-large don't have very much control over the contraction of single muscles and are not really conscious of them as single units. When we learn to play an instrument, a multitude of complex muscle

contractions and hand movements are taking place completely below the level of conscious thought.

While complex unconscious processes go into the initial establishment of learned motor patterns, in some cases such as speech and walking, there is probably also a complicated interaction of developmental processes with signals generated in response to environmental stimuli. As mentioned above, in the early stages of many types of motor learning there is conscious involvement, the need for which disappears over time as part of the learning process. The circuitry and cellular mechanisms underlying motor learning are quite complex, involving the motor cortex, basal ganglia including the neostriatum, and cerebellum.

The site of memory storage for most types of motor memory involve or have access to the principal circuits which mediate the behavioral motor pattern, such as the motor cortex, basal ganglia, and spinal cord motor neurons. A discussion of these systems is presented in Chapter 2 as part of the discussion of human memory systems.

Some motor memories are subject to limited conscious recall, but in most cases trying to replay a motor memory with too much conscious control simply messes things up. This is likely a component of the common "choking" component of sports, although stress-induced release of modulatory neurotransmitters which affect performance is also certainly a factor. It is interesting that the unconscious aspect of motor recall has made it into popular sports lingo. When an athlete is at the top of his or her game they are typically referred to as being "unconscious."

C. Unconscious Learning and Subject to Conscious Recall

The forms of learning we have talked about so far are non-associative. In habituation, sensitization, etc., nothing is learned about the relationship or association of one event with another. We next move on to a more complex form of learning where a predictive relationship is learned—an animal learns that one environmental stimulus reliably predicts another.

An important set of nomenclature in this area arose out of the pioneering work of Ivan Pavlov (Figure 12). Pavlov and his co-workers studied *associative conditioning* of the salivary response of dogs—studies indeed so classic that the terms classical conditioning and Pavlovian conditioning are now used synonymously with associative conditioning. Pavlov knew, as does anyone that has ever owned a dog, that when a dog is presented with a food stimulus a strong salivatory response is elicited (see Figure 13). This is a natural response, of course, and this salivation is referred to as the unconditioned response, and correspondingly the food stimulus is referred to as the unconditioned stimulus. Pavlov's breakthrough realization, which he subsequently rigorously documented and studied, was that he could train dogs to associate a neutral stimulus, such as the ringing of a bell, with the food stimulus. Over time the dog would form an association between the bell and the food, and Pavlov found that the bell alone would ultimately cause a salivatory response just like the food did. The bell-elicited salivation was termed the conditioned response, and correspondingly the bell tone was termed the conditioned stimulus (Figure 13).

In associative learning an animal learns the predictive value of one stimulus for another, in Pavlov's

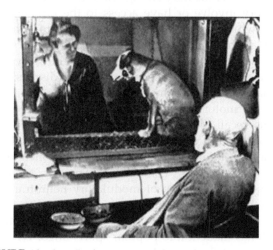

FIGURE 12   Ivan Pavlov pioneered the study of associative conditioning, studying modification of reflex responses in dogs.

example the reliability of a tone for predicting a subsequent food presentation. This type of learning is profoundly important for survival in any natural environment, and for this reason has been robustly selected for in animal evolution. Stated another way, associative learning allows the neural encoding of cause-and-effect relationships. The stable formation of a memory trace, such that an accurate record of cause-and-effect relationships is available for future reference, provides such a pronounced competitive advantage that this form of learning is typically quite vigorous.

The importance of this last point cannot be overstated! Nature has selected for a robust capacity of nervous systems to accurately reflect one of the principal physical laws that govern the real world: cause and effect. Thus, nervous systems of all sorts have evolved to the best of their capacity sophisticated and robust circuit, cellular, and molecular mechanisms to encode these types of information.

Generally associative learning is quite reliable—obviously the accuracy of storing cause-and-effect relationships is of paramount importance and has been selected for evolutionarily. This is one significant factor in the popularity of studying associative learning experimentally—the learned behaviors are observable, relatively rapidly acquired, and reliably expressed. However, this is not to say that associative learning is flawless. Numerous examples exist in the literature and anecdotally of animals having mislearned associations. For example, one of my colleagues who works with Macaque monkeys had a monkey who learned that certain visual stimuli predicted the subsequent

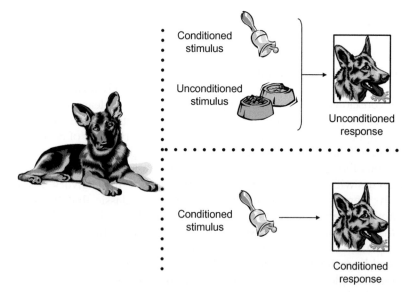

FIGURE 13   Pavlovian associative conditioning of the canine salivary response. Repeated pairings of an auditory cue with food causes the animal to learn the predictive value of one for the other. See text for details.

arrival of a food reward. However, the animal also "learned" that it was necessary to wave his hand in an idiosyncratic way in order for the food reward to be delivered. Of course, in reality the hand movement was entirely superfluous to the task and the reward delivery. B. F. Skinner recorded several similar circumstances in training pigeons in associative learning tasks, where in some cases elaborate but unnecessary motor patterns were executed before the animal pecked an object to receive a food reward. Skinner termed these behaviors "superstitious" behaviors, a somewhat loaded term that is anthropomorphic, but not without appeal. Regardless of the terminology, it is clear that these are examples of associative learning gone awry. Presumably what has happened is that early on in the training, the animal has erroneously associated some movement on their part with the food reward, and formed a lasting but inaccurate memory that executing the movement is necessary to receive the reward. I bring up these examples as indications of the robustness of associative memory, but with the interesting twist that as with all robust systems there is an attendant possibility of error-proneness.

Against this backdrop it is then interesting to consider that associative learning depends on two attributes of the environmental stimuli—*contiguity* and *contingency*. Contiguity refers to the property of the stimuli occurring coincidentally, that is overlapping in time or one immediately after the other in time. This captures Nature's rule of cause and effect. Environmental stimuli are generally perceived simultaneously with or immediately after the events that cause them. Contingency refers to the ordering of the stimuli—that one stimulus consistently precedes the other in onset. This captures the predictive value of one event for the other; that is, in nature the cause will always precede the effect. In the examples of mislearning in the previous paragraph the animals presumably misrepresented contiguous stimuli as also being contingent.

The issue of contiguity in associative conditioning raises the consideration of two basic types of classical associative conditioning: delay conditioning and trace conditioning (see Figure 14). The type of classical associative conditioning we have discussed so far is referred to as delay conditioning. This term derives from the typical timing of this type of associative conditioning protocol experimentally. For example, if one is training an animal to learn that a tone predicts a food reward using a delay conditioning protocol, the tone is started and maintained continuously until the food reward is presented. Thus, the onset of the CS is followed by a delay before the onset of the US. With delay conditioning the CS and US are contiguous and overlapping—in other words the animal receives a US

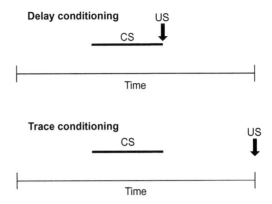

FIGURE 14 Delay and trace conditioning. Associative conditioning falls into two broad categories—delay conditioning, and trace conditioning. In trace conditioning an intervening time interval is introduced between the termination of the CS and the onset of the US. Trace conditioning involves the hippocampus.

simultaneously with a CS after the CS has been presented continuously for some delay period.

Trace conditioning refers to a conditioning protocol where the CS is presented, terminated, and followed after some intervening period by the US. The CS and US never overlap in time, and are temporally contiguous in the sense that they are presented closely in time, but never simultaneously. The term "trace" arises from the fact that some memory trace for the CS must be preserved over time so that it can subsequently be associated with the US.

The distinct use of the two terms "delay conditioning" and "trace conditioning" may seem like scientific hyper-semanticism, because the two protocols seem so similar. However, the reasonably subtle alteration of introducing a brief intervening time span between CS and US brings entirely new neuronal circuits to bear on the cognitive processing involved. Indeed, trace conditioning requires the hippocampus, whereas delay conditioning does not. This hippocampus-dependence of trace associative learning has been largely studied in rodents, but elegant studies in Larry Squire's laboratory have demonstrated that humans with hippocampal lesions also have deficits in trace associative conditioning (7). Thus, delay and trace conditioning differ fundamentally in their underlying anatomy and relevant circuitry, so much so that they indeed are quite different forms of learning. It is for this reason that making the reasonably small move from delay conditioning to trace conditioning progresses us from one category of learning to another entirely.

The recall of trace conditioning has mapped onto it a temporal component as well. Re-experiencing the CS after trace conditioning has occurred allows for conscious recollection of the US, during the "trace" period. For example, let's say that I am trained that a tone precedes a foot shock by five seconds. During testing, when I hear the tone I have five seconds during which I am expecting the foot shock to be delivered. Because of this aspect of the possibility of conscious anticipation, trace conditioning is our first example of learning that can occur unconsciously but can be subject to conscious recall (see Figure 3).

D. Operant Conditioning

Pavlov's dogs were passive participants in their learning experience. They did not have to do anything beyond perceiving the environmental stimulus, after which natural reflexes took over and an unconscious salivatory response occurred. This type of learning is distinct from learning paradigms where a voluntary motor response is elicited. Conditioning where the animal is required to execute a voluntary motor response is referred to as *operant conditioning*. It is important to bear in mind that the distinction is a practical one, based in experimentation. Operant conditioning simply refers to the fact that the experimenter is quantitating a voluntary movement (not a reflex) as the behavioral output indicating that learning has occurred. The examples I used above where monkeys or pigeons were required to push a lever or peck a button are examples of operant conditioning. Over the years there has been debate over whether operant conditioning will use different mechanisms from classical associative conditioning, and whether operant and classical conditioning should really be considered as distinct categories. We don't have the final answer to this question, but suffice it to say that it appears that operant conditioning will not require unique cellular or molecular mechanisms—likely the mechanistic differences will be confined to the types of neuronal circuitry involved.

E. Currently Popular Associative Learning Paradigms

Two associative learning paradigms that are used extensively in the modern laboratory for studying learning are conditioned fear (8–9) and conditioned taste aversion (10). In both paradigms, animals learn an association between a neutral conditioned stimulus and an aversive unconditioned stimulus. Both serve as powerful examples of classical Pavlovian conditioning, and both result in robust, long-lasting memory after even a single CS-US pairing. These two behavioral paradigms are also accommodating to researchers because the neuroanatomical pathways underlying the learning are fairly well-established.

One specific example of fear conditioning involves the delivery of an innocuous acoustic cue (CS) paired with a mild foot shock (US) within a novel environment (see Figure 15). When tested 24 hours after training, rats, mice, and other rodents exhibit marked fear, measured by freezing behavior or other reflex fear responses, in response to representation of either the context (*contextual fear conditioning*) or the auditory CS delivered in a different context (*cued fear conditioning*). Both cued and contextual fear conditioning have been shown to be dependent upon the amygdala, whereas contextual fear conditioning also involves the hippocampus. We will return to these two forms of learning in Chapter 4, where we discuss rodent behavioral models of learning in more detail.

Conditioned taste aversion is another form of associative learning; in this case, an animal learns to associate the novel taste of a new foodstuff (CS) with subsequent illness (US) resulting from ingestion of some toxic agent (see Figure 16). The adaptiveness of this form of learning should be apparent; by preventing subsequent ingestion of poisonous foods survival is greatly enhanced. This is obviously a form of learning that is not very forgiving of multiple training trials; not surprisingly, animals learn after a single pairing of novel taste and toxin to avoid that taste in future encounters.

One interesting aspect of conditioned taste aversion learning is the long CS-US interval. Unlike other associative conditioning paradigms, such as fear conditioning or eye-blink conditioning where the CS-US interval is typically on the order of seconds, with conditioned taste aversion the system can tolerate delays of hours between the CS taste and US toxin. This suggests that there are cellular and biochemical events initiated by the taste stimulus alone that are likely to be long-lasting. Indeed, novel tastes alone trigger memory formation automatically, as can be measured by increased food consumption upon representation of a foodstuff (Figure 16). This phenomenon is referred to as attenuation of neophobia (11).

Finally, comparing and contrasting fear conditioning with conditioned taste aversion raises a final general attribute of associative conditioning, referred to as *salience*. We discussed above that contingency and contiguity are two hallmarks of associative conditioning, and salience is a term used to refer to the third general property. Salience refers to the fact that animals do not in general learn to associate conditioned stimuli and unconditioned stimuli that are not typically paired in their natural environment. For example, nausea-inducing stimuli are by far much more robust producers of taste aversion than are generic painful stimuli that may robustly support other types of aversive conditioning. Similarly, pairing nausea

TRAINING

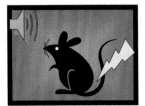

- Animal is placed in novel context
- Hears a tone
- Receives foot shock

CONTEXTUAL TEST

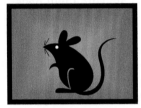

- Animal is returned to same context
- Test for freezing behavior

CUED TEST

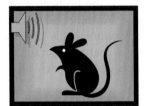

- Animal is placed in modified context
- Hears a tone
- Test for freezing behavior

FIGURE 15 Fear conditioning. Fear conditioning is a form of associative conditioning in which an aversive, fear-evoking stimulus is paired with a novel environmental cue. A wide variety of environmental stimuli can be used for fear conditioning, such as places (contexts), auditory cues, visual cues, odors, etc.

Behavioral procedures used to assess novel taste learning

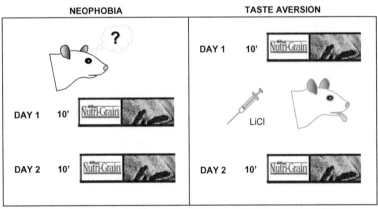

FIGURE 16 Taste learning. Taste learning is a robust and automatic form of learning in animals. Two types of assessments generally used to evaluate taste learning are attenuation of neophobia, in which an animal learns that a taste is not dangerous, and conditioned taste aversion, in which an animal learns that a given taste is dangerous. These can be measured experimentally by giving a single exposure to a novel food on Day 1 (ten minutes of Nutri-grain bar in this case) and monitoring the animal's response to representation of that same stimulus 24 hours later (Day 2). If the animal finds the new food to be non-aversive, consumption of the food will be increased—attenuation of neophobia. If an aversive stimulus is paired with the novel food (e.g., a lithium chloride injection), then the animal will exhibit a decreased consumption of the food on Day 2—conditioned taste aversion. See Chapter 4 for additional details.

with visual stimuli or auditory cues is not very effective at aversive conditioning to these stimuli. Clearly, evolution has operated to select for robust learning of associations that can occur in the natural environment, and a term that is used to describe this is that the stimulus is salient to the animal, in other words, the stimulus is likely to be pertinent to the animal under the given condition.

Thus, in general, it is not the case that unconscious associative learning operates such that any two environmental signals can be associated. This likely arises from a combination of factors. First, there is a degree of anatomical specialization in the CNS such that particular functions are parsed out into particular areas. Thus, as a practical matter, the central processing of two environmental stimuli may never "touch" each other in the brain, and therefore can never be associated. In this instance the stimuli "touching" each other can be taken quite literally in that some anatomical cross-connection must be made. Conversely, for any association to take place the underlying neural circuits processing the environmental information must be able to connect anatomically. It is only possible to draw an associative learning circuit if the two stimuli being paired impinge upon each other at some point.

This probably seems like a statement of something that is intuitively obvious. However, if associative learning requires that two information-processing circuits connect with each other, this must of necessity utilize molecular and chemical processes. A description of these types of processes, in particular molecular mechanisms that can contribute to associative events, is a central theme of later chapters of this book.

Overall, we have seen in this section that various models of associative conditioning have transitioned us from unconscious processes to conscious processes. Many associations can be learned unconsciously and expressed unconsciously. However, various types of associative learning also begin to recruit conscious processes. While learned unconsciously they can be recalled consciously. As a generalization, the transition involves recruitment of the hippocampus into the learning process. In the following section we will transition to even more complex forms of learning that also depend on the hippocampus.

IV. CONSCIOUS LEARNING—SUBJECT TO CONSCIOUS AND UNCONSCIOUS RECALL

A. Declarative Learning

Human declarative learning is what we typically think of when we think of "learning." This is the conscious acquisition of new facts, or the formation of memories for events that occur in our lives, which are available for subsequent recall at will. The extent to which you remember what you read in this book will depend upon the processes of conscious declarative learning. Of course, the extent to which you remember

this book will also depend on a large number of other factors, such as motivation, attention, level of arousal, etc. Thus, human declarative learning, and likely most analogous forms of learning in animals, is subject to a wide variety of modulatory factors.

For example, particularly robust memory for single events is typically referred to as "flashbulb" memory in humans. There are several examples of this type of memory that many Americans have shared, the most recent example being the terrorist destruction of the Twin Towers in New York City. Like most people, I remember vividly how I learned of the attacks, and I am sure I will never forget seeing live on television the second tower collapse. Flashbulb memories are usually associated with a high state of arousal or a high level of emotional valence—an example of the strong modulatory influences that learning is subject to.

As are the other types of conscious learning we will discuss in this section, declarative learning is dependent on the hippocampus—in later sections of the book we will return to the importance of modulatory influences on hippocampus-dependent learning, and discuss some likely molecular mechanisms underlying this effect.

It is difficult to model declarative learning in non-human animals, because the behavioral output for these types of memories is actually quite subtle and in most cases it is not even clear what are relevant type of learning might be in lower animals (see Box 5). Partly for this reason most of what we know about declarative learning comes from human studies, in particular studies of patients with hippocampal lesions. These studies will be described in more detail in Chapter 2 (see also references 12–13). Suffice it to say for our purposes that a number of classic studies of humans with hippocampal lesions led to the dissociation of declarative from non-declarative forms of memory in humans.

Declarative memory is that type of memory that is lost when a human suffers hippocampal damage—this includes the capacity to form memories for facts, names, places, and personal experiences (Figure 3). Hippocampal damage results in *anterograde amnesia* for these types of memories—that is, there is a loss of the capacity to form new memories. Old memories (more than about one year) are largely spared, i.e., there is relatively little *retrograde* amnesia. Non-declarative forms of memory such as sensitization, motor learning, delay classical conditioning, etc., are spared in humans with hippocampal lesions.

A final comment on declarative learning is that it is generally associative, although not in the sense of classical associative conditioning where a cause-and-effect

BOX 5

A RODENT MODEL OF DECLARATIVE MEMORY?

It is difficult to imagine a rodent model for declarative memory, but there is one potentially parallel type of learning in rodents that I will mention briefly. Because toxic plants and other poisonous foodstuffs coexist with most animals, as described above conditioned taste aversion evolved to protect animals from being poisoned out of the gene pool. However, avoidance of something that is toxic is not possible if it has been ingested in lethal quantities, so a supplementary behavior has also evolved to protect animals from toxic foods. *Neophobia* is the characteristic fear of novel foods, and ensures that animals ingest only small quantities, as if to sample the food to determine if it is safe to eat. If the animal develops illness, a conditioned taste aversion results, and this foodstuff will be avoided on future encounters. If no illness results and assuming the food is reasonably palatable, animals will increase their intake on subsequent exposures.

This is readily demonstrated in the laboratory: when rats or mice are presented with highly palatable solutions of novel tastes, such as saccharin or sucrose, they will consume small amounts on the first exposure; on subsequent exposures, the animals consume more (see Figure 16). This attenuation of neophobia is a behavioral measure of memory for the novel taste, and is part of a process of familiarization to the formerly novel taste. There is a fairly clear consensus that the insular cortex is the primary site of learning and memory for novel tastes, so this form of learning is clearly not strictly analogous to human declarative learning. However, it does depend on the cerebral cortex as its storage site, as is likely in human declarative memory. Furthermore, it is reasonably analogous to a human learning a "fact," in this case what something tastes like, and having that information available for conscious recall.

relationship is learned. Most declarative learning does not take place in a cognitive vacuum, but items are typically learned in the context of other related facts or objects. A good example of this for illustrative purposes is learning someone's name. Learning a name is certainly a declarative learning event, and you can list off the names of all the people you know well as a reiteration of a list of "facts." However, each name also serves as a descriptor of an individual and is associated with that person, their face, their house, etc. This type of multiple association for learned facts (i.e., declarative learning) is the rule rather than the exception. It is likely that most declarative learning occurs as learning something within a variety of contexts: other facts or places with which the fact is associated. This point is important to keep in mind as we begin to explore the molecular basis for declarative learning. It is certainly possible that many of the molecular mechanisms that are discovered as subserving what we have defined as *associative* conditioning may translate directly as mechanisms contributing to declarative learning. Stated more strongly, at this point it is appropriate to hypothesize that associative molecular mechanisms will be part of the molecular infrastructure of declarative learning.

B. Spatial Learning

A final example of hippocampus-dependent learning in both humans and lower animals is spatial learning. Obviously animals must learn to navigate their environment, and learn to associate particular places with particular items or events. This type of learning has been the classically defined learning system in which involves the hippocampus. A wide variety of different studies have shown that molecular or anatomical lesions of the hippocampus lead to spatial learning deficits, in both humans and lower animals. Also, direct measurements of a wide variety of molecular and physiologic changes have been shown to correlate with spatial learning. These topics will be discussed in greater detail in the next chapter.

V. SUMMARY

This chapter has described a number of basic attributes of learning and memory, based largely on the psychological study of these phenomena. We also have introduced and discussed a number of terms related to memory and its study. Mastery of these basic terms and an understanding of their utilization will be critical for your comprehension of the remainder of this textbook.

There are a number of basic take-home messages for this chapter.

1. Memory is not monolithic—there are many different types of learning and memory, most of which are subserved by different anatomical areas of the nervous system. This principle is distilled in the *multiple memory systems* concept.
2. Almost all forms of memory have both short-term and long-term forms.
3. The mechanisms underlying short-term memory are distinct from those underlying long-term memory. In general, brief forms of short-term memory are sustained by repetitive or reverberating action potential firing, while long-term forms of memory are sustained by persisting molecular and cellular modifications.
4. Memory can be broadly subdivided into non-declarative and declarative forms, and similarly into unconscious and conscious forms.
5. Both unconscious and conscious forms of learning can be manifest in many different ways, for example associative and non-associative forms, operant forms, etc. These subtypes vary depending on the particular sensory inputs that trigger the learning, and depending on the behavioral output that manifests the memory.

Further Reading

Baddeley, A. (2001). "Is working memory still working?" *Am. Psychol.* 56:849–864.

Eichenbaum, H. (2002). *The Cognitive Neuroscience of Memory*. New York: Oxford University Press.

Eichenbaum, H., Yonelinas, A. P., and Ranganath, C. (2007). "The medial temporal lobe and recognition memory". *Annu. Rev. Neurosci.* 30:123–152.

Gold, P. E. (2004). "Coordination of multiple memory systems". *Neurobiol. Learn. Mem.* 82(3):230–242.

LeDoux, J. E. (2001). *Synaptic Self: How Our Brains Become Who We Are*. New York: Viking.

McDonald, R. J., Devan, B. D., and Hong, N. S. (2004). "Multiple memory systems: the power of interactions". *Neurobiol. Learn. Mem.* 82(3):333–346.

McDonald, R. J., and White, N. M. (1993). "A triple dissociation of memory systems: hippocampus, amygdala, and dorsal striatum". *Behav. Neurosci.* 107(1):3–22.

McNaughton, B. L., Battaglia, F. P., Jensen, O., Moser, E. I., and Moser, M. B. (2006). "Path integration and the neural basis of the 'cognitive map'". *Nat. Rev. Neurosci.* 7(8):663–678.

Milner, B., Squire, L. R., and Kandel, E. R. (1998). "Cognitive neuroscience and the study of memory". *Neuron* 20(3):445–468.

Shiffrin, R. M., and Atkinson, R. C. (1969). "Storage and retrieval processes in long-term memory". *Psychological Review* 76:179–193.

Squire, L. R. (2004). "Memory systems of the brain: a brief history and current perspective". *Neurobiol. Learn. Mem.* 82(3):171–177.

Squire, L. R., and Kandel, E. R. (2008). *Memory: From Mind to Molecules*, 2nd ed. New York: Roberts and Company.

Tronson, N. C., and Taylor, J. R. (2007). "Molecular mechanisms of memory reconsolidation". *Nature Reviews Neuroscience* 8:262–275.

Journal Club Articles

Bechara, A., Tranel, D., Damasio, H., Adolphs, R., Rockland, C., and Damasio, A. R. (1995). "Double dissociation of conditioning and declarative knowledge relative to the amygdala and hippocampus in humans". *Science* 269(5227):1115–1118.

Knowlton, B. J., Mangels, J. A., and Squire, L. R. (1996). "A neostriatal habit learning system in humans". *Science* 273(5280): 1399–1402.

Packard, M. G., and McGaugh, J. L. (1996). "Inactivation of hippocampus or caudate nucleus with lidocaine differentially affects expression of place and response learning". *Neurobiol. Learn. Mem.* 65(1):65–72.

For more information—relevant topic chapters from: John H. Byrne (Editor-in-Chief) (2008). *Learning and Memory: A Comprehensive Reference*. Oxford: Academic Press (ISBN 978-0-12-370509-9). (1.02 Roediger, H. L. III, Zaromb, F. M., and Goode, M. K. *A Typology of Memory Terms*. pp. 11–24; 1.03 Capaldi, E. J., and Martins, A. *History of Behavioral Learning Theories*. pp. 25–39; 1.04 Nadel, L. *Multiple Memory Systems: A New View*. pp. 41–52; 3.01 Eichenbaum, H. *Introduction and Overview*. pp. 1–8; 3.02 White, N. M. *Multiple Memory Systems in the Brain: Cooperation and Competition*. pp. 9–46.)

References

1. Squire, L. R., and Kandel, E. R. (1999). *Memory: From Mind to Molecules* (distributed by W. H. Freeman and Co.). New York: Scientific American Library.
2. Eichenbaum, H. (2001). "The hippocampus and declarative memory: cognitive mechanisms and neural codes". *Behav. Brain Res.* 127:199–207.
3. Kandel, E. R., and Squire, L. R. (2000). "Neuroscience: breaking down scientific barriers to the study of brain and mind". *Science* 290:1113–1120.
4. Eichenbaum, H., and Cohen, N. J. (2001). *From Conditioning to Conscious Recollection: Memory Systems of the Brain*. Upper Saddle River, NJ: Oxford University Press.
5. Vianna, M. R., Szapiro, G., McGaugh, J. L., Medina, J. H., and Izquierdo, I. (2001). "Retrieval of memory for fear-motivated training initiates extinction requiring protein synthesis in the rat hippocampus". *Proc. Natl Acad. Sci. USA* 98:12251–12254.
6. Nader, K., Schafe, G. E., and LeDoux, J. E. (2000). "The labile nature of consolidation theory". *Nat. Rev. Neurosci.* 1:216–219.
7. Clark, R. E., and Squire, L. R. (1998). "Classical conditioning and brain systems: the role of awareness". *Science* 280:77–81.
8. LeDoux, J. E. (2001). *Synaptic Self: How Our Brains Become Who We Are*. New York: Viking.
9. Quirk, G. J., Repa, C., and LeDoux, J. E. (1995). "Fear conditioning enhances short-latency auditory responses of lateral amygdala neurons: parallel recordings in the freely behaving rat". *Neuron* 15:1029–1039.
10. Berman, D. E., and Dudai, Y. (2001). "Memory extinction, learning anew, and learning the new: dissociations in the molecular machinery of learning in cortex". *Science* 291:2417–2419.

11. Swank, M. W., and Sweatt, J. D. (2001). "Increased histone acetyltransferase and lysine acetyltransferase activity and biphasic activation of the ERK/RSK cascade in insular cortex during novel taste learning". *J. Neurosci.* 21:3383–3391.

12. Eichenbaum, H. (1999). "The hippocampus and mechanisms of declarative memory". *Behav. Brain Res.* 103:123–133.

13. Milner, B., Squire, L. R., and Kandel, E. R. (1998). "Cognitive neuroscience and the study of memory". *Neuron* 20:445–468.

14. Kandel, E. R. (2001). "The molecular biology of memory storage: a dialogue between genes and synapses". *Science* 294: 1030–1038.

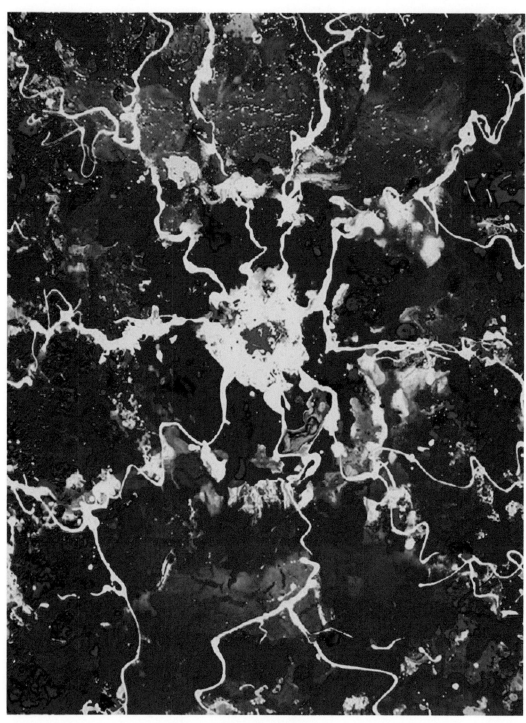

Medium Spiny Neuron
J. David Sweatt, acrylic on canvas, 2008–2009

Studies of Human Learning and Memory

I. INTRODUCTION—HISTORICAL PRECEDENTS WITH STUDIES OF HUMAN SUBJECTS

In the history of memory studies it is likely that rats have been the subjects most often experimented on. This contrasts with humans, who have been the most studied but not the most experimented on. The distinction here is that a scientist has freedom to manipulate a rat for many types of experimental designs, while ethical and moral considerations largely limit scientists to studying (i.e., simply observing) humans without much freedom to lesion, drug, dissect, or otherwise manipulate them. Against this backdrop it is striking, then, that two of the most profound conceptual advances in the history of the memory field have initially come from studies of human subjects.

These two conceptual advances are the idea of memory consolidation, and the idea of multiple memory systems. These two concepts will be discussed in this chapter. The important historical precedence of human studies of basic memory mechanisms as a prelude to later understanding using animal studies is why this chapter on human studies is near the beginning of this book on memory mechanisms. This arrangement of the book content is by design—this order of presentation is historically accurate and the remaining chapters of the book focusing on animal studies owe a great debt to the pioneering work done using observations of human patients. In a sense, the animal studies provide the continuing narrative of the story of scientists' pursuit of understanding memory.

A. Amnesias

Amnesia is both frightening and fascinating to contemplate, so much so that Hollywood has turned to amnesia as a plot device on many occasions (see Table 1).

TABLE 1   Movies Using Amnesia as a Plot Device

Movie	Director (plus notable actors)	Year
Anterograde amnesia		
Memento	Christopher Nolan (Guy Pearce)	2001
Finding Nemo	Andrew Stanton (Animated—Ellen DeGeneris as Dory)	2003
50 First Dates	Peter Segal (Adam Sandler)	2004
Retrograde amnesia		
The Bourne Identity	Doug Liman (Matt Damon)	2002
Total Recall	Paul Verhoeven (Arnold Schwarzenegger, Sharon Stone)	1990
Spellbound	Alfred Hitchcock (Ingrid Bergman, Gregory Peck)	1945
Eternal Sunshine of the Spotless Mind	Michel Gondry (Jim Carrey, Kate Winslet)	2004
The Forgotten	Joseph Ruben (Julianne Moore)	2004
Men in Black	Barry Sonnenfeld (Tommy Lee Jones, Will Smith)	1997
Not sure		
Mulholland Drive	David Lynch (Michael J. Anderson, Diane Baker)	2001

Here are some personal comments, for what they are worth. *Memento* and *Finding Nemo*: outstanding movies that, without a doubt, are the most scientifically accurate movies ever made involving a character with a memory disorder. *50 First Dates:* I have to admit I couldn't stand to watch more than about 10 minutes of this—a chick-flick all the way. *The Bourne Identity, Total Recall, Spellbound:* pretty good action-type films. The disclaimer here is that these are probably the male equivalent of a chick-flick, whatever that's called. *Eternal Sunshine of the Spotless Mind:* pretty creepy sci-fi for something that basically is a chick-flick. *The Forgotten*: the amnestic angry-mother variant of a chick-flick. *Men in Black*: OK, not much amnesia really, but at least it's not a chick-flick. *Mulholland Drive*: Classic David Lynch, and if any movie qualifies as the antithesis of a chick-flick, this is it—seriously. If anybody understands what the heck was going on in this movie, please tell me. Product Liability Warning—never, ever try to watch *Memento* and *Mulholland Drive* in the same night—your brain will probably explode.

The term amnesia is derived from *mnemos*, which is the Greek root for memory. Mnemos is derived from Greek mythology—Mnemosyne was one of the mythological Titans, and she was the goddess of recollection or remembrance—it was she who gifted humans the capacity for memory. Mnemosyne was one of Zeus' lovers, and she gave birth to the nine muses. The muses are the source of inspiration for music, poetry, and stories. They also invented the combining of letters, i.e., writing, arguably the most useful technological development in the history of information storage.[1]

Thus, based on its Greek language roots, amnesia literally means "no memory." As a clinical syndrome, amnesia is referred to as being either *retrograde* or *anterograde*. Retrograde amnesia is a loss of previously formed memory. Thus, it is the loss of memories that

were formed before the memory-damaging insult. The term retrograde amnesia is reserved for profound loss of memory, and is distinct from normal forgetting. Retrograde amnesia is the classic plot device wherein the character wakes up and can't remember who or where he is. Retrograde amnesia can result from injury, disease, or profound psychological trauma.

As a practical matter, it is extremely difficult to distinguish whether retrograde amnesia results from a loss of memory storage or a loss of the capacity for memory recall. We will return to this issue later on in Chapters 4 and 5 where we will discuss experimentally-induced amnesias.

Anterograde amnesia is a loss of the capacity to form new memories. Anterograde amnesia results from a lesion or deficit in the anatomical, cellular, or molecular mechanisms necessary to acquire and store information in the nervous system. In its purest form, anterograde amnesia leaves every previously formed memory still intact and available for recall. Individuals with anterograde amnesia typically have intact short-term memory, but lack the capacity to form long-term memories. Sadly, these individuals live a moment-to-moment existence because they are unable to remember anything that has happened to them for more than a few minutes.

B. Memory Consolidation

Studies with amnestic human subjects have identified a process that we now refer to as memory consolidation. Briefly stated, the idea of memory consolidation is captured in the theory that memory formation and stabilization proceeds as a time-dependent process, and that with time memories get stronger, i.e., less susceptible to disruption. The theory of memory consolidation is now ancient by modern scientific standards. One of the first observations to suggest memories need be consolidated came over a hundred years ago, using human subjects, where distraction and interference immediately after a training session could disrupt long-term memory formation, whereas the same distractions long after a training session had limited effects (1).

Physicians also had noted that patients that had an epileptic seizure could often experience a loss of memory for events immediately preceding the seizure, or that head trauma cases might experience the same effect. In a more recent and systematic study of this effect, Larry Squire and his colleagues studied retrograde memory effects (amnesia) in patients that had been given electroconvulsive shock, which triggers epileptic seizures. Note that the seizures in this case are triggered specifically, safely, and therapeutically—electroconvulsive therapy (ECT) is used clinically in

---

[1] I am not considering language a technology, because its use does not require an implement.

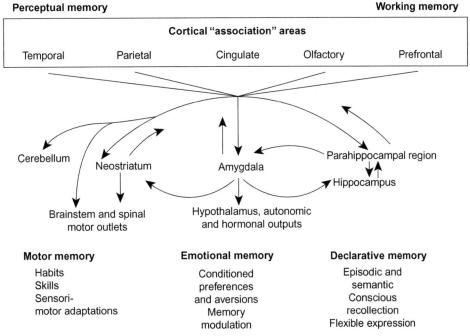

FIGURE 1   A current conception of the major memory systems in the brain. Adapted from *Fundamental Neuroscience, Learning and Memory: Brain Systems*, Howard Eichenbaum. Copyright Elsevier 2003.

cases of severe intractable depression. This iatrogenically-induced type of seizure allowed a unique opportunity to study retrograde amnesia in humans in a prospective and controlled memory study. Because the patients had the seizures at a predefined time, and were available both before and after the ECT treatment, this allowed Squire and his colleagues to systematically evaluate the retrograde amnestic effects of seizure (2). Their finding was that memories less than two years old were much more susceptible to seizure-associated transient loss than older memories. These findings were particularly compelling because the investigators were able to test memory *in the same individual* both before and after seizure. These findings and many others like them provide a compelling case that memories are differentially susceptible to disruption, depending on how old they are. The mechanistic implications of this are critically important—the finding implies that older memories are stored or recalled using different cellular/molecular mechanisms than newer memories. There is no other way they could be differentially susceptible to disruption.

We will return to animal studies of memory consolidation as a cellular and molecular process many times in this book, but human studies were the first to suggest the existence of the phenomenon. It should not escape your attention that the human studies also demonstrate the clinical relevance of understanding amnestic mechanisms.

Multiple Memory Systems

The modern conceptualization of memory in humans is that memory is subserved by multiple memory systems. We now think of human memory not as a single monolithic process, but rather as a complex multi-component, multi-output process. The multiple components are, in most cases, at least partially interacting and in some instances can be completely independent. The multiple components largely map onto discrete anatomical subregions of the central nervous system (CNS)—these subregions and their associated memory systems are summarized in Figure 1 and Table 2.

Most of the human neuroanatomical regions that are associated with specific memory systems have been identified using clinical approaches (see Figure 2). Historically, most of the relevant brain regions were first identified by studying patients who had identifiable brain lesions restricted to particular subregions, or in some cases diseases that exerted their effects in a brain subregion-selective manner. For example, the cytopathological effects of Parkinson's and Huntington's disease are largely limited to the basal ganglia, and these patients have deficits in the acquisition of new motor skills. In another example, patients with lesions to the occipital cortex due to localized strokes can have deficits in word priming. Finally, the classic cases that led to the paradigm shift of thinking about humans as having multiple memory systems came from studies of patients having hippocampal

TABLE 2   Multiple Memory Systems in the Human Central Nervous System

Memory Subtype	Corresponding Central Nervous System Subregion
Working memory	Prefrontal cortex, contributions from caudate nucleus
Declarative, episodic, and spatial memory	Medial temporal lobe system including the hippocampus, dentate gyrus, entorhinal and perirhinal cortices
Habits, motor skills, procedural memory	Striatum (caudate nucleus and putamen), globus pallidus,* and cerebellum
Priming	Occipital cortex, neocortex in general
Aversive associative conditioning	Amygdala
Motoric associative conditioning	Cerebellum
Olfactory and taste conditioning	Olfactory bulb, insular cortex, nucleus tractus solitarius (NTS), positive and negative reinforcement systems (amygdala or nucleus accumbens)
Sensitization, habituation	Spinal cord, brainstem nuclei, amygdala
Circadian rhythm	Hypothalamus—suprachiasmatic nucleus (SCN)
Reward, positive reinforcement, addiction	Nucleus accumbens, ventral tegmental area (VTA)

*Collectively the caudate nucleus, putamen, and globus pallidus are referred to as the basal ganglia.

and temporal lobe lesions, and the associated deficits in declarative, episodic, and spatial memory.

Human clinically-based studies have been particularly compelling in motivating the multiple memory systems concept because there have been many instances that allowed a *double dissociation* of memory systems. For example, a patient with an occipital cortex lesion may have pronounced deficits in word-stem priming. However, that same individual may have no deficits in declarative memory, such as memorizing word lists. In contrast, a patient with a hippocampal lesion will have pronounced declarative memory deficits, but their word-stem priming can be completely normal. Considering these findings from the two patients as one unit of evidence provides a double dissociation between priming and declarative memory. One patient has deficits in system A but not system B, while the other has deficits in system B but not system A. It is very difficult to rationalize this double dissociation as reflecting anything other than two separate and distinct memory systems. There is evidence for these types of double dissociations in human patients for almost all of the different memory systems listed in Table 2.

II. THE HIPPOCAMPUS IN HUMAN DECLARATIVE, EPISODIC, AND SPATIAL MEMORY

As described in the first chapter of this book, the prototypical role of the hippocampus in humans is to allow declarative, episodic, and spatial memory. We will discuss this in more detail in this section, organized

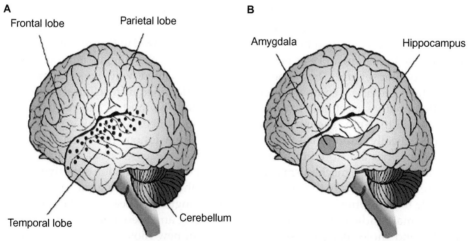

FIGURE 2   Illustrative drawing of the major brain regions and temporal lobe system in the human brain. (A) Anatomical sites, marked by black dots, within the temporal lobe where electrical stimulation evolved memory-like responses in human patients in experiments by Penfield. These studies were some of the first implicating the temporal lobe system in human memory. (B) The location of the hippocampus and amygdala inside the temporal lobe. Adapted from *Basic Neurochemistry, Learning and Memory*, Joe Tsien, Academic Press. Copyright Elsevier 2006.

as follows. First, I will briefly review the anatomy of the hippocampal formation, as this is a necessary foundation for this section and many subsequent chapters in the book. Then we will discuss early studies that highlighted the necessity of proper hippocampal function for memory formation, although this section will be brief because this area has been covered extensively in the literature already and is given adequate treatment in a number of standard textbooks and reviews in the area (see Further Reading).

A. Anatomy of the Hippocampal Formation

As shown in Figure 3, the hippocampus is both downstream and upstream of essentially all the cortical association regions of the CNS (3). This fact in itself suggests that the hippocampus is part of a multimodal sensory integration system in the CNS. We will review the anatomical structure of the hippocampal formation in the following section. This anatomical information will be further strengthened by a variety of functional data that will be reviewed in the last three parts of this section.

Figure 3 illustrates that raw sensory information gathered by the various sensory organs procedes via the thalamus to the cerebral cortex. Sensory information from the various cortical sensory areas is funneled down to the hippocampus via the perirhinal and

entorhinal cortices; these are the cortical areas in the immediate anatomical vicinity of the hippocampus near the rhinal fissure in the temporal lobe. The outputs of the perirhinal and entorhinal cortices then project to the dentate gyrus and the hippocampus proper (these two are referred to jointly as the hippocampal formation).

The hippocampus proper is also known in old-style anatomical nomenclature as *Cornu Ammonis* (Ammon's Horn, after the ram's horn-sporting Greek god) because of its shape. Hippocampus is Greek for sea-horse, which is a term coined by anatomists to describe the overall shape of the anatomical structure. The Cornu Ammonis (CA) terminology leads to four anatomical subdivisions of the hippocampus: areas CA1; CA2; CA3; and CA4. Areas CA1 and CA3 are the largest and most easily identified (Figure 3). The principal neurons in the CA regions are called pyramidal neurons because of the shape of their cell body—they comprise about 90% of all the neurons in the CA regions of the hippocampal formation (see Figure 4). The output neurons of the hippocampus are the CA1 pyramidal neurons—their axons are glutamatergic, and it is via these axons that information leaves the hippocampus proper. The axons of CA1 neurons project predominantly to the ipsilateral and contralateral entorhinal cortices, but additional direct outputs of CA1 neurons project to the contralateral hippocampus via the fornix (see Figure 5). Secondary efferents

Hippocampal Connectivity in the CNS

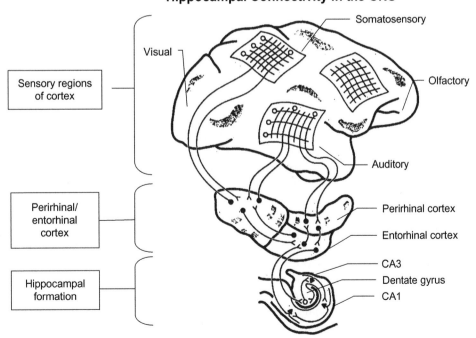

FIGURE 3 Hippocampal connectivity in the CNS. Illustration of the pathway from sensory perceiving regions of the cortex through the perirhinal and entorhinal cortices to the hippocampal formation. Figure adapted from Squire and Zola-Morgan (3). Copyright American Association for the Advancement of Science.

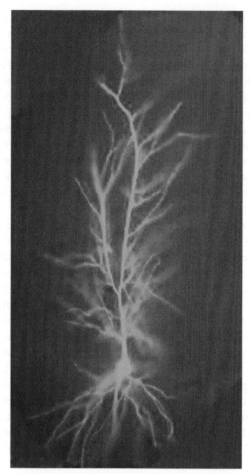

FIGURE 4 A hippocampal pyramidal neuron. This photo illustrates the cell body and dendritic tree of a single hippocampal pyramidal neuron. In this image, the neuron is filled with fluorescent dye to allow visualization. Image courtesy of Shigeo Watanabe and Daniel Johnston.

of CA1 pyramidal neurons via the subicular neurons also project to subcortical regions, including the ventral striatum and mammillary bodies.

We will return to the synaptic structure of the hippocampus in more detail in Chapters 6 and 7. For now suffice it to say that the hippocampus proper, comprising areas CA1–CA4 plus the dentate gyrus, form one functional and anatomical unit involved in information processing and memory consolidation. Exactly how this happens is still a mystery, but current ideas about the cellular and molecular basis of this processing are, of course, the focus of this textbook.

Thus, we can see that information goes out of the hippocampus and ultimately back up into the cortex in its principal pathway, back-tracking its way once again through the entorhinal and perirhinal cortices. I emphasize this because it is important to remember that these cortical areas immediately adjacent to the hippocampal formation are functionally an extension of the hippocampus (and *vice versa*). This is worth

noting because, although I will frequently use the term "hippocampus-dependent," any phenomenon thus described might equally well be described as entorhinal cortex-dependent or perirhinal cortex-dependent. The hippocampal formation and its adjacent cortical regions function in tandem in both memory formation and cognitive processing (4).

Before leaving the topic of cortical inputs into the hippocampus, it is worth emphasizing specifically that the prefrontal cortex and hippocampus are functionally interconnected (5). On the hippocampal input side this connection is from the prefrontal cortex to the entorhinal, perirhinal, and parahippocampal cortices, and thence on to the hippocampus proper. The existence of these connections has, in part, led to the general view of the prefrontal cortex as part of a sensory–motor–limbic integration system. Consistent with this view are the reciprocal connections from the hippocampus back to the prefrontal cortex. These fall into two broad categories. First are the projections from the CA1 pyramidal neurons and subicular neurons to the entorhinal and perirhinal cortices, which then provide efferent innervation back to the prefrontal cortex. A second, more direct route is a projection from CA1 pyramidal neurons onto prefrontal cortex neurons themselves (6).

This integration of hippocampus and prefrontal cortex is important as one considers a potential role for the hippocampus in cognition in general, and schizophrenia in particular, given the widely recognized involvement of dysfunction of the prefrontal cortical areas in schizophrenia (see Table 3). As the hippocampus is one unit that interacts with the prefrontal cortex, dysfunction in each area might precipitate or exacerbate dysfunction in the other.

Finally, note that as is shown in Figure 5 and Table 4, the hippocampus receives a wide variety of extrinsic inputs of various neuromodulatory neurotransmitters. These include projection fibers that are serotonergic, dopaminergic, cholinergic, and noradrenergic. There also are intrinsic interneurons in the hippocampus that are GABAergic, and numerous peptide neuromodulators including reelin, BDNF, NGF, etc., that are all present in the hippocampus. The intrinsic connections between pyramidal neurons in the hippocampus are glutamatergic. I list these neurotransmitter systems to point out the wide variety of neuromodulators hypothesized to be involved in, and important for, hippocampal function.

Although there is not room to go into the function of these various transmitters and neuromodulators in detail, in general these neurotransmitters and neuromodulators help optimize hippocampal function. For example GABA, acetylcholine, norepinephrine, and serotonin all participate in synchronizing hippocampal neuron firing patterns by various mechanisms, effects which are associated with both memory formation and

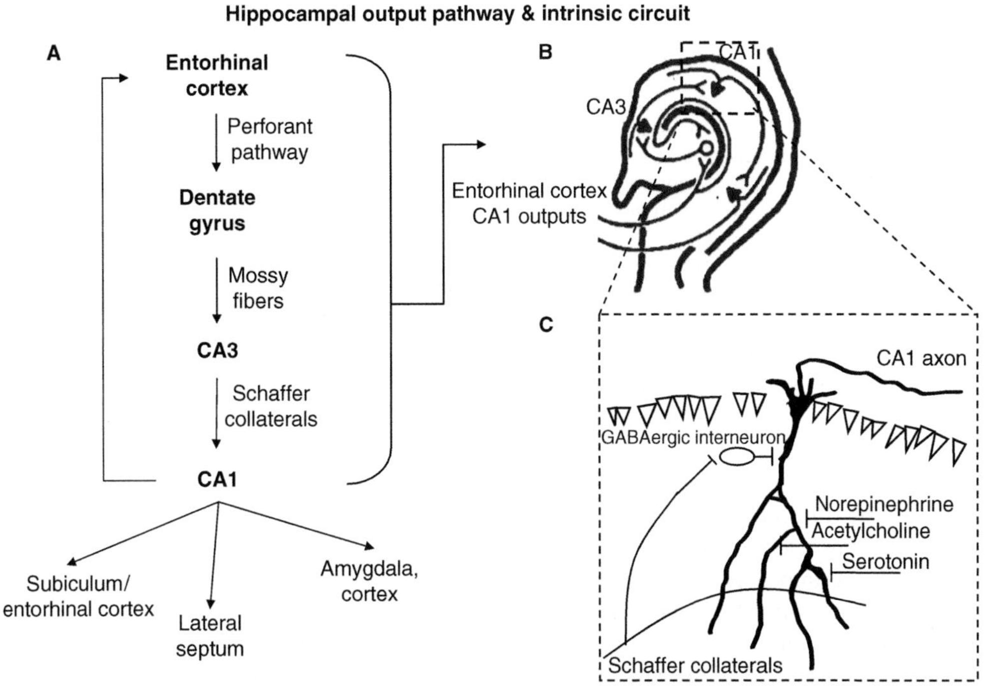

Hippocampal output pathway & intrinsic circuit

FIGURE 5 Hippocampal intrinsic circuit and output pathways. Schematic and illustration of the principal pathway through the hippocampus. On the left is a schematic of the structures through which the sensory signal travels within the hippocampal formation. Top right is a more realistic drawing of these structures (1). Bottom right shows the signaling occurring in area CA1 of the hippocampus, focusing on the cellular connections.

TABLE 3   Memory-Associated Cognitive Dysfunction in Humans

Disease or Syndrome	Type of Memory Affected or Involved*	Likely Anatomical Locus
Schizophrenia	Working memory	Prefrontal cortex
Major depression	Declarative memory	?
Aging-related dementias	Long-term declarative and episodic memory	Temporal lobe hippocampal system
Korsakoff's Syndrome (alcoholism, malnutrition)	Long-term declarative and episodic memory	Mamillary bodies, limbic system, thalamus
Huntington's Disease and Parkinson's Disease	Motor learning, habit learning	Nigro-striatal system
Attention deficit	Generalized or specific learning	Frontal lobes?
hyperactivity disorder (ADHD)	disabilities, dyslexia	Basal ganglia?
Post-traumatic stress disorder* (PTSD)	Aversive associative conditioning, lack of extinction	Amygdala, hippocampus

This is a partial listing of human diseases or syndromes that are associated with certain types of learning and memory deficits. Please note that not all disease characteristics and anatomical regions affected are listed. In addition, learning disabilities and Alzheimer's disease are subjects of entire later chapters of the book. Major depression has been found to be associated with a variety of memory deficits including declarative memory, although the basis for this is unclear.

*PTSD is unique on this list in that it is a disorder caused by excessively robust (or inappropriate) memory, as opposed to a disorder associated with an inability to form memories.

cognitive processing. BDNF and reelin, while typically thought of as trophic factors, also have acute effects on synaptic function in the adult hippocampus. Both these large peptides function as neuromodulators controlling the likelihood of triggering long-lasting changes in hippocampal synaptic function. Of course, the function of glutamate receptors, including the NMDA receptors integral to long-term synaptic plasticity in the hippocampus, is necessary for proper function of the hippocampus and attendant cognitive processing.

As mentioned above, the general roles of the hippocampus and nearby associated cortices appear to be

at least two-fold. One role is to process information of a wide variety of sorts, which we will discuss in other sections of this chapter. The second general function is to download information into the cortex for storage as long-term memory, which we will discuss in the next section.

B. Lesion Studies in Human Memory Formation

As we have already discussed, consolidation is the general term for the process by which memories are rendered stable and lasting. Its existence as a

TABLE 4   Major Neurotransmitters in the Hippocampus

Neurotransmitter	Abbreviation, synonym	General role
Serotonin	5HT, 5-hydroxytryptamine	neuromodulation
Dopamine	DA	neuromodulation
Acetylcholine	ACh	neuromodulation
Norepinephrine	NE	neuromodulation
Gamma-amino butyric acid	GABA	inhibitory transmission
Glutamate	Glu	excitatory transmission

Principle neurotransmitter systems in the hippocampus

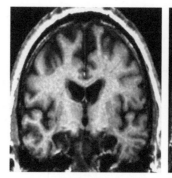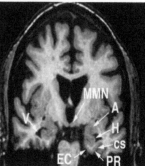

FIGURE 6   (Left) Magnetic resonance imaging scan showing the removal of medial temporal lobe structures in patient H. M. The lesion included all of the entorhinal cortex, most of the perirhinal cortex and amygdala, and about half of the hippocampus. (Right) Scan of a normal control subject showing the structures removed in H. M. A, amygdala; cs, collateral sulcus; EC, entorhinal cortex; H, hippocampus; MMN, medial mammillary nucleus; PR, perirhinal cortex. From Corkin et al. (9). Copyright Elsevier 2003.

phenomenon has been reliably demonstrated by many investigators using many different learning paradigms over a span of four decades. Despite its long history of investigation, however, certain aspects of the process are quite mysterious. For example, it is not clear if consolidation is a process whereby a short-term memory is rendered long-lasting, i.e., a process of serial conversion of short-term to long-term memory, or if short-term and longer-term memories of a given event are consolidated entirely separately.

A few things are clear, however. Consolidation clearly is not a unitary process. There are consolidation processes that subserve different types of learning (explicit versus implicit, for example), that at a minimum utilize different brain areas. There are also distinct consolidation processes for short-term, intermediate-term, and long-term memories that probably are different—we will return to this in the next chapter of the book. There is also a clear distinction between the consolidation of memory versus the storage of memory. Brain lesions to specific areas can lead to a selective disruption of consolidation of new memories without affecting storage and recall of old memories.

The classic studies illustrating this distinction involve patient "H. M." The story of H. M. has been told and analyzed repeatedly in the learning and memory literature, so I will only briefly review the case here. The first studies of H. M. and his memory deficits are landmarks in the field, and helped unequivocally establish the existence of memory consolidation as a distinct process (7–9).

H. M. was (Henry Gustav Molaison, deceased 2008) an unfortunate victim of human neurosurgical experimentation. H. M. initially presented in the early 1950s with epilepsy that was effectively untreatable by any of the drugs or procedures of the day. His seizures were profound and debilitating. His physicians hypothesized that his seizures originated in the hippocampus, a known and common locus of seizure generation. A neurosurgeon named William Scoville performed a bilateral

medial temporal lobe resection on his patient, in an admittedly desperate attempt to control the seizures. This procedure removed most of H. M.'s hippocampi on both sides along with the adjacent cortical tissue, and the amygdala (see reference 9). Figure 6 shows an MRI of patient H. M.'s CNS, illustrating his hippocampal lesions compared to a control subject. Figure 7 illustrates the analysis of the MRI of H. M., compared to the original surgeon's estimate of the extent of his lesions.

This iatrogenic lesion partially treated the epilepsy, and essentially completely destroyed H. M.'s capacity for long-term memory consolidation. H. M.'s prior memories were mostly intact for his lifetime up to several years predating the surgery. However, after the time of the surgery H. M. was essentially completely unable to form any new long-lasting declarative and episodic memories. He lived a minute-to-minute existence for his last 50 years. His only new memories were of facts that he had been exhaustively exposed and re-exposed to.

Testing of H. M. unambiguously demonstrated the existence of consolidation processes in human memory. He had preservation and stability of a large number of pre-existing memories, and a clear capacity to recall them consistently. What he did not have was the capacity to make any new memories that lasted for more than a few seconds without continuous rehearsal.

There has been a general tendency to ascribe this deficit to loss of the hippocampus, which is consistent with a wide variety of animal lesion studies and indeed with the memory consolidation deficits of other patients with more selective hippocampal lesions. However, it is important to remember that H. M. had lesions of the surrounding perihippocampal cortices and the amygdala, which likely contribute to the particularly pronounced nature of his deficits (Figure 7).

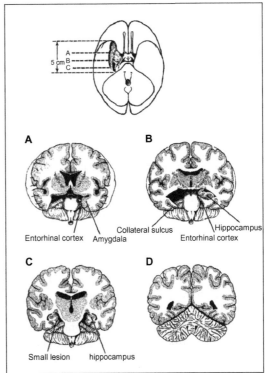

FIGURE 7   MRI of patient H. M.'s brain lesions. (Left) Scan showing the removal of medial temporal lobe structures in H. M. The lesion included all the entorhinal cortex, most of the perirhinal cortex and amygdala, and about half of the hippocampus. (Right) Scan of control subject. A, amygdala; cs, collateral sulcus; EC, Entorhinal cortex; H, hippocampus; MMN, medial mammillary nucleus; PR, perirhinal cortex. Reproduced from Corkin et al. (9).

Also, given what we discussed earlier in this chapter about the role of the hippocampus in multimodal cognitive processing, one wonders about generalized cognitive deficits in H. M. I am not referring to a loss of intelligence, but rather to the possibility of a general inability to process information about his surroundings, correlations among items and events, etc. These problems may also have contributed to his cognitive problems and his long-term memory deficits. These considerations do not negate the conclusion of a deficit in memory consolidation in H. M., but simply point out that interpreting the basis of H. M.'s cognitive deficits should take into consideration modern ideas about the important role of the hippocampus in information processing as well as memory consolidation.

The role of the hippocampus in memory consolidation that was identified in the initial landmark studies of H. M. have been confirmed and extended in a wide variety of hippocampal lesion studies in experimental animals. Obviously, animal experimentation allows a much more detailed and controlled experimental approach than human studies and a number of attributes of hippocampus-dependent memory consolidation have become clear. For example, inhibitors

of protein synthesis block memory consolidation when they are applied after training. Consolidation is known to be a process that requires several hours after training. Hippocampus-dependent long-term memory consolidation is also dependent on altered gene expression. Activation of the NMDA subtype of glutamate receptor is involved, as are a number of signal transduction mechanisms and neuromodulatory neurotransmitter systems. Overall, a quite wide variety of studies using many different approaches have demonstrated that involvement in memory consolidation is a central attribute of hippocampal function. We will spend much of the rest of the book discussing the cellular and molecular particulars of this process. In brief, the hippocampus serves as an intermediate-term memory store that ultimately downloads information to the cortex for longer-term storage. The basis for this process is mysterious, but one thing that is clear is that the hippocampus must be able to hold a memory trace for some appreciable period of time—hours to days or weeks at least.

In Chapter 7 we will talk about a cellular mechanism likely to be critical to allowing the hippocampus to serve as this sort of memory buffer—*long-term*

BOX 1

STUDIES IN NON-HUMAN PRIMATE MODELS

Human patient studies have provided compelling evidence for multiple memory systems, and indeed have fundamentally changed scientific thinking about how memory works. Careful and ethically-conscientious studies of human subjects have both improved our basic understanding of mechanisms of memory and allowed the development of new medical and behavioral approaches to improving function in patients with cognitive disorders. However, studies with human subjects are, of necessity, limited by ethical and moral considerations.

Studies with non-human primates represent a powerful additional approach to understanding memory and cognitive processing in complex nervous systems that closely resemble the human CNS anatomically. Studies in non-human primates, of course, allow different kinds of experimental approaches that are not practicable in humans. Many sophisticated and elegant studies of memory function in non-human primates have supported the basic models of memory systems that we have been discussing in this chapter, at the anatomical, functional, cellular, and behavioral levels. However, animal studies have led to significant refinements of our thinking about the role of medial temporal lobe structures in primate (including human) memory. These "refinements" can be briefly summarized as:

Thinking of human declarative, episodic, and spatial memory as exclusively hippocampus-dependent is too great an oversimplification. Many medial lobe anatomical structures are involved in these forms of memory, including the perirhinal, parahippocampal, and entorhinal cortices, and likely even the amygdala and its adjacent cortical areas are involved in a modulatory capacity.

Lesions to the hippocampus provoke greater retrograde amnesia than was initially thought, based on studies of patients like H. M. Sophisticated studies in monkeys demonstrated that hippocampal lesions result in retrograde amnesia for items learned weeks or months before. Indeed, recent studies using human subjects have indicated that hippocampal damage results in partial retrograde amnesia for events occurring up to several years previously (22). At a minimum, these various studies imply that the hippocampus-dependent memory consolidation period in primates extends much longer than is apparent from most studies of simpler animal models.

Detailed descriptions of the experimental basis for these brief generalizations are presented in reviews by Mishkin et al. (1998), Cipolotti and Bird (2006), and Zola and Squire (2001), listed in Further Reading.

---

potentiation (LTP). Long-lasting synaptic potentiation of this sort is also likely involved in the precise formation and maintenance of hippocampal place cell firing patterns. We also will touch on shorter-lasting forms of synaptic plasticity that may be involved in short-term storage of information and information processing in the hippocampus; phenomena such as post-tetanic potentiation (PTP) and short-term potentiation (STP) that may be involved in the "timing" aspect of hippocampal processing of CS-US contingencies over the period of a few seconds.

Characterization of the memory deficits in H. M. provided a turning point in the history of cognitive neuroscience. For example, it became clear that H. M. had selective deficits in certain types of memory. Some memory systems were still intact, and thus hippocampus-independent. Studies of H. M. and patients like him with hippocampal lesions led to a new classification system for different types of memory in the human—the multiple memory systems concept that we

discussed at the beginning of the chapter. Declarative memories, facts and personal experiences, are dependent on the hippocampus and medial temporal lobe for their formation. Many other types of memories, including motor learning and many types of associative conditioning, are hippocampus-independent.

C. Imaging Studies

A clear prediction of the hypothesis that the hippocampus is involved in memory formation is that measurable hippocampal activation should be associated with long-term memory formation. The availability of functional imaging technologies that allow one to test the CNS structures that are activated with various tasks, using non-invasive techniques on living, breathing, thinking humans (see Box 2), has made testing the hypothesis a practical possibility. Indeed, a wide variety of different *in vivo* imaging experiments using human subjects have explored the idea

BOX 2

MRI, fMRI, AND PET

The capacity to probe the structure and function of the human CNS, non-invasively, and in an awake, behaving human is one of the most phenomenal technological steps forward in recent history. The three most commonly used approaches in this area for human studies are: magnetic resonance imaging (MRI); functional MRI (fMRI); and positron emission tomography (PET).

The order of this list also generally reflects their ease of use and the breadth of their availability.

MRI was originally referred to as nuclear magnetic resonance (NMR) imaging. NMR is actually a more accurate term to describe the physical basis of MRI—MRI is a sophisticated technology based on the capacity to detect subtle changes in the orientation of atomic

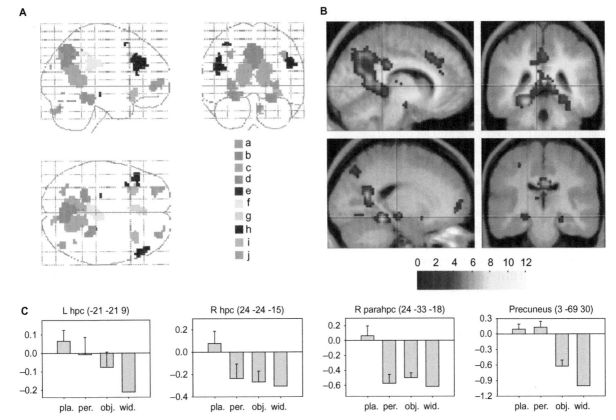

BOX 1 Functional neuroimaging of the retrieval of the spatial context of an event. (A) Areas activated in the place condition relative to the perceptual control condition width are shown in color on a "glass brain" and include: (a) posterior parietal; (b) precuneus; (c) parieto-occipital sulcus and retrosplenial cortex; (d) parahippocampal gyrus; (e) hippocampus; (f) midposterior cingulate; (g) anterior cingulate; (h) dorsolateral prefrontal cortex; (i) ventrolateral prefrontal cortex; and (j) anterior prefrontal cortex ($p < 0.001$ uncorrected for multiple comparisons). (B) Activations in place-width shown on the averaged normalized structural MR images of the subjects, with threshold $p < 0.01$ uncorrected for multiple comparisons. Coronal and saggital slices through the left retrosplenial cortex (above) and left hippocampus (below) are shown. (C) Level of activation in four regions across all conditions place (pla), person (per), object (obj), and width (wid), shown as estimated percent signal change relative to background activation (i.e., when the subject is moving between questions). The name of the regions and x, y, and z coordinate of location (the voxel of peak response) is given above each graph. Note the strongly spatial response of right (R) hippocampal (hpc), and parahippocampal (parahpc) areas. The left parahippocampus (not shown) shows a similarly spatial pattern, whereas the responses estimate for that condition and the parameter estimate for the width condition. Figure adapted from Burgess et al. (2001b). Copyright Elsevier 2002.

Continued

BOX 2—cont'd

MRI, fMRI, AND PET

nuclei when they are placed in a powerful magnetic field and probed with electromagnetic pulses. The resonance of nuclei in the atoms and molecules in tissue is the fundamental property being measured by an MRI machine. Due to differences in the magnetic resonance properties of different types of tissues and fluids in the human body, highly detailed anatomical images can be generated by quantitating these differences and displaying them as an anatomical picture.

MRI is thus a powerful tool to image anatomical structures in living humans, without hurting the subject under study. MRI is typically used to define normal anatomy, and lesions, pathologies, and breakages. When NMR imaging began to be widely applied to human patients, the "nuclear" was dropped from the name in order to make the process sound less frightening. The 2003 Nobel Prize in medicine was awarded to Paul Lauterbur and Sir Peter Mansfield for developing MRI for clinical use.

Metabolic changes in brain cells of course trigger chemical changes in fluids surrounding the tissue, especially secondarily to the use of oxygen for metabolic purposes. These chemical changes trigger local changes in blood flow in order to compensate for oxygen usage—specifically, oxygen is dumped from hemoglobin and local blood flow rate increases to compensate. This causes a change in the magnetic resonance properties of the hemoglobin in the blood that is detectable with MRI. Functional MRI measures these metabolic changes in real-time, and is used as an index of functional activity. An fMRI (blood flow) signal can be mapped onto a corresponding

anatomical MRI (see Figure) to localize regions of the CNS that are activated under specific conditions, such as learning a list of names. This is an experiment in real-time, in a behaving human, which gives insights into the anatomical structures involved in CNS function. The principal limitations of fMRI are the relatively slow rate of real-time analysis (minutes instead of seconds) because of the need for averaging signals, and the fact that fMRI is measuring a signal (indirectly, oxygen usage) that is many mechanistic steps removed from neuronal activity *per se*. Nevertheless, fMRI is an extremely powerful approach for studying the neuroanatomical basis of human cognitive function and dysfunction.

PET imaging is less widely used, because it involves the use of radioactive materials injected into the subject. For PET, materials that can tag a tissue or cell type of interest are labeled with a radioactive atom and the anatomical distribution of the radioactive material is determined with tomography techniques. How does one tag the tissue or cell of interest? You might look for metabolically active cells using labeled glucose derivatives, for example, or use labeled specific ligands that bind to receptors on certain cells to localize those types of cells. In PET scanning, the distribution of the radioactive material is compared to an anatomical image produced by MRI or X-ray-based methods. This allows the accurate anatomical localization of the molecule of interest. The PET term comes from the fact that when the radioactive material decays it results indirectly in positron emission, and the anatomical distribution is determined with tomography.

that hippocampal activation should be correlated with memory formation, using either PET or fMRI-type imaging. Unfortunately, so far there has not been a great deal of consistency in the results among these types of studies, therefore it has not been unambiguously demonstrated that hippocampal activation is clearly associated with memory formation.

Part of the reason for the inconsistent results is probably the fact that *in vivo* imaging technologies in humans are fairly new, and there likely has been inconsistent application of the technology across studies. Also, new technologies, of necessity, bring with them a period of time when the various technical and theoretical approaches are being refined; this has certainly been the case with human imaging studies

in memory. Therefore, at this point in the development of the field not many definitive statements can be made concerning the role of the hippocampus in human memory formation, based on the approach of human imaging. However, I would like to make a few general comments to indicate some of the interesting ideas that are beginning to emerge.

One interesting idea that has been supported by numerous studies is that there is lateralization of hippocampal function in humans. Lateralization simply means that the left hippocampus does something different from the right hippocampus. In general, the right hippocampus (in humans) appears to be more involved in visual and spatial learning and memory, while the left hippocampus appears to be more

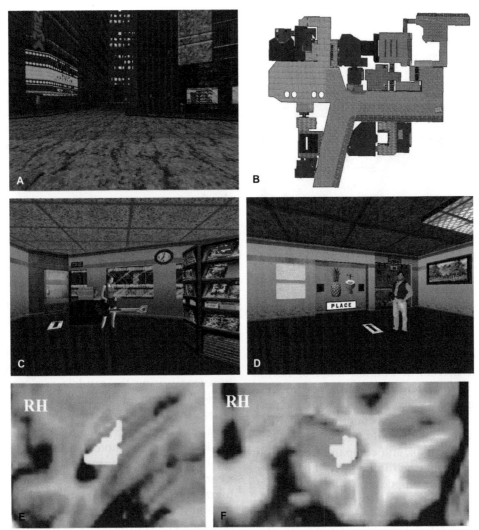

FIGURE 8   The virtual reality town used in functional neuroimaging and neurophysiological studies of topographical and episodic memory. (A) A view from within the town, as seen by a subject. (B) Aerial view of the area used for testing navigation in neuropsychological studies. This view was never seen by subjects. (C) Receiving an object in the episodic memory test. (D) Answering a "place" question in the episodic memory test. (E and F) Activation of the right hippocampus correlates with accuracy of navigation in the virtual reality (VR) town. The loci of significant correlation are shown superimposed on the structural template to which all scans were normalized (r = 0.56); significant correlation was also found in the right inferior parietal cortex. Adapted from Burgess et al. (2002). *Neuron* 35:625–642. Copyright Elsevier 2002.

involved in verbal and narrative memory. Another interesting finding that appears with reasonable consistency in the literature is that the hippocampus is reliably activated with memory retrieval. This is, of course, not a prediction that necessarily arises out of the hypothesis that the hippocampus is involved in memory consolidation.

This is not to say that the hippocampus has not been found to be activated with memory acquisition—that is also the case. For example, the hippocampus has been found to be activated when human subjects learn to navigate a "virtual town." In these studies human subjects in an fMRI scanner can learn to navigate a computer-based virtual town, and the activity of the hippocampus be imaged simultaneously (see Figure 8

and reference 10). Studies of this sort, along with other studies of memory acquisition, have in many instances supported a role for the hippocampus in memory acquisition, and also in spatial navigation. Along similar lines, various studies have reported hippocampal activation, using both PET and fMRI approaches, when subjects are presented with novel stimuli. The activation of the hippocampus with novel stimuli may both represent the use of the hippocampus as a memory comparator for identifying novel stimuli, and the use of the hippocampus to encode and form memories for new items or places.

Finally, one of the more fascinating human imaging studies investigating the function of the hippocampus involved studying London taxi drivers. The layout of

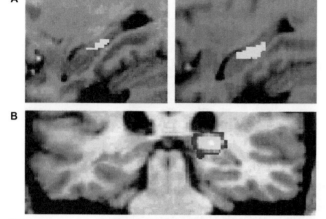

FIGURE 9 (A) Voxel based morphometry indicates increased posterior hippocampal volume bilaterally in licensed London taxi drivers compared with control subjects. (B) Amount of time spent taxi driving (corrected for age) was positively correlated with volume increase in the right posterior hippocampus. Adapted from Maguire et al. (2000a). Copyright Elsevier 2002.

the streets of London is notoriously convoluted, and experienced taxi drivers in London must of necessity have undertaken extensive learning and memorization of navigational cues and street relationships. Hence, Maguire and colleagues undertook structural MRIs of the brains of licensed London taxi drivers, analyzed their hippocampi, and compared them with those of control subjects who did not drive taxis. They found that the posterior hippocampus (bilaterally) of taxi drivers was significantly larger relative to that of control subjects (see Figure 9 and reference 11). In addition, hippocampal volume correlated with the amount of time they had spent as a taxi driver. These findings suggest the interesting idea that the posterior hippocampus is involved in storing a spatial representation of the environment, and that this particular brain region can grow to accommodate a need for this capacity in people with a high dependence on navigational skills. Overall, these data are also consistent with a role for the hippocampus in spatial navigation and spatial memory formation.

III. MOTOR LEARNING

One cannot help but be awed when watching an accomplished gymnast, professional athlete, or virtuoso guitarist in action (Figure 10). The human capacity for learning and executing finely-tuned motor patterns is the product of millions of years of evolutionary refinement through natural selection. Indeed, it's fairly easy to imagine how the three examples I gave in the first sentence may translate into an improved

likelihood of survival of the species. The capability to perform an acrobatic maneuver might mean escaping a predator. The capacity to throw a round object with great velocity and accuracy might mean putting dinner on the table. The capacity to rapidly and precisely move your fingers on a six-stringed instrument might mean … er …, uhm … OK, maybe my father was right and I wasted my time learning how to do that. Regardless, the human capacity for motor learning is amazing.

A. Anatomy

There are two basic anatomical systems involved in human motor performance and motor learning (see Figure 11). The first is the cerebellar system, which we will discuss in more detail in Chapter 5 where we will talk about cerebellum-dependent associative memory. The second is the basal ganglia-dependent (striatal) system, which I will briefly outline here.

The term "basal ganglia" refers to a collection of interacting CNS structures and neuronal nuclei (see Figures 12 and 13). The basal ganglia are the striatum (comprising the caudate nucleus, putamen, and nucleus accumbens), and the globus pallidus. The striatum is the principal input nucleus for this pathway, and it receives afferents from essentially every cortical area, both motor and sensory. Other parts of the basal ganglia are the subthalamic nucleus, which interacts with the globus pallidus, and the substantia nigra, which contains dopaminergic neuron cell bodies and modulates striatal function. The output of the basal ganglia is principally to the ventral anterior and ventrolateral nuclei of the thalamus. There is very little output of these thalamic nuclei to the brain stem or spinal cord motor nuclei—instead they project back up into the cortex to the motor and premotor cortices (along with the prefrontal association cortex).

This basic and simplified wiring diagram (see Figure 13) illustrates that the basal ganglia are part of a signal-processing recurrent loop that downloads information from the cortex, processes it, and returns it to the cortex. The upshot of all this wiring is that the basal ganglia do not directly control movement—they coordinate motor programs. Thus, it is very important to note that the striatal system does not perform learning operations independently. As is suggested by the anatomical wiring described above, the motor cortex and premotor cortex also are integrally involved in striatum-dependent learning.

In addition, it is important to note that the basal ganglia are also involved in goal-oriented behavior. Reward systems involving the nucleus accumbens and the substantia nigra dopaminergic system are important for positively motivated learning (12–14).

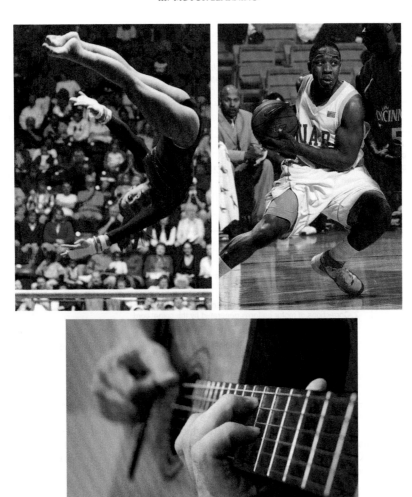

FIGURE 10 Examples of excellence in human motor learning and memory: University of Alabama gymnast (photo courtesy of Dusty Compton), a University of Alabama at Birmingham basketball player (image courtesy of the UAB Athletic Department), and a University music student playing guitar.

This system can also be "hijacked" in order to promote drug addiction (see Box 3). Finally, recent findings suggest that the striatal system is also likely involved in learning certain non-motor cognitive tasks that involve repetition—a good example is becoming facile with reading mirror-images of words (15). The basal ganglia system may indeed be involved in language learning and cognition in general, although this is fairly speculative at this point in time (16).

B. Habits

This striatum-associated system is involved in learning several different subtypes of memorized responses that involve motor responses as an output. One category is habits—for example you might always turn left after you get off the elevator, in order to get to your laboratory. With time this will become a simple ingrained motor response that you execute automatically. Habits are generally not consciously perceived unless the parameters change—for example when someone changes laboratory locations and needs to turn right instead of left when they get off the elevator. For a while after the laboratory moves locations they may keep "accidentally" turning left when they get off the elevator, until they reform a new appropriate habit.

C. Stereotyped Movements

Another category of striatum-dependent learning is the learning of stereotyped movements. A classic example of this from animal behavioral studies is memory involving stereotyped motor movements, such as bar-pressing for food rewards. Normal human stereotyped movements can be fairly complex and based on contingencies—for example "step on the gas when the stoplight turns green." One may perform

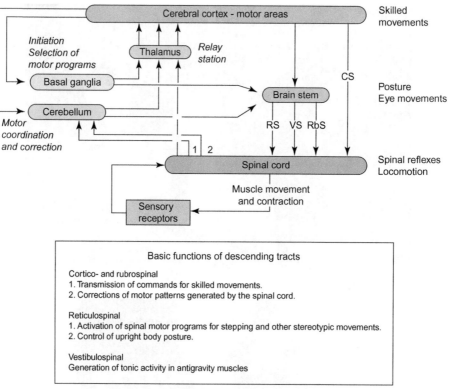

FIGURE 11 Summarizing scheme of the interaction between different motor centers. The different major compartments of the motor system and their main pathways for interaction are indicated. The basic functions of the different compartments and descending tracks are summarized on and below the scheme. CS, corticospinal; RbS, rubrospinal; VS, vestibulospinal; RS, reticulospinal. Adapted from *Fundamental Neuroscience, Fundamentals of Motor Systems*, Sten Grillner. Copyright Elsevier 2003.

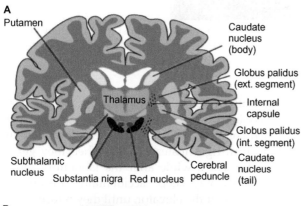

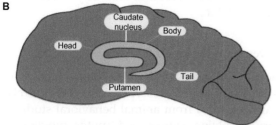

FIGURE 12 Location of basal ganglia in the human brain. (A) Coronal section. (B) Parasagittal section. Figure from *Fundamental Neuroscience: The Basal Ganglia*, Jonathan Mink. Copyright Elsevier 2003.

this stereotyped response many times every day, in an unconscious fashion. This unconscious stereotyped movement might cause someone to accidentally step on the gas when the left-hand turn arrow turns green, while their lane still has a red light.

The term stereotyped, when applied to behaviors, can also refer to non-learned behaviors. Psychologists and ethologists used the term stereotyped to refer to innate behaviors that are developmentally programmed. In the clinical literature, stereotyped also refers to unlearned repetitive motor behaviors that are associated with certain diseases and pathologies. For example, girls with Rett's Syndrome exhibit stereotyped repetitive hand-wringing as part of the disorder. Tourette's Syndrome can involve stereotyped tics and even extensive involuntary limb movements.

D. Sequence Learning

A third category of striatum-dependent learning is the learning of sequenced movements. A good example of this is dialing telephone numbers. If you think of a telephone touch-pad as a 3×4 matrix, dialing a phone number is a motor sequence involving serially touching specific spots on the matrix. How long does

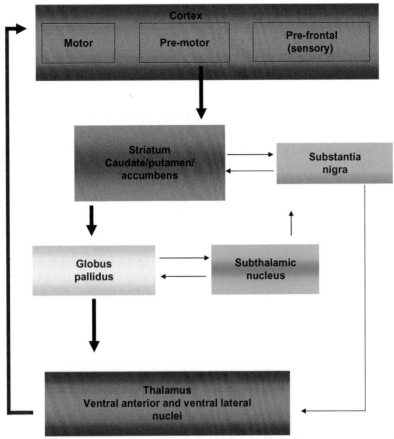

FIGURE 13 The striatal motor learning system. The principal anatomical interconnections of the system are illustrated. Figure by J. David Sweatt and Felecia Hester.

BOX 3

DRUG ADDICTION AND REWARD

Addiction manifests itself as a compulsive drive to obtain and use various substances. Drugs of abuse include such compounds as cocaine, amphetamine, methamphetamine, phencyclidine (PCP or angel dust), ecstacy, heroin or its derivatives, and nicotine. Drug addiction manifests itself as altered behavior, and this altered behavior is acquired via experiencing specific environmental and endogenous cues. Altered behavior in response to environmental signals—sound familiar? Sounds like memory.

Indeed, recent discoveries have highlighted two striking commonalities between memory and addiction. Both commonalities are mechanistic. First, addiction and positively reinforced learning and memory have in common their utilization of the dopaminergic reward system in the CNS. Many drugs of abuse act either directly or indirectly on ventral tegmental area-based (VTA) dopaminergic neurons, and other reward circuitry in the CNS, in order to reinforce their administration. Thus, many drugs of abuse "hijack" the reward system used in normal memory formation. Thereby, memory and drug addiction share a common anatomical and cellular substrate. In part, addiction "sounds like memory," because it in fact uses some of the same mechanisms used for normal memory formation. The dopaminergic reward system contributes to the reinforcing effects of acute administration of many drugs, and to the cognitive and psychological drive to consume those drugs again in the future.

Memory and addiction also have a second commonality. At the molecular level they use many of the same signal transduction and gene transcription pathways to

Continued

BOX 3—cont'd

DRUG ADDICTION AND REWARD

trigger their lasting effects. There is a striking conservation of molecular signaling pathways that have been discovered to be operating in drug addiction versus normal memory formation. This is perhaps not surprising in retrospect, because molecular pathways that trigger lasting changes in one situation and in one set of cells are likely to be involved in triggering lasting changes in other situations and in other sets of cells. Nevertheless, many of the specific molecular mechanisms for learning and memory that we will be discussing in the remainder of this book are also implicated in drug addiction.

One final point is not a commonality between addiction and memory, but is also a point worth emphasizing.

Drugs of abuse are usually repeatedly administered. Over time this leads to down-regulation of both the reward system and molecular pathways activated by the drug. This situation leads to tolerance of the drug, a diminution of its effects. This sets up a vicious cycle with the addict needing increasing doses of the drug over time to achieve the same rewarding effects. This exacerbates an already bad situation. Moreover, the down-regulation of the drug-stimulated pathways, in cells both inside and outside of the CNS, contributes to physical dependency on the drug. That is, the person's overall physiology, having adapted to the chronic presence of the drug, no longer operates normally in its absence.

---

it take you to dial a 10-digit phone number the first time you dial it? How long does it take you to dial a number you call all the time? It almost certainly takes noticebably less time for you to dial a very familiar number. But think about it—the motor task *is the same* for both numbers—hit 10 spots on a 3×4 matrix in a particular order. Your facility with dialing a familiar number is due to your having learned a particular motor sequence.

Sequence learning of this sort involves the striatal motor memory system. Interestingly, the caudate nucleus appears to be involved in sequence learning that involves voluntary processing, while the putamen may underlie "incidental" or unconscious sequence learning. These types of sequence learning are likely modules also contributing to the learning of more complex overall motor patterns. The striatal learning system allows humans to produce the examples of skilled motor learning with which we began this discussion, e.g., gymnastics, sports, and playing musical instruments.

IV. PRODIGIOUS MEMORY

A. Mnemonists

A mnemonist is a person with a prodigious memory capacity. It also is common to refer to these individuals as having a photographic memory, or total recall.

The experimental psychologist A. R. Luria has written an excellent brief exposition of one of his subjects—S,[2] who had an apparently limitless capacity for memorization (17). Limitless is used here in a literal sense—Luria was never able to experimentally saturate or confound S's capacity for memorization. S could also accurately recall long, random, arbitrary lists of items for years without any intervening rehearsal.

As a young person S worked as a newspaper writer. He came to Luria's attention because S's editor noticed that he never needed to take any notes concerning the long list of daily reporting assignments he was given. Naturally, his editor was curious. When the editor inquired concerning his lack of need for note-taking, he expressed surprise that his memory capacity was anything unusual. The editor sent S to Luria, a prominent psychologist in Moscow at the time (the 1920s). Luria characterized S's prodigious capacity for memorization and documented his results in the scientific literature.

It is interesting to consider how S's memorization process worked. Luria determined through interviews that his capacity for memorization was not automatic—he had developed techniques to facilitate his memory. For example, when memorizing lists he would mentally place the serial components of the list along a geographical or architectural substructure. For

---

[2] S's real name was Solomon Veniaminovich Shereshevskii—no wonder Luria abbreviated it.

example, he might memorize a list by assigning each component serially to a specific place along a familiar city street. Item A would be assigned to the corner shop, Item B to the next shop in line, Item C, to the next, and so on. This is similar to a memory-enhancement technique that many individuals still practice today. In essence what this does is allow multiple associations to be formed for each item in a list that needs to be remembered. There are multiple memory-recall cues available for individual items.

S also manifested the phenomenon referred to as *synesthesia*. With synesthesia, individual sensory stimuli also simultaneously trigger other multiple sensory impressions. For example, with synesthetics seeing the color green may also automatically trigger a specific taste perception and the perception of hearing a particular tone. In S's case the recruitment of these multiple sensory modalities as part of the memory-forming process gave him additional associations, automatically, every time he presented himself with items to memorize.

We might well be envious of individuals like S who have such a comprehensive and total capacity for memorization. However, one must be careful what they wish for. In S's case he was in fact fairly dysfunctional in terms of daily living. His synesthesia, for example, made it very difficult for him to maintain his thoughts while trying to read. Random words in a sentence might trigger horrendous sensations or associations, completely distracting him from the topic at hand. Sadly, S lived out the later years of his life as a carnival and stage performer, demonstrating feats of memorization. His idiosyncrasies precluded him from being able to maintain employment in more traditional careers.

Another more recent example of someone possessing a prodigious memory is Rajan Srinavasen Mahadevan (who pursues his side-career as a mnemonist simply using the name Rajan, see Figure 14). Rajan memorized over 30,000 digits worth of the numerical value of the mathematical constant π (pi). You may be lucky to remember π as 3.14159 …, and likely recall that pi is a numerically undefined geometrical ratio and continues infinitely with no repetition. In other words, memorizing pi to almost 32,000 decimal places is no small feat (see Figure 15). Rajan's capacity to recall and work with his memorized value for pi is not limited to simply repeating it back. For example, if you present Rajan with a string of digits, within a few seconds he can accurately determine whether or not the string appears in his memorized value for pi. Within about 10 seconds he can also recall any specific digit within the first 10,000 digits of pi—for example, that spot number 6,482 in the sequence is the number 3 (or whatever it is).

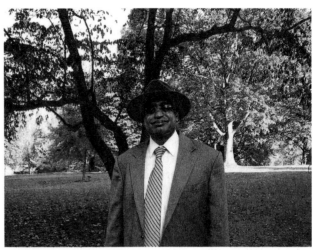

FIGURE 14   Rajan. Photo courtesy of Dr Rajan Mahadevan.

3.141592653589793238462643383279502884197169399375105820974944592307816406286208998628034825342117067982148086513282306647093844609550582231725359408128481117450284102701938521105559644622948954930381964428810975665933446128475648233786783165271201909145648566923460348610454326648213393607260249141273724587006606315588174881520920962829254091715364367892590360011330530548820466521384146951941511609433057270365759591953092186117381931926117931051185480744623799627495673518857527248912279381830119491298336733624406566430860021394946395224737190702179860943702770539217176293176752384674818467669405132000568127145263560827785771342757789609173637178721468440901224953430146549585371050792279689258923542019956112129021960864034418159813629774771309960518707211349999998372978049951059731732816096318595024459455346908302642522308253344685035261931188171010003137838752886587533203881420617177669147303598253490428755468731159562863882353787593751957781857780532171226806613001927876611195909216420198 9....

FIGURE 15   1000 decimal places of pi. Memorization of the mathematical constant pi (π), which extends infinitely without repetition, has been used to demonstrate impressive mnemonic capacity in individual humans. Several people have been documented to have accurately memorized pi to thousands of decimal places. For illustrative purposes, 1000 digits of pi are shown above.

Systematic studies of Rajan's memory capacity have given a couple of additional insights. First, it is notable that Rajan's memory capacity for numbers is based on a "matrix" technique that he developed, that is, a specific mental assistance device that he devised. Rajan developed the matrix technique as part of about a thousand hours of practice memorizing the numerical value of pi. In part for this reason, Rajan's exceptional memory capability extends to memorizing various lists of numbers, but does not generalize to other categories of memorization such as spatial memorization (18–19).

B. Savant Syndrome

A savant is a learned person, a scholar, a polymath. If you are reading this book you likely aspire to be a savant. However, in some cases exceptional capacities in one realm are associated with severe disabilities in another. For example, an individual with severe learning disabilities and mental retardation may still have astounding abilities in a single pursuit, such as music, calculation or memorization. An oxymoronic and outdated term for this condition is "idiot savant." More modern usage refers to this as savant syndrome, or in some cases autistic savant where diagnosable autism is present.

Savant syndrome has fascinated humans throughout history. Many of you have probably seen the movie *Rain Man*, starring Dustin Hoffman as Raymond (Rain Man) Babbit. The Rain Man character is very loosely based on a real person, Kim Peek, a man possessing both prodigious memory and an amazing capacity for performing mental mathematical calculations (Figure 16).

Although Peek has a number of specific learning disabilities and some fairly restrictive problems with motor coordination, he is able to work as a book-keeper, utilizing his exceptional skills (memory and the capacity for rapid calculation) in that endeavor. Peek has undergone both extensive psychological testing and neuro-imaging (20). Neuro-anatomically he has cerebellar abnormalities, accounting for the diminished motor coordination, and he also lacks a corpus callosum.

Peek's memory capacity is truly astounding, and is the type we commonly think of when we think of a photographic memory (also referred to as eidetic memory). Peek can read a book from cover to cover, taking about 8–10 seconds per page—for your reference that means he could read this entire book in a little over an hour. After reading a book once, he has the contents completely memorized and available for rapid and very accurate recall. Thus far he has memorized over 10,000 books. This suggests that his memory capacity is essentially inexhaustible.

Like other savant syndrome patients that have been studied, Peek has great facility in associating specific calendar dates (past or future) with days of the week. This capacity has been associated with prodigious memory, and the two phenomena may be causally linked (21). This conclusion is based on a case study with PET imaging studies of a human subject, which demonstrated that the hippocampus and other temporal lobe memory-associated systems are activated when an autistic savant "computes" the days of the week associated with specific calendar dates. However, it is important to note that this aspect of savantism could be related to prodigious mathematical capacity as well, or involve both calculating and memorization.

C. You are a Prodigy

While we have spent the last few sections discussing mnemonists and savants, just regular memory is

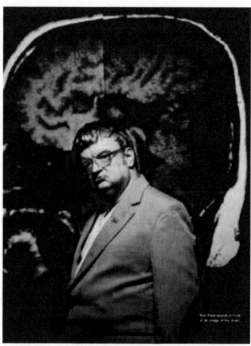

FIGURE 16 Kim Peek. Photo courtesy of Darold Treffert, Wisconsin Medical Society (2006). *Scientific American Mind* 17(3):50–55. Copyright Scientific American 2006.

prodigious enough when you think about it. Things you take for granted in your everyday life require an extremely accurate and capacious memory system for you to execute. You can recognize hundreds of faces and scenes with an astounding degree of accuracy. Your vocabulary comprises thousands of words. You can remember hundreds of anecdotes and stories about your experiences. The memories for these items and episodes can last a lifetime without being subject to significant corruption. The normal human capacity for memory could be described with the term "prodigious" for the majority of individuals. It is just that our memory capacity is so familiar that we take it for granted, and words like prodigious are reserved to denote the exceptions and rarities.

But, before moving on to our continuing discussion of memory mechanisms in further chapters, I want to reinforce this notion of the impressiveness of the durability and fidelity of normal human memory. After all, we are interested in understanding normal memory, not just exceptional memory. As memory scientists we really only look at exceptional memory in order for it to give us insights into normal memory; in the following few paragraphs I will review a set of studies that suggest that normal human memory may be closer to "prodigious" than you might first think.

An important insight into this issue arose from Wilder Penfield's studies with stimulating human cortex during surgery to treat epilepsy—stimulating the cortex in particular areas appeared to trigger recall of specific memories (see Figure 2). These findings are part of what has led to the broadly held hypothesis that the cerebral cortex is the site of storage of declarative and episodic memories in humans and other animals.

However, we will consider Penfield's discovery in a different light. When Penfield stimulated a patient's cortex, in many instances he evoked vivid and highly detailed recollections. The degree of detail involved was beyond anything that might be available for normal deliberately evoked conscious recall; in other words, a degree of detail beyond what was normally available to the human subject under study. This suggests that recall, not storage, might be the normal rate-limiting process for human memory. All of us might have prodigious memory storage, just not prodigious capacity for recall.

I do not wish to focus on the limitations of recall; I want to focus your attention on the implication of these observations concerning the normal human capacity for memory formation and storage. Penfield's observations suggest that the average human may have a vast array of highly-detailed memories stored in their cerebral cortex. These memories are stored there for years, decades or a lifetime. They apparently are stored with high fidelity and accuracy. This tells us something fundamental about normal human memory—there must exist in our CNS the cellular and molecular machinery that allows storage of huge amounts of information, which is stored with high fidelity and for all practical purposes permanently, as long as we are alive and healthy. The rest of this book will be a summary and description of our current state of understanding of these cellular and molecular processes.

Finally, I would like to emphasize that it is becoming clear that the hippocampus is involved in much more than just its well-established role in long-term memory consolidation. Experimental results over the last several years have demonstrated that the hippocampus is involved in moment-to-moment processing of a wide variety of environmental signals, and in forming a cohesive construct and unified representation of the outside world within the CNS. This new understanding has emerged largely from studies of hippocampal pyramidal neuron firing patterns recorded *in vivo* in behaving rodents, studies that will be the basis for Chapter 6.

In Chapter 6, I will describe work from several laboratories that followed the patterns of firing of hippocampal pyramidal neurons while animals executed a number of different behavioral tasks, including exploring mazes, learning that some environmental cues reliably predict others, while processing complex environmental signals. These studies have led to a new appreciation of the role of the hippocampus in moment-to-moment cognitive processing, and in forming a cohesive construct of the animal's surround. It is important to remember that this level of cognitive processing also is dependent on the hippocampus, in addition to the processes of long-term memory consolidation that will be the focus of this section.

V. SUMMARY

The capacity for high-fidelity lifelong memory is indeed impressive and fascinating. In the next chapter we will begin to discuss molecular and cellular investigations into the mechanisms underlying such memory. In doing this we begin a fascinating journey that will take us through the rest of the book, exploring in detail the biochemical and neurophysiological mechanisms that underlie memory formation and storage.

However, in considering several basic aspects of human memory, several highlights from this chapter are important.

1. Studies of human subjects provided insights into two fundamental aspects of memory: that there are multiple memory systems and that long-term memory requires consolidation.
2. The hippocampus and associated temporal lobe system are critical for long-term declarative and episodic memory formation.
3. The basal ganglia system is integrally involved in human motor learning and in reward-based learning.
4. Humans possess an awe-inspiring capacity for memorization.

Further Reading

Burgess, N., Maguire, E. A., and O'Keefe, J. (2002). The human hippocampus and spatial and episodic memory. *Neuron* 35:625–641.

Carey, B. H. M. (2008). An Unforgettable Amnesiac Dies at 82. New York Times, (Obituary) Dec 4.

Cipolotti, L., and Bird, C. M. (2006). Amnesia and the hippocampus. Curr Opin Neurol. 2006. 19:593-8.

Corkin, S. (2002). What's new with the amnesic patient H.M.?. *Nat. Rev. Neurosci.* 3(2):153–160.

Corkin, S., Amaral, D. G., Gonzalez, R. G., Johnson, K. A., and Hyman, B. T. (1997). H. M.'s medial temporal lobe lesion: findings from magnetic resonance imaging. *J. Neurosci* 17:3964–3979.

Eichenbaum, H., and Cohen, N. J. (2001). *From Conditioning to Conscious Recollection.* New York: Oxford University Press.

Graybiel, A. M. (2005). The basal ganglia: learning new tricks and loving it. *Curr. Opin. Neurobiol.* 15(6):638–644.

Hyman, S. E., Malenka, R. C., and Nestler, E. J. (2006). Neural mechanisms of addiction: the role of reward-related learning and memory. *Annu. Rev. Neurosci.* 29:565–598.

Kreitzer, A. C., and Malenka, R. C. (2008). Striatal plasticity and basal ganglia circuit function. *Neuron* 60(4):543–554.

Luria, A. R. (2000). *The Mind of a Mnemonist.* Cambridge, MA: Harvard University Press.

Milner, B., Squire, L. R., and Kandel, E. R. (1998). Cognitive neuroscience and the study of memory. *Neuron* 20:445–468.

Mishkin, M., Vargha-Khadem, F., and Gadian, D. G. (1998). Amnesia and the organization of the hippocampal system. *Hippocampus* 8:212–216.

Nishino, H., Hattori, S., Muramoto, K., and Ono, T. (1991). Basal ganglia neural activity during operant feeding behavior in the monkey: relation to sensory integration and motor execution. *Brain Res. Bull.* 27(3–4):463–468.

Schacter, D. L. (1997). The cognitive neuroscience of memory: perspectives from neuroimaging research. *Philos. Trans. R. Soc. Lond. B. Biol. Sci.* 352(1362):1689–1695.

Schacter, D. L. (2002). *The Seven Sins of Memory: How the Mind Forgets and Remembers*. New York: Houghton Mifflin.

Schacter, D. L., and Slotnick, S. D. (2004). The cognitive neuroscience of memory distortion. *Neuron* 44(1):149–160.

Schultz, W. (1999). The primate basal ganglia and the voluntary control of behaviour. *J. Conscious Stud.* 6:31–45.

Thompson, R. F. (2005). In search of memory traces. *Annu. Rev. Psychol.* 56:1–23.

Wiltgen, B. J., Law, M., Ostlund, S., Mayford, M., and Balleine, B. W. (2007). The influence of Pavlovian cues on instrumental performance is mediated by CaMKII activity in the striatum. *Eur. J. Neurosci.* 25:2491–2497.

Zola, S. M., and Squire, L. R. (2001). Relationship between magnitude of damage to the hippocampus and impaired recognition memory in monkeys. *Hippocampus* 11:92–98.

Zola-Morgan, S., and Squire, L. R. (1993). Neuroanatomy of memory. *Annu. Rev. Neurosci.* 16:547–563.

Journal Club Articles

Clark, R. E., and Squire, L. R. (1998). Classical conditioning and brain systems: the role of awareness. *Science* 280:77–81.

Corkin, S., Amaral, D. G., Gonzalez, R. G., Johnson, K. A., and Hyman, B. T. (1997). H. M.'s medial temporal lobe lesion: findings from magnetic resonance imaging. *J. Neurosci* 17:3964–3979.

Maguire, E. A., Gadian, D. G., Johnsrude, I. S., Good, C. D., Ashburner, J., Frackowiak, R. S., and Frith, C. D. (2000). Navigation-related structural change in the hippocampi of taxi drivers. *Proc. Natl. Acad. Sci. USA* 97:4398–4403.

Scoville, W. B., and Milner, B. (2000). Loss of recent memory after bilateral hippocampal lesions. 1957. *J. Neuropsychiatry Clin. Neurosci.* 12:103–113.

For more information—relevant topic chapters from: John H. Byrne (Editor-in-Chief) (2008). *Learning and Memory: A Comprehensive Reference*. Oxford: Academic Press (ISBN 978-0-12-370509-9). (1.05 Urcelay, G. P., and Miller, R. R. *Retrieval from Memory*. pp. 53–73; 1.13 Dalton, P., and Spence, C. *Attention and Memory in Mammals and Primates*. pp. 243–257; 1.14 Kensinger, E. A., and Corkin, S. *Amnesia: Point and Counterpoint*. pp. 259–285; 1.16 Fischer, J. *Transmission of Acquired Information in Nonhuman Primates*. pp. 299–313; 1.24 Sara, S. J. *Reconsolidation: Historical Perspective and Theoretical Aspects*. pp. 461–475; 1.36 Ostlund, S. B., Winterbauer, N. E., and Balleine, B. W. *Theory of Reward Systems*. pp. 701–720; 2.02 Mulligan, N. W. *Attention and Memory*. pp. 7–22; 2.03 Cowan, N. *Sensory Memory*. pp. 23–32; 2.04 Gathercole, S. E. *Working Memory*. pp. 33–51; 2.11 McNamara, T. P., Sluzenski, J., and Rump, B. *Human Spatial Memory and Navigation*. pp. 157–178; 2.14 Marsh, E. J., Eslick, A. N., and Fazio, L. K. *False Memories*. pp. 221–238; 2.29 Ross, B. H., Taylor, E. G., Middleton, E. L., and Nokes, T. J. *Concept and Category Learning in Humans*. pp. 535–556; 2.32 Perruchet, P. *Implicit Learning*. pp. 597–621; 2.34 Lee, T. D., and Schmidt, R. A. *Motor Learning and Memory*. pp. 645–662; 2.42 Anders Ericsson, K. *Superior Memory of Mnemonists and Experts in Various Domains*. pp. 809–817; 2.44 Neuschatz, J. S., and Cutler, B. L. *Eyewitness Identification*. pp. 845–865; 3.03 Burwell, R. D., and Agster, K. L. *Anatomy of the Hippocampus and the Declarative Memory System*. pp. 47–66; 3.04 Squire, L. R., and Shrager, Y. *Declarative Memory System: Amnesia*. pp. 67–78; 3.06 Nyberg, L. *Structural Basis of Episodic Memory*. pp. 99–112; 3.07 Martin, A., and Simmons, W. K. *Structural Basis of Semantic Memory*. pp. 113–130; 3.13 Buchsbaum, B. R., and D'Esposito, M. *Short-Term and Working Memory Systems*. pp. 237–260; 3.14 Ranganath, C., and Blumenfeld, R. S. *Prefrontal Cortex and Memory*. pp. 261–279; 3.15 Chiba, A. A., and Quinn, L. K. *Basal Forebrain and Memory*. pp. 281–301; 3.17 Knowlton, B. J., and Moody, T. D. *Procedural Learning in Humans*. pp. 321–340; 3.21 Nudo, R. J. *Neurophysiology of Motor Skill Learning*. pp. 403–421; 3.22 Sanes, J. N. *Cerebral Cortex: Motor Learning*. pp. 423–439; 4.12 Winstanley, C. A., and Nestler, E. J. *The Molecular Mechanisms of Reward*. pp. 193–215.)

References

1. Mueller, G. E., and Pilzicker, A. (1900). Experimental contributions to the science of memory. (Translated from German). *Z. Psychology* 1:1–288.

2. Squire, L. R., Slater, P. C., and Chace, P. M. (1975). Retrograde amnesia: temporal gradient in very long term memory following electroconvulsive therapy. *Science* 187:77–79.

3. Squire, L. R., and Zola-Morgan, S. (1991). The medial temporal lobe memory system. *Science* 253:1380–1386.

4. Lanenex, P., and Amaral, D. G. (2000). Hippocampal-neocortical interaction: a hierarchy of associativity. *Hippocampus* 10:420–430.

5. Burwell, R. D., and Amaral, D. G. (1998). The cortical afferents of the perirhinal, postrhinal, and entorhinal cortices of the rat. *J. Comp. Neurology* 398:179–205.

6. Swanson, L. W. (1981). A direct projection from Ammon's horn to prefrontal cortex in the rat. *Brain Research* 217:150–154.

7. Scoville, W. B., and Milner, B. (2000). Loss of recent memory after bilateral hippocampal lesions. 1957. *J. Neuropsychiatry Clin. Neurosci.* 12:103–113.

8. Milner, B., Squire, L. R., and Kandel, E. R. (2000). "Cognitive neuroscience and the study of memory." *Neuron* 1998, 20:445–468.

9. Corkin, S., Amaral, D. G., Gonzalez, R. G., Johnson, K. A., and Hyman, B. T. (1997). H. M.'s medial temporal lobe lesion: findings from magnetic resonance imaging. *J. Neurosci.* 17:3964–3979.

10. Burgess, N., Maguire, E. A., and O'Keefe, J. (2002). The human hippocampus and spatial and episodic memory. *Neuron* 35:625–641.

11. Maguire, E. A., Gadian, D. G., Johnsrude, I. S., Good, C. D., Ashburner, J., Frackowiak, R. S., and Frith, C. D. (2000). Navigation-related structural change in the hippocampi of taxi drivers. *Proc. Natl. Acad. Sci. USA* 97:4398–4403.

12. Adcock, R. A., Thangavel, A., Whitfield-Gabrieli, S., Knutson, B., and Gabrieli, J. D. (2006). Reward-motivated learning: mesolimbic activation precedes memory formation. *Neuron* 50(3):507–517.

13. Graybiel, A. M. (1995). Building action repertoires: memory and learning functions of the basal ganglia. *Curr. Opin. Neurobiol.* 5:733–741.

14. Schultz, W., Dayan, P., and Montague, P. R. (1997). A neural substrate of prediction and reward. *Science* 275:1593–1599.

15. Poldrack, R. A., and Gabrieli, J. D. (2001). Characterizing the neural mechanisms of skill learning and repetition priming: evidence from mirror reading. *Brain* 124(Pt 1):67–82.

16. Doupe, A. J., Perkel, D. J., Reiner, A., and Stern, E. A. (2005). Birdbrains could teach basal ganglia research a new song. *Trends Neurosci.* 28(7):353–363.

17. Luria, A. R. (2000). *The Mind of a Mnemonist*. Cambridge, MA: Harvard University Press.

18. Biederman, I., Cooper, E. E., Fox, P. W., and Mahadevan, R. S. (1992). Unexceptional spatial memory in an exceptional memorist. *J. Exp. Psychol. Learn Mem. Cogn.* 18(3):654–657.

19. Ericsson, K. A., Delaney, P. F., Weaver, G., and Mahadevan, R. (2004). Uncovering the structure of a memorist's superior 'basic' memory capacity. *Cognit. Psychol.* 49(3):191–237.

20. Treffert, D. A., and Christensen, D. D. (2005). Inside the mind of a savant. *Sci. Am.* 293(6):108–113.

21. Boddaert, N., Barthelemy, C., Poline, J. B., Samson, Y., Brunelle, F., and Zilbovicius, M. (2005). Autism: functional brain mapping of exceptional calendar capacity. *Br. J. Psychiatry*, 187:83–86.

22. Bayley, P. J., Hopkins, R. O., and Squire, L. R. (2006). The fate of old memories after medial temporal lobe damage. *J. Neurosci.* 26:13311–13317.

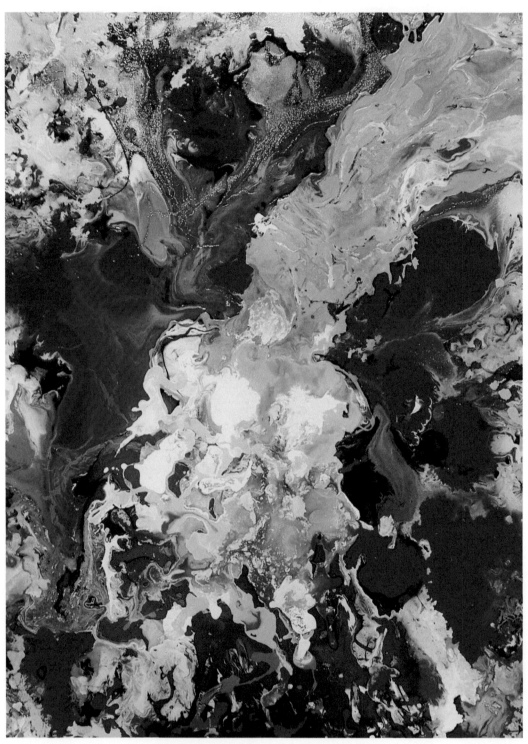

Cytoskeletal Rearrangement in Synaptic Plasticity
J. David Sweatt, acrylic on canvas, 2008–2009

Non-Associative Learning and Memory

I. INTRODUCTION—THE RAPID TURNOVER OF BIOMOLECULES

Almost no human has a good intuitive grasp of the ephemeral nature of biomolecules. Proteins and metabolic intermediates turn over at amazingly fast rates in a mammalian cell, including in a neuron in the CNS. Biochemical bonds are generally quite labile things, and the ongoing breakdown and resynthesis of the constituent molecules of the cells of your body occurs at what is, relatively speaking, breakneck speed. It is difficult to truly grasp this fact in the face of what appears to be such stability and consistency of both our bodies and our minds.

Neuroscientists are not immune to this lack of intuition. The apparent stability of synapses, cells, behavioral patterns, and CNS morphology in our everyday experiments tends to deceive us in our thinking about neuronal function. Activity-induced changes in neuronal and synaptic function can be long-lasting and stable over the course of days and weeks. Memories

are measurably preserved over a significant fraction of an animal's lifetime. This constancy and durability of CNS-based phenomena obscures the underlying rapid turnover of most of the constituent molecules that provide their molecular underpinnings.

I will use one example from my own experiments to illustrate my point of rapid molecular turnover in cells, although the biochemistry and signal transduction literature is full of thousands of similar examples. Biochemists commonly use radioactive tracer compounds to track specific molecular events in cells. A typical experimental design is, for example, to introduce ^{32}P labeled inorganic phosphate ($^{32}PO_4^-$) into the culture medium surrounding a neuron maintained *in vitro*, which is then taken up and incorporated into phosphate-containing molecules in the cell. This radioactive label can then be used to measure the extent of phosphate incorporation into cellular proteins by measuring their level of radioactivity. This is a direct measure of protein phosphorylation by kinases in the cell or, more accurately stated, a direct measure of the steady-state ratio of kinase to phosphatase activity acting on a specific substrate at a specific time point.

The control experiment that one has to do in order to validate this type of approach is to demonstrate that the ^{32}P isotope has reached *isotopic equilibrium* in the cell. This simply means that the ^{32}P-PO$_4$ must have completely dispersed itself throughout all the relevant pools of phosphate that already existed in the cell which, of course, are not radioactive to start with. One needs to know that a change in radioactive content is truly a reflection of a change in phosphate content in, e.g., a substrate protein. The way one demonstrates this is by showing experimentally that the ^{32}P has reached isotopic equilibrium, i.e., the labeled compound has come to a random distribution throughout all the non-radioactive phosphate that was previously there. Thus, a change in ^{32}P content is truly a reflection of a change in phosphate content in a protein.[1]

There are several ways to demonstrate that the cells have reached isotopic equilibrium in the pool of molecules one is investigating. The simplest, if one is interested in protein phosphorylation, is to show that the total ^{32}PO$_4$ in cellular proteins has reached a plateau level (see Figure 1). This means that the incorporation of label into cellular proteins has achieved a steady-state level—the rate of increase in label in proteins has now been matched by the rate of decrease in label in proteins. The radiolabel has reached equilibrium, and is no longer showing either a net increase or a net decrease. One can also specifically measure the ^{32}PO$_4$ content of cellular ATP, ADP, and AMP, and show that they are also at a steady-state level. This means that the phosphates in the alpha, beta, and gamma positions of all these adenine nucleotides has undergone turnover at least once, and the net rate of ^{32}P incorporation is matched by the net rate of ^{32}P loss.

To further refine your control experiment you can show that if you stimulate the cell, with a neurotransmitter for example, there is no additional increase in overall phosphate content in all the cellular proteins or in cellular ATP. This means there is no hidden pool of phosphate in the cell that is only accessed under the conditions of stimulation.

I did these types of experiments as part of studies in Eric Kandel's lab when we studied substrate protein phosphorylation in *Aplysia* sensory neurons, which we maintained *in vitro* and labeled with ^{32}PO$_4$ (1). How long does it take for ^{32}P-phosphate to reach isotopic equilibrium in an *Aplysia* sensory neuron? The answer is less than 24 hours, a number which is typical for neurons in culture and mammalian cells in general, when maintained at 37°C.

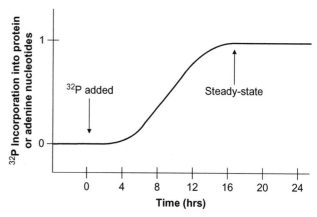

FIGURE 1 Hypothetical graph of ^{32}P-PO$_4$ reaching steady-state. Steady-state is the point at which the rate of incorporation of the radioactive label equals the rate of breakdown of phosphate bonds in labeled proteins, RNA or DNA. Isotopic equilibrium is the point at which all phosphate-containing molecules throughout the cell have achieved steady-state labeling. See text for additional discussion.

But think about the implications of this number. It means that essentially every phosphate bond at all three positions in the entire cellular ATP pool, and essentially every phosphate moiety in every cellular phosphate-containing protein, has been broken down and resynthesized in a one-day time period! As a first approximation, every day all the phospho-proteins in your brain have had their phosphate removed and replaced. If one is considering protein phosphorylation as a mechanism contributing to information storage for any appreciable period of time, one must remember that there is continual breakdown and resynthesis of the basic molecular structure underlying the memory.

This high rate of turnover is not limited to phosphorylation events. Protein constituents of neurons are also broken down and resynthesized at a rapid rate. One particular type of potassium channel that has been studied in the context of memory is the Kv4.2 potassium channel: its half-life in a cell is about four hours. This means that, roughly speaking, the entire cellular content of this potassium channel is broken down and resynthesized over a one-day period. Studies of AMPA-type glutamate neurotransmitter receptors have shown that the half-life for this protein in neurons is approximately 30 hours (see Figure 2 and reference 2). These investigations specifically measured the AMPA receptor cell surface pool, which are the functional receptors on the surface of neurons. The implication of this finding is that the total pool of neuronal cell surface AMPA receptor proteins in your brain is completely broken down and resynthesized from scratch over the course of one week.

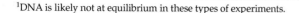

[1]DNA is likely not at equilibrium in these types of experiments.

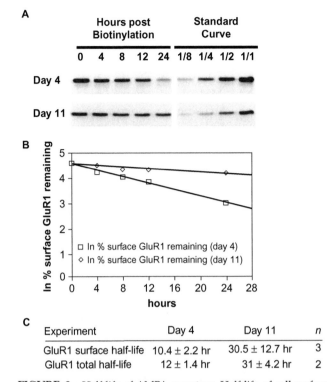

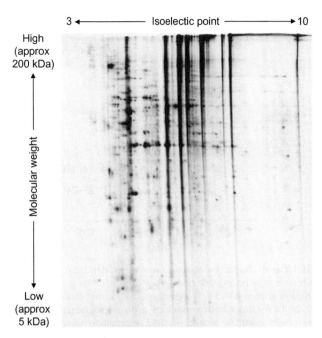

FIGURE 3 Rapid rate of protein turnover. In this experiment, (Sweatt and Kandel, unpublished) two-dimensional gel analysis of ^{35}S-methionine labeled proteins from area CA1 of guinea pig hippocampus reveals rapid and extensive labeling of proteins over a very short time period. This implies a fairly rapid breakdown and resynthesis of the labeled proteins. See text for additional explanation of the experiment.

FIGURE 2 Half-life of AMPA receptors. Half-life of cell-surface GluR1 in spinal cord neuronal cultures at Day 4 and Day 11 *in vitro*. Cell surface molecules were selectively labeled by reacting them with biotin. Plates of spinal cord neurons were biotinylated at Day 4 and Day 11 and recultured for 0–24 hours, at which time cell extracts were harvested, sonicated, and frozen. Subsequently, these samples were thawed and incubated with streptavidin-linked beads, and the streptavidin-precipitated material was loaded onto gels. (Streptavidin selectively binds biotinylated proteins with very high affinity.) (A) A standard curve including serial dilutions of the t = 0 streptavidin-precipitated material was included on each gel for purposes of quantitation. After transfer, gels were probed with a GluR1-reactive antibody in order to quantitate the amount of glutamate receptor remaining from the initial labeling with biotin. (B) The natural log of the percent of remaining surface GluR1 was plotted against time, and half-lives were calculated from the regression slopes of the resulting lines. (C) Summary of half-life and percent of receptor on surface experiments. A paired t test demonstrated a significant increase in the half-life of surface GluR1 from Day 4 to Day 11 (p < 0.05). Data and figure legend adapted from Mammen, Huganir, and O'Brien (2).

A rapid rate of protein turnover is the rule rather than the exception. This is illustrated by the simple experiment shown in Figure 3. In this experiment guinea pig hippocampal slices were prepared and labeled *in vitro* with ^{35}S-methionine for just 30 minutes. Thus, any protein that is labeled with ^{35}S was synthesized *de novo* from precursor amino acids over the course of this half-hour time-frame or even less, because the precursor methionine was added to the extracellular medium and had to cross the cell membrane and be incorporated into methionyl-tRNA

before it could be incorporated into a cellular protein. After the labeling period, area CA1 was dissected out and cellular proteins were separated on the basis of charge and molecular weight using 2-dimensional gel electrophoresis. As you can see in Figure 3, at least a couple of hundred different protein spots were labeled sufficiently to be detectable using autoradiography of this 2-D gel. Thus, hundreds of proteins in hippocampal area CA1 are being synthesized at a sufficiently rapid rate that they show up using this brief, 30-minute period of pulse-labeling. It is reasonable to infer that since the cell is at steady-state, i.e., the cells are not growing larger, that the rate of breakdown of these same proteins is matching their high rate of synthesis. These data are just a specific example from the hippocampus of what is generally known about protein synthesis—protein half-lives in the cell range from about 2 minutes to about 20 hours, and half-lives of proteins typically are in the 2-to-4 hour time range.

Okay, you say, that's fine for proteins but what about "stable" things like the plasma membrane and the cytoskeleton? Neuronal membrane phospholipids also turn over with half-lives in the minutes-to-hours range (3–4). The vast majority of actin microfilaments in dendritic spines of hippocampal pyramidal neurons turn over with astonishing rapidity—the average

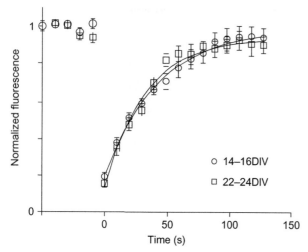

FIGURE 4 Rapid basal actin turnover in dendritic spines. The turnover of actin in dendritic spines from neurons grown for 14–16 days *in vitro* (DIV) was indistinguishable from those grown for 22–24 DIV. Under both conditions actin microfilaments undergo essentially complete breakdown and reformation about every two minutes. Actin turnover was assessed using fluorescent actin and monitoring recovery from photobleaching. Adapted from Star, Kwiatkowski, and Murthy (5).

However, the memory biologist must overcome this cognitive dissonance and come to grips with the rapid turnover of individual molecular components in the nervous system, in order to really be able to begin to understand memory storage. In this chapter we will begin to think about memory processes from this perspective, focusing on experiments investigating one of the simplest forms of learning, long-term sensitization.

Thus, we will begin to think about memory as a product of biochemical reactions that subserve persisting changes of varying durations. We will develop a generalized chemical categorization of the types of chemical reactions that underlie memory storage. In this vein we will discuss three types of memory-storing reactions: short-term reactions mediated by transient changes in second messenger levels; long-term reactions mediated by biochemical species with long half-lives; and ultralong-term or *mnemogenic* reactions that can store memory indefinitely, even in the face of ongoing turnover of the molecules involved (7). Using this framework I will give some specific examples of the various types of chemical reactions that may and must underlie memory storage in biological systems.

turnover time for an actin microfilament in a dendritic spine is 44 seconds (see Figure 4 and reference 5). These considerations apply equally well to anatomical structures. Direct measurements of fractional breakdown rates of skeletal muscle protein indicate that human muscle mass is broken down and resynthesized at about 3–4%/day (6). Development puts everything in its right place, but maintaining anatomical structures is an active process and the component molecules are turning over with surprising rapidity.

There is an extremely important take-home message here. A single phosphorylation event or the synthesis of a new protein or the insertion of a membrane receptor or ion channel, or even the formation of a new synapse is not capable of storing memory for any appreciable period of time. As a first approximation the *entirety* of the functional components of the CNS are broken down and resynthesized over a two-month time span. This should scare you. Your apparent stability as an individual is a perceptual illusion.

The fact of the complete turnover of cellular signaling constituents on the time-frame we are talking about flies completely in the face of our perception. The facts are at odds with the apparent stability that we perceive in ourselves and others. Our memories last. Our behavior is consistent. Our facial features stay the same. However, our intuition based on our day-to-day perceptions is directly at odds with the available experimental data.

II. SHORT-TERM, LONG-TERM, AND ULTRALONG-TERM FORMS OF LEARNING

For this chapter we will focus on examples from the *Aplysia* model system. This is because in many ways the details of the specific molecular mechanisms underlying short-, intermediate-, and long-term memory are better understood in this system than in any other. This is particularly true as relates to the mechanisms for transitioning from one memory phase to the next, while preserving the same cellular read-out. As part of this discussion we will talk about specific chemical reactions involved in memory in *Aplysia*, and begin to investigate some details of the specific molecules involved in memory formation and storage.

Aplysia has a long, storied, Nobel Committee-approved status in the memory field. No textbook on memory mechanisms would be complete without some description of studies using this preparation. In the next few sections I will give a brief introduction to the *Aplysia* model (see Figure 5) to set the framework for the more detailed molecular biological description that will follow (see Further Reading and references 8–11).

As we discussed in the first chapter, essentially all forms of learning including sensitization in *Aplysia* exhibit themselves in either short-term or long-term forms. Indeed, with only a few exceptions, the duration of the memory for a learned event depends on the

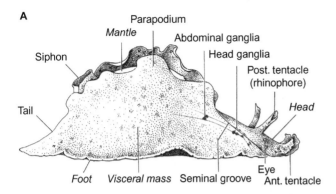

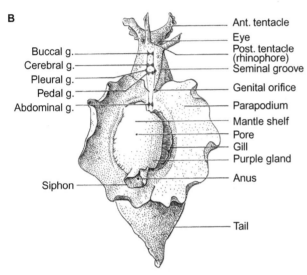

FIGURE 5 *Aplysia californica.* (A) Side view illustrating head, mantle, visceral mass, and foot. The major ganglia of the nervous system are superimposed in the relative position they have inside the animal. (B) Dorsal view. The parapodia have been retracted and the mantle is partially exposed. The outline of the nervous system has again been superimposed to indicate the relative positions of the various ganglia. Figure from Eric Kandel, *Cellular Basis of Behavior.* WH Freeman & Co. Copyright 1976.

number of times an animal experiences the behavior-modifying stimulus. In *Aplysia* a single sensitizing stimulation may elicit sensitization that lasts only a few minutes, whereas repeated stimulation results in sensitization lasting hours to days (see Figure 1 in Chapter 1). Repeated presentations of multiple training trials can elicit sensitization lasting for even more prolonged periods, in many cases memories that last a significant fraction of the animal's lifetime. Thus, the acquisition of memory is a *graded* phenomenon. It is intriguing to wonder how repeated presentations of the identical stimulus can uniquely elicit a long-lasting behavioral alteration, especially when one considers that the behavioral output (e.g., enhanced responsiveness) is identical in the short- and long-lasting forms.

III. USE OF INVERTEBRATE PREPARATIONS TO STUDY SIMPLE FORMS OF LEARNING

Starting in the 1960s, the answers to intriguing questions such as this began to be worked out at the cellular and biochemical level. Part of this watershed of new understanding of the basis of learning and memory came about as a result of the insight to capitalize on easily-studied, simple forms of learning in special preparations that lent themselves to experimental investigation at the cellular level. In particular, the work of Eric Kandel and his colleagues allowed enormous progress in our understanding of the cellular basis of behavior, and learning and memory specifically. Kandel, along with Jack Byrne, Tom Carew, the late Jimmy Schwartz, and many others, have used the simple marine mollusk *Aplysia californica* to great effect to study the behavioral attributes and cellular and molecular mechanisms of learning and memory.

Much (but by no means all) of the work in *Aplysia* has been geared toward understanding the basis of sensitization in this animal. *Aplysia* has on its dorsum a respiratory gill-and-siphon complex, which is normally extended when the animal is in the resting state (Figure 6). If the gill or siphon is lightly touched (or experimentally, squirted with a Water-Pic), this elicits a defensive withdrawal reflex in order to protect the gill from potential damage. The animal's tail also exhibits a similar defensive withdrawal reflex when stimulated. These defensive withdrawal reflexes can undergo both habituation (by repeated modest stimuli) and sensitization. Sensitization occurs when the animal receives an aversive stimulus, for example a tail-shock (see Figure 7). After sensitizing stimulation, the animal exhibits a more robust, longer-lasting gill withdrawal in response to the identical light touch or water squirt. As was illustrated in Chapter 1, acquisition of this sensitization response is graded; repetitive sensitizing stimuli can give sensitization lasting minutes to hours (one to a few shocks), or weeks (repeated training trials over a few days).

Progress in beginning to understand this memory system came by way of mapping certain aspects of the neuronal circuitry underlying the defensive withdrawal reflex and the associated modulatory inputs from the tail. One appeal of the *Aplysia* experimental system was the relatively simple nervous system in the animal, allowing the tracing of significant parts of the circuitry underlying the behavior using electrophysiology techniques. This circuit tracing was greatly facilitated by the enormous (relatively speaking) size of the neurons in *Aplysia*, allowing for easy microelectrode recording from specific, identified neurons in the animal's CNS. Ironically, the critical locus for the memory of sensitization resides for the most part in the smallest neurons in the animal.

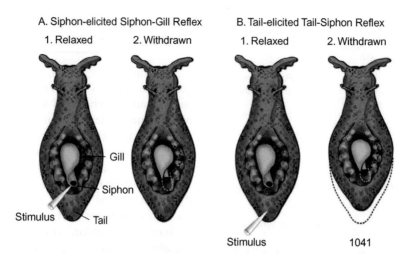

FIGURE 6   Siphon-gill and tail-siphon withdrawal reflexes of *Aplysia*. (A) Siphon-gill withdrawal. Dorsal view of *Aplysia* (1) Relaxed position. (2) A stimulus (e.g., a water jet, brief touch, or weak electric shock) applied to the siphon causes the siphon and the gill to withdraw into the mantle cavity. (B) Tail-siphon withdrawal reflex. (1) Relaxed position. (2) A stimulus applied to the tail elicits a reflex withdrawal of the tail and siphon. Adapted from Fioravante et al. *Learning and Memory: A Comprehensive Review*, Volume 4, Chapter 3. Copyright Elsevier 2008.

A. The Cellular Basis of Synaptic Facilitation in *Aplysia*

Greatly simplified diagrams of the circuitry underlying sensitization of the gill-and-siphon withdrawal reflex and the tail withdrawal reflex in *Aplysia* are given in Figure 8. The touch to the gill-and-siphon complex stimulates siphon sensory neurons, which make direct and indirect (via interneurons) connections to gill motor neurons. The gill motor neurons stimulate muscles in the gill-and-siphon complex that mediate the defensive withdrawal reflex. The tail shock impinges on this circuit by way of tail sensory neurons that make direct contacts (and indirect contacts by way of interneurons) with the pre-synaptic terminals of the siphon sensory neurons.

It was soon realized that plasticity at the siphon sensory neuron/gill motor neuron synapse is one critical locus contributing to sensitization in the animal—one of the first demonstrations of the importance of *synaptic plasticity* in learning and memory. A predominant component of plasticity at this synapse is increased neurotransmitter release from the gill-and-siphon sensory neurons. Thus, tail shock and the attendant activity in tail sensory neurons and associated interneurons leads to release of modulatory neurotransmitters onto the siphon sensory neuron pre-synaptic terminal, increasing the release of neurotransmitter from these cells and augmenting the defensive withdrawal reflex (Figure 9). These observations highlighted the role of pre-synaptic facilitation of neurotransmitter release as a mechanism for memory in this system. The excitatory neurotransmitter whose release is increased at the gill-and-siphon sensory neuron-motor neuron synapses is glutamate.

Although all of the modulatory neurotransmitters involved in pre-synaptic facilitation in *Aplysia* sensory neurons are not yet identified, one important player is serotonin. Serotonin (5-hydroxytryptamine or 5HT) is released onto a subset of the siphon sensory neurons by a serotonergic tail sensory neuron stimulated by tail shock. In fact, serotonin application to siphon sensory neurons elicits the vast majority of the physiologic responses contributing to pre-synaptic facilitation of neurotransmitter release and sensitization in the animal. This type of modulation of neurotransmitter release from one neuron, triggered by release of a modulatory agent (like serotonin) from another neuron, is referred to as "hetero-synaptic facilitation."

Once it was realized that hetero-synaptic facilitation of neurotransmitter release from gill-and-siphon sensory neurons (hereafter referred to simply as "sensory neurons") was an important component of sensitization in the animal, and that serotonin could mimic the effects of sensitizing stimulation on sensory neuron physiology, it became clear that an effective model system for studying sensitization in *Aplysia* was to study the cascade of events elicited by serotonin application to sensory neurons. This model system has been exploited to characterize the cellular, electrophysiologic, and biochemical mechanisms operating to achieve enduring pre-synaptic facilitation in these cells.

Another type of sensitization that has been extensively studied in *Aplysia* involves defensive withdrawal of the tail. Just like sensitization of the gill-and-siphon withdrawal reflex, *Aplysia* can be trained to exhibit

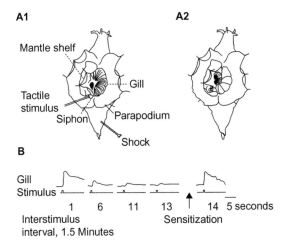

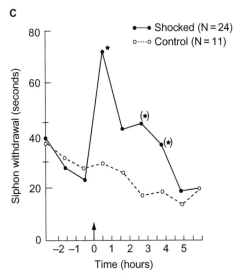

FIGURE 7 Short-term sensitization of the gill-withdrawal reflex in *Aplysia*. (A) 1. Experimental arrangement for behavioral studies in the intact animal showing the gill in a relaxed position. A gill-withdrawal reflex is elicited by a water jet (tactile) stimulus to the siphon. The sensitizing stimulus is a noxious mechanical or electrical stimulus to the neck or tail. 2. Gill after withdrawal. The relaxed position is indicated by the dotted lines. (B) Photocell recordings showing sensitization and habituation of the gill-withdrawal reflex. After 13 stimuli, the reflex response was reduced to less than 30 percent of its initial value. Arrow: noxious sensitizing (electrical) stimulus applied to the tail (arrow). (C) Time course of sensitization after a single strong electrical shock to the tail. The siphon-withdrawal reflex was tested once every 0.5 hour, and the mean of each two consecutive responses is shown. Even this low rate produced some habituation. After the third siphon stimulus, the experimental group received a single shock to the tail (arrow). After this sensitizing stimulus the experimental animals had significantly longer withdrawals than controls for up to four hours. Figure and legend adapted from Kandel and Schwartz, (1982). *Science* 218:433–443. Figure courtesy of Dr Eric Kandel. Reprinted with permission from AAAS. Copyright 1982.

enhanced defensive withdrawal of their tail (and siphon) in response to touch. Again, experimentally the sensitizing stimulus is mild electric shock to the tail. The behavioral parameters, underlying neuronal

circuitry and molecular mechanisms subserving tail withdrawal sensitization have been extensively investigated in Jack Byrne's laboratory, and are illustrated in Figures 8 and 9.

Sensitization in *Aplysia* exhibits both short-term and long-term forms. Similarly, in sensory neurons involved in gill-and-siphon and tail withdrawal sensitization, serotonin application can lead to either short-term or long-term facilitation of glutamate release from the sensory neuron. Single (5 minute) applications of serotonin give facilitation that lasts only a few minutes: repeated (5×5 minutes over the course of an hour) applications give facilitation lasting at least 24 hours. This is, of course, very reminiscent of the durations of behavioral sensitization in response to single or multiple presentations of tail shock stimuli.

Physiologic Effects of Serotonin

The cellular substrates affected in response to serotonin application to sensory neurons are varied, involving proteins controlling both the electrical properties of the sensory neuron cell membrane and mechanisms involved in the process of neurotransmitter release. The overall result of serotonin application is an orchestrated set of changes leading ultimately to increased neurotransmitter release from the sensory neuron. In the next few paragraphs I will describe some of the known targets of serotonin neuromodulation in *Aplysia*.

In attempting to understand how serotonin-induced pre-synaptic facilitation in *Aplysia* sensory neurons occurs, it is worth considering the mechanisms normally operating to produce baseline neurotransmitter release. First, stimulation of siphon sensory neuron nerve endings in the gill-and-siphon complex (for example by light touch) leads to membrane depolarization and generation of an action potential. Invasion of the action potential into the pre-synaptic terminal causes the opening of voltage-gated calcium channels, which are open for a period of time proportional to the duration of the action potential. Of course, the invasion of multiple action potentials will also elicit additional calcium influx. This calcium signal triggers activation of the molecular machinery, leading to fusion of neurotransmitter-containing vesicles with the sensory neuron pre-synaptic membrane, resulting in release of neurotransmitter into the synaptic cleft.

By and large, pre-synaptic facilitation is achieved by modulation of three sites in the cascade of events resulting in neurotransmitter release, sites which I will now describe. (Please note that additional sites are likely involved, see Figure 10.) One site is closure of "S"-channels, or serotonin-sensitive potassium channels

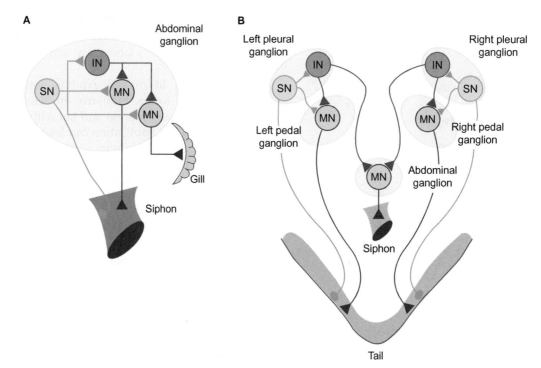

FIGURE 8 Simplified circuit diagrams of the siphon-gill (A) and tail-siphon (B) withdrawal reflexes. Stimuli activate the afferent terminals of mechanoreceptor sensory neurons (SN), the somata of which are located in central ganglia (abdominal, pedal, and pleural). The sensory neurons make excitatory synaptic connections (triangles) with interneurons (IN) and motor neurons (MN). The excitatory interneurons provide a parallel pathway for excitation of the motor neurons. Action potentials elicited in the motor neurons, triggered by the combined input form the SNs and INs, propagate out peripheral nerves to activate muscle cells and produce the subsequent reflex withdrawal of the organs. Modulatory neurons (not shown here), such as those containing serotonin (5-HT), regulate the properties of the circuit elements and, consequently, the strength of the behavioral responses. Figure and legend adapted from Brown et al. *From Molecules to Networks*, Chapter 18. Copyright Elsevier 2004.

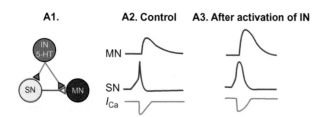

FIGURE 9 Model of hetero-synaptic facilitation of the sensorimotor connection that contributes to short-term sensitization in *Aplysia*. (A) 1. Sensitizing stimuli activate facilitatory interneurons (IN) that release modulatory transmitters, one of which is 5-HT. The modulator leads to an alteration of the properties of the sensory neuron (SN). 2, 3. An action potential in a SN after the sensitizing stimulus results in a greater transmitter release, and hence a larger postsynaptic potential in the motor neuron (MN) than an action potential prior to the sensitizing stimulus. For short-term sensitization the enhancement of transmitter release is due, at least in part, to broadening of the action potential and an enhanced flow of Ca^{2+} in to the sensory neuron. Adapted from Fioravante et al. *Learning and Memory: A Comprehensive Review*, Volume 4, Chapter 3. Copyright Elsevier 2008.

($g_{K,S}$ in Figure 10). A second site is modulation of Ikv, or voltage-sensitive potassium channels ($g_{K,V}$ in Figure 10). Finally, there is modulation of the responsiveness of the neurotransmitter release machinery to the action

potential-associated calcium influx. In the following sections, I will briefly describe the impact of the alterations of each of these sites.

S-channels

The S-channel achieved fame as one of the first ion channels discovered to be modulated by a phosphorylation event (12). The S-channel is what is referred to as a "leak" potassium channel, i.e., it is normally open at rest and thus contributes to establishing the resting membrane potential. The cAMP-dependent protein kinase (PKA) phosphorylates and closes the S-channel. Closure of this channel has several effects on the electrical properties of the sensory neuron cell membrane. First, as the channels are closed there is less resting potassium current flowing across the membrane, resulting in a modest depolarization of the membrane. This brings the resting membrane potential closer to the threshold for action potential generation, and increases the likelihood of action potential firing. In addition, the closure of S-channels leads to decreased spike-frequency accommodation, such that the cell is more likely to fire multiple action potentials with prolonged stimulation. Finally, the S-channel makes

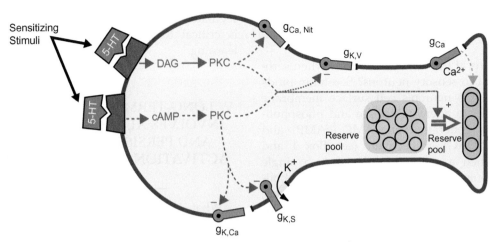

FIGURE 10   Molecular events in *Aplysia* sensory neuron short-term facilitation. 5-HT released from the facilitatory interneuron (see Figure 9) binds to at least two distinct classes of receptors on the outer surface of the membrane of the sensory neuron, which leads to the transient activation of two intercellular second messengers: DAG and cAMP. These second messengers, acting through their respective protein kinases, affect multiple cellular processes, the combined effects of which lead to enhanced transmitter release when a subsequent action potential is fired in the sensory neuron. Adapted from Fioravante et al. *Learning and Memory: A Comprehensive Review*, Volume 4, Chapter 3. Copyright Elsevier 2008.

a modest contribution to repolarizing the membrane after an action potential, so closure of voltage-gated calcium channels contributes to a prolongation of the action potential duration, allowing increased duration of calcium influx through voltage-gated calcium channels. (In fact, an additional component of the effect of serotonin is a direct effect on these calcium channels ($g_{Ca, Nif}$ in Figure 10), augmenting their responsiveness to depolarization.) Thus, closure of the S-channel overall leads to increased likelihood of triggering one or more action potentials, and to increased calcium influx in response to the action potential.

Ikv

Work in Jack Byrne's laboratory has been instrumental in the discovery of the modulation of this channel as a mechanism for pre-synaptic facilitation in *Aplysia* sensory neurons (9). Ikv is a voltage-sensitive potassium channel that opens in response to the membrane depolarization caused by the arrival of the action potential, and after opening the potassium current flowing through this channel contributes substantially to returning the membrane potential to its resting level. Therefore, in contrast to the S-channel, the voltage-sensitive potassium channel Ikv is a major player in repolarizing the cell membrane after the arrival of an action potential, and modulation of this channel is a potent mechanism for prolonging action potential duration. Both the PKA and protein kinase C (PKC) cascades impinge on this mechanism, leading to inhibition of Ikv function, action potential

prolongation, and an attendant increase in calcium influx with each action potential.

Modulation of the Release Machinery and Synaptic Vesicle Pools

A third, less well-understood mechanism recruited by the PKA and PKC pathways is direct augmentation of the responsiveness of the neurotransmitter release machinery to the action potential-associated calcium influx. This is quite a robust effect recruited by serotonin to contribute to pre-synaptic facilitation, however at present our mechanistic understanding of this process is incomplete. This mechanism likely involves mobilization of synaptic vesicles from a reserve pool to a readily releasable pool, and possibly augmentation of the synaptic vesicle fusion machinery as well.

IV. SHORT-TERM FACILITATION IN APLYSIA IS MEDIATED BY CHANGES IN THE LEVELS OF INTRACELLULAR SECOND MESSENGERS

One very active area of *Aplysia* research over the last 25 years has been dissecting the biochemical cascades operating to cause these short- and long-term physiologic effects, in particular trying to understand how the different durations of effects are achieved. In the following sections I will briefly describe the molecular mechanisms that have been discovered to play a role in short-, intermediate-, and long-term facilitation of neurotransmitter release in *Aplysia* sensory neurons.

What happens at the biochemical level when serotonin is applied to sensory neurons? Serotonin binds to receptors in the neuron's cell surface membrane that are coupled to adenylyl cyclase and phospholipase C, which generate cyclic AMP (cAMP) and diacylglycerol (DAG), respectively (see Box 1 and Figure 10). When a sensory neuron sees a single pulse of serotonin, adenylyl cyclase and phospholipase C are activated, cAMP and DAG levels increase, and the activities of the cAMP-dependent protein kinase (PKA) and protein kinase C (PKC) are greatly enhanced. These kinases phosphorylate intracellular targets, including those described above—potassium channels and the vesicle release machinery, increasing glutamate release into the synapse. As long as serotonin is present, the PKA and PKC enzymatic activities remain elevated, their targets have their phosphorylation increased, and glutamate release is increased.

However, once serotonin is removed, metabolic enzymes in the sensory neuron return the cell to its resting state. In this case, cAMP phosphodiesterase breaks down cAMP, diacylglycerol lipase breaks down DAG, and protein phosphatases dephosphorylate the protein kinase substrates. Thus, the duration of facilitation in response to a single application of serotonin is determined by the amount of time serotonin is present, the rate of breakdown of the second messengers, and the rate of reversal of the effects of the protein kinases after serotonin is removed. After a single application of serotonin these effects are rapidly reversed—usually within a few minutes, therefore, a single application of serotonin gives only short-lasting facilitation.

Reaction Category 1—Altered Levels of Second Messengers

Thus, *Aplysia* short-term facilitation of neurotransmitter release provides an example of our first category of memory-forming chemical reaction: transient, stimulus-mediated changes. In this case the duration of the memory is essentially dependent on continued release of 5HT onto the neuron.

It is an interesting thought experiment to consider the effects in this system if the breakdown enzymes were removed. Over time second messengers and phosphorylated proteins would accumulate, eventually driving the system to saturation. Then, whenever a sensory neuron received a serotonin signal, it would be unable to modulate its intracellular milieu appropriately, and no alteration in synaptic efficacy could be achieved. This thought experiment serves to illustrate an important point; it is the capacity to *dynamically*

regulate the molecular messengers in a system that is critical to the synaptic plasticity that underlies learning.

V. LONG-TERM FACILITATION IN *APLYSIA* INVOLVES ALTERED GENE EXPRESSION AND PERSISTENT PROTEIN KINASE ACTIVATION—A SECOND CATEGORY OF REACTION

What happens when the sensory neuron sees repeated applications of serotonin, which elicit long-lasting synaptic facilitation? Repeated applications of serotonin lead to sustained elevation of second messengers, and this sustained elevation elicits activation of a unique and elaborate cascade of biochemical events. Although, so far, many mechanistic details have not yet been worked out, several key steps in this cascade have been identified. The long-lasting elevation of cAMP leads to PKA activation and subsequent phosphorylation of the transcription factor CREB. Activation of the ERK MAP Kinase cascade (see Boxes 2 and 3) is also involved as a modulator of CREB activation, specifically acting through disinhibition via repression of negative regulators of CREB (see Figure 11). Through mechanisms that have not been entirely worked out, CREB activation leads to altered gene expression and subsequent regulation of protein breakdown. Specifically, the *ubiquitin* system is recruited to cause the proteolytic degradation of one subunit of PKA, the PKA regulatory subunit (see Figure 11).

An understanding of the consequences of this stimulus-induced loss of PKA regulatory subunits becomes clear on review of the normal control of this enzyme. The cAMP-dependent protein kinase is a tetramer comprising two regulatory and two catalytic subunits (Figure 12). The two identical regulatory subunits each contain one cAMP binding site; when cAMP binds the regulatory subunits dissociate from the two (identical) catalytic subunits. The free catalytic subunits are then enzymatically competent and able to phosphorylate their downstream effector proteins. Therefore, proteolytic loss of regulatory subunits results in a decrease in the overall ratio of regulatory to catalytic subunits, promoting an excess of free, active catalytic subunits, and increased phosphorylation of PKA substrates.

In this manner, PKA is persistently activated. Even after cAMP returns to its resting level after serotonin is removed, the excess catalytic subunits remain free of regulatory subunits and active in the sensory neuron. By this clever mechanism a chain of events is set

BOX 1

COUPLING OF RECEPTORS TO INTRACELLULAR MESSENGERS

Neurotransmitters that act by binding to receptors on the cell surface can elicit a wide variety of biochemical effects inside a neuron. How does a signal at the cell's surface manage to alter the activities of enzymatic processes intracellularly? In many cases this is achieved by virtue of the neurotransmitter receptor coupling to and altering the catalytic activity of second messenger-generating enzymes on the inner leaflet of the cell membrane. The second messengers thus produced typically activate downstream protein kinases, which are enzymes that regulate the activity of a wide variety of intracellular proteins by attaching phosphate groups to (phosphorylating) specific amino acids in the protein's sequence.

Typically, coupling of the receptor to the effector enzyme is mediated by G proteins, or guanine nucleotide binding proteins. G proteins are themselves enzymes that bind GTP and hydrolyze it to GDP. Receptors activate G proteins by causing an allosteric change in the protein that causes an exchange of GTP onto the protein, replacing the GDP that is there in the inactive state. The GTP-bound version of the G protein is active and interacts with second messenger generating enzymes (or ion channels in some cases), greatly increasing their catalytic rate and producing elevations of the intracellular levels of the second messengers. Once the G protein has hydrolyzed GTP to GDP, the G protein relaxes back to its inactive state, where it can remain unstimulated or once again be activated by the neurotransmitter/receptor complex.

Why does this elaborate machinery exist? Why not have the receptor directly interact with the second messenger-generating enzyme? One answer to this question lies in the kinetics of the GTP hydrolysis reaction. On the kinetic scale at which enzymes typically operate, G proteins are notably slow. This means that once receptor stimulates the exchange of GTP onto the G protein, the G protein will stay in the GTP-bound, active conformation for a relatively extended period of time, on the order of a few minutes. However, once GTP is bound, the G protein quickly dissociates from the ligand/receptor complex. The ligand-occupied receptor can then proceed to activate additional G protein molecules. The net effect of the G protein involvement, then, is both amplification and prolongation of the neurotransmitter-stimulated event. Overall, the cell trades energy (in the form of GTP hydrolysis) for the benefit of augmented signal transduction across the membrane.

There are two well characterized second messenger generating enzymes that are activated by G proteins: adenylyl cyclase and phospholipase C. Adenylyl cyclase converts ATP to adenosine 3', 5'-cyclic monophosphate, using magnesium as a cofactor. cAMP is known to activate two downstream effectors: the cAMP-dependent protein kinase (PKA) and certain types of cyclic nucleotide-gated ion channels. The activity of phospholipase C results in the production of two different second messengers. Phospholipase C hydrolyzes the membrane

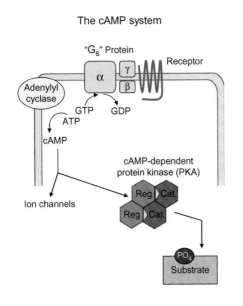

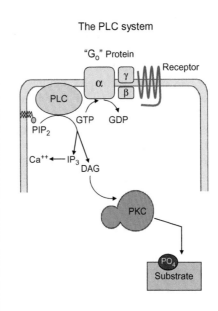

Continued

BOX 1—cont'd

COUPLING OF RECEPTORS TO INTRACELLULAR MESSENGERS

phospholipid phosphatidylinositol 4,5-bis phosphate at the linkage between the glycerol backbone and the phospho-head group, liberating diacylglycerol (DAG) and inositol 1,4,5-tris phosphate (IP_3). Both of these compounds serve as second messengers. DAG binds to and activates the downstream effector protein kinase C (PKC). IP_3 binds to an intracellular receptor in the endoplasmic reticulum that is a calcium channel, leading to calcium mobilization from intracellular stores. Calcium, of course, is a pluripotent messenger in its own right and can activate a wide variety of intracellular proteins and enzymes, including the calcium-and-calmodulin activated kinase CaMKII.

As second messengers are such powerful agents, regulation of their levels is carefully controlled. In cells there are specific enzymes for the breakdown of each of these messengers, which keep the levels of the compounds low in the resting cell. Phosphodiesterase is an enzyme that hydrolyzes cAMP into the inactive product 5′-AMP. Similarly, DAG lipase hydrolyzes DAG into its component parts, a glycerol molecule and two free fatty acids. DAG can also be inactivated by phosphorylation to phosphatidic acid, via the actions of DAG kinase. IP_3 is further metabolized by a very elaborate enzymatic system. IP_3 can be both broken down by phosphatases, leading ultimately to production of free inositol, or phosphorylated at additional sites by various kinases, eventually leading to the production of additional signaling molecules.

BOX 2

MAPKs, SIGNAL INTEGRATORS CONTROLLING ION CHANNELS, AND GENE TRANSCRIPTION IN NEURONS

Mitogen-activated protein kinases, or MAPKs, were originally discovered as critical controllers of cell division, as the name implies. Extracellular-signal regulated kinases (ERKs) are a specific subtype of MAPK that have been extensively linked to regulation of synaptic plasticity and memory formation in many systems. Regulation of the ERK cascade is complex, but this complexity allows for some interesting possibilities in terms of biochemical information processing and neuronal coincidence detection. The ERK cascade, like MAPK cascades in general, is distinguished by a characteristic core cascade of three kinases (see Figure). The first kinase in the sequence is Raf-1 (or B-Raf), which activates the second kinase, MEK, by serine/threonine phosphorylation. MEKs are "dual specificity" kinases, which means that they phosphorylate both a threonine and tyrosine side chain in their substrates. Via this dual phosphorylation they activate a downstream MAP kinase (p44 MAPK = ERK1, p42MAPK = ERK2). One important feature of the cascade is that ERK (both ERK1 and ERK2)

activity is exclusively regulated by MEK—dual phosphorylation by MEK is both necessary and sufficient for ERK activation. This allows the use of MEK inhibitors to selectively block activation of the ERKs.

Several second messenger-regulated kinases have been shown to activate the ERK/MAPK cascade in neurons. Stimulation of protein kinase C produces a robust activation of ERK2, and activation of the cAMP cascade also leads to secondary activation of MAPK (see Figure). In mammalian systems such as the hippocampus, activation of β-adrenergic receptors (βARs) leads to MAPK activation, an effect attenuated by PKA inhibition. Metabotropic glutamate receptors, muscarinic acetylcholine receptors, DA receptors, alpha7 nicotinic acetylcholine receptors, and serotonin receptors all also lead to ERK activation in neurons in general and the hippocampus in particular. Moreover, regulation of ERK activation in the hippocampus is not limited to neurotransmitter receptors. One of the most widely studied activators of

BOX 2—cont'd

MAPKs, SIGNAL INTEGRATORS CONTROLLING ION CHANNELS, AND GENE TRANSCRIPTION IN NEURONS

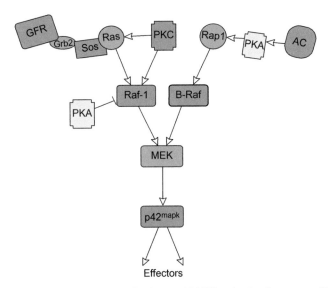

Effectors

BOX 2 Potential signal transduction routes leading to MAPK activation in neurons. While regulation of cell proliferation is the best-studied function of the ERK MAPK cascade, it is now known that hippocampal ERK activation is necessary not only for *Aplysia* long-term facilitation, but also for hippocampal LTP and a wide variety of forms of hippocampus-dependent memory formation. It is interesting to consider that this cascade so critical for normal development is utilized for memory formation in the adult, suggesting a generalized mechanistic conservation between development and adult learning. Abbreviations: RAS, the low molecular weight G protein ras; GEF, guanine nucleotide exchange factor; PKA, cAMP-dependent protein kinase; GFR, growth factor receptor; RSK, ribosomal S6 kinase; CREB, cAMP response element binding protein; Rap-1, RAF, MEK, and ERK are all components of the extracellular signal-regulated kinase (ERK) cascade, a subfamily of the mitogen-activated protein kinases. Reproduced from (13).

hippocampal ERKs is BDNF; BDNF receptors couple to ERK activation, and the ERK activation contributes to BDNF-induced synaptic plasticity in the hippocampus. Other intriguing possible regulators of ERK include a novel GTPase activating protein, SynGAP, which potentially links Ca^{2+}/calmodulin activation to ERK stimulation, and reactive oxygen species including superoxide, that can lead to ERK activation in the hippocampus.

This wide variety of upstream regulators of ERK suggests that this signal transduction cascade may serve to integrate diverse cell-surface signals into a coherent intracellular response. Especially intriguing is the possibility that this signal integration may not simply serve to sum up signals, but rather in some cases serve to allow synergistic effects or coincidence detection. Recent important results from Tom O'Dell's laboratory suggest that this type of information processing is indeed

occurring. For example, Tom O'Dell's research group has observed synergistic activation of hippocampal ERKs by convergent activation of β-adrenergic receptors and muscarinic acetylcholine receptors. These data suggest that the ERK cascade can serve as a coincidence detector in its own right.

In considering a role for the ras/raf/MEK/ERK pathway in learning and memory it certainly warrants emphasis that this pathway has been implicated in learning and memory in a wide variety of species. Studies in *Aplysia*, *Lymnaea*, *Hermissenda*, *C. elegans*, crayfish, Zebra Finch, *Drosophila*, mice, and rats have all directly or indirectly implicated a role for this cascade in learning and memory. Recent studies of human gene mutations associated with learning and memory deficits also suggest that it is appropriate to add the human to this list (13).

BOX 3

REGULATION OF RAS BY GAPS AND GEFS

Ras is a low molecular weight GTP-binding protein (G protein) classically studied as a target for particular receptor tyrosine kinases. Ras acts as a critical relay in signal transduction by cycling between an active conformational state when bound to GTP, and an inactive state when bound to GDP (see Figure). The GTPase, or turn-off activity of Ras, is dependent on the opposing effects of two distinct classes of regulatory ras-binding molecules; GAPs (GTPase activating proteins) and GEFs (Guanine nucleotide exchange factors). GAPs promote formation of the GDP-ras complex through increasing ras GTPase activity, and thus inactivate ras. GEFs act by catalyzing the exchange of GTP for GDP, causing ras activation. The best-known GEFs fall into two major classes; the son of sevenless class (SOS) and the ras-guanine-nucleotide releasing factor (ras-GRF) class.

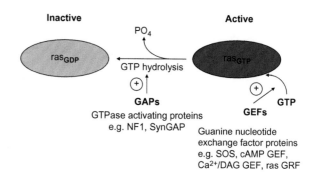

It also is important to note that there are three different isoforms of ras: H, N, and K. These different ras types likely have similar functions, but they exhibit distinct tissue distributions—all are found in the brain.

in motion whereby a biochemical effect is established in the cell that outlasts the initial, triggering elevation of the second messenger cAMP. The PKA will remain activated until compensatory resynthesis of new regulatory subunits occurs, or until the catalytic subunit is degraded. Interestingly, although the mechanism has not yet been worked out, the DAG-responsive effector PKC is also persistently activated after serotonin stimulation of sensory neurons.

Persistent kinase activation is one powerful mechanism contributing to long-lasting facilitation of neurotransmitter release in sensory neurons. Available evidence indicates that the persistent activation of PKA underlies a stage of facilitation lasting on the order of many hours after the triggering applications of serotonin are finished. Interestingly, pioneering work on this mechanism was performed using sensitization training in animals, emphasizing the strong likelihood of this mechanism contributing to the underlying cellular basis for the change in the animal's behavior *in vivo*.

Reaction Category 2—Generation of Long Half-Life Molecules

Aplysia long-term facilitation of neurotransmitter release provides an example of our second category of memory-forming chemical reaction: generation

of long half-life signaling molecules. In this case, the duration of the memory subserved by this mechanism is essentially dependent on the half-life of the free PKA catalytic subunit and other specially modified proteins. Reversal of the persisting event is dependent on the half-life of the protein or the rate of synthesis of regulatory protein subunits.

It is interesting to note how the short- and long-term mechanisms manage to achieve the same final common output of increased synaptic strength. The elegant solution to this problem is inherent in the mechanisms themselves. As both short-term mechanisms and longer-term mechanisms ultimately result in activation of the same kinases, PKA and PKC, the final read-out is the same: increased phosphorylation of PKA and PKC substrates. However, the mechanisms to achieve the kinase activation are distinct and of different durations, leading to different durations of potentiation.

Intermediate-Term Facilitation in Aplysia

Tom Carew and his co-workers, along with Kandel and colleagues, have also identified a form of synaptic facilitation (and associated sensitized gill withdrawal behavior) that is intermediate in duration between short-term and long-term facilitation. This intermediate-term facilitation (ITF) lasts on the order

A *Aplysia*

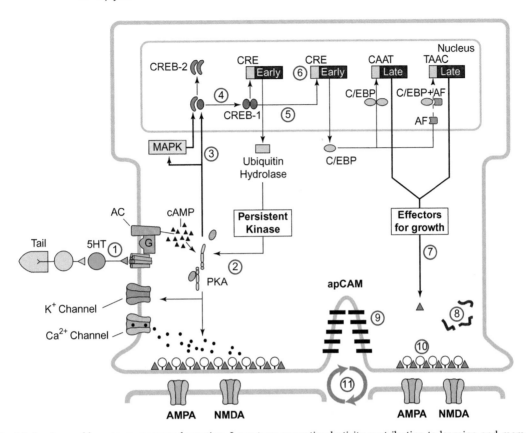

FIGURE 11 Mechanisms of long-term memory formation. Long-term synaptic plasticity contributing to learning and memory in *Aplysia* involves a sequence of cellular and molecular mechanisms including: (1) neurotransmitter release and short-term strengthening of synaptic connections; (2) equilibrium between kinase and phosphatase activities at the synapse; (3) retrograde transport from the synapse to the nucleus; (4) activation of nuclear transcription factors; (5) activity-dependent induction of gene expression; (6) chromatin alteration and epigenetic changes in gene expression; (7) synaptic capture of newly-synthesized gene products; (8) local protein synthesis at active synapses; (9) synaptic growth and the formation of new synapses; (10) activation of pre-existing silent synapses; and (11) self-perpetuating mechanisms and the molecular basis of memory persistence. The location of these events, which may act in part to stabilize some of the changes that occur during short- and intermediate-term plasticity, moves from the synapse (1–2) to the nucleus (3–6) and then back to the synapse (7–11). Adapted from Bailey et al. *Learning and Memory: A Comprehensive Review*, Volume 4, Chapter 2. Copyright Elsevier 2008.

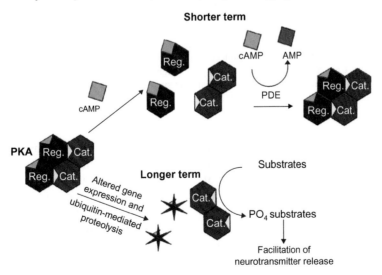

FIGURE 12 The Schwartz and Kandel model of short-term and long-term regulation of PKA in *Aplysia* sensory neurons. See explanation of pathway in text. PKA shown as tetramer of two regulatory (Reg.) and two catalytic (Cat.) subunits. Catalytic site is shown in yellow. PDE = Phosphodiesterase.

A   *Aplysia*

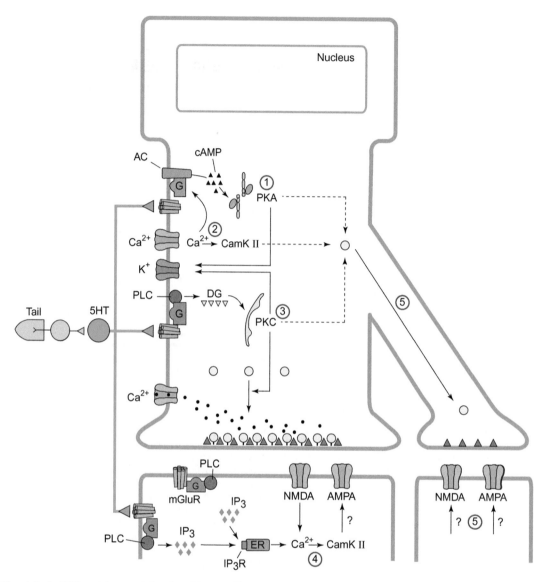

FIGURE 13   *Aplysia*. Different forms of short- and intermediate-term synaptic plasticity contributing to learning and memory in *Aplysia* involve different combinations of pre- and post-synaptic molecules including: (1) pre-synaptic cyclic adenosine monophosphate-dependent protein kinase; (2) pre-synaptic Ca^{2+} and CamKll; (3) pre-synaptic protein kinase C; (4) post-synaptic Ca^{2+} and CamKll; and (5) recruitment of pre- and possibly post-synaptic molecules to seed potential new synaptic sites. Adapted from Bailey et al. *Learning and Memory: A Comprehensive Review*, Volume 4, Chapter 2. Copyright Elsevier 2008.

of 90 minutes, and is subserved by several molecular mechanisms distinct from those involved in short-term facilitation. For example, ITF, which itself has at least two distinct forms and underlying mechanisms, involves altered protein synthesis and persistent activation of protein kinase C.

One additional notable difference is that post-synaptic mechanisms triggered in the follower motor neuron are involved in the induction and maintenance of ITF, as demonstrated by David Glanzman and his colleagues. Thus, ITF is distinct from short-term facilitation

in involving mechanisms in the post-synaptic cell. Specifically, glutamate receptors in the post-synaptic membrane are involved in triggering activation of the calcium/calmodulin-dependent protein kinase II (CaMK II), which causes increased trafficking and insertion of AMPA subtype glutamate receptors into the post-synaptic membrane (see Figure 13). The increased glutamate receptor expression post-synaptically contributes to synaptic facilitation by increasing the sensitivity of the motor neuron to synaptic glutamate released from the pre-synaptic sensory neuron.

VI. LONG-TERM SYNAPTIC FACILITATION IN *APLYSIA* INVOLVES CHANGES IN GENE EXPRESSION AND RESULTING ANATOMICAL CHANGES

We have already discussed that long-term facilitation in *Aplysia* involves persistent activation of PKA. However, after the persistent kinase activation has decayed, what then maintains the strengthened connection between the siphon sensory neurons and their follower motor neurons? Strikingly, continued augmentation of the defensive withdrawal reflex is based on morphological changes in the circuit (see Figure 14). Sensitization lasting on the order of 24 hours or more is mediated by an actual increase in the number of synaptic contacts between siphon sensory neurons and follower motor neurons (Figure 14). Thereby stimulation of the siphon sensory neuron elicits a greater response in gill withdrawal, because a greater number and density of excitatory connections are made between the two cells.

Studies into long-term effects of serotonin on sensory neurons strongly suggests that these morphological changes are a result of a pathway involving cAMP- and MAPK-mediated changes in gene expression, resulting in increased synthesis of some proteins, down-regulation of others, and an overall remodeling of the zones of contact between sensory and motor neurons (Figure 11). The dissection of these molecular cascades is an active area of research at present.

One final comment is that pioneering work in *Aplysia* demonstrated that long-lasting habituation of the gill-and-siphon withdrawal response was associated with a decreased number of synaptic contacts between siphon sensory neurons and gill motor neurons. Both long-term inhibition and enhancement of behavior therefore have in common an underlying anatomical basis. Although our understanding of the molecular mechanisms underlying these types of anatomical changes is incomplete at present, these observations about long-term sensitization and long-term habituation serve to illustrate that structural rearrangements of synaptic connections are likely to be a powerful and general mechanism underlying long-lasting behavioral changes.

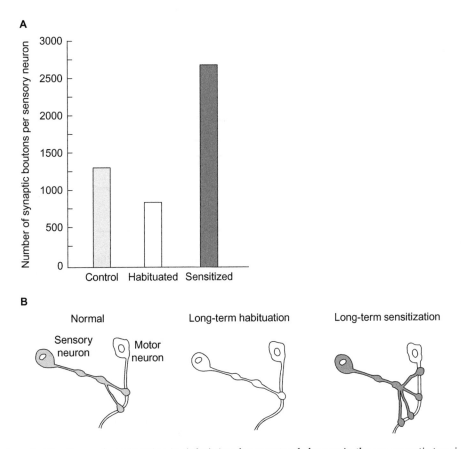

FIGURE 14 Long-term habituation and sensitization in *Aplysia* involve structural changes in the pre-synaptic terminals of sensory neurons. Adapted from Bailey and Chen (1983). (A) When measured one day or one week after training, the number of pre-synaptic terminals is highest in sensitized animals (about 2800) compared with control (1300) and habituated animals (800). (B) Long-term habituation leads to a loss of synapses and long-term sensitization leads to an increase in synapses. Figure and legend from Eric Kandel, *Principles of Neural Science*. Copyright McGraw-Hill 2000.

BOX 4

HABITUATION AND SYNAPTIC INHIBITION

As was described in the first chapter, habituation is perhaps the simplest form of learning and is a diminution of a behavioral response. Habituation occurs in response to repeated stimulation and is manifest as a decreased response to that stimulus over time. As was described in the first chapter and in this one, *Aplysia*

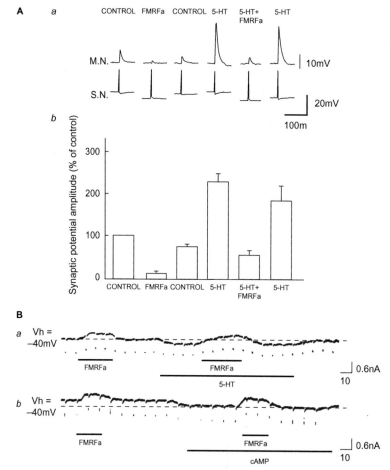

BOX 4 FMRFamide (FMRFa) antagonizes the actions of 5-HT and cAMP. (A). FMRFamide produces pre-synaptic inhibition and antagonizes pre-synaptic facilitation with 5-HT. (A) a. Intracellular recordings of membrane potential from motor neurons (top) and sensory neurons (bottom) in response to brief depolarizing current stimuli to sensory neurons. Action potentials in sensory neurons elicit a fast excitatory post-synaptic potential (e.p.s.p.) in motor neurons. b. Average data from five experiments. Error bars show s.e.m. Application of $10\,\mu m$ FMRFamide alone inhibits the synaptic potential recorded in a follower neuron to 11% of that of the initial control. The same dose ($10\,\mu m$) of 5-HT produces facilitation of the synaptic potential is reduced to a level slightly below that of the control (55%). (B) a. Antagonism by FMRFamide of membrane current response to 5-HT. First application of FMRFamide ($10\,\mu m$) produces a 450 pA increase in outward S-channel current ($V_m = -40\,mV$). Application of 5-HT then produces a 270 pA decrease in outward S-channel current. Subsequent application of FMRFamide in the presence of 5-HT produces a 660 pA increase in outward current, so that net membrane current approaches peak outward level in FMRFamide alone. b. Antagonism of current response to cAMP by FMRFamide. $V_{h.,}$ Holding voltage. First application of FMRFamide produces a 420 pA increase in outward current. Next, application of $200\,\mu m$ chlorophenyl-thio-cAMP causes a 300 pA decrease in outward current. Finally, application of FMRFamide in the presence of cAMP causes a 570 pA increase in outward current. On average, FMRFamide alone causes an increase in outward current of $0.28\,nA \pm 0.06$ ($\pm$ s.d.; n = 6; $V_m = -40\,mV$), whereas cAMP alone causes a mean decrease in outward current of $0.2 \pm 0.04\,nA$ ($\pm$s.d.; n = 6; $V_m = -40\,mV$). In the maintained presence of cAMP, FMRFamide induces a larger increase in outward current of $0.4 \pm 0.007\,nA$ ($\pm$ s.d.; n = 6; $V_m = -40\,mV$). Copyright 1989, Nature Publishing Group, Macmillan Publishers.

BOX 4—cont'd

HABITUATION AND SYNAPTIC INHIBITION

exhibits both short-term and long-term habituation of its gill-and-siphon withdrawal reflex. Behavioral modification of the withdrawal response is not limited to an increased response, sensitization, but also includes a decrement of the response, habituation.

Habituation is thus the opposite and opposing effect to sensitization, and this opposition is also exhibited at the cellular and molecular level. For example, habituation of the gill-and-siphon withdrawal response is associated with decreased synaptic strength at the same sensory neuron–motor neuron synapses that are potentiated with sensitization. Thus, habituation is associated with synaptic inhibition. However, one mechanistic difference between sensitization and habituation is that the decrease in synaptic strength associated with habituation is homo-synaptic—only the pre-synaptic sensory neuron and the post-synaptic motor neurons are involved. No third neuron releasing a modulatory neurotransmitter, such as 5HT in the case of *Aplysia* hetero-synaptic facilitation, is involved.

However, hetero-synaptic inhibition does occur at sensorimotor synapses in *Aplysia*. For example, the peptide neurotransmitter FMRFamide (Phe-Met-Arg-Phe-amide) causes pronounced synaptic inhibition when applied to the sensory neuron–motor neuron synapse (see Figure). Indeed, serotonin and FMRFamide produce opposing modulatory effects on synaptic transmission, on membrane potassium channel function, and on resting membrane potential. When the two neuromodulators are simultaneously present, the effects of FMRFamide dominate, leading to a net synaptic inhibition.

The existence of bidirectional modulation of synaptic strength should come as no surprise. Intuitively, it seems clear that most behavioral responses should be subject to both strengthening and weakening. From a theoretical perspective, synapses subject to only potentiation might in the long-term be driven to saturation and rendered aplastic, negating their utility as components of a dynamic memory system. Figure and legend adapted from reference (1).

Self-Perpetuating Chemical Reactions in Memory Maintenance

While long-term memory is associated with structural anatomical changes, this is not the end of the story. As we discussed at the beginning of this chapter, there is nothing inherently stable about morphological changes or increased synaptic contacts. All the component molecules that make up these structures are being continually broken down and resynthesized. How does the cell solve the problem of maintaining a change in the face of continual loss and replacement of its component molecules?

The theoretical answer to this question is based in a specific category of chemical reactions that Erik Roberson and I have referred to as *mnemogenic*, or memory-forming chemical reactions. The essential descriptor of a mnemogenic chemical reaction is given in Equation 1.

$$X + X^\bullet \rightarrow X^\bullet + X^\bullet \qquad (1)$$

In this reaction, X is a molecule that can exist in either a basal state (X) or an activated or modified form ($X^\bullet$). The initiation of a learning event triggers activation of X by conversion into the $X^\bullet$, or activated form.

$$X \xrightarrow{\text{trigger}} X^\bullet$$

This activated $X^\bullet$ leads to manifestation of the memory phenotype, affecting either directly or indirectly some biochemical process regulating neuronal function, such as synaptic strength or neuronal excitability. The unique feature of the mnemogenic reaction is that the activated molecule, $X^\bullet$, can react with an inactive molecule of X and convert it to the $X^\bullet$ form. This is how levels of $X^\bullet$ are sustained despite molecular turnover. Although the nucleus synthesizes only the inactive form, the activated species at the synapse catalyzes its activation, and thus more active $X^\bullet$ is created, perpetuating the reaction.

Two specific examples of mnemogenic chemical reactions have been identified as potentially maintaining long-lasting synaptic facilitation in *Aplysia*. The first example is based on seminal work in this area by Arnold Eskin, Jack Byrne, and their colleagues (14, 15). Their work seeks to address the question of how an

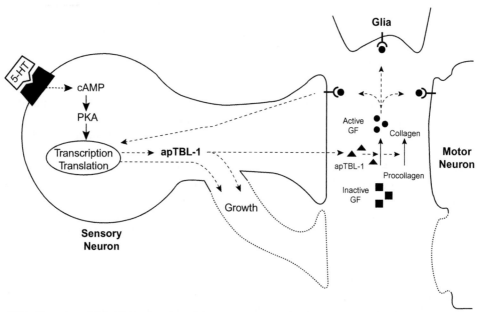

FIGURE 15   The Eskin/Byrne model for the expression of *Aplysia* TBL-1 in *Aplysia* long-term facilitation. This figure presents the Eskin/Byrne model of possible roles of apTBL-1 in long-term pre-synaptic facilitation in *Aplysia* sensory neurons. A sensory neuron, motor neuron, and glial cell are represented schematically. The growth processes of sensory neurons and motor neurons are drawn with dotted lines. 5-HT increases the transcription of the apTBL-1 gene. apTBL-1 protein might remain in the cytoplasm by alternative translation and might play a role as a protease to modify the cytoskeleton structure in the growth process within the sensory neuron. apTBL-1 might also be secreted to modify the extracellular matrix (procollagen) or activate TGF-b-like growth factors. The activated growth factors could bind to Ser/Thr kinase receptors and trigger the signal transduction cascade, leading to the regulation of cell growth. The activated growth factors also might modify the motor neurons to complement the morphological changes in the sensory neurons, or they might activate glial cells to secrete extracellular matrix components that might then help stabilize the morphological changes. Some of the same events elicited by the activation of TGF-b also could be caused by modification of the extracellular matrix component collagen. Figure and legend reproduced from Liu et al. (15).

increased number of synaptic contacts are maintained in the face of continual breakdown and resynthesis of the synaptic molecular infrastructure. They have found that long-term facilitation is associated with increased expression of a Tolloid/Bone Morphogenetic Protein referred to as *Aplysia* TBL-1 (Tolloid/Bone morphogenetic protein-Like protein-1). TBL-1 is (among other things) a protease that is involved in growth factor processing. The current hypothesis is that TBL-1 is induced with serotonin treatment and secreted into the extracellular space, where it converts pro-TGFβ into active TGFβ (Transforming Growth Factor Beta). TGFβ can then bind to its receptors on the cell surface and activate signal transduction cascades that, like serotonin, lead to increased expression of TBL-1 (see Figure 15). In this way a self-reinforcing loop is established that can persist beyond the breakdown and resynthesis of individual component molecules. The increased number of synaptic connections is maintained in this model by having the component molecules for synapse maintenance synthesized in parallel with the TBL-1—a conceptually straightforward mechanism for this is simply to have them read out from the same gene promoters that regulate TBL-1 expression.

This process is an example of a mnemogenic chemical reaction; specifically a variant termed a circular mnemogenic reaction. Mnemogenic reactions are not limited to a single molecule catalyzing production or activation of itself. Interacting sets of molecules can act in series to establish a regenerative molecular circuit. In this case the reactions have the following forms, where X catalyzes activation of Y, and Y in turn catalyzed activation of X:

$$X^{\bullet} + Y \rightarrow X^{\bullet} + Y^{\bullet}$$

$$X + Y^{\bullet} \rightarrow X^{\bullet} + Y^{\bullet}$$

By summing these partial reactions and rearranging to the form of Equation 1, we see that this system creates a sort of double mnemogenic reaction:

$$X + X^{\bullet} + Y + Y^{\bullet} \rightarrow X^{\bullet} + X^{\bullet} + Y^{\bullet} + Y^{\bullet}$$

BOX 5

FORGETTING

Given the continual turnover of the molecular constituents of our CNS it's amazing that we can remember anything at all for any period of time. With this in mind, the emerging recognition of the error-proneness of human memory may come as no surprise.

Forgetting and memory lability come part and parcel with molecular turnover. Even an extremely low error rate as one molecule passes along its information to its successor will accumulate significant retention errors over the course of a lifetime. After all, a long-lived protein in a neuron has a half-life of about 24 hours. It will be broken down and resynthesized from scratch about 50 times over the course of a single year.

Although it is a stretch to go from molecules to cognitive psychology, it is entertaining to think of limitations in memory for which protein turnover may be the underlying culprit. The easiest example is transience. Transience is simply the diminution of a particular memory over time. Your memory for recent events is more robust and detailed for recent events than for those from farther in your past. Memory has a half-life because the molecules that store it have a half-life. In the case of those memories stored using a mnemogenic, self-perpetuating reaction, the memory half-life is basically determined by the error rate of the underlying mnemogenic reaction as it replicates itself.

Other examples of mnemogenic reaction systems such as this have recently been elaborated, based on computer modeling of signal transduction mechanisms operating in synaptic plasticity (16). In the case of the *Aplysia* TBL-1/TGFβ system the interacting cascades produce a bistable molecular state of a synapse that is capable of perpetual memory storage.

The second example of a mnemogenic biochemical reaction proposed to underlie long-term facilitation in *Aplysia* involves a prion protein-like mechanism of positive reinforcement at the synapse. Prion proteins (PrPs) of all sorts undergo a mnemogenic reaction that is not based on covalent modifications, but rather on the self-promoted catalysis of a persisting conformational change (17). PrPs are hypothesized to exist in two conformations, the cellular form that is present normally in cells and a "scrapie" form that is an infectious particle and the cause of various neurodegenerative disorders. One molecule of the scrapie form catalyzes the conversion of a molecule of the cellular form into a second molecule of the scrapie form; a reaction of the type described by Equation 1. Once converted to the scrapie conformation the molecule is essentially irreversibly changed and by promoting the generation of copies of itself the scrapie conformation preserves itself against elimination by proteolytic cellular protein turnover. Thus, PrP is a bistable molecule that can exist either in the cellular form (PrP^C) in which it is synthesized by neurons or the scrapie form (PrP^{Sc}) associated with encephalopathy. Via this mechanism PrP undergoes a mnemogenic reaction in which PrP^{Sc} (X) can induce the conversion of PrP^C (X) into new PrP^{Sc}.

$$PrP^C + PrP^{Sc} \rightarrow PrP^{Sc} + PrP^{SC}$$

By this means, in certain types of encephalopathies the prion proteins effect a type of memory whereby the infection is maintained despite the turnover of the PrP.

Kausic Si, Eric Kandel and colleagues have proposed a prion-protein-like mechanism as being involved in the persistence of potentiation in *Aplysia* synaptic facilitation (see Journal Club Articles). In their initial studies they detected prion-like properties in a neuronal member of the CPEB protein family (CPEB = cytoplasmic polyadenylation element binding protein), a family of proteins that regulate mRNA translation. *Aplysia* neuronal CPEB protein has an N-terminal extension that exhibits characteristics of prion proteins. They hypothesize that conversion of CPEB to a prion-like state in stimulated synapses helps to maintain long-term synaptic changes associated with memory storage. Specifically, they propose that CPEB regulates local protein synthesis and provides a mark at the potentiated synapse that stabilizes the synaptic growth associated with long-term facilitation.

VII. ATTRIBUTES OF CHEMICAL REACTIONS MEDIATING MEMORY

What do these examples of memory mechanisms in *Aplysia* tell us about the chemical reactions that support them? First, there must be chemical reactions with different time courses that mediate short-, long-, and ultralong-term memory. Second, because manifestation of the memory phenotype between shorter-term and longer-term memories is seamless, the various chemical reactions are likely to converge on common effectors. And finally, there must be some unique mechanism to mediate those ultralong-term memories that defeats the problem of molecular turnover.

These studies of *Aplysia* sensitization also support one of the great unifying theories to emerge out of

neuroscience research in the last century, that is, that synaptic plasticity subserves learning and memory. This fundamental principal is nicely illustrated by studies in *Aplysia* described above. Because synapses mediate the neuron–neuron communication that underlies an animal's behavior, changes in behavior are ultimately subserved by alterations in the nature, strength, or number of interneuronal synaptic contacts in the animal's nervous system.

BOX 6

CENTRAL PATTERN GENERATORS

Some of the most striking examples of the use of invertebrate models to investigate the neural mechanisms underlying behavior come from studies of fixed pattern

generators, also known as central pattern generators. There are many examples of animals utilizing fixed patterns of movement, for example in cases where ongoing

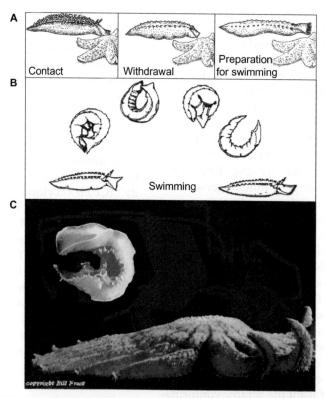

BOX 6 Escape swimming in *Tritonia*, a fixed-action pattern consisting of four stages. (A and B) Stages of *Tritonia* escape. (1) Contact and withdrawal—the relaxed animal with branchial tufts and rhinopores extended contacts a predator. After contact with a starfish the animal withdraws reflexly and bends ventrally. (2) Preparation for swimming—the animal elongates and enlarges the oral veil while bending slightly in the dorsal direction. (3) Swimming—the animal first makes vigorous ventral flexion and then vigorous dorsal flexion. This cycle is repeated several times (adapted from a figure by Tom Prentis). (4) Termination—after a final dorsal flexion the animal returns to an unflexed position with the extremities still withdrawn, oral veil and tail enlarged. One to five dorsal flexions occur before the animal regains its original relaxed posture. (C) Escape response. Photograph by Bill Frost.

BOX 6—cont'd

CENTRAL PATTERN GENERATORS

repetitive movements are utilized subconsciously (walking, for example), or where a rapid but fixed response pattern is required (such as dodging an oncoming object that you don't see until the last second).

Crabs and lobsters have been widely used to study one example of repetitive subconscious movements. The *stomatogastric ganglion* in crustaceans such as these controls a stereotyped pattern of muscle contractions in the animals' digestive systems. The muscle movement pattern is a highly synchronized, coordinated response to food ingestion that serves to provide the smooth movement of foodstuffs down the digestive tract. Many details of the neuronal circuitry and coordinated firing of individual neurons have been worked out for this system, along with an impressive dissection of the underlying cellular physiology.

In some cases, the stereotyped behaviors can be quite elaborate, involving extended, multi-component patterns of movement in the entire animal. One such example is a defensive escape response exhibited by the opisthobranch mollusc *Tritonia*. Predatory starfish feed on *Tritonia*, and a starfish touching *Tritonia* leads to the animal exhibiting a stereotyped response of defensive withdrawal and escape swimming. Again, this pattern of behavior is mediated by the highly coordinated firing of an elaborate network of neurons in the animal's nervous system. Much of the circuitry and cellular physiology of this central pattern generator was worked out in the late Peter Getting's laboratory.

Why do I bring this up in the context of general theories of the chemistry of memory? Because these are classic examples of "hard-wired" behavioral responses. They are seemingly immutable in the absence of injury to the animal or its nervous system. Nevertheless, even highly stable behavioral patterns are mediated by neurons whose molecular constituents are undergoing constant turnover. Self-perpetuating chemical reactions, not anatomy, are what provide the constancy of behavioral output in these "fixed" patterns.

VIII. SENSITIZATION IN MAMMALS

Behavioral sensitization in humans is a complex cognitive process involving multiple levels of processing such as attention, arousal, and emotional state. One simple example of sensitization is that school children are frequently sensitized to the sound of a ringing bell when they are waiting for the end of the school day. You may experience cognitive sensitization when you are waiting for your cell phone to ring when you know someone important is about to call. In extreme cases cognitive sensitization may be involved in such pathological processes as phobias and post-traumatic stress disorders.

However, there are less complex examples of human sensitization that are more analogous to the simple forms of sensory sensitization that we have been discussing thus far in this chapter. In humans, tissue injury results in persistently increased pain sensation to mildly noxious stimuli (hyperalgesia) and pain perception to normally non-noxious stimuli (allodynia).

These two forms of sensitization clearly fit within the definition of learning we are using in this textbook—persisting behavioral modification in response to an environmental signal. However, in the case of tissue injury one mechanism contributing to the altered behavior is persisting production of chemical signals locally at the site of damage, a mechanism that is not a memory event but a persisting change in local sensory function. However, there are also pain-associated central plastic changes that occur in the CNS that also alter perception of constant environmental signals. These mechanisms clearly qualify as CNS-based sensitization of behavioral responses.

Rodent model systems have allowed the delineation of some of the mechanisms underlying persistent pain sensitization after tissue injury. One mechanism is that primary sensory afferents known as Aδ and C fibers conveying peripheral pain signals to the central nervous system become sensitized. Physiologically, this sensitization manifests as a lower stimulus intensity threshold for firing, and possibly increased transmitter release in the primary sensory neurons. Second, and less well understood mechanistically, the central nervous system changes its processing of signals received from the periphery, such that mildly noxious stimuli are coded more intensely and non-noxious stimuli are coded as noxious.

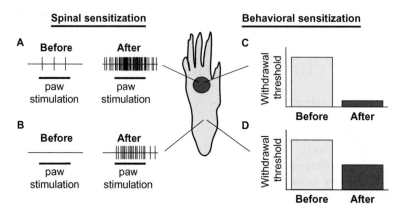

FIGURE 16 Diagrammatic representation of injury-induced spinal and behavioral sensitization. (A, B) Responses of a spinal cord dorsal horn neuron to paw stimulation before and after tissue injury. (A) Responses to stimulation in the injured area (red circle). After tissue injury, dorsal horn neurons exhibit increased responsiveness to a given stimulus. (B) Responses to stimulation in the noninjured area. Before tissue injury, the receptive field of the neuron did not include the stimulated area. After tissue injury, the neuron responds to stimulation in the noninjured area, demonstrating an enlargement of the receptive field (C, D). Paw withdrawal thresholds in response to mechanical stimulation before and after tissue injury. After tissue injury, withdrawal thresholds in response to mechanical stimulation of the injured (C) and noninjured areas (D) decrease. Adapted from Carrasquillo and Gereau, *Learning and Memory: A Comprehensive Review*, Volume 4, Chapter 5. Copyright Elsevier 2008.

Rodents behaviorally exhibit the sequelae of peripheral and central sensitization in a manner analogous to human behavior. Simple reflexive behavior, such as paw withdrawal, allows experimenters to quantify and study responsiveness to stimuli in rodents (see Figure 16). Analogous to human sensations, rodents with tissue injury withdraw their paws when given non-noxious stimuli such as warm heat or a light brush. Rodents thereby provide a model system to dissect out the molecular mechanisms of sensitization through biochemistry and physiology in correlation with simple behavioral assays.

In these types of experiments it has been discovered that one of the main loci for central sensitization is the spinal cord dorsal horn, the first relay station for pain signals arriving from the periphery (see Figure 17). This sensitization involves changes in the coding of noxious signals and minimally involves changes in synaptic strength and neuronal excitability—an interesting parallel to mechanisms of synaptic plasticity that we discussed regarding sensitization in the *Aplysia* system.

IX. SUMMARY—A GENERAL BIOCHEMICAL MODEL FOR MEMORY

Learning and memory have always intrigued those interested in the functioning of the brain. The mammalian CNS has an amazing capacity to store and recall diverse types of information, and learned responses shape to a great degree an animal's behavior. How are memories formed and stored?

Contemporary understanding of this issue highlights the importance of changes in synaptic strength (synaptic plasticity) as the means whereby the nervous system forms and stores memory (see Box 7). But by what means are changes in synaptic strength achieved? The fundamental answer to this question is not a mystery: changes in synaptic strength must of necessity be mediated by chemical changes, i.e., changes in the fundamental properties of the enzymes and other proteins comprising the synapse.

What sorts of chemical changes underlie memory formation and storage? Memory has as its defining characteristic persistence: an environmental stimulus causes a change that greatly outlasts the duration of the triggering signal. Therefore, at the chemical level, memory must have as its hallmark changes in protein functions which are able to persist beyond initial, triggering events. Understanding biochemical reactions that manifest this property will greatly increase our understanding of the mechanisms that must underlie memory.

In this chapter one goal has been to identify and characterize the types and time courses of persisting biochemical reactions underlying learning and memory, where possible highlighting specific, well-documented examples from studies of sensitization in *Aplysia californica*. The types of biochemical reactions underlying information storage fall into three general classes:

Category 1: Short-term changes that are mediated by the presence of extracellular or intracellular messenger molecules and which are subject to fairly rapid removal due to specific breakdown or clearance mechanisms. The prototype example is the acute action of a

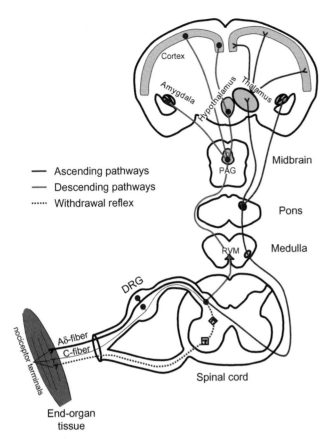

- Ascending pathways
- Descending pathways
- Withdrawal reflex

FIGURE 17 Illustration of anatomical pain pathways. Nociceptive information is transduced in nociceptor terminals located in the skin, muscle, and other end-organ tissues. Small-diameter unmyelinated C-fibers transmit the nociceptive information to the neurons in the dorsal horn of the spinal cord, which in turn project to various brain regions via ascending pathways (solid blue line) that relay in the medulla, pons, and thalamus. Activation of motor neurons (□) by excitatory interneurons (◇) mediates the pain withdrawal reflex (dotted blue line). Descending pathways from the brain (red line), that relay in the periaqueductal gray matter (PAG) and rostroventromedial medulla (RVM), modulate nociceptive transmission in the dorsal horn. DRG, dorsal root ganglia. Adapted from Carrasquillo and Gereau, *Learning and Memory: A Comprehensive Review*, Volume 4, Chapter 5. Copyright Elsevier 2008.

neurotransmitter on cellular biophysical or synaptic properties. In this phase the memory trace resides in the continued presence of the stimulus. The duration of the memory is dependent on ongoing production of the signal, for example the continued release of neurotransmitter into the synaptic cleft.

Category 2: Intermediate- and long-term changes that are mediated by a transient signal producing a persisting chemical memory trace. The generation of the persisting species may be produced by direct covalent modification of a pre-existing molecule, the triggering of an enzymatic modification of a pre-existing molecule, increased synthesis of an active enzyme, or altered gene expression resulting in enzyme activation

or synthesis. In general the duration of the chemical trace is determined by the half-life of the activated protein. The half-life of the protein may be controlled by passive metabolic processes, or alternatively may be regulated by specific control mechanisms. In some cases, the half-lives of the relevant species may be very long and capable of supporting a memory for hours, days, or even weeks, but these memories cannot be stored indefinitely as they remain susceptible in time to degradation of the trace molecule.

Category 3: Lifelong changes that are mediated by mnemogenic chemical reactions. The mnemogenic reaction could be triggered by the transient signal of Category 1, the persisting signal of Category 2, or by a distinct and parallel mechanism. The mnemogenic reaction, being self-perpetuating, does not have a half-life in the normal sense, but potentially can be reversed by a specific triggered mechanism. The activated mnemogenic species maintains the memory trace and results in the expression of memory through impinging on some biophysical, metabolic or structural neuronal component.

While it is certainly lacking in specifics, the general model described above serves as an organizing structure for thinking about various phases of memory, from the perspective of their being subserved by specific subtypes of chemical reactions.

Returning to the conundrum which was raised in the beginning of this chapter: how are robust lifelong memories stored as a biochemical reaction when their constituent molecules are subject to molecular turnover? If memories are stored in a synapse (or any other cellular compartment), how does a sustaining chemical species necessary for the memory render itself immune to degradation or spontaneous decay? This problem is particularly profound when considering examples of lifelong memory that can be induced by a single, transient environmental stimulus. The generic answer to this question has historically been that long-term changes are mediated by "anatomical" or "structural" changes, somehow implying that these changes are somehow protected from degradation. However, the same question of protein turnover applies to anatomical or structural changes. A structural feature does not "develop" and stay that way. It must be preserved (through being restored) on a minute-to-minute basis.

These considerations highlight the fact that preservation of memories is an active, ongoing process at the chemical level, subserved by mnemogenic self-perpetuating biochemical reactions (18–20). A molecule of finite lifetime that is involved in memory storage must somehow pass along its acquired characteristics to a successor molecule, before it is degraded and information is lost.

BOX 7

SUMMARY—SOME UNIFYING THEMES IN MEMORY RESEARCH

In this chapter we have identified six major concepts, concepts which are central to our current understanding of mechanisms of memory:

1. There is a cellular basis to behavior—all behaviors are mediated by underlying cellular mechanisms.
2. Changes in synaptic function are one important basis for memory formation and storage.
3. Synaptic plasticity is bidirectional.
4. Memory is subserved by biochemical reactions of various durations, providing short-, intermediate-, and long-term memories.
5. The different durations of biochemical mechanisms achieve the same final behavioral output by converging on common downstream effectors—effectors of synaptic function and structure in the examples we discussed in this chapter.
6. Permanent memory is sustained in the face of constant turnover of cellular constituents via tightly regulated self-reinforcing positive feedback mechanisms.

Further Reading

Bailey, C. H., Kandel, E. R., and Si, K. (2004). "The persistence of long-term memory: a molecular approach to self-sustaining changes in learning-induced synaptic growth". *Neuron* 44(1):49–57.

Bhave, G., and Gereau, R. W. (2004). "Posttranslational mechanisms of peripheral sensitization". *J. Neurobiol.* 61(1):88–106.

Byrne, J. H., and Kandel, E. R. (1996). "Presynaptic facilitation revisited: state and time dependence". *J. Neurosci.* 16:425–435.

Kandel, E. R. (2007). *In Search of Memory: The Emergence of a New Science of Mind*. New York: W. W. Norton and Co.

Kandel, E. R. (1976). *Cellular Basis of Behavior: An Introduction to Behavioral Neurobiology*. San Francisco, CA: W. H. Freeman.

Kandel, E. R. (2001). "The molecular biology of memory storage: a dialogue between genes and synapses". *Science* 294:1030–1038.

Lisman, J. E. (1985). "A mechanism for memory storage insensitive to molecular turnover: a bistable autophosphorylating kinase". *Proc. Natl. Acad. Sci. USA* 82:3055–3057.

Roberson, E. D., and Sweatt, J. D. (1999). "A biochemical blueprint for long-term memory". *Learn. Mem.* 6:381–388.

Rudy, J. W. (2008). *Neurobiology of Learning and Memory*. New York: Sinauer Associates.

Journal Club Articles

Carrasquillo, Y., and Gereau, R. W. (2007). "Activation of the extracellular signal-regulated kinase in the amygdala modulates pain perception". *J. Neurosci.* 27(7):1543–1551.

Miller, S. G., and Kennedy, M. B. (1986). "Regulation of brain type II Ca^{2+}/calmodulin-dependent protein kinase by autophosphorylation: a Ca^{2+}-triggered molecular switch". *Cell* 44:861–870.

Shuster, M. J., Camardo, J. S., Siegelbaum, S. A., and Kandel, E. R. (1985). "Cyclic AMP-dependent protein kinase closes the serotonin-sensitive K+ channels of *Aplysia* sensory neurones in cell-free membrane patches". *Nature* 313:392–395.

Si, K., Giustetto, M., Etkin, A., Hsu, R., Janisiewicz, A. M., Miniaci, M. C., Kim, J. H., Zhu, H., and Kandel, E. R. (2003). "A neuronal isoform of CPEB regulates local protein synthesis and stabilizes synapse-specific long-term facilitation in *Aplysia*". *Cell* 115(7):893–904.

Si, K., Lindquist, S., and Kandel, E. R. (2003). "A neuronal isoform of the *Aplysia* CPEB has prion-like properties". *Cell* 115(7):879–891.

For more information—relevant topic chapters from: John H. Byrne (Editor-in-Chief) (2008). *Learning and Memory: A Comprehensive Reference*. Oxford: Academic Press (ISBN 978-0-12-370509-9). (1.27 Eisenhardt, D., and Stollhoff, N. *Reconsolidation in Invertebrates*. pp. 529–548; 1.30 Benjamin, P. R., and Kemenes, G. *Behavioral and Circuit Analysis of Learning and Memory in Mollusks*. pp. 587–604; 2.12 Nairne, J. S., and Pandeirada, J. N. S. *Forgetting*. pp. 179–194; 2.32 Perruchet, P. *Implicit Learning*. pp. 597–621; 4.02 Bailey, C. H., Barco, A., Hawkins, R. D., and Kandel, E. R. *Molecular Studies of Learning and Memory in* Aplysia *and the Hippocampus: A Comparative Analysis of Implicit and Explicit Memory Storage*. pp. 11–29; 4.03 Fioravante, D., Antzoulatos, E. G., and Byrne, J. H. *Sensitization and Habituation: Invertebrate*. pp. 31–51; 4.04 Butterfield, M. P., and Rankin, C. H. *Molecular Mechanisms of Habituation in* C. elegans. pp. 53–64; 4.05 Carrasquillo, Y., and Gereau IV, R. W. *Pain Sensitization*. pp. 65–90; 4.23 Colbran, R. J. *CaMKII: Mechanisms of a Prototypical Memory Model*. pp. 469–488; 4.26 Hegde, A. N. *Proteolysis and Synaptic Plasticity*. pp. 525–545; 4.27 Cole, C. J., and Josselyn, S. A. *Transcription Regulation of Memory: CREB, CaMKIV, Fos/Jun, CBP, and SRF*. pp. 547–566; 4.33 Costa-Mattioli, M., Sonenberg, N., and Klann, E. *Translational Control Mechanisms in Synaptic Plasticity and Memory*. pp. 675–694.)

References

1. Sweatt, J. D., and Kandel, E. R. (1989). "Persistent and transcriptionally-dependent increase in protein phosphorylation in long-term facilitation of *Aplysia* sensory neurons". *Nature* 339:51–54.
2. Mammen, A. L., Huganir, R. L., and O'Brien, R. J. (1997). "Redistribution and stabilization of cell surface glutamate receptors during synapse formation". *J. Neurosci.* 17:7351–7358.
3. Chikhale, E. G., Balbo, A., Galdzicki, Z., Rapoport, S. I., and Shetty, H. U. (2001). "Measurement of myo-inositol turnover

in phosphatidylinositol: description of a model and mass spectrometric method for cultured cortical neurons". *Biochemistry* 40:11114–11120.

4. Rapoport, S. I. (2001). "*In vivo* fatty acid incorporation into brain phos-holipids in relation to plasma availability, signal transduction and membrane remodeling". *J. Mol. Neurosci.* 16:243–261, discussion 279–284.

5. Star, E. N., Kwiatkowski, D. J., and Murthy, V. N. (2002). "Rapid turnover of actin in dendritic spines and its regulation by activity". *Nat. Neurosci.* 5:239–246.

6. Zhang, X. J., Chinkes, D. L., Sakurai, Y., and Wolfe, R. R. (1996). "An isotopic method for measurement of muscle protein fractional breakdown rate *in vivo*". *Am. J. Physiol.* 270:E759–E767.

7. Roberson, E. D., and Sweatt, J. D. (1999). "A biochemical blueprint for long-term memory". *Learn Mem.* 6:381–388.

8. Bailey, C. H., Bartsch, D., and Kandel, E. R. (1996). "Toward a molecular definition of long-term memory storage". *Proc. Natl Acad. Sci. USA* 93:13445–13452.

9. Byrne, J. H., and Kandel, E. R. (1996). "Presynaptic facilitation revisited: state and time dependence". *J. Neurosci.* 16:425–435.

10. Frost, W. N., and Kandel, E. R. (1995). "Structure of the network mediating siphon-elicited siphon withdrawal in *Aplysia*". *J. Neurophysiol.* 73:2413–2427.

11. Kandel, E. R. (1976). *Cellular Basis of Behavior: An Introduction to Behavioral Neurobiology.* San Francisco, CA: W. H. Freeman.

12. Shuster, M. J., Camardo, J. S., Siegelbaum, S. A., and Kandel, E. R. (1985). "Cyclic AMP-dependent protein kinase closes the serotonin-sensitive K^+ channels of *Aplysia* sensory neurones in cell-free membrane patches". *Nature* 313:392–395.

13. Sweatt, J. D. (2001). "Protooncogenes subserve memory formation in the adult CNS". *Neuron* 31:671–674.

14. Zhang, F., Endo, S., Cleary, L. J., Eskin, A., and Byrne, J. H. (1997). "Role of transforming growth factor-beta in long-term synaptic facilitation in *Aplysia*". *Science* 275:1318–1320.

15. Liu, Q. R., Hattar, S., Endo, S., MacPhee, K., Zhang, H., Cleary, L. J., Byrne, J. H., and Eskin, A. (1997). "A developmental gene (Tolloid/BMP-1) is regulated in *Aplysia* neurons by treatments that induce long-term sensitization". *J. Neurosci.* 17:755–764.

16. Weng, G., Bhalla, U. S., and Iyengar, R. (1999). "Complexity in biological signaling systems". *Science* 284:92–96.

17. Li, L., and Lindquist, S. (2000). "Creating a protein-based element of inheritance". *Science* 287:661–664.

18. Crick, F. (1984). "Memory and molecular turnover". *Nature* 312:101.

19. Lisman, J. E. (1985). "A mechanism for memory storage insensitive to molecular turnover: a bistable autophosphorylating kinase". *Proc. Natl. Acad. Sci. USA* 82:3055–3057.

20. Lisman, J. E., and Fallon, J. R. (1999). "What maintains memories?". *Science* 283:339–340.

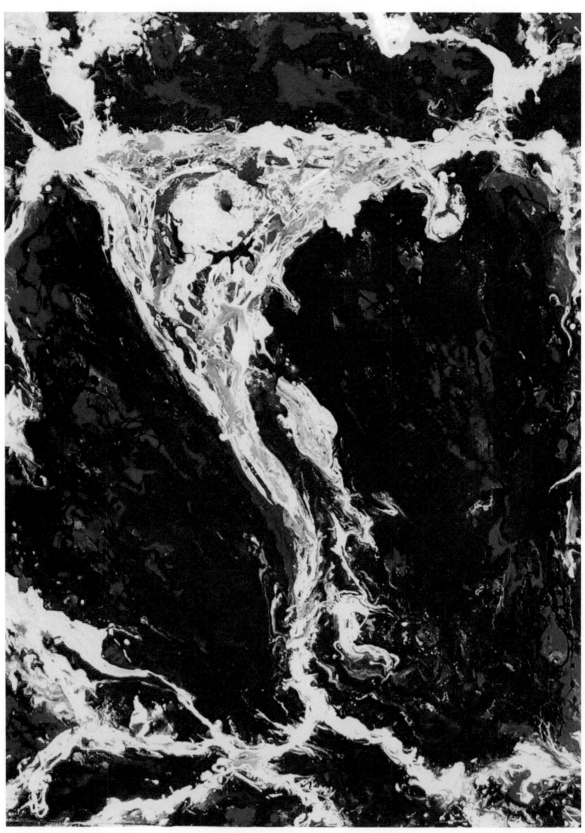

Hippocampal Pyramidal Neuron
J. David Sweatt, acrylic on canvas, 2008–2009

4

Rodent Behavioral Learning and Memory Models

I. INTRODUCTION

The study of learning and memory requires the development and use of experimental model systems that can be utilized both to characterize the fundamental behaviors associated with memory and to explore the underlying mechanisms. In the last chapter we discussed the *Aplysia* model system and studies of the cellular and molecular basis of sensitization in that "simple" system. In this chapter we will transition into a discussion of mammalian systems used experimentally to investigate the cellular and molecular basis of learning and memory, and will focus on behavioral experimental systems as a prelude to more detailed discussions of cellular and molecular mechanisms in subsequent chapters. We will limit our discussion to rodent model systems, particularly those involving rats and mice, because essentially all the cellular and molecular studies that we will discuss in the rest of the book utilize rats and mice.

We also will focus largely on learned behaviors that involve the hippocampus, although some other paradigms for assessing amygdala- and cerebellum-dependent learning will also be described. We will focus on the hippocampus because this sets the stage for our subsequent discussions in the book of many examples of hippocampal cellular plasticity that have been extensively studied and that are hypothesized to be involved in hippocampus-dependent learning and memory. In addition, the next chapter will focus on associative learning paradigms that involve the amygdala and cerebellum, so those forms of memory will subsequently be given a more detailed treatment.

Our current approaches to behavioral assessments related to learning and memory are based on a foundation laid many years ago. During the beginning and middle of the last century studies by a number of experimental psychologists led to an explosive advancement of our understanding of the basics of learned behaviors. Classic studies carried out by Ivan

Pavlov, B. F. Skinner, and Karl Lashley, to name but a few who used non-human models, laid the foundation for much of the modern laboratory memory research. These studies even received a reasonable degree of public recognition—there's a line from a Rolling Stones song that goes "Yeah, when you call my name, I salivate like Pavlov's dog ..." How many experiments have ever reached that level of popular recognition? These studies have also reached the level of iconism; running rats through mazes is now symbolic in the public eye of neuroscience studies in general.

Of course, rat maze learning is but the tip of the iceberg of modern rodent behavioral research. In this chapter we will discuss a number of specific examples of contemporary rodent behavioral paradigms used to study learning and memory. In reviewing these models it is important to always keep in mind that when one does a memory experiment at least three things are happening with the animal over the time-course of the experiment: they are learning (i.e., forming a memory); they are generating a stable record of the event (a memory); and they are recalling the memory in order to produce a detectable read-out. The complexity of these processes is in many ways obscured by the apparent simplicity of the learning behaviors themselves. At any given point in time during the experiment any one or all of these processes may be occurring, each with their own distinct underlying cellular and molecular mechanisms.

For the remainder of this chapter I will describe rodent behavioral assessment paradigms that are utilized in modern learning and memory studies. I will begin with a description of behavior tests that are used to assess basic behaviors such as baseline activity, motor coordination, and sensory systems. I will then describe more complicated tests that are used to assess learning and memory *per se*. Finally in this chapter I will provide a brief overview of the basics of experimental design, focusing on their application to behavioral, cellular, and molecular assessments of learning and memory mechanisms.

II. BEHAVIORAL ASSESSMENTS IN RODENTS

A. Assessing General Activity and Sensory Perception

Open Field Analysis and Elevated Plus Maze Performance

Open field analysis is utilized to measure the level of spontaneous motor activity and exploratory behavior in an animal. The open field apparatus can also be used to assess habituation to the novel environment:

over an extended period of time in the open field apparatus (see Figures 1 and 2) the spontaneous motor behavior decreases, a manifestation of habituation.

In a typical open field experiment animals are placed in an open field chamber (e.g., a $40 \times 40 \times 30$ cm box) for 5–30 minutes in standard room-lighting conditions. Activity in the open field is monitored by light beams and photoreceptors on each side of the chamber, or with a camera mounted over the open field, and activity is analyzed using a computer-operated system. With this test, general activity levels are evaluated by measurements of horizontal activity (movement across and through the field), vertical activity (e.g., rearing up onto the hind legs), and total distance traveled during a test session (see Figure 2). These types of data are used to screen for normal motor activity, hypo- and hyperactivity. Either hypo- or hyperactivity can be a complication to the subsequent assessment of many different types of learned behaviors.

Animals in an open arena or box exhibit *thigmotaxis* when they are anxious or fearful. Thigmotaxis is "wall-hugging" behavior—this behavior is frequently exhibited by humans when they get into an elevator with strangers, for example. In an open field experiment rodents will typically exhibit less thigmotaxis as they become acclimatized to the chamber (see Figure 2A). By quantitating this change in behavior the open field test can also be used to measure anxiety levels. This is assessed by taking the ratio of the time (or distance traveled) the animal spent in the center of the open field, relative to the total time in the maze (or total distance traveled). In other words, quantitating the amount of time the animal spent exploring the open center part of the field, versus the total area including that part next to the walls. Anxious or fearful animals will spend less time in the center of the field and more time next to the walls, yielding a decreased center-to-total time ratio.

The open field assessment is often used in conjunction with the elevated plus maze as an anxiety index (see Figure 3). The elevated plus maze task quantitates the amount of time an animal spends in the protected arms of a raised plus-shaped maze, relative to the time spent exploring the two other limbs of the plus maze that are open on each side. Similar to the open field assessment, in the elevated plus maze assessment an anxious or fearful animal will spend proportionally less time in the open arms and more time in the walled, protected arms.

Rotating Rod Performance—Coordination and Motor Learning

The rotating rod task is commonly used to assess behavioral parameters related to cerebellar function. In this test, an animal is required to maintain its balance after being placed on a rotating rod, as the

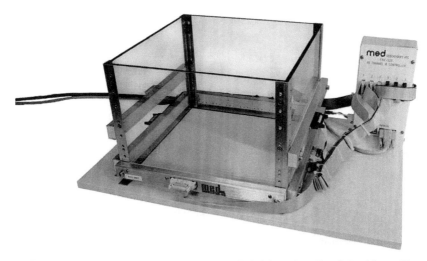

FIGURE 1   Open field apparatus. Image courtesy of Med Associates Inc., Saint Albans, Vermont.

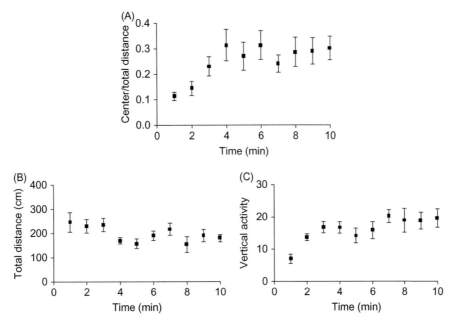

FIGURE 2   Open field behavior. Animals were placed in the open field apparatus and activity monitored using automated recording equipment. (A) Total distance traveled per minute for a 10-minute period. (B) Vertical activity (number of rearings per minute) over a 10-minute period. (C) Ratio of center distance to total distance traveled for each minute over a 10-minute period. The data in (A) and (B) are taken as indices of general activity; the data in (C) is taken as an index of anxiety. Results shown are for C57Bl6 animals, mean ± SEM for n = 10 animals. Data courtesy of Coleen Atkins.

name implies. Over the course of a five-minute trial, the speed of the rotating rod (commonly called a "rotarod") accelerates from 4 to 40 rpm (see Figure 4). The amount of time before the animal falls off the rod is measured as the behavioral index in this test. In a typical experiment, animals undergo four rotarod trials per day, separated by an hour rest period, for two consecutive days.

Initial trials are used to assess the animal's coordination; the amount of time an animal can stay on a rotating rod is an index of its general level of motor abilities, reflexes, balance, and overall motor coordination. These behaviors are all dependent on proper cerebellar function. In addition, motor coordination is an important component of most behavioral assessments of learning and memory, where complicated motor output is necessary for successful execution of a learned task.

The rotating rod task is also used as a measure of motor learning. Mice and rats improve their performance with repeated training over several trials

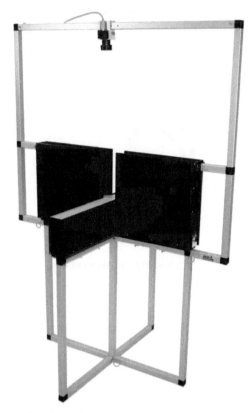

FIGURE 3 Elevated plus maze. Image courtesy of Med Associates Inc., Saint Albans, Vermont.

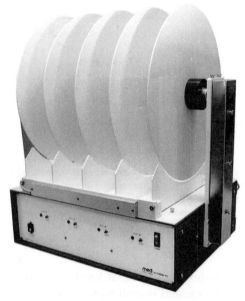

FIGURE 4 Roto Rod. Image courtesy of Med Associates Inc., Saint Albans, Vermont.

(see Figure 5), which is an indicator of motor learning and memory. Thus, motor skill acquisition can be assessed in its own right by using the rotating rod test and determining the rate of improvement on the task on repeated trials.

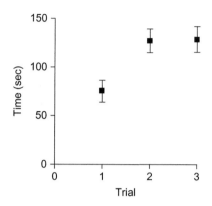

FIGURE 5 Rotating rod behavior. Total time the animals remained on the rotating rod was measured for each training period. Three training trials were given in a single day. The increase in time the animal remained on the rod is taken as an index of motor learning. Results shown are for C57Bl6 animals, mean ± SEM for n = 10 animals. Data courtesy of Coleen Atkins.

Acoustic Startle and Prepulse Inhibition

Just like humans, mice and rats normally exhibit a startle response to a loud noise. Interestingly, if a modest noise is presented immediately preceding the loud noise, the startle response is significantly attenuated (see Figure 6) in mice, rats, and humans. This phenomenon is referred to as prepulse inhibition. To test acoustic startle and prepulse inhibition, animals are typically placed within a sound-insulated testing chamber with a 70 dB background noise level, and left undisturbed for a five-minute acclimatization period. Acoustic startle is then measured by quantitating the animal's motor response to a brief, 120 dB sound burst. Prepulse inhibition, the phenomenon whereby the acoustic startle response is reduced on presentation of a sound (or prepulse) just prior to the startle stimulus, is also assessed in the same chamber. For prepulse inhibition, in addition to the single acoustic startle stimulus, there are also prepulse stimulus trials where prepulse sounds of lower dB intensities are presented 100 milliseconds before the startle stimulus. The diminution of the startle response due to the presentation the prepulses is quantitated as prepulse inhibition.

In rats and mice prepulse inhibition can be used to assess the animal's general reflexes (startle), and it also serves as a very sensitive and quantitative assessment of the animal's hearing. Normal mice, for example, exhibit prepulse inhibition with a threshold around 70 dB, and reliably give quantitatively different responses to prepulses varying by only a few dB (see Figure 6). Of course, hearing assessment is a critical control for auditory cued learning paradigms and prepulse inhibition can be used in this fashion.

Prepulse inhibition is also used as an assessment of sensory–motor gating, which is disrupted in

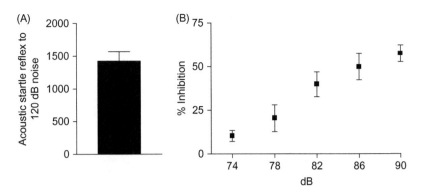

FIGURE 6 Acoustic startle and prepulse inhibition. (A) Acoustic startle in response to a 120 dB noise, assessed as the force exerted on an underlying footplate. (B) Effect of a pre-tone (sound intensity given in dB) to diminish the magnitude of acoustic startle. Results are given as percent diminution of the force of the subsequent 120 dB startle response. Results shown are for C57Bl6 animals, mean ± SEM for n = 10 animals. Data courtesy of Coleen Atkins.

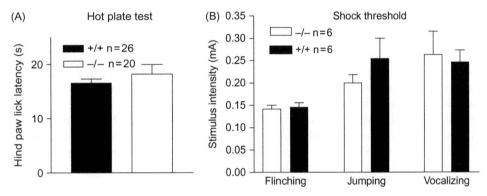

FIGURE 7 Nociception behavior. (A) A hot plate test was used to compare PKC beta knockout animals (□) versus wildtype (■) sensitivity to a noxious stimuli. Thermal nociception was measured on a 55°C hot plate as the latency to hind paw lick. (B) As an additional control to the hot plate test, the shock threshold test was used to compare sensitivity to foot shock measured by the extent of flinching, jumping or vocalization to increasing foot shock intensities. Data courtesy of Coleen Atkins.

schizophrenic patients. Schizophrenics do not exhibit prepulse inhibition, suggesting a disruption of this normal sensory filtering mechanism. Prepulse inhibition in rodents is therefore also used to model this aspect of schizophrenia.

Nociception

Nociception is an animal's sensory perception of aversive or noxious stimuli. One index of nociception is assayed by placing the animals on a 55°C hot plate, a temperature that is hot to the touch but will not burn the animal. Latency to lick the hind paw is measured (see Figure 7) as an index of the animal's ability to perceive the aversive stimulus. After animals lick their hindpaw they are of course immediately removed from the hot plate.

Thermal sensory thresholds in rats and mice can also be determined using an apparatus known as a Hargreave's radiant heat apparatus. In this test, the animals are allowed to move freely in small enclosures on an elevated glass plate. After a one-hour acclimitization period, radiant heat is applied locally to one

paw via a visible light source. The animals are not restrained, and thus when they feel discomfort, they withdraw the stimulated paw. The latency from onset of the stimulus to paw withdrawal is recorded as an index of sensory perception and sensitization. In a conceptually similar test electric shock threshold sensitivity can be measured by scoring animals for flinching, vocalizing, and jumping behavior in response to small incremental increases in foot shock intensity.

In many learning and memory behavioral training paradigms aversive sensory stimuli are utilized. In this context, with assessments of learning and memory, it is frequently necessary to have control data that animals are capable of normally perceiving aversive stimuli such as mild foot shock. Finally, it is important to note that it is almost universally the case that modest aversive stimuli are much more effective for training animals than are painful stimuli.

Vision Tests—Light–Dark Exploration and Visual Cliff

Overall, available visual tests for rodents are not very sensitive or sophisticated. Two common tests

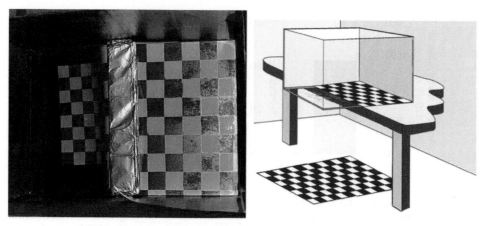

FIGURE 8   Visual cliff. Image courtesy of Jason White.

of vision are light–dark exploration and the "visual cliff." Light–dark exploration is used to asses an animal's ability to perceive light and dark. One typical variation consists of a polypropylene chamber unequally divided into two chambers by a black partition containing a small opening. The large chamber is open and brightly illuminated while the small chamber is closed and dark. Animals are placed into the illuminated side and allowed to move freely between the two chambers for several minutes—normal animals spend a majority of their time in the darkened chamber, as is expected for dark-preferring, nocturnal animals.

A second visual assessment paradigm is the visual cliff (see Figure 8). In this task animals are placed on a see-through surface, such as glass or plexiglass. This solid platform has a solid surface underneath it on one half, and air-space above the floor on the other half. Thus, a seeing animal perceives that one half of the chamber is a solid surface while the other half appears to be the open space above a large drop-off. In this test animals are placed on the "solid" surface and animals that can see rarely venture over the edge of the cliff. Non-seeing animals, of course, are unable to discern one area from the other as the tactile stimulus is a continuous smooth sheet.

In many learning tasks visual perception is an important variable. It is important to note that many inbred strains of rodents have poor vision, and that in general rats and mice are not particularly "visual" creatures (limited stereopsis, for example).

Summary

The variety of behavioral experiments described above can be combined into a general assessment battery consisting of open field test, rotating rod, acoustic startle, prepulse inhibition, hot plate, shock threshold, and visual assessment tasks. This battery of tests is quantitative and an excellent general screen for a wide variety of behaviors and sensory responses. Also typically included as control data are assessments of general physical parameters such as weight, temperature, coat appearance, basic reflexes, etc. Taken together, these tests also serve as useful controls for experiments in which anatomical or molecular lesions are being used to probe for the role of specific structures or molecules in rodent behavioral learning and memory (1, 2).

B. Fear Conditioning

One popular behavioral model system with which to study learning and memory is a robust learning paradigm that capitalizes on the capacity of mammals, including rodents, to associate environmental cues with a mild aversive stimulus. This type of learning, generally called fear conditioning, is an example of classical associative conditioning similar to Pavlovian conditioning. Some aspects of the neuronal circuitry underlying this behavior have been worked out and it is clear that the amygdala is involved in memory formation in this behavior (see references 3 and 4, for example). In addition, the fear conditioning paradigm has been quite fruitful as a model in which to study cellular and molecular mechanisms underlying learning and memory, as we will return to in detail in the next chapter. One final reason for the high level of enthusiasm for pursuing this behavioral paradigm is its potential relevance as a model system for human anxiety disorders.

Cue-plus-Contextual Fear Conditioning

Cue-plus-contextual fear conditioning is one variation of fear conditioning that is widely used in studies of rodent learning and memory. A typical cue-plus-contextual fear conditioning experiment proceeds

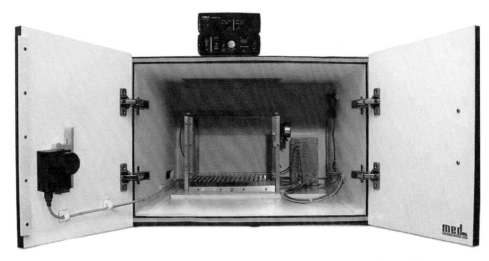

FIGURE 9   Fear conditioning chamber. Image courtesy of Med Associates Inc., Saint Albans, Vermont.

as follows. Animals are placed in a fear conditioning apparatus (see Figure 9) for about two minutes, then a 30 second acoustic CS (tone or preferably white noise, but light cues can also be used) is delivered. During the last two seconds of the tone, a mild foot shock (US) is applied to the floor grid of the apparatus. This pairing protocol can be repeated with a brief intervening period (e.g., two minutes) between pairings. The stimulus strength and number of training pairs are typically chosen based on pilot experiments to optimize learning without overtraining the animals. When trained in this fashion, the animals learn at least two things. One thing they learn is that the training chamber is bad news; that is, that the context in which they are trained is a place to be feared. Another thing that they learn is that the noise or light CS predicts an upcoming foot shock, and thus it also is to be feared. These two components of the learning are referred to as contextual and cued fear conditioning, respectively (see Figure 10).

Cued Fear Conditioning

Cued fear learning is assessed by quantitating the amount of fearful behavior exhibited by the animal following representation of the CS, when the CS is presented in a different context from that in which the training took place. This use of a different context is important to isolate the cued conditioning from the contextual conditioning: a variation is to habituate the animal to the fear conditioning apparatus (i.e., the training context) before presenting the CS-US pairing (see reference 5, for example).

Increased fearful behavior on later representation of the CS is an indication of the animal having formed a lasting association between the CS cue and the fear-evoking stimulus. To assess cue learning, animals are

A Cue-plus-contextual fear conditioning

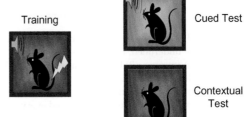

Training   Cued Test

                                                                     Contextual
                                                                     Test

B   Context alone conditioning
Training

                                                                     Contextual
                                                                     Test

C   Context discrimination
                                                        Test

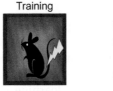

            Train   Context 1

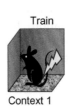

                                                                     Context 2
Context 1

FIGURE 10   Variants of fear conditioning in rodents. See text for details.

placed in a context different from the training context (e.g., novel odor, cage floor, and visual cues or alternatively a context similar to the home cage), and baseline behavior is measured for a few (e.g., three)

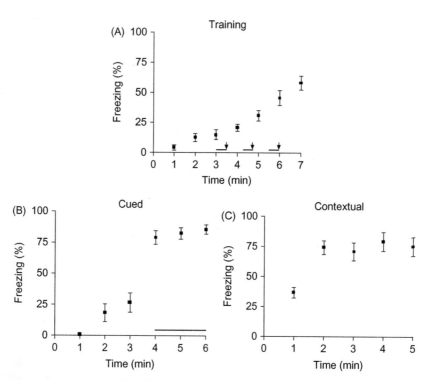

FIGURE 11 Cued-plus-contextual fear conditioning. (A) Freezing behavior on the day of training. The white noise CS is presented for the three periods of time underlined. Foot shocks are presented at the arrows. Stereotyped freezing posture is scored visually and expressed as percent of time spent freezing. (B) Freezing in response to CS presentation on Day 2 after training. For these experiments the animals are in a different context than that in which they were trained. The period of white noise (CS) presentation is indicated by the line. (C) Freezing in response to replacement in the training context. The animal is placed in the context at t = 0. All panels: results shown are for C57Bl6 animals, mean ± SEM for n = 10 animals. Freezing is scored every five seconds and averaged over one-minute epochs. Data from Weeber et al. (6).

minutes. Then the acoustic CS is presented for about three minutes and learning is assessed by measuring fearful behavior (see Figure 11).

To assess short-term cue learning, the animals are typically placed in the non-training context 1–2 hours following the completion of the training session, and fear assessed in response to representation of the acoustic or light CS. Long-term cue learning can be tested 24 hours to several weeks later.

How does one assess the fearful behavior indicative of learning? There are two basic ways to assess fear in rodents: freezing and startle potentiation. Freezing is a stereotyped immobile posture exhibited by rats and mice when they are fearful, which is readily recognizable to a trained human observer. In this case the scorer of the behavioral experiments should, of course, be blind in reference to whether the animal is a control or an experimental animal. Alternatively, computer-assisted video monitoring systems have been developed recently that can score freezing behavior automatically. The other variation for assessing fear in rodents is measuring fear-associated potentiation of their normal startle response, which can be quantitated automatically using a variety of devices. Potentiation of the animal's normal startle response to a loud noise, by representation of the CS (light for example) is one

of the standard indices of cue-evoked fear. Anyone who has ever watched a Hollywood "slasher" movie is familiar with fear-potentiated startle.

Contextual Fear Conditioning

To assess contextual learning, the animals are placed back into the training context post-training and scored for fear behavior for a short period of time, typically a few minutes, to minimize extinction of their fear of the context (see Figures 10–12). Similar to cued fear conditioning, contextual fear conditioning exhibits short-term and long-term forms.

It also is possible to train animals using a context-alone variant (see Figures 10 and 12). The procedures are essentially the same as the context-plus-cued paradigm described above, but no visual or auditory cue is delivered when the animal is trained. With this procedure the animal learns to fear the training context—on replacement into the training context the animal exhibits marked freezing.

Good evidence exists indicating that contextual fear conditioning is hippocampus-dependent, mostly based on lesioning studies, selective infusion of pharmacological agents into the hippocampus, and animals genetically engineered to have hippocampal deficits.

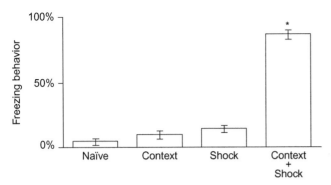

FIGURE 12 Contextual fear conditioning in rats. Rats were placed in the fear conditioning chamber for two minutes, then a one second shock (1.5mA) was delivered to the floor grid. This protocol was repeated for a total of five shocks with two minutes between each shock. Following the fifth shock, the subject remained in the training chamber for one minute and was removed to its home cage. Results shown are an assessment of fear conditioning 24 hours after training. Freezing behavior was measured every 10 seconds for five minutes, 24 hours after exposure to the contextual fear conditioning paradigm. One control group of animals ("Context") was exposed to the conditioning chamber for the same amount of time as the fear conditioned group, but did not receive any shocks. A second control group ("Shock") was shocked (five seconds, 1.5mA) immediately on placement into the conditioning chamber and immediately removed. "Naïve" animals were not exposed to the fear conditioning chamber, nor did they receive an electric shock. Exposing animals to the contextual fear conditioning paradigm significantly enhanced freezing behavior in animals 24 hours after training that paired the context and electric shock, but did not affect freezing behavior of animals that received either the context or shock alone, relative to naïve animals (Figure 4A; F[3,24] = 226.6, p <0.0001). Data from Levenson et al. (7).

However, there is some controversy on the point of the hippocampal dependence of contextual fear conditioning. A certain amount of controversy is perhaps not surprising given the ill-defined nature of the "context." Generally what is meant by "context" is a multimodal representation of the training environment. Of course, an individual animal may simply be associating a single aspect of the training environment with the foot shock, in essence converting contextual conditioning into cued conditioning for a single visual or olfactory cue in the training apparatus. To help get around this problem, a variant of contextual fear conditioning called "context discrimination" has been developed (8). In this variant an animal is tested in the training environment and also in another environment that shares some of the same cues as the training environment. The testing thus allows one to determine if the animal has learned to distinguish two similar environments from each other. The available evidence indicates that context discrimination is very sensitive to hippocampal deficits.

In experiments where one is looking for learning deficits in an experimental animal, a variety of behavioral control experiments are necessary to bolster any conclusion that animals are deficient in learning or

memory versus simply having derangements of normal sensory or motor function. Some of these types of control experiments for sensory and motor responses were described in the first part of this chapter. However, one simple control is to monitor animals during the training phase of fear conditioning, for example by assessing the freezing of the animal in response to presentation of the foot shock (see Figure 11). Normal animals exhibit a freezing response to foot shock presentation. Normal freezing by an experimental animal during training indicates that they are able to at least sense the foot shock and to freeze normally.

As an additional control in experiments where a learning deficit is indicated, one can undertake a retraining experiment. Thus, one can simply retrain the same animals that exhibited a learning deficit using a more vigorous training protocol in order to assess whether they are capable of fear conditioning at all. The goal in retraining experiments is to control for the potential confound that an apparent fear conditioning deficit is simply due to an inability of experimental animals to exhibit the freezing or fear-potentiated startle that is being quantitated as an index of learning. With retraining or overtraining, if the animal ultimately learns one can conclude that at least they are capable of exhibiting the learned behavior. It is also reasonable to infer that they are capable of sensing the environmental stimuli, although one possible explanation for a necessity for overtraining is that the animal has sensory deficits.

Passive avoidance training can also be used as a "control" for cued fear conditioning, although it also is a learning model in its own right. In this test (see the next section and Figure 4) animals learn to suppress their normal dark-seeking reflex because their entry into a dark chamber is paired with a foot shock. This control is particularly appealing because it can be set up to use the identical aversive sensory stimulus (foot shock) as cued fear conditioning. Passive avoidance is not as well suited as a control for contextual fear conditioning, because both tasks are likely to involve the hippocampus and share some underlying mechanisms, although manipulations have been found that can lead to selective deficits in passive avoidance versus contextual fear conditioning (see reference 6, for example).

In summary for this section, fear conditioning is a robust form of classical conditioning exhibited by rodents. Cued conditioning can be used as an index of general associative learning that is amygdala-dependent but hippocampus independent. Context-dependent conditioning is a variant to assess a likely hippocampus-dependent form of learning. The initial responses of the animal during and immediately after the training period also serve as a good screen for sensory responses to the foot shock and for the ability of the animal to exhibit fearful behavior.

Extinction of Fear Conditioning

After an animal is trained using a fear conditioning protocol, what happens if the CS is subsequently presented in the absence of the US? Of course, initially the animals exhibit a fearful response. However, with repeated presentations of CS alone the animals' conditioned fear response will be extinguished. This is also referred to as "extinction" of the memory. Extinction of conditioned fear is a unique memory process that is studied in its own right, and indeed most types of associative conditioning will exhibit extinction with repeated CS-alone presentations. In effect extinction is a reversal or "unlearning" of a previously learned association.

It is important to emphasize that extinction is *not* forgetting; nor is it erasure of the previously learned association. Extinction is its own type of learning, and is a relearning of a different contingency than the previously learned one. With extinction, animals learn that a CS does not reliably predict the US that it previously predicted. The fact that extinction does not involve forgetting or erasure of the prior memory is nicely illustrated by the following observation. If a fully extinguished animal is given a "reminder" the memory comes back fully expressed, without extensive retraining. For example, a fully extinguished contextual fear memory will come back, expressed as a robust, context-specific long-term memory, if the animal is given a single foot shock in a novel context. The foot shock in the novel context is clearly not retraining the animal—the context is different from the original training context. However, the experience of sensing a single foot shock in a different place is sufficient to drive reinstatement of the original conditioned response. This observation emphasizes the fact that the prior CS-US association is a latent memory still stored in the CNS. However, extinction training leads to the original memory being overridden and not expressed.

C. Avoidance Conditioning

In the passive avoidance learning paradigm, rodents learn to suppress their natural tendency to seek out dark areas over well-lit areas. This behavioral change is triggered by training the animal using the pairing of a mild foot shock with the animals' passage into the dark area from the well-lit one. One typical variation is referred to as the *step-through passive avoidance task* (see Figures 13 and 14). Animals are placed in a conditioning chamber separated into two compartments, one illuminated (e.g., by a 75 watt light bulb) and one dark. The two sides are separated by a guillotine-type partition. On the training day, animals are placed into the illuminated side of the conditioning apparatus and the amount of time it takes to move into the dark compartment, called the step-through latency, is measured. Once a subject has passed into the dark chamber, the partition is lowered and the animal receives a foot shock through the grid floor. After 10 seconds or so in the dark compartment, the animal is removed and returned to its home cage. Various periods of time later, animals are tested for associating the darkened chamber with the foot shock by measuring their step-through latency on replacement into the lit side of the conditioning chamber. The animal having learned the contingency is manifest as an increased latency to cross over to the dark side of the chamber.

Another variation of passive avoidance is referred to as *step-down avoidance*. During one-trial step-down avoidance training, animals are placed on an elevated platform and given a mild foot shock when they step off the platform onto the grid below. Memory is then assessed by the latency to step off the platform following training—trained animals avoid stepping off the platform. Both step-down avoidance and step-through avoidance learning are subject to disruption with hippocampal lesions.

Avoidance and Operant Conditioning

Much more elaborate avoidance conditioning paradigms that involve active avoidance on the part of the animal have also been developed. As specific directed behavior on the part of the animal is required, active avoidance is, of course, an example of operant conditioning. In one popular active avoidance paradigm, an apparatus called a *shuttle-box* is used. In the shuttle-box paradigm animals are trained to move from one side of the apparatus to the other in order to avoid foot shock. The trigger for movement can be linked to various CS cues, such as light or sound, or the animal can simply learn that it must periodically change sides within a given time period. Interestingly, several different types of operant learning, such as active avoidance in a shuttle box, are actually enhanced by hippocampal lesions.

One popular behavioral assessment paradigm for assessing operant conditioning involves lever-pressing for a reward. In a typical lever-press operant conditioning paradigm animals are trained in a specialized apparatus (see Figure 15). Animals learn to associate their lever-pressing behavior with the delivery of a positive reinforcer, such as a food pellet or liquid reward. (Alternatively the lever-press may avert the delivery of a negative reinforcer, such as a foot shock.) In a more complicated variation of the lever-press operant design, the availability of the reward may also be cue-dependent; for example, the animal may be required to learn that an auditory (sound)

Passive avoidance

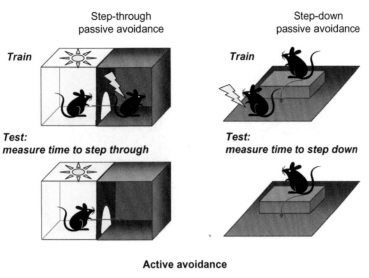

Active avoidance

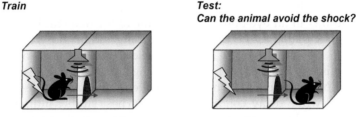

FIGURE 13   Passive and active avoidance paradigms. See text for details.

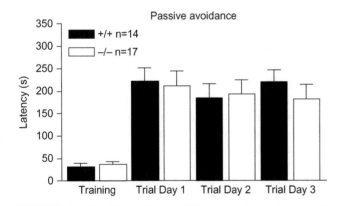

FIGURE 14   Passive avoidance. This test utilizes the natural tendency for mice to retreat from a lit area to a darker area during the training session. On entering the dark area a mild foot shock is given, and learning is assessed as the avoidance of the dark area following the training session. Passive avoidance was tested by measuring step-through latencies from a lit compartment to a dark compartment when the animals are replaced in the avoidance chamber. Results are shown as step-through latency during trial sessions one, two or three days following training for PKCβ deficient mice (□) or wildtype mice (■), mean ± SEM. Data from Weeber et al. (6). Both control and knockout animals successfully learned to avoid the darkened half of the chamber.

or visual (light) cue must be present in order for the lever-press to trigger delivery of the reward.

Another form of operant conditioning is *conditioned place preference*. In this procedure the animal learns, for example, that half of a divided box (with distinct contextual cues) is always associated with a reinforcer. The animal manifests its having learned that the one particular place is associated with the reinforcer by spending a greater proportion of its time in the reinforced chamber, even when delivery of the reinforcer is discontinued. Conditioned place preference is frequently used in studies of drug-seeking and drug addiction. For example, animals exhibit conditioned place preference for contexts in which they receive cocaine or other types of addictive drugs.

D. Eye-Blink Conditioning

Classical conditioning of the eye-blink response is typically performed using rabbits as the experimental animal, although the procedure can also be utilized with rats and mice. Eye-blink conditioning uses the association of a neutral stimulus, such as tone or light CS, paired with a nociceptive US, such as an air

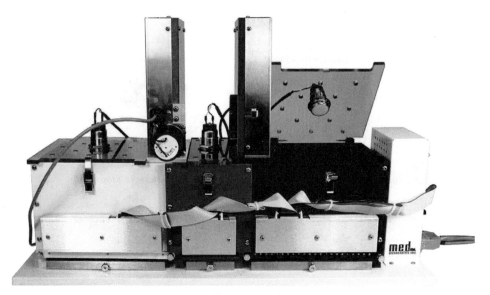

FIGURE 15 Bar press operant and/or conditioned place preference apparatus. Image courtesy of Med Associates Inc., Saint Albans, Vermont.

puff delivered to the eye or a mild periorbital shock. Representation of the CS results in an eye-blink conditioned response (CR) in anticipation of the US (see Figure 16).

Trace eye-blink conditioning (CS followed by an intervening time delay) is a hippocampus-dependent form of associative learning, while delay conditioning (no intervening time delay) is hippocampus-independent. Sophisticated neuroanatomical studies have mapped much of the relevant neuronal circuitry underlying this behavior. In addition, an elegant series of studies has implicated a role for long-term synaptic depression (LTD) in the cerebellum in eye-blink conditioning. We will return to these studies in more detail in the next chapter, where we will discuss molecular and cellular mechanisms, and the general role of synaptic plasticity, in associative learning.

E. Simple Maze Learning

The study of maze learning in rodents has always played a prominent role in experimental psychology, so much so that in some ways it can be considered the archetypal experiment in the field. From a historical perspective this can be illustrated nicely by Karl Lashley's use of maze learning in his studies to try to find the anatomical locus of the *engram*—the engram being defined as the finite locus for memory storage in the CNS. Lashley undertook a number of studies of maze learning in rats, and of memory storage for previously learned mazes. His basic experiment was to induce lesions of the cerebral cortex and evaluate the subsequent effects on memory in rats learning or remembering the location of food rewards in mazes of

increasing complexity. These pioneering studies were some of the first studies to illustrate the complexity of learning and memory, for Lashley found that no single cortical locus for learning or memory could be found using this approach. At best, memory loss could be related in a general sense to the extent of the lesioned area. These studies ultimately led to the currently held view that complex memories are held in (or at least accessed by) broadly distributed loci in the CNS.

Fast-forwarding to the current day, a wide variety of mazes containing food rewards are still employed in behavioral studies of rodent learning and memory. Popular variations include "T"-shaped mazes of various sorts (see Figure 17), and four- and eight-armed radial mazes. Most applications of these types of mazes are fairly ethological, in the sense that they capitalize on rodents' natural foraging tendencies and involve food rewards. There is a wide variety of applications of mazes for rats and mice learning placements of food rewards in various limbs of the maze, and quantitation generally involves counting errors, i.e., the animal entering places in the maze where they should know, based on prior experience, that no food is available. Also, manipulating the delay period between training and testing is commonly used to parse short-term memory from long-term memory, and variations in the use of distal spatial cues can assess the role of this type of information in the learning process.

Overall, maze learning has been widely used to probe for the role of the hippocampus in rodent learning and memory, using a wide variety of types of lesions to the CNS. Also, maze learning has lent itself well to studies where hippocampal cellular responses

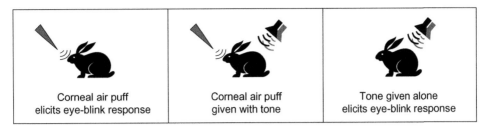

FIGURE 16 Eye-blink conditioning in rabbits. Animals are trained in a Pavlovian conditioning paradigm to learn that a tone predicts a puff of air to the eye surface. Over time the animals learn to blink in response to the tone alone.

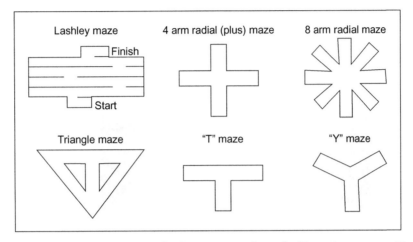

FIGURE 17 Types of mazes. A few representative types of rodent mazes are shown for illustrative purposes. Most of these mazes are used in conjunction with food rewards located at specific positions in the maze.

are recorded *in vivo* in real-time as the animal learns and remembers. Using these approaches along with others, hippocampal "place cells" have been identified, that is, hippocampal pyramidal neurons that fire specifically when an animal occupies a particular spatial location. We will also discuss these experiments in more detail in a later chapter of this book.

F. Spatial Learning

The Morris Maze

Richard Morris has developed a "water" maze that is now a classic test of spatial learning in rodents (9). The Morris water maze is a hippocampus-dependent spatial learning task in which mice or rats are required to learn to locate an escape platform in a pool of water using visual cues surrounding the maze (see Figure 18). The basic set-up is a circular shallow pool full of opaque water with an escape platform hidden just under the surface of the water, so that it is not visible to the animal. Animals are placed in the pool at either constant or varying starting positions and forced to swim because the water is just deep enough that they cannot touch the bottom. Similarly, the walls of the pool are high enough that they cannot climb out. Rodents, while they are generally

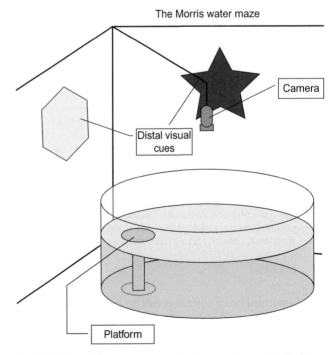

FIGURE 18 Morris water maze. A diagram illustrating the basic components of the Morris water maze system, including visual cues on the walls, a monitoring camera, pool with opaque water, and hidden platform.

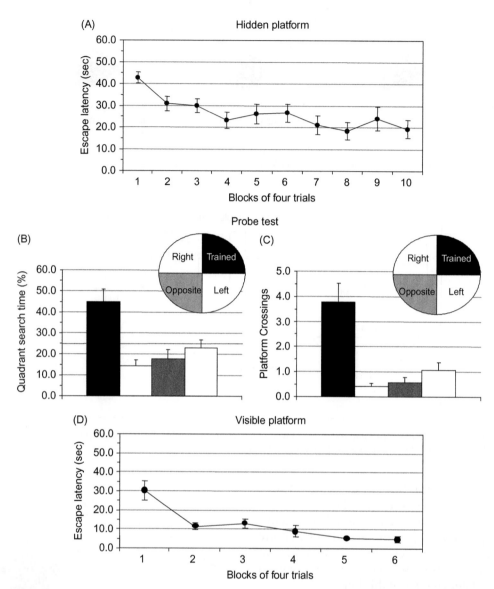

FIGURE 19 Experimental results for various aspects of the Morris water maze. (A) Average escape latency (i.e., the time taken to find the hidden platform) was assessed during training on the hidden platform task. Performance for mice ($n = 13$) improved over the course of the training, indicating learning of the task and the location of the hidden platform. Animals were trained using 10 blocks of four training trials, over a five-day period. (B) and (C) Probe tests are used to assess whether the animal has used a selective spatial strategy in learning the task. A selective search strategy is indicated by the subject spending significantly more time searching in the trained quadrant than in the other three quadrants when they are placed in the tank after the hidden platform has been completely removed (see text). The subject also crosses the area where the platform had been during the training sessions significantly more often than they cross the corresponding areas in the other quadrants. During the probe trials on Days 4 and 5, mice ($n = 13$) spent significantly more time searching in the trained quadrant (B), and crossed the platform area in the trained quadrant more frequently than in any of the alternate quadrants (C). (D) Average escape latency during training on the visible platform task. Performance for mice ($n = 5$) improved during training in this non-spatial variant of the Morris water maze task. Data and figure courtesy of Joel Selcher (10).

good swimmers, of course prefer to be on a stable platform out of the water. In initial training trials, by random chance most animals bump into the hidden platform and can thus escape the water. Those who don't find the platform by luck (usually swims are limited to a one-minute duration) are retrieved from the water by the experimenter and manually placed on the platform.

For the hidden platform version of the task, a typical training protocol generally consists of two blocks of four training trials a day with an interblock interval of approximately one hour (see Figure 19). Subjects are released into the pool from one of four starting positions, and the location of the platform remains constant throughout training. The training is given for about 6–10 consecutive days. Time to find the escape platform is measured. Mice and rats display significant improvement in their performance in locating the hidden platform over the several blocks of training trials (Figure 19A), as assessed by the animals' escape latencies (i.e., the time taken to locate the escape platform).

To determine if animals are using a spatial learning strategy to locate the escape platform, they are subjected to "probe" trials after training (see Figure 19B,C). In the probe test, the platform is removed and animals are allowed to search the pool for 60 seconds. Quadrant search time and platform crossings are assessed to characterize a subject's search behavior during the probe trial. The quadrant search measure is obtained by conceptually dividing the pool into four equal quadrants, then measuring the amount of time that the subject spends searching in each quadrant. The platform crossing measure is the number of times a subject crosses the exact place where the platform had been located during training. For comparison, the number of times a subject crosses the equivalent location in the other quadrants is determined. Animals that have learned the (now presumed) location of the underwater platform spend significantly more time searching in the trained quadrant than in each of the other three quadrants (Figure 19B). They also cross the place where the platform had been located during training significantly more often than the corresponding place in the other quadrants (Figure 19C). Thus, animals that have learned the location of the platform selectively search in the correct quadrant.

Modern automated monitoring systems also allow the acquisition of additional control data during the probe trials. For example, one can monitor the swimming behavior of each animal during the probe trials to determine general mobility. Thus, one can assess total path length and swim velocity for individual mice (see Figure 20).

It is generally held that data acquired during the probe trial is the best indicator of the animals using a spatially-biased search strategy to locate the platform during training and performance. Data acquired during training (i.e., measurement of escape latencies) may be less informative, and in some instances can be dissociated from the performance during the probe trail.

To control for motivational factors and perceptual and motor abilities, animals are tested in the visible platform version of the Morris water maze task (Figure 19D). In this variant of the task, the escape platform is clearly indicated by placement of a visible colored marker directly above the escape platform, and the location of the platform remains constant throughout training. Training typically consists of two blocks of four trials a day for three consecutive days. Escape latencies are determined for each trial, and

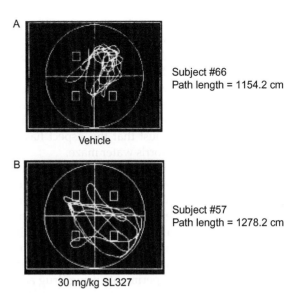

Subject #66
Path length = 1154.2 cm

Vehicle

Subject #57
Path length = 1278.2 cm

30 mg/kg SL327

FIGURE 20   Path tracking in the probe test. Representative probe trial of a mouse in the Morris water maze task. Upper panel: the swim path trace shown here provides an excellent example of a selective search. This particular subject was trained with the platform located in the northeast quadrant. During the probe trial, this mouse spent 56% of the time in the correct quadrant and crosses the exact area where the platform had been nine times. Adult male 129S3/SvImJ mice (formerly 129/Sv-$^{+p+Tyr-c+Mgf-Sl}$/J; Jackson Laboratory, Bar Harbor, ME) were used in these experiments and those in Figure 19. The lower panel shows the path of an animal whose learning during training was blocked with an inhibitor of MAP kinase activation. The animal swims randomly throughout the tank. Data and figure courtesy of Joel Selcher (10).

animals quickly learn to swim to the marked platform in order to escape the water. These visible platform data serve as a useful control for any impairment seen in the hidden platform version. If differences in controls versus experimentals are seen in the hidden platform version, but not the visible platform version, one can conclude that the difference is likely not due to changes in motivation to escape the pool or to changes in the motor abilities necessary to execute the task.

The Morris water maze task has been used extensively since its introduction, and in many ways it has been the "gold standard" of spatial learning tasks for the last two decades. It has been used many times in order to probe the involvement of specific anatomical structures and specific molecules in hippocampus-dependent spatial learning. It is important to keep in mind that Richard Morris himself has demonstrated that the task overall is cognitively quite complex, and can be experimentally dissociated into at least two components. One component is learning the task, i.e., that there is a platform, that spatial cues are relevant, etc. A second component is learning the specific location of the escape platform. Some types of lesions can lead to a loss in an animal's ability to learn the task, while not affecting the ability of the animal to learn a specific platform location, for example. These considerations do not limit the utility of the task, but rather point out the importance of considering the complexity of the task when interpreting the resulting data. For example, a deficit may not be due to a deficit in spatial learning *per se*, but rather due to a deficit in learning the parameters of the task. Of course, this caveat applies to learning tasks in general; it's just that this aspect has been best explored with the Morris water maze.

The principal practical limitations of the water maze are that it requires a fairly large dedicated room, is messy (in the housekeeping sense), and the training and testing periods are fairly long. Thus, in contrast to a single-training-trial task, such as fear conditioning, there is no temporally well-defined period of learning. This can present some practical difficulties when trying to design experiments using drug administration, or where one is trying to measure learning-associated biochemical or physiological changes.

Another practical limitation to the water maze is that it is a fairly rigorous and demanding task physically for the animals under study. This consideration is most pronounced when undertaking experiments on old or otherwise infirm animals. However, in these circumstances an alternative is available, commonly referred to as the Barnes maze.

The Barnes Maze

Carol Barnes has had a long-standing interest in aging-related memory decline, and developed a circular hole-board maze task to use as an assessment of spatial learning (11). This task is applicable in circumstances where the strength and stamina of the animals under study may be limiting, because it involves only mild locomotor activity. In addition, the measured parameter is errors, not time to complete the task, so the speed at which the animal completes the task is not a factor.

The Barnes maze is essentially a well-lit round table with many holes around the periphery (see Figure 21). Rodents find open, well-lit spaces aversive and they will search around the platform trying to find a safe, dark haven. All the holes around the periphery but one lead simply to a drop-off to the floor. However, one hole leads to an escape chamber that is a darkened box secured under the hole. On locating this hole, animals will enter the chamber to escape the lit surface.

The spatial learning in the task involves visual cues placed on the four walls around the table top. The escape hole is always located in a constant place relative to these spatial cues, and much like the water maze the animal must use these cues to learn the location of the escape hole. Performance can be quantitated in its simplest form by simply counting the number of errors

The Barnes maze

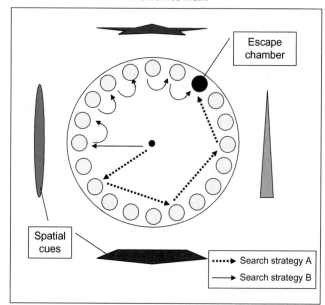

FIGURE 21 Diagram of the basic components of the Barnes maze. Animals learn to locate an escape chamber using visual cues placed on the walls of the room. Learning is assessed as a decrease in the number of errors an animal makes in locating the escape chamber.

an animal makes before they finally find the escape hole. An error is, of course, defined as an attempt to enter a non-escape hole. In one of the first examples of the use of this task, aged rats displayed impairment in the rate of acquisition of spatial memory involving navigation around the circular platform (11).

G. Taste Learning

Taste learning and *conditioned taste aversion* are fascinating behavioral phenomena that have only relatively recently begun to be studied mechanistically in rodents. One reason for being interested in these forms of learning is that they are clearly cortex-dependent, and may represent the closest rodent homolog to high-order human learning of factual information. Regardless of whether this last speculation is correct, taste learning is without a doubt one of the most robust and ethologically relevant forms of rodent learning currently under study.

Conditioned Taste Aversion

Conditioned taste aversion is a form of associative learning; in this case, an animal learns to associate the novel taste of a new foodstuff (CS) with subsequent illness (US) resulting from ingestion of some nausea-inducing agent. The adaptive value of this form of learning is clear; by preventing subsequent ingestion of sickening foods, survival is enhanced. For this

Conditioned taste aversion

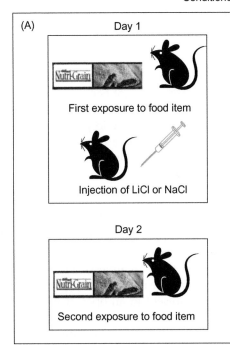

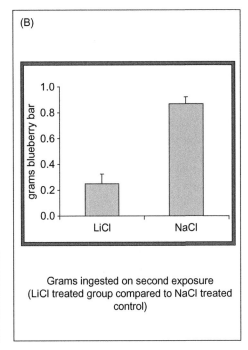

FIGURE 22 Conditioned taste aversion. Mice all received 10 minute access to a blueberry bar, a novel taste stimulus, followed by injection of LiCl or NaCl. Pairing solid novel food with LiCl, which produces nausea, produces a conditioned taste aversion (CTA). CTA is indicated by the observation that mice injected with LiCl following access to blueberry bar consume significantly less than NaCl-injected controls when tested for food consumption 24 hours later (***$p < 0.001$ by one-way ANOVA). Data and figure courtesy of Mike Swank (12).

reason evolution has selected for robust learning under these conditions, and animals learn after a single pairing of a novel taste with a nausea-inducing agent to avoid that taste in the future. This single-trial learning is also quite robust in that there can be a rather long delay—often measured in hours—between the novel taste and toxin.

A typical conditioned taste aversion paradigm is to pair a novel taste with intraperitoneal injection of a malaise-inducing agent such as LiCl (see Figure 22). Pairing intake of a novel taste with LiCl significantly suppresses subsequent intake of that taste, either as a solid food or in drinking water. In these experiments the effect of LiCl is typically compared to NaCl injected controls.

Conditioned taste aversion is selective for novel tastes. If an animal has experienced a taste previously, it is no longer successful in serving as a CS in conditioned taste aversion. Behavioralists term this phenomenon *latent inhibition*. A "latent" memory for the taste is formed, inhibiting subsequent formation of an association with the toxic agent. Again, ethologically this makes sense—if a foodstuff has been previously tried and found non-aversive, it should thereafter be taken out of consideration as a toxic agent. This aspect of taste learning is particularly fascinating and still mysterious.

The implications of latent inhibition of taste aversion are two-fold. First, somewhere in the taste processing centers of the CNS is a novelty detector—a system that is able to tag a taste as something that has never been experienced by the animal before. If you take a few minutes to consider this it will become apparent what a conundrum this is. How can you know that something is an unknown? Is there a recorded list somewhere in the brain that contains every taste ever experienced by the animal, against which every subsequent taste is compared throughout the animal's lifetime? Or is there a system present that has a prearranged matrix of every conceivable potential taste combination that an animal will ever experience, from which tastes are scratched off after they are first experienced? It is food for thought, so to speak. The second implication is that every novel taste experience is a learning experience. Automatically, when a taste is first experienced it forms a memory trace that is perpetuated for the lifetime of the animal. This second consideration brings us to our next form of taste learning—novel taste learning and neophobia.

Novel Taste Learning and Neophobia

Neophobia is the characteristic fear of novel foods, and ensures that animals ingest only small quantities of new foodstuffs. If no illness results from consumption of the new food, and assuming that the food is reasonably palatable, animals will increase their intake on subsequent exposures. This is readily demonstrated in the laboratory: when rats or mice are presented with highly palatable solutions of saccharin or sucrose, they will consume small amounts on the first exposure; on subsequent exposures, the animals drink more. In these types of experiments, animals are usually maintained on water deprivation so that they are motivated to drink.

There also is a variation of this procedure that uses solid food in non-deprived mice (see Figure 23 and reference 12). In using this taste learning paradigm in one series of studies in my laboratory we found that Kellogg's Nutri-Grain blueberry breakfast bars are readily consumed by rodents, and that their consumption of this food is easy to measure. During a single 10-minute exposure to the novel blueberry bar, mice will consume around 200–300 mgs (see Figure 23). On subsequent exposures, the mice will double their intake, thus demonstrating an attenuation of the initial neophobia. This attenuation of neophobia is a behavioral measure of memory for the novel taste.

One very appealing aspect of these simple taste learning paradigms is that the learning is robust and automatic. The learning is a simple single-trial experience (simply exposure to a novel taste) that results in lifelong memory. Also, there is a fairly clear consensus that the insular cortex is the primary site of learning and memory for novel tastes, so the relevant brain region in rodents has also been identified. While taste learning has not been nearly as extensively studied as the spatial learning tasks described above, these types of paradigms hold great promise for future use. They represent one of the most tractable experimental models for measuring cortically-dependent learning in rodents.

H. Novel Object Recognition

Novel object recognition is a hippocampus-dependent memory test based on the natural tendency of mice to investigate a novel object rather than a familiar object, when both objects are simultaneously present in an open field (see Figure 24). This test does not involve primary reinforcement such as food or electric shocks, making it comparable in some

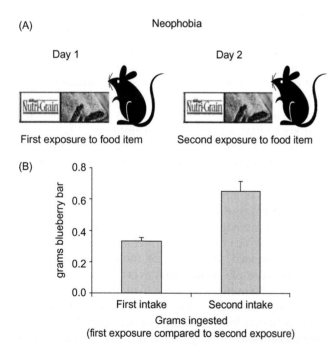

(A) Neophobia

FIGURE 23 Neophobia. Neophobia during first access to a novel solid food is attenuated on second exposure. Mice were given 10-minute access to a novel taste, Nutri-Grain blueberry bar, and intakes recorded. Ten-minute intakes on the second day are significantly higher, demonstrating attenuation of neophobia through familiarization (*p <0.05 by one-way ANOVA). Data and figure courtesy of Mike Swank (12).

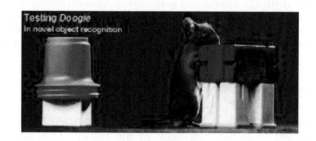

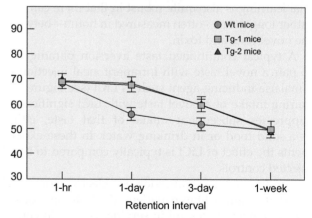

FIGURE 24 Novel object recognition. A genetically-engineered mouse (the "Doogie" mouse) is performing the novel object recognition task. This task allows researchers to measure the amount of time the animal spent on exploring either the old toy (in orange on the left) or new one (the red one on the right). If the mouse remembers the old toy, it tends to spend more time playing with the new one. The graph shows the transgenic NR2B mice are capable of remembering for at least three days, whereas the wildtype littermates retain the memory for only one day (modified from Tsien, J. Z. (2000). *Scientific American* 282:62–68) Copyright 2006 American Society for Neurochemistry.

ways to recognition memory tests currently used in humans. Novel object recognition is a fairly complex task to execute in the laboratory, and many laboratories utilize special variations of the procedures. Below I will describe one version of the task to introduce the basics of how it is used.

In the example I will use, novel object recognition training and testing is performed over three consecutive days. During the first day the rat or mouse is placed in an empty arena, typically an open field apparatus, for 10 minutes. During the second training day the animal is placed in the arena with two different novel objects, typically small children's toys. Object recognition memory is assessed on the third day by placing the animal in the arena with one familiar and one new object. The number of visits to and the amount of time spent exploring each object is recorded. A normal animal spends more time investigating the novel object than the object leftover from the day before, indicating a memory for the familiar, leftover object. Object recognition learning indices are expressed as the amount of time spent exploring the novel object versus the amount of time exploring the familiar object (see Figure 24).

As simple as this test may sound, it likely investigates one of the most cognitively complex behaviors exhibited by small rodents. Perhaps because of

this, there is typically a large degree of variability in learning indices among individual animals in a group.

I. Studying Memory Reconsolidation Using a Fear Conditioning Protocol

Memories, when retrieved or recalled, can become labile and susceptible to disruption, which implies the necessity of a process for restabilizing previously formed memories. This process is commonly referred to as memory reconsolidation. For example, as described above in the rodent contextual fear conditioning paradigm, a novel context (training chamber) is paired with a foot shock, and after this training event a long-term memory for this association is formed. After memory formation, re-exposing the animal to the training chamber triggers memory retrieval. Re-establishment of the contextual conditioned fear memory is subject to disruption through inhibition of protein synthesis, or when signaling cascades such as the ERK/MAPK or the NF-κB transcription regulation cascade are inhibited (see Figure 25, for example).

On the basis of experiments like this, it has now been clearly established that a memory can be interfered with, at least temporarily, by application of various inhibitors immediately after retrieval. Recent

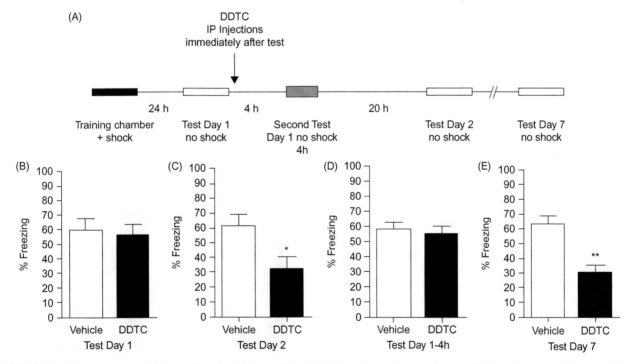

FIGURE 25 Memory reconsolidation: effect of inhibition of the NF-κB signaling pathway on reconsolidation of contextual fear conditioning after context re-exposure. (A) Diagram outlines the experimental design used with data presented below in (B)–(E) (vehicle, $n = 10$; DDTC, $n = 9$). (B) Freezing behavior on Test Day 1. (C) Freezing behavior during re-exposure on Test Day 2. (D) Short-term memory test, assessed four hours after re-exposure to chamber. (E) Freezing behavior on Test Day 7. DDTC is an inhibitor of NFκB signaling. Figure and legend adapted from (13). Copyright Elsevier 2007.

interest in memory reconsolidation was revived by the work of Joe LeDoux and Karim Nader, who took a targeted, molecular approach similar to experiments performed over 30 years earlier by Susan Sara's research group (see Nader et al. in Journal Club Articles). Memory reconsolidation is not a universal or monolithic attribute of all forms of memory. The amnestic effect produced by this type of interference can be either long-lasting or, alternatively, subject to spontaneous recovery. These differences have led to an ongoing, largely unresolved, debate concerning whether reconsolidation interference represents an erasure of the memory trace (in the case of long-lasting amnesia) or a retrieval deficit (in the case of spontaneous recovery of the memory).

An additional important point is that it can now be said with a fair amount of certainty that reconsolidation is not a recapitulation of the mechanisms underlying initial consolidation, despite what the term "reconsolidation" may suggest. Thus, reconsolidation does not simply occur by a reiteration of the initial consolidation process, but rather utilizes its own unique mechanisms (Box 1).

III. MODERN EXPERIMENTAL USES OF RODENT BEHAVIORAL MODELS

Having briefly described several of the basic rodent learning paradigms in common use, we now turn

---

BOX 1

OF MICE AND RATS

Rats have been the prototype animal for learning studies, although recently great effort has been expended to adapt these procedures to mice. This is because the recent advent of transgenic mouse technologies has generated substantial optimism concerning the development of murine models for human learning disorders and memory dysfunction, as well as optimism for their application to understanding the basic molecular mechanisms of memory itself. Moreover, the potential applicability of transgenic animal approaches in mice gives great promise for the discovery of new gene products involved in behavior in general. Against this backdrop it has been important to develop standardized protocols for behavioral characterization of transgenic animals that are widely adaptable for laboratory use. Jean Wehner at the University of Colorado, Jackie Crawley at the NIMH, and Richard Paylor at Baylor College of Medicine have been leaders in adapting the historically used rat behaviors into the modern situation of mouse characterization. Much of what is described in this chapter in terms of applying rodent behavioral paradigms in mice is based on their research (1, 2, 14–15).

It is also important to note that while the behaviors we are discussing are exhibited by both rats and mice, there are significant interspecies differences in learning behavior. In general, these differences can be summed up by saying that rats are a lot smarter than mice. In fact, in the early days there was some discussion of whether mice could even learn to perform some of the standard

rat behavioral paradigms, although fortunately this concern was unfounded.

Finally, it is important to point out that in addition to interspecies differences there are also appreciable interstrain differences in learning behavior. Learning in outbred strains of rats and mice is typically much more robust than in inbred strains. Different inbred strains of rats and mice also have different, specific deficits that affect their learning and memory. Many of these differences are described in reference (1) by Crawley et al. at the end of this chapter.

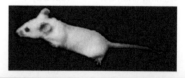

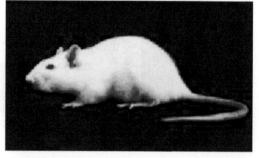

our attention to thinking about their application in cellular and molecular studies. By way of introduction to this topic I think it is useful to step back and review some of the basics of experimental design. In the next section we will consider the basics of hypothesis testing. We will then proceed to considering how the fundamentals of experimental design are applied in the modern era in extending behavioral studies into the cellular and molecular realm. A more thorough and detailed treatment of the concepts and principles of experimental design is presented separately as an Appendix at the end of this book. However, a brief introduction is necessary at this point in order to provide a foundation for the terminology used in the remainder of this book.

A. The Four Basic Types of Experiments

In general there are four basic types of experiments that any scientist can perform. I refer to them as "block, measure, mimic, and determine" experiments. I have found this categorization a useful mnemonic device throughout my career as a scientist, and I strongly encourage any young scientist who reads this book to incorporate them into their thinking about experimental design. It is important to develop a framework for thinking about experimental design, because what we do as scientists is test hypotheses and the testing of any hypothesis is much stronger if a variety of independent lines of evidence are available to support the conclusions reached.

What follows is a brief description of each of these four types of experiments (see Figure 26). A more detailed description is presented in the Appendix.

The "determine" experiment is not really an experiment at all. The determine approach is to perform a basic characterization of the system or molecule at hand, independent of any experimental manipulation. Examples of this type of pursuit are determining the amino acid sequence of a protein, sequencing a genome, determining the crystal structure

of an enzyme or determining the structure of the DNA double helix. Determinations of this sort are not experiments, in that no manipulation of the system is attempted—to do an experiment you tweak the system to see what happens. If you mutate a residue in a protein and see what effect that has on the structure, then you have done an experiment. The basic determination of the structure is not an experiment in and of itself.

"Block," "measure," and "mimic" are experiments, and they are all specific types of approaches to test different predictions of a hypothesis. For the following discussion we will take the simple case of testing the hypothesis "A causes C by activating B" (see Figure 26). We will illustrate the application of the basic types of experiments in the context of molecular and cellular studies of memory, studies which widely utilize the behavioral procedures we discussed earlier in this chapter.

Mimic Experiments

The mimic experiment tests the prediction that "if B causes C, then if I activate B artificially I should see C happen as a result." An example that we will return to later is: if I hypothesize that a particular protein kinase causes synaptic potentiation, then applying a drug that activates that protein kinase should elicit synaptic potentiation. The mimic terminology arises from the fact that you are trying to mimic with a drug (etc.) an effect that occurs with some other stimulus (potentiation-inducing synaptic stimulation in this example). The principal limitation of the mimic experiment is that B may be able to cause C, but that in reality A acts independently of B to cause the same effect. B causing C and A causing C may be true, true, and unrelated.

At the current state of understanding and experimental sophistication, mimic experiments are just about impossible to execute in the context of mammalian learning and memory. This is because an enormous amount of fundamental understanding of the system is necessary, along with the capacity for very subtle manipulation, in order for the experiment to work. For example, suppose I hypothesize that a synaptic potentiation underlies learning. In theory, the mimic experiment is to put an electrode in the brain, cause synaptic potentiation, and then the animal will have an altered behavior identical to that caused by a training session. Of course, doing this experiment requires that I know exactly which synapses to potentiate so that I can selectively achieve the right behavioral output—this is beyond the level of understanding for essentially all mammalian behaviors at this point.

Four types of experiments

Hypothesis: **A→B→C**

Experiment	Prediction
• Determine	• None (**A** makes **C** happen)
• Block	• Blocking **B** should block **A** causing **C**
• Mimic	• Activating **B** should cause **C**
• Measure	• **A** makes **B** happen

FIGURE 26 The four basic types of experiments. See text for discussion.

Measure Experiments

The "measure" experiment tests the prediction that "A should cause activation of B." Using our example of kinases in synaptic potentiation, the measure experiment predicts that the physiologic potentiating stimulus should cause an increase in the activity of the kinase. This is, of course, determined by measuring the activity of the kinase as directly as possible, hence the measure terminology. The measure experiment has been applied in a variety of different ways in the memory field, ways that we will discuss at various points throughout the book including looking for anatomical, physiologic, and molecular changes in the nervous system in association with learning. The principal theoretical limitation of the measure experiment is that it is correlative. One can show that A causes activation of B, but that does not demonstrate that activation of B is necessary for C to occur.

Block Experiments

This brings us to the "block" experiment. The block experiment tests the prediction that "if I eliminate B then A should not be able to cause C." In our working example, this means that a kinase inhibitor should block the ability of the physiologic potentiating stimulus to cause potentiation. At present, the vast majority of investigations into mechanisms of memory involve this approach, and we will make many references to this type of experiment throughout the book. All of the behavior protocols that we discussed earlier in this chapter have been widely and extensively used in these types of "block" experiments. Specific examples include assessing the effects of anatomical lesions, drug infusion studies, and genetic manipulations to test the roles of specific circuits, physiologic processes, and molecules in memory formation.

The principal theoretical limitation of the block experiment is that it does not distinguish whether *activation* of B is necessary for C, versus whether the *activity* of B is necessary for C. For example, suppose that B provides some tonic effect on C that is necessary for it to occur. Inhibiting B will block the production of effect C, when in fact A never has any effect on B whatsoever. In behavioral terms for learning experiments this is referred to as a performance deficit—the animal is simply unable to execute the behavioral read-out necessary to exhibit the fact that they have learned.

In summary, then, the mimic experiment tests sufficiency, the block experiment tests necessity, and the measure experiment tests whether the event does in fact occur. Each type of experiment has its strengths and weaknesses. Positive outcomes, in testing each of these three predictions for any hypothesis make for clear, strong support of the hypothesis.

B. Use of Behavioral Paradigms in Block and Measure Experiments

As has already been alluded to, the behavioral paradigms I have been discussing in this chapter have, by and large, been used in two ways in the modern cellular-and-molecular era. The first application is as a stimulus in measure experiments; the second is as a read-out in blocking experiments (see Shalin et al. in Journal Club Articles). For our present purposes I would like to briefly describe some examples of the use of behavioral paradigms in these two types of experiments. This is because the specific examples will help to introduce some refinements of the procedures that are necessary for some applications, and also to introduce some of the sorts of behavioral control experiments that are used to shore up the conclusions that are reached in executing the experiments.

Using Behavioral Paradigms as a Stimulus in Measure Experiments

In these types of experiments the behavioral paradigms we have reviewed are used to train the animal using a set of defined and optimized environmental signals that are known to elicit learning and memory. The behavioral read-out of the learned behavior is really only used as confirmation that the animal has learned—in essence control data that the procedure has been effective. What is really of interest in these types of experiments is determining what has gone on inside the animal's CNS while or after it learned.

There are several prominent examples of great successes in measuring physiologic changes in the brain with behavioral training paradigms. The best-established paradigm is measuring alterations in hippocampal pyramidal neuron firing with rodent spatial learning. These elegant experiments use implanted recording electrodes to monitor neuronal responses *in vivo* in the behaving animal. These experiments led to the identification of hippocampal "place" cells and variations thereof: these experiments will be described in more detail in later chapters.

Somewhat of a "holy grail" experiment in learning and memory has been to obtain data demonstrating that long-term potentiation of hippocampal synaptic transmission occurs with learning in rodents. To date this approach has recently met with success as pertains to the hippocampus (see Whitlock et al. in Further Reading), and there have been landmark findings in this area from the LeDoux and Shinnick–Gallagher laboratories, utilizing fear conditioning and amygdala recordings of synaptic transmission. We will return to these observations in later chapters, where I will review the data supporting a role for LTP in learning.

Finally, there have been nice demonstrations of alterations of hippocampal neuron excitability that occur with learning. Both Matt Wilson's and John Disterhoft's laboratories have found alterations in hippocampal pyramidal neuron excitability with spatial learning and trace eye-blink conditioning, respectively. These alterations, for which there is indirect and direct evidence suggesting involvement of altered potassium channel function, will be addressed in more detail in later chapters.

Using Behavioral Paradigms as an Assay of Learning in Block Experiments

This is by far the most common use of rodent behavioral assessment paradigms such as those we have been discussing. In these experiments the behavioral paradigms we have reviewed are used to assess whether an animal has a learning or memory deficit when a particular process is blocked. The behavioral read-out of the learned behavior is used to assess whether the animal has learned. A memory variation commonly used is to assess animals behaviorally to determine if an experimental treatment causes a faster decrement of learned behavior over time.

The three most common examples of experimental manipulations in the application of the block approach to behavior, roughly in historical order, are: anatomical lesions; drug infusion studies; and more recently gene manipulation experiments. What is of interest in these types of experiments is determining what structures or molecules are necessary for an animal to learn, remember, and recall a learned event.

We will be returning to a great many specific examples of these types of experiments later in the book, experiments that have implicated specific molecules and categories of molecules in learning and memory and synaptic plasticity. Thus, for the present I will discuss these types of experiments only in general terms. Of course, there are a great many caveats in the interpretation these types of experiments, and we will focus our discussion here on five general considerations that must be kept in mind in interpreting them. I review them here in general terms so that I can avoid repeating them throughout the book when we discuss specific experiments. They also illustrate the necessity of undertaking a comprehensive behavioral assessment (see Box 2 and references 1–2) as part of performing experiments to determine if a particular manipulation leads selectively to learning and memory deficits. Indeed, most of the baseline sensory and motor behavioral assessments described at the beginning of the chapter are utilized as control experiments when undertaking block experiments.

The first consideration in behavioral block experiments is that there may have been non-specific effects of the manipulation, as is always the case with inhibitors or lesions of any sort. The drug may not be specific for the molecule of interest, the knockout animal may not have developed a normal CNS, or the anatomical lesion may have destroyed fibers of passage connected to distal brain regions. This limitation is practical in nature and in general has received a great degree of attention in the literature. The specifics also vary greatly depending on the experiment under consideration, so we will not address this point further at present.

The second limitation is largely conceptual. In behavioral learning experiments one is training an animal using environmental signals and measuring at some later time point a complex behavioral read-out. Many things are occurring during the training, learning, memorizing, recalling, and execution of the read-out. It is fundamentally difficult with the basic block experimental design to distinguish among effects on learning, memory or recall. Imagine the simplest case where an animal has a molecular deficit throughout the experiment—it is clear that no conclusion can be drawn concerning whether the animal has a deficit in learning, memory or recall.

Two basic variations of the block experiment are used to try to begin to distinguish between these possibilities. A transient inactivation experiment, where a structure or molecule is inhibited for a limited period of time, allows one to begin to parse effects on learning/memory versus recall, for example. However, it is still difficult with the transient inactivation design to distinguish between effects on learning versus effects on early memory consolidation. This brings us to the second variation, where memory is assessed at short time points versus long time points. If an animal with a molecular or anatomical deficit is able to perform normally at short time periods after training and has a selective deficit at longer time periods, this implies that learning has occurred but that there is a loss of longer-term memory. The principal limitation to this approach is that it assumes that the learning mechanisms for short-term memory are identical to the mechanisms used for long-term memory.

A third consideration that must be kept in mind in interpreting block experiments is that compensation may have occurred, acutely or chronically. For example, the loss of a brain structure or molecule may force the CNS to utilize an ancillary mechanism that is capable of doing the job, but that normally is never brought into play. From a hypothesis-testing perspective this leads to a false negative result—we conclude that molecule or structure X is not necessary, but in fact it *is* necessary under normal circumstances. The enormous plasticity of the CNS in general makes this a particularly bothersome concern. I will use Lashley's

---

BOX 2

CHARACTERIZING A GENETICALLY-ENGINEERED MOUSE

The recent advent of transgenic mouse engineering technologies has generated the opportunity for the development and utilization of murine models for understanding memory mechanisms and for making mouse models of human memory disorders. Therefore, studies of memory in genetically-engineered mice have been a significant growth area in neurobiology over the past 10 years. The following is a brief description of a "typical" series of tests used to assess baseline behaviors and memory performance in genetically-engineered mice.

OPEN FIELD ANALYSIS AND ELEVATED PLUS MAZE PERFORMANCE

Open field analysis is utilized to measure the level of spontaneous motor activity, exploratory behavior, and habituation of the animals to an open area. This task is typically used in conjunction with the elevated plus maze as an index of anxiety.

ROTATING ROD PERFORMANCE

The rotating rod task is used to assess two parameters related to cerebellar function. Initial trials are used to assess the animal's general coordination, and the task is used to evaluate motor skill acquisition by determining the rate of improvement on the task on repeated trials.

ACOUSTIC STARTLE AND PREPULSE INHIBITION

This task is used to assess the animal's general reflexes and sensory–motor gating. While prepulse inhibition is utilized as a type of screen as a phenotype related to certain types of psychiatric disorders such as psychosis, it also serves as a very sensitive and quantitative assessment of the animal's hearing. This is a critical control for auditory cued fear conditioning, for example.

FEAR CONDITIONING

Fear conditioning is used to test classical conditioning. Auditory cued (white noise) conditioning is used as an index of general associative learning that is amygdala-dependent but hippocampus independent. Context-dependent conditioning is used as a variant to assess a likely hippocampus-dependent form of learning. The initial responses of the animal also serve as a good screen for sensory responses to foot shock. Passive or active avoidance is also frequently used as an adjunct to (or substitute for) fear conditioning in characterizing mice.

MORRIS WATER MAZE

The Morris water maze is the now-classic test of hippocampus-dependent spatial learning in rodents. The use of this task allows an assessment of the animal's capacity to use spatial cues to locate a hidden underwater platform. The visible platform task is also used to assess the animal's ability to navigate using non-spatial cues, and as an assessment of general motor skill (swim rate).

This behavioral assessment battery is quantitative and an excellent general screen for a wide variety of behaviors and sensory responses. It is important to note in this context that a typical behavioral testing battery includes learning paradigms to evaluate cerebellar, amygdalar, and hippocampal function. This is in addition to tests for sensory system function and motor coordination. Also typically included, but not listed above, are assessments of general physical parameters such as weight, temperature, coat appearance, basic reflexes, etc.

---

classic lesioning experiments to illustrate this point, precisely because they have been so important in shaping modern thinking about memory. Lashley trained rats in mazes, and made post-training cortical lesions in order to try to localize the maze memory trace anatomically. Lashley observed that, by and large, no single lesion could erase a memory, but rather that maze performance declined in relation to

the overall extent of cortical lesioning. Thus, Lashley concluded that it was likely that memories are "distributed" throughout the cortex and that there was no discrete memory trace. The caveat is that there may have been multiple, redundant, memory traces and that only when the last one was destroyed was there an appreciable decline in maze perfomance. Unfortunately there is very little that can be done in

BOX 3

SUMMARY—BEHAVIORAL TESTS COMMONLY USED IN RODENTS

Test Name	Measurement	Index of:
Open field analysis	Distance moved over time	Activity
Elevated plus maze	Time spent in open arms	Anxiety
Rotating rod	Time to fall off	Coordination and motor learning
Acoustic startle	Force of jump	Hearing
Prepulse inhibition	Suppression of startle	Sensorimotor gating
Hot plate	Time to lick paw	Nociception
Hargreave's apparatus	Time to lift paw	Nociception
Light–dark exploration	Time in lit chamber	Vision
Visual cliff	Suppression of movement	Vision
Fear conditioning: cued	Freezing or startle	Auditory associative learning
Fear conditioning: contextual	Freezing or startle	Spatial associative learning
Passive avoidance	Time spent in lit chamber	Spatial associative learning
Active avoidance	Time spent in cued chamber	Operant conditioning
Lever-press	Number of bar presses	Operant conditioning
Conditioned place preference	Time spent in one chamber	Operant conditioning
Eye-blink conditioning	Blink in response to cue	Associative conditioning
Simple maze learning	Errors or time to completion	Spatial learning, working memory
Morris water maze	Quadrant time, platform crossings	Spatial memory
Barnes maze	Errors	Spatial memory
Conditioned taste aversion	Food or taste avoidance	Taste learning
Novel taste learning	Attenuation of neophobia	Taste learning
Novel object recognition	Time spent with object	Recognition memory

the way of control experiments to clearly address this general limitation—for the most part it must simply be left as a caveat to the interpretation.

The fourth and fifth overall considerations in interpreting block behavioral experiments are at least well-defined enough that control experiments can be brought to bear—these are performance deficits and sensory processing deficits. In hypothesis-testing terms both of these limitations lead to potential false positive results.

In many of the types of memory paradigms we have been discussing, fairly sophisticated control experiments can be executed to rule out these limitations. However, the biology has to be working to your advantage, and of course you have no control over that. One of my favorite examples is finding a selective

deficit in contextual versus cued fear conditioning. If a lesioned animal performs normally in cued fear conditioning, but has a deficit in contextual fear conditioning, you can make a reasonable interpretation that the animal can feel the foot shock (thus no sensory deficit for foot shock) as well as exhibit freezing behavior (no performance deficit in freezing). Another favorite is selective effects on long-term versus short-term memory—if short-term memory is intact then it is reasonable to conclude that the lesioned animal both perceived the environmental stimuli and is capable of performing the necessary behavioral read-out of memory. A final example is that an experimental manipulation might lead to a selective deficit in trace versus delay conditioning. In general, these examples illustrate the point that in some instances two different types of learned behaviors might utilize exactly the same training stimuli and behavioral output—in that case a selective deficit in one versus the other form of learning allows an investigator to rule out generalized deficits in sensation or performance.

In many cases, however, the biology does not work to your advantage and these types of sophisticated control experiments cannot be used. In that case, more indirect measures must be employed to bolster your case that the experimental manipulation has not led to general deficits in overall health or motivation, perception, or motor performance. In this case the motor and sensory behavioral experiments outlined in Section II.A can be brought to bear as controls.

IV. SUMMARY

In this chapter we have discussed the wide variety of specific behavioral paradigms applicable to assessing learning and memory in rodents (see Box 3). Understanding these procedures is important for two general reasons. First, these procedures have been used historically as basic experiments to characterize the fundamental attributes of learning and memory behaviorally. Second, in the modern era these procedures are used in literally thousands of separate studies investigating the anatomical, cellular, and molecular basis of learning and memory. We will be discussing the results of many of these experiments in more detail throughout the rest of the book. Having a firm grasp on the basics of rodent behavioral paradigms is key to understanding the design, interpretation, and limitations of modern cellular and molecular investigations into memory formation in mammalian model systems. Thus, we have dedicated a reasonable amount of time to considering the design of these experiments, their attendant caveats, and the necessary control experiments that go along with them.

A second theme of this chapter has been the basics of hypothesis testing. We covered in an abstract sense the four fundamental types of experiments that one has available for testing various predictions of a hypothesis. We will return to these basic experimental types many, many times throughout this book. While we will discuss them specifically as pertains to studies of learning and memory and their attendant cellular and molecular mechanisms, mastery of the basic concepts of hypothesis testing is crucial for students, whatever their ultimate field of endeavor. Working through their application in the context of learning and memory will undoubtedly be useful as a mental exercise, helpful beyond the specifics of their application in one scientific subdiscipline.

Further Reading

Berman, D. E., and Dudai, Y. (2001). Memory extinction, learning anew, and learning the new: dissociations in the molecular machinery of learning in cortex. *Science* 291(5512):2417–2419.

Crawley, J. N. (2007). *What's Wrong With My Mouse? Behavioral Phenotyping of Transgenic and Knockout Mice*, 2nd ed. Hoboken, NJ: Wiley-Interscience.

Crawley, J. N., and Paylor, R. (1997). A proposed test battery and constellations of specific behavioral paradigms to investigate the behavioral phenotypes of transgenic and knockout mice. *Horm. Behav.* 31:197–211.

Crawley, J. N., Belknap, J. K., Collins, A., Crabbe, J. C., Frankel, W., Henderson, N., Hitzemann, R. J., Maxson, S. C., Miner, L. L., Silva, A. J., Wehner, J. M., Wynshaw-Boris, A., and Paylor, R. (1997). "Behavioral phenotypes of inbred mouse strains: implications and recommendations for molecular studies." *Psychopharmacology* (Berl) 132:107–124.

Grant, S. G., O'Dell, T. J., Karl, K. A., Stein, P. L., Soriano, P., and Kandel, E. R. (1992). Impaired long-term potentiation, spatial learning, and hippocampal development in fyn mutant mice. *Science* 258(5090):1903–1910.

LeDoux, J. E. (1993). Emotional memory systems in the brain. *Behav. Brain Res.* 58(1–2):69–79.

McCormick, D. A., Clark, G. A., Lavond, D. G., and Thompson, R. F. (1982). Initial localization of the memory trace for a basic form of learning. *Proc. Natl. Acad. Sci. USA* 79(8):2731–2735.

Miller, C. A., and Marshall, J. F. (2005). Molecular substrates for retrieval and reconsolidation of cocaine-associated contextual memory. *Neuron* 47(6):873–884.

Silva, A. J., Paylor, R., Wehner, J. M., and Tonegawa, S. (1992). Impaired spatial learning in alpha-calcium-calmodulin kinase II mutant mice. *Science* 257(5067):206–211.

Silva, A. J. (2007). "The science of research: the principles underlying the discovery of cognitive and other biological mechanisms." *J. Physiol.* (Paris) 101(4–6):203–213.

Whitlock, J. R., Heynen, A. J., Shuler, M. G., and Bear, M. F. (2006). Learning induces long-term potentiation in the hippocampus. *Science* 313(5790):1093–1097.

Journal Club Articles

McCormick, D. A., and Thompson, R. F. (1984). Cerebellum: essential involvement in the classically conditioned eyelid response. *Science* 223(4633):296–299.

Morris, R. (1984). Developments of a water-maze procedure for studying spatial learning in the rat. *J. Neurosci. Methods* 11:47–60.

Nader, K., Schafe, G. E., and Le Doux, J. E. (2000). Fear memories require protein synthesis in the amygdala for reconsolidation after retrieval. *Nature* 406(6797):722–726.

Shalin, S. C., Hernandez, C. M., Dougherty, M. K., Morrison, D. K., and Sweatt, J. D. (2006). Kinase suppressor of Ras1 compartmentalizes hippocampal signal transduction and subserves synaptic plasticity and memory formation. *Neuron* 50(5):765–779.

For more information—relevant topic chapters from: John H. Byrne (Editor-in-Chief) (2008). *Learning and Memory: A Comprehensive Reference*. Oxford: Academic Press (ISBN 978-0-12-370509-9). (1.06 Jozefowiez, J., and Staddon, J. E. R. *Operant Behavior*. pp. 75–101; 1.09 Bouton, M. E., and Woods, A. M. *Extinction: Behavioral Mechanisms and Their Implications*. pp. 151–171; 1.11 Lazareva, O. F., and Wasserman, E. A. *Categories and Concepts in Animals*. pp. 197–226; 1.18 Domjan, M. *Adaptive Specializations and Generality of the Laws of Classical and Instrumental Conditioning*. pp. 327–340; 1.20 Stephens, D. W., and Dunlap, A. S. *Foraging*. pp. 365–383; 1.21 Fortin, N. *Navigation and Episodic-Like Memory in Mammals*.

pp. 385–417; 1.22 Kamil, A. C., and Gould, K. L. *Memory in Food Caching Animals.* pp. 419–439; 1.23 Salwiczek, L. H., Dickinson, A., and Clayton, N. S. *What Do Animals Remember about Their Past?* pp. 441–459; 1.26 Salas, C., Broglio, C., Duran, E., Gomez, A., and Rodriguez, F. *Spatial Learning in Fish.* pp. 499–527; 3.09 Alvarado, M. C., and Bachevalier, J. *Animal Models of Amnesia.* pp. 143–167; 3.13 Buchsbaum, B. R., and D'Esposito, M. *Short-Term and Working Memory Systems.* pp. 237–260; 3.18 Packard, M. G. *Neurobiology of Procedural Learning in Animals.* pp. 341–356; 3.19 Poulos, A. M., Christian, K. M., and Thompson, R. F. *Procedural Learning: Classical Conditioning.* pp. 357–381; 3.20 Cullen, K. E. *Procedural Learning: VOR.* pp. 383–402; 3.24 Maren, S. *Emotional Learning: Animals.* pp. 475–502; 3.25 Juraska, J. M., and Rubinow, M. J. *Hormones and Memory.* pp. 503–520; 3.26 McGaugh, J. L., and Roozendaal, B. *Memory Modulation.* pp. 521–553; 3.27 Gold, P. E. *Memory-Enhancing Drugs.* pp. 555–575.)

References

1. Crawley, J. N., Belknap, J. K., Collins, A., Crabbe, J. C., Frankel, W., Henderson, N., Hitzemann, R. J., Maxson, S. C., Miner, L. L., Silva, A. J., Wehner, J. M., Wynshaw-Boris, A., and Paylor, R. (1997). "Behavioral phenotypes of inbred mouse strains: implications and recommendations for molecular studies." *Psychopharmacology* (Berl) 132:107–124.

2. Crawley, J. N., and Paylor, R. (1997). A proposed test battery and constellations of specific behavioral paradigms to investigate the behavioral phenotypes of transgenic and knockout mice. *Horm. Behav.* 31:197–211.

3. Quirk, G. J., Repa, C., and LeDoux, J. E. (1995). Fear conditioning enhances short-latency auditory responses of lateral amygdala neurons: parallel recordings in the freely behaving rat. *Neuron* 15:1029–1039.

4. Cahill, L. (2000). Modulation of long-term memory storage in humans by emotional arousal: adrenergic activation and the amygdala. In *The Amygdala: A Functional Analysis*, Aggleton, J. P. (Ed.), 2nd ed. Oxford, New York: Oxford University Press, pp. 425–445.

5. Impey, S., Smith, D. M., Obrietan, K., Donahue, R., Wade, C., and Storm, D. R. (1998). Stimulation of cAMP response element (CRE)-mediated transcription during contextual learning. *Nat. Neurosci.* 1:595–601.

6. Weeber, E. J., Atkins, C. M., Selcher, J. C., Varga, A. W., Mirnikjoo, B., Paylor, R., Leitges, M., and Sweatt, J. D. (2000). A role for the beta isoform of protein kinase C in fear conditioning. *J. Neurosci.* 20:5906–5914.

7. Levenson, J., Weeber, E., Selcher, J. C., Kategaya, L. S., Sweatt, J. D., and Eskin, A. (2002). Long-term potentiation and contextual fear conditioning increase neuronal glutamate uptake. *Nat. Neurosci.* 5:155–161.

8. Frankland, P. W., Cestari, V., Filipkowski, R. K., McDonald, R. J., and Silva, A. J. (1998). The dorsal hippocampus is essential for context discrimination but not for contextual conditioning. *Behav. Neurosci.* 112:863–874.

9. Morris, R. (1984). Developments of a water-maze procedure for studying spatial learning in the rat. *J. Neurosci. Methods* 11:47–60.

10. Selcher, J. C., Atkins, C. M., Trzaskos, J. M., Paylor, R., and Sweatt, J. D. (1999). A necessity for MAP kinase activation in mammalian spatial learning. *Learn. Mem.* 6:478–490.

11. Barnes, C. A. (1979). Memory deficits associated with senescence: a neurophysiological and behavioral study in the rat. *J. Comp. Physiol. Psychol* 93:74–104.

12. Swank, M. W., and Sweatt, J. D. (2001). Increased histone acetyltransferase and lysine acetyltransferase activity and biphasic activation of the ERK/RSK cascade in insular cortex during novel taste learning. *J. Neurosci.* 21:3383–3391.

13. Lubin, F. D., and Sweatt, J. D. (2007). The IkappaB kinase regulates chromatin structure during reconsolidation of conditioned fear memories. *Neuron* 55(6):942–957.

14. Paylor, R., and Crawley, J. N. (1997). "Inbred strain differences in prepulse inhibition of the mouse startle response." *Psychopharmacology* (Berl) 132:169–180.

15. Paylor, R., Baskall-Baldini, L., Yuva, L., and Wehner, J. M. (1996). Developmental differences in place-learning performance between C57BL/6 and DBA/2 mice parallel the ontogeny of hippocampal protein kinase C. *Behav. Neurosci.* 110:1415–1425.

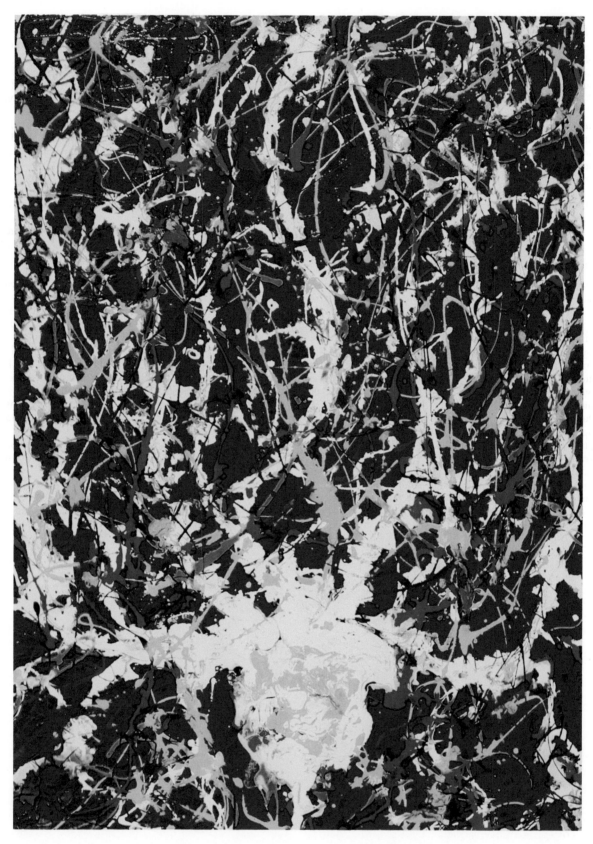

Purkinje Neuron
J. David Sweatt, acrylic on canvas, 2008–2009

5

Associative Learning and Unlearning

I. INTRODUCTION

Associative conditioning is the simplest form of learning that the average person tends to think of as "real" learning. It begins to capture the types of higher-order, relational, cognitive function that the general public generally equates with human learning and memory capacity. In this chapter we will explore various forms of associative conditioning. We will review both aversive conditioning and conditioning by positive reinforcement. We also will discuss examples of how a previously learned association can be "unlearned," and an example of how future associative conditioning can be prevented by prior experience.

Moreover, in two specific instances, fear conditioning and eye-blink conditioning, we will begin to discuss

cellular and molecular mechanisms underlying mammalian long-term memory. We will focus on these two examples because they are the two forms of associative conditioning that are best-understood in mechanistic detail, including at the cellular and molecular levels.

In this chapter we also will begin an exploration of the role of *synaptic plasticity* in mammalian memory. The general role of synaptic plasticity as a mechanism contributing to most forms of memory was discussed in Chapter 3, as was the unifying concept that learning and memory are subserved by lasting changes in the function of intercellular connections in the nervous system. Two prominent and important forms of mammalian synaptic plasticity will be introduced in this chapter: long-term synaptic potentiation (LTP) and long-term synaptic depression (LTD). This chapter

---

BOX 1

INVERTEBRATE MODEL SYSTEMS FOR STUDYING ASSOCIATIVE CONDITIONING

While this chapter focuses on associative learning in vertebrate species, the adaptive power of being able to learn cause-and-effect relationships has led to the evolution of the capacity for associative conditioning in most animals. This manifestation of associative learning and memory at many phylogenetic levels in the animal kingdom has allowed memory scientists to pursue many diverse, colorful, and interesting animal model systems outside of the vertebrate realm.

A detailed exploration of the cellular and molecular mechanisms underlying associative conditioning in invertebrate species is beyond the scope of this book, but in a series of text boxes in this chapter we will explore some interesting and intriguing examples of associative conditioning in invertebrates. These are examples of powerful systems for exploring the mechanistic basis of associative conditioning. These examples also provide a sample of the rich history of cleverly-designed studies of ethologically relevant memory behaviors across the animal kingdom. Thus, in many cases in these studies the development of useful laboratory approaches to study associative conditioning in these species required a deep understanding of which stimuli and responses are relevant to the species in their natural environment. These ethologically-relevant stimuli and behavioral responses were then imported into the laboratory in order to be able to effectively train and monitor the behavior of the invertebrate species under study.

---

will provide a snapshot of these two phenomena, which will be discussed in much greater detail in several subsequent chapters of the book. For now, we will focus on introducing the basic phenomena of LTP and LTD, and provide a context for their importance by describing an instance for each of them wherein they have been strongly linked to memory function in mammals. This provides a foundation and rationale for subsequent more detailed discussions of their molecular and cellular mechanisms.

A. Classical Associative Conditioning

At the outset it is important to explain some terms that will be used repeatedly throughout this chapter, which indeed you have already been introduced to when we discussed Pavlov training his dogs (see Figure 1). During classical associative learning, an animal is taught to associate a neutral conditioned stimulus (CS) with an aversive or reinforcing unconditioned stimulus (US). From the very outset even before training the US elicits an instinctive, reflexive, or previously learned baseline response, the unconditioned response (UR). After training by pairing CS and US, the animal responds to the CS with a conditioned response (CR) which behaviorally is indistinguishable from the pre-existing unconditioned response.

For example, classical conditioning of the eye-blink response in rabbits uses the association of a neutral CS

Stimulus or response term	Abbreviation	Actual stimulus or response by the dog in Pavlov's experiments
Conditioned stimulus	CS	A ringing bell
Unconditioned stimulus	US	Food
Unconditioned response	UR	Salivation
Conditioned response	CR	Salivation

FIGURE 1 The terminology of associative conditioning, as illustrated by the classic experiments of Pavlov. A number of terms that arise out of the basic design of associative conditioning will be used repeatedly in this chapter, as well as in the literature. For convenience, this figure provides a ready reference to the terms as applied to the well-known classical conditioning studies of Ivan Pavlov that were briefly discussed in Chapter 1, Section III. Pavlov trained dogs using a classical associative conditioning paradigm. In these experiments Pavlov trained a dog to associate a neutral conditioned stimulus (CS, a ringing bell) with a positive reinforcement unconditioned stimulus (US, food). From the very outset the US elicits a reflexive baseline response, the unconditioned response (UR, salivation). After training by pairing CS and US, the dog will respond to the CS with a conditioned response (CR, also salivation). While behaviorally the CR is indistinguishable from the pre-existing unconditioned response, the CR now uniquely occurs on presentation of the CS where it did not before training.

BOX 2

HERMISSENDA

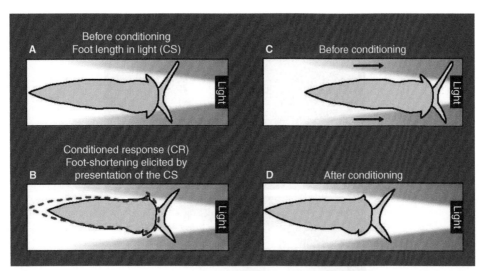

BOX 2 Pavlovian conditioning of foot-shortening and phototaxic inhibition in *Hermissenda*. (A) Foot length in light (CS) before conditioning. (B) CR foot-shortening elicited by the CS. Red outline indicates foot length in light before conditioning. (C) Light-elicited ciliary locomotion toward a light source (phototaxis) assessed before conditioning. (D) Inhibition of light-elicited ciliary locomotion detected after Pavlovian conditioning. Random or pseudorandom presentations of the CS and US do not produce either inhibition of ciliary locomotion or CS-elicited foot-shortening. Figure adapted from Crow, T. (2004). "Pavlovian conditioning of *Hermissenda*: Current cellular, molecular, and circuit perspectives." *Learn. Mem.* 11:229–238. Copyright Elsevier 2008.

The small, brightly colored marine mollusk *Hermissenda crassicornis* (see Box 4 in Chapter 1) has been utilized to investigate associative conditioning at the anatomical, cellular, and molecular levels. While historically studies of the other main mollusk memory model, *Aplysia*, focused on non-associative learning paradigms like sensitization, from the outset *Hermissenda* studies focused on mechanisms of associative conditioning.

The Pavlovian conditioning paradigm in *Hermissenda* focuses on behavioral conditioning of the animal's natural light-seeking behavior. *Hermissenda* exhibit a natural phototaxic response, meaning that reflexively they will crawl toward light. Training is achieved by repeated

pairing of light with an aversive stimulus—water turbulence is typically used as the aversive stimulus, which mimics a naturally occurring aversive stimulus in the ocean. Training results in a suppression of the phototaxic response and indeed even a reversal of the baseline behavior such that the animal now retreats from light (see Figure). Although this might seem to be a fairly simple conditioning paradigm, in fact this form of learning in Hermissenda exhibits a necessity for contiguity and contingency in the CS-US pairing, manifesting the capacity for triggering both short-term and long-term memory, and exhibiting selective extinction with repeated CS presentations after training.

stimulus, such as a tone or light, with an aversive US, such as an air puff delivered to the eye. The air puff to the eye, as you might expect, elicits a defensive reflex, an eye-blink—this is the baseline UR. After an animal has been effectively trained by repeated CS-US pairings, representation of the CS by itself results in an

eye-blink. The eye-blink in response to the CS is the conditioned response (CR). The ethological relevance of this behavioral modification is that the eye-blink in response to the CS provides a protective response that can be triggered in anticipation of the US, before the US actually arrives. Indeed, many forms of associative

THE POND SNAIL *LYMNAEA*

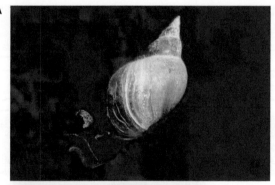

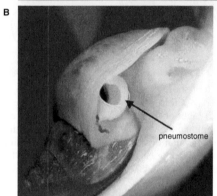

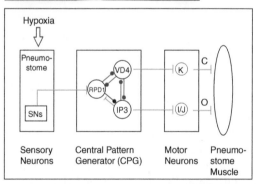

BOX 3 (A) The snail *Lymnaea stagnalis* sinks from the water surface to the ground of the pond. Photo by Kathrin Spöcker. (B) The snail *Lymnaea stagnalis* and the neuronal network underlying respiratory behavior. Upper panel: *Lymnaea stagnalis* with opened pneumostome (arrow). From Lukowiak, K., Sangha, S., Scheibenstock, A., et al. (2003). "A molluscan model system in the search for the engram." *J. Physiol.* 69–76. Lower panel: Schematic drawing of the central pattern generator (CPG). A chemosensory stimulus (here hypoxia) activates sensory neurons (SNs) in the pneumostome area, which in turn provide excitatory input (green line) to the right pedal dorsal 1 interneuron (RPeD1). Once stimulated, RPeD1 activates the input 3 interneuron (IP3) via a biphasic effect (inhibition followed by excitation) (blue line) and inhibits visceral dorsal 4 interneuron (VD4) (red line). IP3 in turn excites both RpeD1 and the I/J motor neurons involved in pneumostome openings (O). IP3 also produces an inhibitory effect on VD4, and after release from this inhibition, VD4 fires, resulting in pneumostome closure (C). Tactile stimulation of the pneumostome area evokes closure of the pneumostome, and the aerial respiratory behavior stops. Figure and legend from Eisenhardt, D., and Stollhoff, N. *Learning and Memory: A Comprehensive Reference*, Volume 1. Copyright Elsevier 2008.

BOX 3—cont'd

THE POND SNAIL *LYMNAEA*

The lowly pond snail *Lymnaea stagnalis* (see Figure A) has a capacity that many humans might envy—it can breathe both underwater and in the air. Underwater it achieves oxygenation passively through its skin. However, when oxygen tension in the water is too low for this mechanism to be effective, it has an alternative. It can rise to the surface of the pond and respire through a lung under its shell, via a mouth-like *pneumostome* (see Figure B). This rise-to-the-surface reflex is referred to as the *aerial respiration response*, and its ethological relevance and value in promoting survival of the species is obvious.

Components of this aerial respiration response are subject to associative conditioning. Animals are trained by delivering a modest tactile aversive stimulation when they open their pneumostome for breathing air. The baseline behavior is triggered in the laboratory by exposing the animals to hypoxic conditions. With repeated training trials the animals suppress pneumostome opening and the aerial respiration response, even in the hypoxic conditions. This suppression is a manifestation of associative conditioning because the animals have made an association between the aversive tactile stimulus and pneumostome opening, and suppressed this behavior. In fact, this is also an example of operant conditioning, because the training is contingent on the animal performing an act—in this case opening their pneumostome.

Lymnaea behavioral modification is not limited to operant conditioning of the aerial respiration response. *Lymnaea* also exhibit both aversive and reward-based classical conditioning of feeding behavior, along with non-associative forms of learning such as sensitization and habituation. Thus, the diversity of learned behaviors in such a simple species is actually fairly astounding.

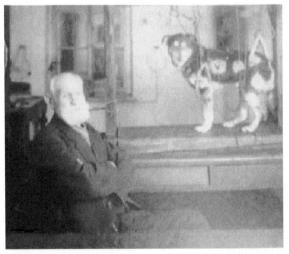

FIGURE 2 Ivan Pavlov and one of his canine subjects. Classical conditioning is frequently referred to as Pavlovian conditioning, in recognition of Ivan Pavlov's pioneering studies in this area.

conditioning follow this general rubric, that is, they are of adaptive value because they allow newly-learned protective or defensive responses to novel environmental stimuli.

It is also important to observe the fact that the conditioned response is a brand new behavior for the animal. There has been a fundamental change in the animal's behavioral repertoire. Never before has the animal responded to the CS in the way it now does. True, the animal previously exhibited the basic behavior, the UR (for example the eye-blink in the case of eye-blink conditioning). But never before had the CS triggered that basic response. Thus, the CR is a novel behavior for the animal in the sense that it is now a behavioral output in response to the CS, whereas it never was before. The UR and the CR are the identical behavior, but the larger behavioral pattern of the CS triggering the UR/CR behavior is completely new.

One final point is that the fact that the UR and the CR are the same behavior is the defining characteristic of classical (or Pavlovian) conditioning (see Figures 1 and 2). The term classical conditioning is reserved for those forms of associative conditioning where the UR and the CR are identical behavioral outputs. This is not the case for all forms of associative conditioning, so classical conditioning is a subset of the broader category, associative conditioning.

BOX 4

APLYSIA ASSOCIATIVE CONDITIONING

In Chapter 3 we discussed extensively the utility of the *Aplysia* model system for studies of short-term and long-term non-associative conditioning, especially the sensitization response. However, *Aplysia* exhibit a much broader range of memory behaviors including a capacity for aversive classical conditioning, appetitive (food-based) classical conditioning, and operant conditioning of food-seeking behavior.

Studies of these classical conditioning paradigms in *Aplysia* were largely pioneered by Tom Carew and his co-workers. Their studies mapped out many of the circuit, cellular, and molecular mechanisms underlying

associative conditioning in *Aplysia*. While we will not go into details of these studies here, one of the most fascinating aspects of their work is that both non-associative and associative memory mechanisms in *Aplysia* utilize many of the same underlying mechanisms, including a role for neuromodulation by serotonin and an involvement of synaptic facilitation at sensory–motor synapses (see Chapter 3). The striking implication of these findings is that evolutionarily speaking, the development of the capacity for associative memory may have "piggy-backed" onto pre-existing simpler mechanisms underlying non-associative conditioning.

II. FEAR CONDITIONING AND THE AMYGDALA

The most extensively studied form of mammalian associative conditioning is fear conditioning. Fear conditioning is a classical conditioning paradigm where a neutral CS is paired with a fear-evoking US. After training, the previously neutral CS now evokes a fear response on its own; the conditioned response. Fear conditioning, as you might imagine, is readily inducible in humans with a wide variety of stimuli in the laboratory setting (see Figure 3). Typical conditioned stimuli are things like brief soft noise cues, colored cards or lights that can be flashed on and off, tactile stimuli, or contexts such as specific chairs, desks or even whole rooms. USs are typically aversive stimuli like a mild electric shock to the skin, or the delivery of loud noxious noises, or even airblasts delivered to various body parts.

Any laboratory assessment of fear conditioning requires a way to measure the behavioral fear output, in order to be able to quantitate the UR and the CR. Investigators using human subjects have developed a number of clever ways to assess human fear responses objectively, several of which can be used in combination. A fearful human typically exhibits an increased respiratory and heart rate, for example. An additional component of the reflexive human fear response is an increased galvanic skin response, which is a fancy way of saying increased skin electrical conductivity due to the presence of sweat. Fear-induced

potentiation of the acoustic startle response is also frequently used in human fear conditioning studies. In this case, the fearful mental state of the subject is manifest as an exaggerated response to an unexpected loud noise.

A fundamental neuroanatomical component of the fear conditioning circuit in mammals including humans is the amygdala. Amygdala is Greek for "almond," and indeed in humans the amygdala is an almond-shaped structure residing in the medial temporal lobes. Numerous studies have implicated the amygdala specifically in human fear conditioning, and moreover the amygdala is implicated in human emotional behavior in general. Human patients with temporal lobe damage that includes the amygdala are deficient in fear conditioning memory. Human fMRI studies have also directly implicated the amygdala in fear conditioning, as this area is activated during the training process (see Figure 4). These human studies have been complemented by decades of very sophisticated work using laboratory animals that clearly demonstrate a critical role for the amygdala in fear conditioning.

Animal studies have led to a great degree of understanding of the neuroanatomy of the amygdala and how the neural circuits of this structure contribute to fear conditioning. The fundamental circuitry of the amygdala-based fear system, its inputs and outputs, and how it maps onto a typical cued fear conditioning paradigm is shown in Figure 5. In overview, the amygdala receives diverse sensory input from various

A

B

C

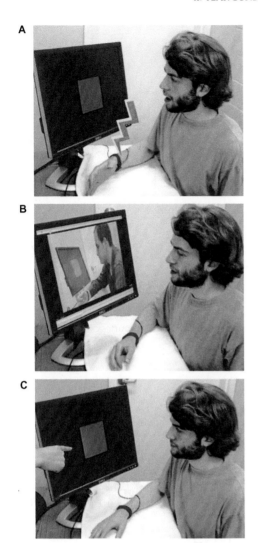

FIGURE 3 Non-social and social fear learning in humans. An individual learns to fear a CS through its pairing with: (A) an electric shock to the wrist (fear conditioning); (B) a learning model's expression of distress (observational fear learning); and (C) verbal information about its aversive qualities (instructed fear). Figure adapted from Olsen and Phelps (2007). *Nature Neuroscience* 10(9). Reprinted by permission from Macmillan Publishers, Ltd, *Nature Neuroscience*, copyright 2007.

A

B

C

D

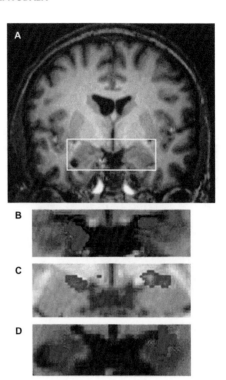

FIGURE 4 Fear learning in the human amygdala. (A) The outlined box contains the area of the medical temporal lobe that includes the bilateral amygdala. (B)–(D) Amygdala activation to the CS is seen bilaterally after fear conditioning (B) and observational fear learning (C), and unilaterally (D) in the left amygdala after instructed fear. Figure courtesy of Andreas Olsson and Elizabeth Phelps (2007). *Nature Neuroscience* 10(9). Reprinted by permission from Macmillan Publishers, Ltd. *Nature Neuroscience*, copyright 2007.

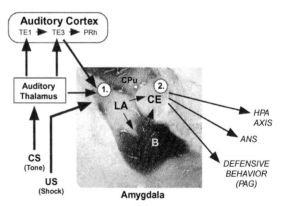

FIGURE 5 Anatomy of the fear system. (1) Auditory fear conditioning involves the transmission of CS sensory information from areas of the auditory thalamus and cortex to the lateral amygdala (LA), where it can converge with incoming somatosensory information from the foot shock US. It is in the LA that alterations in synaptic transmission are thought to encode key aspects of the learning. (2) During fear expression, the LA engages the central nucleus of the amygdala (CE), which projects widely to many areas of the forebrain and brain stem which control the expression of fear CRs, including freezing, hypothalamic-pituitary-adrenal (HPA) axis activation, and alterations in the cardiovascular activity. CPu, caudate/putamen; B, basal nucleus of amygdala; ANS, autonomic nervous system; PRh, perirhinal cortex; PAG, periaqueductal gray. Figure courtesy of G. E. Schafe and J. E. Le Doux. Adapted from *Learning and Memory: A Comprehensive Review*, Volume 4. Copyright Elsevier 2008.

cortical regions including the visual, somatosensory, and auditory cortices, as well as direct inputs from thalamic nuclei that are involved in processing sensory information. Outputs of the amygdala project to subcortical and hypothalamic regions of the CNS to allow them to precipitate the wide variety of motor, vascular, and hormonal manifestations of fear.

Within the amygdala itself the three main subregions (see Figure 5) are the lateral nucleus (LA), the basolateral nucleus (BLA), and the central nucleus (CE). As a first approximation, the LA receives sensory input, the BLA is involved in sensory and associative processing in association with the LA, and the CE is involved in mediating output from the amygdala.

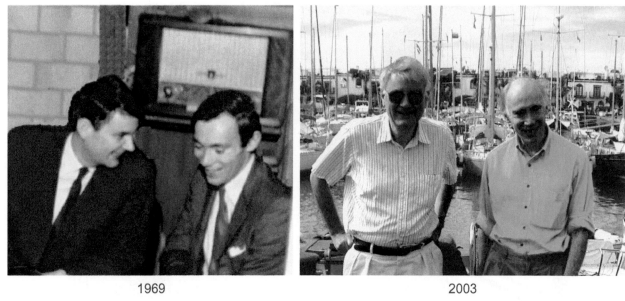

1969   2003

FIGURE 6   Terje Lomo and Tim Bliss, the co-discoverers of long-term potentiation. Photos courtesy of Tim Bliss.

A. Long-Term Potentiation in Cued Fear Conditioning

In Chapter 3 focusing on long-term synaptic facilitation in *Aplysia*, I introduced a unifying concept that is broadly applicable concerning memory mechanisms— the concept that lasting changes in synaptic function underlie information storage in the CNS. We will now discuss an example of this principle that occurs at central synapses in the mammalian brain, focusing on the role of long-term potentiation (LTP) in amygdala-dependent fear conditioning. Indeed, LTP in the amygdala has received prominent attention as a mechanism contributing to auditory cued fear conditioning. The role of LTP in amygdala-dependent fear conditioning, in fact, is the area for which the strongest case can be made for a direct demonstration of a behavioral role for LTP in a mammalian model.

Plasticity of synaptic function, including phenomena such as LTP and long-term depression (LTD), is the rule rather than the exception for most forebrain synapses. LTP is a long-lasting, activity-dependent increase in synaptic strength that is a leading candidate as a cellular mechanism contributing to memory formation in mammals in a very broadly applicable sense. LTP was first discovered and characterized by Tim Bliss and Terje Lomo working in the hippocampus, work they performed in Per Anderson's laboratory in Oslo, Norway (see Figure 6). We will return to a much more detailed description of hippocampal LTP and its cellular and molecular mechanisms later in this

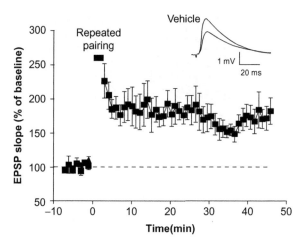

FIGURE 7   Long-term potentiation in the amygdala. This figure shows "pairing-induced" LTP in neurons of the basolateral nucleus of the amygdala. The plot shows mean ± SE percent EPSP slope (relative to baseline) in cells treated with 0.1% DMSO vehicle (black squares) before and after LTP induction. Traces from an individual experiment before and 40 min after induction are shown in the inset. Traces are averages of five responses. Adapted from Schafe et al. (1).

book. For now we will simply focus on LTP as a basic physiologic change, i.e., a lasting increase in synaptic strength.

LTP not only occurs in the hippocampus, but also occurs widely throughout excitatory glutamatergic synapses in the mammalian CNS including glutamatergic synapses in the amygdala (see Figure 7). It is important to bear in mind throughout your reading of

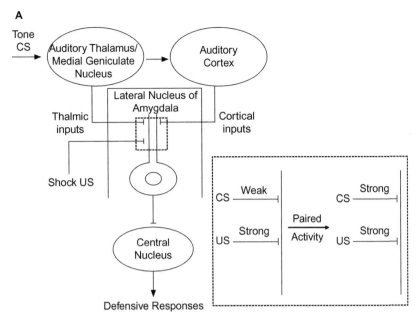

FIGURE 8 Diagram of the principal circuit of the amygdala. Model adapted from Blair et al. (4).

the rest of the book, that amygdalar LTP exhibits some mechanistic differences from the NMDA receptor-dependent LTP that we will be focusing on later. However, the basic physiologic phenomenon, which is what we will be discussing in this chapter, is the same—a long-lasting increase in synaptic strength that is induced by synaptic activity.

In the following few paragraphs I will briefly review the considerable and impressive data linking LTP with cued fear conditioning as an example of a situation where LTP likely plays a role in a specific form of mammalian memory.

The broad hypothesis that LTP is involved in learning makes the prediction that one should be able to see LTP happen within the CNS when an animal learns. (This is what we have referred to as the "measure" experiment.) In 1997 two groups broke through a long-standing barrier by directly demonstrating the occurrence of LTP in association with behavioral training in animals (2–3). These studies were particularly compelling, because in this system there is appreciable understanding of the structure of the relevant circuits and how they map onto the behavior, as we discussed above (see Figure 8). The hypothesis that was tested by both groups was that fear conditioning would be associated with LTP of synaptic connections in the lateral nucleus (LA) of the amygdala, specifically synaptic connections to the principal neurons of that nucleus. The prediction was that the connections of CS (thalamic) inputs to these neurons would be strengthened after the CS-US training of fear conditioning, such that the CS input pathway would make

a stronger connection to the lateral nucleus neurons after training.

The behavioral system under study by both groups was auditory cued fear conditioning in rats, a popular rodent learning paradigm we discussed in the last chapter. In these experiments animals were trained to associate an auditory cue CS with an aversive foot shock US. The US normally elicits a spectrum of defensive, fear-associated behaviors such as immobile posture (freezing), tachycardia, and increased startle responses—these are the unconditioned responses (URs) in this paradigm. Both groups confirmed that after fear conditioning training the auditory cue elicits the same spectrum of defensive and physiologic responses as the foot shock did previously, including startle potentiation for example (see Figure 9A).

The relevant anatomical connections and circuit pathways underlying auditory cued fear conditioning in the amygdala are well-established. The tone CS is transduced to the lateral nucleus of the amygdala via both thalamic and cortical relays (see Figure 8). The shock pathway also triggers activity in the lateral nucleus via a strong input, the pathway that mediates triggering the reflexive defensive and fear behaviors. It is known that pairing of the cue with the US somehow allows the CS to co-opt the reflex pathway, and trigger the defensive responses on its own.

How does this happen? Is it mediated by LTP in amygdala synapses? Both Pat Shinnick-Gallagher's group and Joe LeDoux's group have performed fascinating experiments indicating that pairing of the strong US signal with the weaker CS input to the lateral

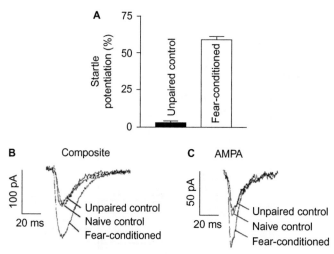

FIGURE 9　Fear conditioning results in potentiation of evoked EPSCs in the amygdala. (A) Plot of percent startle potentiation in fear-conditioned and unpaired control animals. (B) Composite EPSCs in amygdala neurons in trained and untrained animals, evoked with constant input stimulations of 9 V. (C) AMPA Receptor-mediated EPSCs evoked with input stimulations of 9 V. Reproduced from McKiernan and Shinnick-Gallagher (2).

nucleus of the amygdala leads to LTP of the CS input (2–3, 5). This LTP results in the augmentation or unmasking of a latent circuit—the CS is now able to trigger the entire spectrum of defensive behaviors because the CS input is potentiated and now sufficiently strong to trigger a behavioral output via the central nucleus of the amygdala (see Figures 9 and 10). This strong CS input is able to activate the lateral nucleus cells and trigger the conditioned response.

The key findings by both groups involved directly measuring LTP production in the amygdala in response to behavioral training. The two groups took distinct and complementary approaches to looking for LTP in response to fear conditioning training. McKernan and Shinnick-Gallagher used an *ex vivo* approach (2). These investigators trained animals and assessed the presence of LTP in amygdala slices prepared acutely, using electrical stimulation of synaptic inputs to the lateral nucleus from the medial geniculate nucleus (see Figure 9). LeDoux's colleagues used *in vivo* recording techniques with implanted electrodes (see Figure 10 and reference 3). They monitored field responses from the amygdala in response to presentation of the tone cue—directly monitoring population neuronal responses to an environmental signal. Both approaches yielded the same conclusion—synaptic potentiation of CS inputs into the amygdala is occurring with fear conditioning training.

Subsequent work by several groups has indicated that the relevant LTP is probably of a mixed etiology. It appears that both NMDA receptor-dependent and independent LTP is involved. Moreover, a number of sophisticated molecular studies are underway probing the biochemical basis of LTP in the amygdala in the context of memory formation. These studies also demonstrate an excellent correlation between the molecular mechanisms activated in the amygdala by fear conditioning and molecular mechanisms known to be involved in LTP at those synapses.

Overall this work suggests that LTP at the CS pathway–lateral nucleus synapses is sufficient to mediate the alteration in behavior. The papers are landmark publications in the history of the learning and memory field—the first clear demonstrations of LTP triggered *in vivo* by environmental signals. Important conclusions from these studies are that LTP can happen *in vivo*, with endogenously occurring, natural patterns of neuronal firing, triggered by salient environmental signals, at synapses relevant for the memory of those environmental signals.

III. EYE-BLINK CONDITIONING AND THE CEREBELLUM

A second major form of associative conditioning that has been extensively studied at the circuit, synaptic, and molecular levels is eye-blink conditioning. Most studies of the molecular and cellular basis of classical conditioning of the eye-blink response have used rabbits as the experimental animal. As we discussed in Chapter 4, classical conditioning of the eye-blink response in rabbits uses delivery of a neutral stimulus, such as a tone, paired with a mild aversive stimulus, such as an air puff delivered to the surface

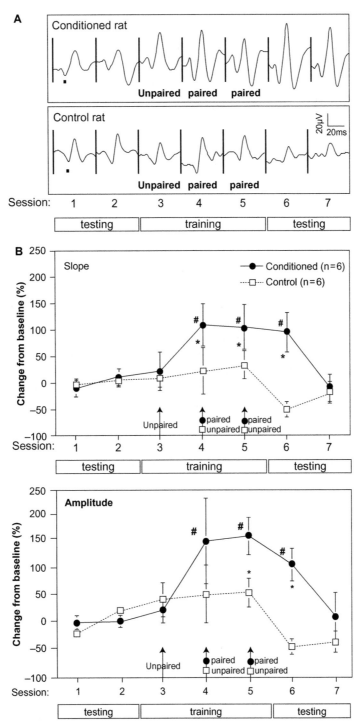

FIGURE 10 The effect of paired and unpaired training on CS-evoked field potentials. Sessions are numbered 1–7; one session occurred per day, except that sessions 3 and 4 occurred on the same day. (A) CS-evoked field potentials from a conditioned rat (top) and a control rat (bottom), covering the full time-course of the experiment. Quantitative analysis was performed on the first negative (downward)-going deflection (dot). Previous studies of these waveforms have concentrated on this feature as it has the shortest latency, is reliably present, coincides with local evoked unit activity, shows experience-dependent plasticity, and reflects transmission from the auditory thalamus to the amygdala. The other components of the waveform visible in these examples are not reliably present across trials and subjects, and little is known about their origin and mechanisms. (B) Fear conditioning increases the slope and amplitude of CS-EPs, but unpaired training does not. Slope and amplitude of the negative-going potential are normalized as a percentage of the mean values before training (sessions 1 and 2). The normalized slope and amplitude of the evoked potentials were evaluated statistically with two-factor ANOVAs with group (conditioned, control) as the between-subjects factor and experimental session as within subject factor. A significant group-session interaction was observed for both measures ($P < 0.05$). Significant differences of *post hoc* analyses are indicated ($P < 0.05$). Error bars = s.e.m. Reproduced from Rogan, Staubli, and LeDoux (3).

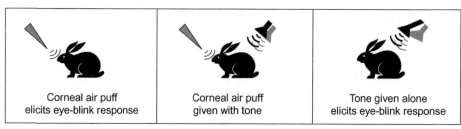

| Corneal air puff elicits eye-blink response | Corneal air puff given with tone | Tone given alone elicits eye-blink response |

FIGURE 11 Eye-blink conditioning in rabbits. Animals are trained in a Pavlovian conditioning paradigm to learn that a tone predicts a puff of air to the eye surface. Over time, the animals learn to blink in response to the tone alone. See text for additional details.

BOX 5

ADAPTATION OF THE VESTIBULO-OCULAR REFLEX

While eye-blink conditioning may seem somewhat outside the range of typical human experience, the function of the cerebellar cortex has been demonstrated to play a role in another important form of learned behavior that is of clinical relevance in humans: adaptation of the vestibulo-ocular reflex (VOR). Adaptation of the VOR is more complicated than eye-blink conditioning (see Further Reading), but I will illustrate the VOR with the following example. Shake your head back and forth while you are looking at this word. Notice that you are amazingly good at keeping your eyes pointed at exactly the right spot as your head goes back and forth. This seems to be simple, but remember that you are precisely moving both your left and right eyes to counterbalance your head movements. The VOR is what allows this to happen. To get a feel for what it would be like to live without a VOR, hold your finger out at arm's length and stare at your fingertip. Now rotate your entire upper body back and forth—quite a difference! Without a VOR your image of the world would move like this every time you moved your head.

The VOR detects signals from your vestibular system semicircular canals (that read-out head movement) and allows triggering of the appropriate eye muscle contractions to hold the eye position constant in space. To complicate matters further, this reflex is of necessity subject to adaptation. If your eye movements are not holding the visual field constant for some reason (e.g., damage to your oculomotor system or to the eye muscles themselves, or even a new pair of eyeglasses that change your focal point), the system adapts to the change and modifies the VOR to make it appropriate for your new state. This depends on complicated signals from the visual cortex that provide information concerning constancy of the visual percept—obviously not a trivial matter.

---

of the eye (Figure 11). With repeated pairings animals learn that the tone predicts the air puff and they will learn to blink when the tone is delivered by itself; a learned protective response involving co-opting a reflex pathway.

Eye-blink conditioning sounds simple, but is actually fairly complex. For example, the "blink" is really more than a blink; it is an elaborate programmed motor response involving a number of muscle groups that cause eyeball retraction and closure of the eyelid. The animals can also learn precisely the temporal relationship between tone and air puff. They automatically adjust their blink to slightly precede the air puff delivery.

Trace eye-blink conditioning where the CS is followed by a time delay is hippocampus-dependent, while delay conditioning (no intervening time delay) is hippocampus-independent. Both forms of eye-blink conditioning depend on the function of the cerebellum, both the cerebellar cortex and the underlying deep brainstem nuclei such as the nucleus interpositus. Sophisticated neuroanatomical studies have mapped much of the relevant neuronal circuitry underlying this behavior, which is shown in Figure 12 (reviewed in references 6–7). Importantly, synaptic plasticity within this cerebellar circuit has been implicated as one of the components mediating eye-blink conditioning.

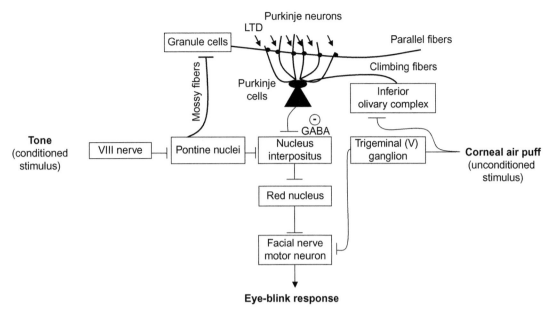

FIGURE 12 A simplified diagram describing the neural circuit underlying eye-blink conditioning. See text for discussion.

Clearly, synaptic plasticity at a single type of synapse cannot account for all of the elaborate behavioral changes underlying eye-blink conditioning. However, a wide variety of evidence from pharmacologic, genetic, lesioning, and physiologic recording studies has indicated an important role in eye-blink conditioning for long-term synaptic depression at parallel fiber-to-Purkinje cell synapses in the cerebellar cortex. This LTD in the cerebellar cortex has been extensively studied, and in the following section I will highlight a few of its properties and present a simplified version of how it might participate in eye-blink conditioning.

These findings represent our second major example of a role for synaptic plasticity in mammalian memory. However, in contrast to the work done in the amygdala described above, these studies illustrate a role for long-lasting *decreases* in synaptic strength as a mediator of memory. This consideration highlights the important point that it is *plasticity* of synapses that is important in memory, not the specifics of whether the change is an increase or a decrease in synaptic connectivity.

Parallel fiber LTD in the cerebellum is a persistent, input-specific decrease in the efficacy of synaptic transmission between the parallel fibers and Purkinje cells in the cerebellar cortex (see Figure 12). It is induced by low-frequency coactivation of climbing fibers and parallel fiber inputs to Purkinje neurons. Climbing fibers are highly potent inputs onto Purkinje neurons—a single climbing fiber matches to only one Purkinje neuron, and its activation is sufficient to trigger

an action potential in its specific follower Purkinje neuron. Climbing fibers originate in brainstem nuclei and are involved in processing sensory signals, such as sending a signal to the cerebellar cortex that an eye-blink has been triggered by a puff of air on the cornea. Parallel fibers originate from cerebellar granule cells, which are a major cell type in the cerebellum. Parallel fibers carry information such as auditory signals—for example information that an auditory cue has been received. Thus, via this part of the circuit a coincidence of auditory cue (parallel fibers) and air puff (climbing fibers) can lead to a depression of parallel fiber inputs onto the Purkinje neurons. This is activity-dependent synaptic plasticity, manifest as a synaptic weakening.

How does this synaptic depression translate into a behavioral change? The Purkinje neurons are the only output neurons from the cerebellar cortex—they provide the net output of the cerebellum and are involved in modulating a wide variety of motor movements, including those involved in eye movement and the eye-blink. Purkinje neurons use gamma-amino butyric acid (GABA) as their neurotransmitter, thus they are inhibitory. LTD at their parallel fiber inputs leads to a net loss of inhibitory output onto motor pattern generators downstream. In the case of eye-blink conditioning, this loss of inhibition causes a net enhancement of a pre-existing connection between tone-activated neurons and follower neurons that when unmasked can trigger an eye-blink (see VIIIth nerve inputs in Figure 12). This connection is normally inhibited in a feed-forward fashion by the Purkinje cell output from the cerebellar cortex, and thus is inactive. Loss of the Purkinje cell inhibitory input allows unmasking of the connection between the tone-activated cells and the blink pattern generator cells. Thus, the tone is then able to trigger the eye-blink response on its own. The conditioned stimulus (tone) now triggers the conditioned response (eye-blink), in classical conditioning parlance.

It is important to keep in mind that this is a great oversimplification of the cellular basis of eye-blink conditioning. Nevertheless, it allows us to make several important points. First, this is a specific example of the generalization that associative learning involves the unmasking of latent circuits, ones already in existence in the CNS but that become effective in triggering behavior due to plasticity of their synaptic inputs (the same can be said of the latent circuit that is unmasked in auditory cued fear conditioning). Second, it illustrates that learning does not have to be dependent on strengthening synapses—depressing synapses is an equally effective mechanism for memory formation. A positive or negative behavioral change can be mediated by either a positive or negative change in synaptic strength; it all simply depends on the circuit in which the neuron is embedded.

IV. POSITIVE REINFORCEMENT LEARNING

The examples of associative learning and memory that we have discussed so far have involved negative

---

BOX 6

THE FRUITFLY

The fruitfly *Drosophila melanogaster* (see Figure A) has been a workhorse of genetic studies since its introduction to the field 100 years ago by Thomas Hunt Morgan. Morgan's studies of inheritance in *Drosophila* led to his discovery of the chromosome as the basis for Mendelian inheritance, and to his being awarded a Nobel Prize in 1933 for these studies.

The intellectual descendants of Morgan have capitalized on the rich trove of information concerning *Drosophila* genetics in order to probe the role of specific genes in learning and memory in this species. The principal associative learning paradigm used for studies of *Drosophila* is an aversive olfactory conditioning paradigm (see Figure B). In this paradigm a fly is trained by exposing it to a specific odor paired with an electric shock. Repeated pairings of odor and shock lead to a long-lasting associative memory in the animal, and in subsequent testing a trained animal will exhibit an avoidance of the trained odor. Typically odor avoidance is assessed by giving animals a choice between being in the presence of the trained odor versus being in the presence of a novel untrained odor.

The *Drosophila* olfactory training and testing paradigm is amenable to being used to train and test batches of 100 flies at once, allowing for rapid screening of large populations of flies. This factor, combined with the rapid generation time for flies and the presence of sophisticated genetic engineering approaches in this animal make for a powerful system in which to test genetic and molecular influences on memory. Moreover, the availability of this convenient assay system for screening large numbers of flies simultaneously made it possible in early studies to screen large groups of flies for genetic mutants that exhibited selective defects in learning and memory. Studies in *Drosophila* have been among the most powerful experimental studies available for investigating the roles of genes in behavior.

Traditionally, scientists who discover a new *Drosophila* mutant get to name the mutant fly line; moreover, this scientific community has taken the approach that the discoverers can have some fun coming up with the name. This has led to a colorfully named group of *Drosophila* learning and memory mutant lines such as *dunce, rutabaga, amnesiac, radish, crammer,* and *tequila. Dunce* and *rutabaga,* the first *Drosophila* learning/memory mutants characterized, were discovered to have defects in the cAMP signaling cascade. These studies, along with pioneering studies in the *Aplysia* system, were the first to implicate a specific molecular cascade in memory formation.

BOX 6—cont'd

THE FRUITFLY

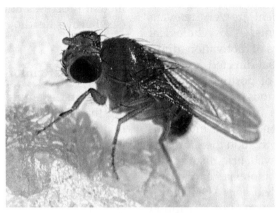

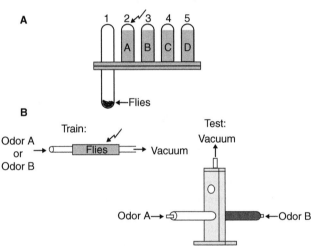

BOX 6   (A) Olfactory learning in *Drosophila*. A schematic diagram of the apparatus used for olfactory operant conditioning. Flies are placed in a start tube and coaxed up the tube by attraction to a bright light. The
five tubes on the top of the apparatus can be slid horizontally so that anyone of them is in register with
the start tube. Training begins by allowing the flies to walk into the tube containing odor A and electric
shock for 30 seconds. The flies are then tapped back into the start tube and allowed to walk into the tube
containing odor B for 30 seconds. After this training, the animals are tested by first allowing them to walk
into a fresh tube containing odor A without shock (tube 4), and the fraction of the flies that avoid the odor
is recorded. Finally, the flies are tested with odor B in the last tube. Selective avoidance, after training, of
the tube containing odor A, but not the tube containing odor B, is taken as an index of performance. (B) A
schematic diagram of the apparatuses used for olfactory classical conditioning. Flies are sequestered in a
tube and odors are drawn through the tube in an air current. Electric shock is delivered when only one of
the two odors is presented to the flies in the tube. After training, the animals are tested in a T-maze runway
in which they must choose to avoid odor A or odor B, the odors being carried to the choice point in air currents. Adapted from *Progress in Neurobiology* 76:328–347. Copyright Elsevier 2005.

reinforcers or aversive conditioned stimuli. Of course positive reinforcement and reward-based learning are also powerful phenomena. This is particularly notable in the case of human behavior, where much goal-directed behavior is based on positive reinforcement and reward. In this section we will discuss reward-based associative learning by providing a few examples of this phenomenon in the laboratory setting.

A. Reward and Human Psychopathology

At the outset it is important to note the great human clinical relevance of systems related to reward, positive reinforcement, and goal-directed behavior. Several examples are particularly notable. First, reward and positive reinforcement are very relevant to depression in human patients. A psychological component of depression is a loss of motivation, diminution of desire to manifest goal-directed behavior, and a decrease in the seeking of positive reinforcement. An inability to find various sensory stimuli and experiences rewarding is a fundamental aspect of clinical depression. Understanding the underpinnings of reward learning and motivation therefore has great relevance to this major psychiatric disorder. In addition, the clinical syndromes anorexia nervosa and attention deficit/hyperactivity disorder (ADHD) also likely involve at least some component of disruption of the reward system. A final compelling example is drug addiction. In this case humans express an exceptional and deleterious desire for agents that they perceive as rewarding. At a very basic level, many aspects of drug addiction involve a drug usurping the fundamental processes underlying normal reward learning (see Further Reading).

B. Positive Reinforcement Learning

The first example of positive reinforcement learning that we will address is conceptually very similar to the negative reinforcement paradigms we have already discussed. In this example the US is a rewarding stimulus such as food, and it is paired with any typical CS, such as light. With repeated pairings associative conditioning occurs, such that the CS now triggers a conditioned response. Indeed, the landmark

---

BOX 7

THE HONEYBEE

In my estimation the honeybee (*Apis mellifera*) is the Einstein of the invertebrate world—they manifest an amazing diversity of learned behaviors and innate skills. Honeybees are social insects that operate within a hive community, and they have the capacity to communicate with each other. They are foraging animals with exceptional spatial navigation skills and place memory. They even practice a form of economics where they maximize their foraging efficiency by visiting the most nectar-laden flowers with greater frequency.

Perhaps their most amazing behavioral ability is the capacity to communicate newly learned information to their hive-mates. This behavior is manifest as the *waggle dance*. On a single foraging expedition from the hive a single bee might have either found very little food (in the form of nectar from flowers, for example) or have learned of a particularly rich source of nutrition in a specific place (for example a field full of nectar-laden flowers). A bee that finds a rich source of food has the capacity to communicate the location of the food to other bees in its hive using the waggle dance. The waggle dance (see Figure A) allows a bee to tell its hive-mates both the *vector heading* and *distance* to the food! This is an extremely impressive capacity to convey newly-learned information to other individuals.

While the waggle dance is fascinating, other simpler forms of associative learning in bees have been more extensively studied in the laboratory. For example, bees can be trained in operant conditioning experiments to fly toward specific visual stimuli using positive or negative reinforcement, and the cellular and circuit basis of this behavior has been investigated. Likely the most extensively studied form of associative conditioning in honeybees is conditioning of the *proboscis extension reflex*, commonly abbreviated to PER. When the antennae, a main sensory organ of the bee, are touched with a sucrose solution, the animal reflexively extends its proboscis. The proboscis is a tongue-like feeding tube used to suck up nectar during nectar-gathering. If sucrose application is repeatedly paired with specific, previously neutral, olfactory cues, over time associative conditioning develops and the olfactory cue alone will begin to elicit the PER (see Figure B). This is clearly a form of associative conditioning, and in the natural setting is likely used so that the animal can efficiently forage in nectar-laden flowers based on their smell alone. The neuroanatomical and cellular basis of this form of learning has been extensively studied.

BOX 7—cont'd

THE HONEYBEE

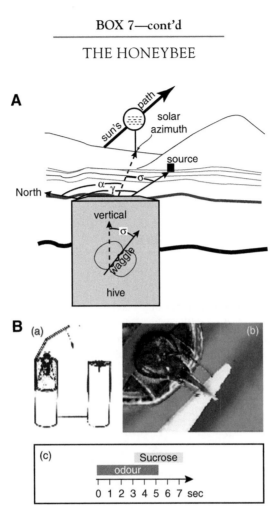

BOX 7 (A). In the waggle dance, the returned forager circles in alternate directions from one waggle run to the next, forming a figure of eight. The angle of the repeated waggle runs, relative to vertical, indicates the solar bearing of the source from which the forager has returned. The number of waggles indicates its distance. α = the solar azimuth, its compass direction; σ = the solar bearing of the source, its relative to the direction of the sun; γ = the compass direction of the source. Note that the compass direction of the source is the sum of the solar azimuth and the solar bearing: $\gamma = \alpha + \sigma$. (B). The honeybee *Apis mellifera*: olfactory conditioning of the proboscis extension response. (a) Single honeybees are restrained in small tubes to condition the proboscis extension response (PER). Adapted from Bitterman, M. E., Menzel, R., Fietz, A., and Scahfer, S. (1983). "Classical conditioning of proboscis extension in honeybees (*Apis mellifera*)." *J. Comp. Psychol.* 97:107–119. (b) Honeybees reflexively elicit their proboscis when the antennae and the proboscis are touched with sugar water. Here a toothpick that is moistened with sucrose solution is used to touch the honeybee's proboscis. After the PER is elicited, the honeybee licks sucrose solution from the toothpick. (c) Schematic diagram of the olfactory conditioning of the PER. An odor (conditioned stimulus) is presented for five seconds; after three seconds the PER is elicited with sucrose solution (unconditioned stimulus), and the honeybee is allowed to lick the sucrose solution for four seconds. Figure and legend from Gallistel, C. R. *Learning and Memory: A Comprehensive Reference*, Volume 1. Copyright Elsevier 2008.

studies of Ivan Pavlov where he presented food paired with an auditory cue are the archetype of this form of positive reinforcement learning.

However, further consideration of this example begins to reveal some additional interesting aspects of positive reinforcement learning. For example, food only works as an effective US in a non-satiated animal. A fully-fed animal is very unlikely to be effectively trained with a food reward, and indeed in the case of over-consumption, food can serve as an aversive stimulus.

This illustrates the subjective nature of positive reinforcers—their reward value is contingent on the psychological state of the animal. This consideration must be carefully taken into account when designing experiments utilizing positive reinforcement.

C. Operant Conditioning of Positive Reinforcement

Positive reinforcement is also frequently and very effectively used in operant conditioning paradigms in the laboratory. Operant conditioning, you will recall, by definition involves deliberate action on the part of the experimental subject. The classic example of operant conditioning in laboratory rats is training the animal to lever-press for food. In the simplest example of this type of operant conditioning an animal is trained by presenting it with a food reward every time it presses a lever. This particular variation of operant conditioning is also referred to as instrumental conditioning, because it involves a mechanical manipulation on the part of the subject.

BOX 8

BIRDBRAINS

Avian species have been utilized in a large number of learning and memory-related studies, starting with early pioneering studies of operant conditioning in pigeons by B. F. Skinner (see Figure). A few examples of interesting avian memory-related behaviors that are currently studied in the laboratory are listed below. As you can see from the list, the pejorative "birdbrain" should be used with caution.

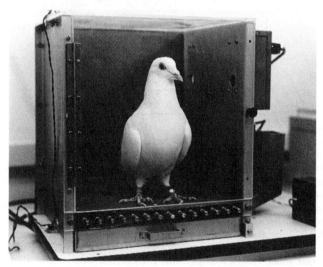

BOX 8   A pigeon in a "Skinner Box"—note that the left-hand indicator is lit, indicating that the animal should peck that spot. Photo courtesy of Robert W. Allen, Lafayette College, Easton, PA.

Species	Behavior	Type of Learning/Memory
Pigeon	Pecking, bar-pressing	Operant conditioning
Chicken (hatchling) (a feeding instinct)	Instinctive bead-pecking	Conditioned taste aversion
Canaries, Finches	Song learning	Declarative memory? Language?
Chickadees, Nutcrackers, Blue Jays	Seed caching	Spatial memory
Barn Owls	Visual system adaptation	Motor adaptation learning
Crows	Tool making	Motor learning, instrumental learning

Bar press = Reward — CUED

Bar press = No reward — UNCUED

FIGURE 13 Auditory cue reward learning. In this example of operant conditioning with positive reinforcement, the presentation of the auditory cue signals the animal that a food reward will be obtained when they press the lever in the cage.

However, there is an interesting variation of this procedure where the experimenter makes the food reward in response to the lever-press contingent on the presence of another distinct CS. Thus, for example, the animal can be trained that whenever an auditory (tone) CS is presented, lever-pressing results in the delivery of a food or sugar reward, while lever-pressing in the absence of the auditory CS yields no reward (see Figure 13). In other words, the animal is trained that lever-pressing results in reward delivery if, and only if, the CS is present.

However, consider the new components that this type of conditioning introduces. The learning process still involves the Pavlovian association between the auditory CS and the food reward. However, in addition there is now an association on the part of the animal between the auditory CS and the lever-pressing, and an association between the lever-pressing and the food reward. Overall this is a much more complex set of contingencies than simple Pavlovian conditioning, and these new contingencies introduce additional cognitive aspects to the task.

For example, the original tone CS–food association allows the tone CS to take on some of the rewarding components of the food. Thus, the tone can subsequently serve as a positive reinforcer in its own right, and after conditioning the animal will lever-press to trigger the tone coming on in the absence of the food reward. In this case the tone has become a *conditioned reinforcer*, wherein the auditory CS is essentially taking the place of the food as an effective reinforcer all by itself.

Principal brain areas involved in motivation, reward and positive reinforcement learning include the frontal cortex, the amygdala, and the nucleus accumbens. These three brain subregions are components of the limbic-corticostriatal loop (see Figure 14). In broad outline the frontal cortex processes sensory input,

the amygdala contributes to determining the positive or negative valence of the reinforcing stimulus, and the nucleus accumbens is involved in rewarding and reinforcing specific motor responses.

V. MEMORY SUPPRESSION—FORGETTING VERSUS EXTINCTION, AND LATENT INHIBITION

Associative conditioning instantiates a memory for a cause-and-effect relationship between the CS and the US, that is, it establishes a memory that the CS reliably predicts the upcoming occurrence of the US. In the natural setting, knowledge of a predictable relationship between environmental stimuli has great adaptive advantage. However, consider the situation in which the CS-US relationship changes such that the CS no longer reliably predicts the US. An animal would then be responding inappropriately to the CS, for example fleeing when unnecessary or worse, yet not fleeing because it thought the CS indicated a non-threatening situation. Clearly these types of behaviors would not be advantageous. These considerations bring up the issue of the necessity of memory systems to be able to "undo" a previously learned association. This undoing of associative memory can take one of two forms: *forgetting* and *extinction*.

Forgetting is the dissipation over time of a previously-formed memory. Forgetting conceptually can be due to a failure in the fidelity of the memory storage process, or a failure of recall mechanisms such that they can no longer trigger effective retrieval of the memory.

Extinction is the specific override of a prior memory in response to a new set of contingencies. In the context of associative conditioning, extinction is triggered by the situation that the CS no longer predicts the US. In the laboratory setting, extinction of learned associations is generally triggered by repetitive presentation of the CS without a subsequent presentation of the US. Over time, with repeated CS-alone presentations, the prior CS-US association is extinguished.

Learned associations generally are quite robust, and it is not unusual for extinction of an association to require many more CS-alone presentations than were required for the initial learning of the original CS-US contingency.

As was emphasized previously in this book, extinction is *not* forgetting. Nor is it a manifestation of an obliteration of the previously learned association. Experimentally, this can be demonstrated by delivering a "reminder" presentation of a CS-US pairing to a fully-extinguished animal. Generally, after a single

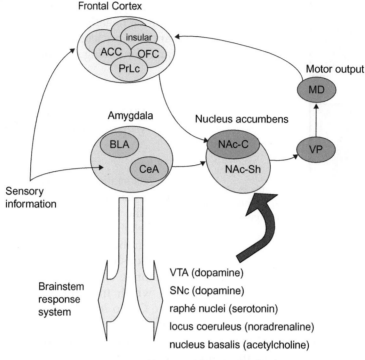

FIGURE 14 Simplified diagram of the limbic corticostriatal loop. (Abbreviations: ACC, anterior cingulated cortex; OFC, orbitofrontal cortex; PrLC, prelimbic cortex; BLA, basolateral amygdala; CeA, central amygdala; VTA, ventral tegmental area; SNc, substantia nigra pars compacta; NAc-C, nucleus accumbens core; NAc-Sh, nucleus accumbens shell; VP, ventral pallidum; MD, mediodorsal thalamus). The frontal cortex is functionally heterogeneous, and several frontal regions are involved in different aspects of instrumental responding. As discussed in the text, the PrLC, part of the medial prefrontal cortex, is involved in detecting the instrumental action-outcome contingency and is essential for the maintenance of goal-directed behavior. The functions of ACC are complex and are not described in detail here, but involve resolving response conflict and error detection, whereas the insular cortex, containing the primary gustatory cortex, encodes the primary sensory qualities of specific foods. The OFC plays a role in integrating changes in the incentive value of a reward with representations of the expected outcome, a function which is thought to depend on its connections with the BLA. The BLA is one of the primary structures involved in encoding CS-US associations and is necessary for the presentation of a CS to trigger retrieval of the motivational value of its associated US. It can work in concert with the CeA to influence brainstem function, arousal, and neurotransmitter release. As the "limbic-motor interface," the NAc combines information from both frontal and amygdala systems, as well as from other inputs, to generate motivational drive. The NAc-Sh signals the motivational properties of unconditioned (primary) reinforcers, whereas the NAc-C has a more pronounced role in mediating the motivational impact which Pavlovian conditioned stimuli have on behavior. Figure and legend from C. A. Winstanley and E. J. Nestler, *Learning and Memory: A Comprehensive Review*, Volume 4. Copyright Elsevier 2008.

reminder trial the CS-US association comes back as a fully manifest, robust response. In other words, a single CS-US pairing is sufficient to drive reinstatement of the original conditioned response. This observation emphasizes the fact that the prior CS-US association is a latent memory still stored in the CNS. However, extinction training leads to the original memory being overridden, and not expressed.

The existence of extinction as a unique cognitive process illustrates that memory recall or retrieval is not simply a passive process that does not impact the CNS. Rather, recall in many instances also sets in motion its own set of processes that allow the capacity for relearning of new contingencies alongside the previously learned ones. As has already been pointed out, the necessity for memories to be reconsolidated after retrieval (see Box 9) also illustrates the complex

and unique events set in motion during and after a memory recall episode.

Finally, there is one additional example of a suppressive form of memory that has already been discussed in an earlier chapter, latent inhibition. Latent inhibition refers to the capacity of prior experience to suppress (inhibit) new learning. The "latent" in latent inhibition refers to the attribute that the process is experimentally not observable or demonstrable until one observes a failure of learning in a subsequent test. Regarding associative conditioning paradigms, latent inhibition is generated by repeated presentations of CS alone without a subsequent contingent US presentation. The repeated CS-alone presentations diminish or completely block the subsequent capability of the animal to learn a CS-US association when they experience CS-US training trials.

BOX 9

RECONSOLIDATION OF MEMORIES

What if every time you recalled a memory you made that memory subject to erasure? A frightening thought, certainly. The idea also seems somewhat at odds with our perception of consistency in our own memories—recalling them seems to make them stronger, not weaker. Nevertheless, recent provocative studies have suggested that every time we recall a specific memory, we make it necessary for that memory to be re-established. The word used to describe this attribute of memory is "reconsolidation" in reference to the well-known attribute that long-term memories, when initially formed, are labile and subject to disruption over a period of hours. It appears that previously established long-term memories also are subject to disruption, specifically during that period immediately after each time they are recollected.

The most definitive recent experiment concerning memory reconsolidation was performed by Karim Nader and Glenn Schafe in Joe LeDoux's laboratory (8), although important work in this area has also been performed by the laboratories of Susan Sara, Yadin Dudai, and Alcino Silva, among others. Nader et al. studied memory reconsolidation using cued fear conditioning in rats which, as we discussed in this chapter, is an amygdala-dependent process. Basically, Nader et al. found that when an animal is re-exposed to a conditioned stimulus (an auditory cue in this case), which of course elicits recollection of a prior CS-US pairing, restorage of that memory can be disrupted by inhibiting protein synthesis in the amygdala. The same memory is impervious to an equivalent period of protein synthesis inhibition as long as the animal is not stimulated to recall the CS-US pairing during that time. The implication of these studies is that reactivated memories must be put back into long-term storage via a protein synthesis-dependent process similar to that used during the initial consolidation period; hence, the use of the term reconsolidation.

There are of course a great number of questions raised by these studies. Is the reconsolidation mechanism identical to the initial consolidation mechanism? Are all long-term memories subject to reconsolidation after each recollection, or is this mechanism restricted to particular brain areas or memory types? Might disruption of this process contribute to memory pathologies such as aging-related memory loss? Could pharmacologic means be used as a therapeutic intervention in "pathologic" memory such as post-traumatic stress disorder? Future studies will hopefully lead to new insights into these and other questions concerning this fascinating phenomenon.

VI. SUMMARY

In this chapter we have discussed various aspects of associative, operant, and instrumental conditioning. We have seen that these types of learning can be promoted by either positive or negative reinforcement. In two instances, cued fear conditioning and eye-blink conditioning, we have been able to explore the circuit and cellular basis of associative conditioning in the mammalian CNS. In a series of inset boxes, the rich variety of ethologically relevant associative learning paradigms that have been studied using invertebrate animal models were described. These various model systems and studies of associative conditioning allow several broad conclusions to be drawn.

1. Both increases and decreases in synaptic strength can subserve memory. Increased synaptic strength *does not* necessarily imply learning, and decreased synaptic strength *does not* necessarily imply forgetting or extinction.

2. Associative conditioning relies on the unmasking of a latent circuit. Moreover, the two relevant pathways, the CS pathway and the US pathway, must intersect somewhere in the nervous system in order for an association to be formed between the two stimuli.

3. Associative conditioning can be mediated by both positive and negative reinforcers, and in the case of the reward system the psychological state of the animal may determine whether a given stimulus is perceived as a positive or negative stimulus.

4. Despite their apparent simplicity, invertebrate animals exhibit an impressive array of capacities for associative learning. The adaptive power and survival value of associative conditioning is illustrated by its widespread presence in the animal kingdom.

5. Learned associations can be unlearned. The mechanisms for this unlearning are unique and rarely involve erasure of the prior memory trace; rather, the prior memory is overridden by a newly-acquired dominant trace.

Further Reading

Baxter, D. A., and Byrne, J. H. (2006). "Feeding behavior of *Aplysia*: a model system for comparing cellular mechanisms of classical and operant conditioning." *Learn. Mem.* 13(6):669–680.

Berry, J., Krause, W. C., and Davis, R. L. (2008). "Olfactory memory traces in *Drosophila*." *Prog. Brain Res.* 169:293–304.

Bolhuis, J. J., and Gahr, M. (2006). "Neural mechanisms of birdsong memory." *Nat. Rev. Neurosci.* 7(5):347–357.

Christian, K. M., and Thompson, R. F. (2003). "Neural substrates of eyeblink conditioning: acquisition and retention." *Learn. Mem.* 10(6):427–455.

Crow, T. (2004). "Pavlovian conditioning of *Hermissenda*: current cellular, molecular, and circuit perspectives." *Learn. Mem.* 11(3):229–238.

du Lac, S., Raymond, J. L., Sejnowski, T. J., and Lisberger, S. G. (1995). "Learning and memory in the vestibulo-ocular reflex." *Annu. Rev. Neurosci.* 18:409–441.

Ito, M. (2002). "The molecular organization of cerebellar long-term depression." *Nat. Rev. Neurosci.* 3(11):896–902.

Ito, M. (2000). "Mechanisms of motor learning in the cerebellum." *Brain Res.* 886(1–2):237–245.

Kelley, A. E. (2004). "Memory and addiction: shared neural circuitry and molecular mechanisms." *Neuron* 44(1):161–179.

Lang, P. J., Davis, M., and Ohman, A. (2000). "Fear and anxiety: animal models and human cognitive psychophysiology." *J. Affect. Disord.* 61(3):137–159.

LeDoux, J. E. (2000). "Emotion circuits in the brain." *Annu. Rev. Neurosci.* 23:155–184.

Lukowiak, K., Sangha, S., Scheibenstock, A., Parvez, K., McComb, C., Rosenegger, D., Varshney, N., and Sadamoto, H. (2003). "A molluscan model system in the search for the engram." *J. Physiol. Paris.* 97(1):69–76.

Medina, J. F., Repa, J. C., Mauk, M. D., and LeDoux, J. E. (2002). "Parallels between cerebellum- and amygdala-dependent conditioning." *Nat. Rev. Neurosci.* 3(2):122–131.

Menzel, R. (2001). "Searching for the memory trace in a mini-brain, the honeybee." *Learn. Mem.* 8(2):53–62.

Myers, K. M., and Davis, M. (2007). "Mechanisms of fear extinction." *Mol. Psychiatry.* 12(2):120–150.

Phelps, E. A., and LeDoux, J. E. (2005). "Contributions of the amygdala to emotion processing: from animal models to human behavior." *Neuron* 48(2):175–187.

Rodrigues, S. M., Schafe, G. E., and LeDoux, J. E. (2004). "Molecular mechanisms underlying emotional learning and memory in the lateral amygdala." *Neuron* 44(1):75–91.

Journal Club Articles

Krupa, D. J., Thompson, J. K., and Thompson, R. F. (1993). "Localization of a memory trace in the mammalian brain." *Science* 260(5110):989–991.

McKernan, M. G., and Shinnick-Gallagher, P. (1997). "Fear conditioning induces a lasting potentiation of synaptic currents *in vitro*." *Nature* 390:607–611.

Rogan, M. T., Staubli, U. V., and LeDoux, J. E. (1997). "Fear conditioning induces associative long-term potentiation in the amygdala." *Nature* 390:604–607.

For more information—relevant topic chapters from: John H. Byrne (Editor-in-Chief) (2008). *Learning and Memory: A Comprehensive Reference*. Oxford: Academic Press (ISBN 978-0-12-370509-9). (1.06 Jozefowiez, J., and Staddon, J. E. R. *Operant Behavior*. pp. 75–101; 1.10 Blaisdell, A. P. *Cognitive Dimension of Operant Learning*. pp. 173–195; 1.17 Marler, P. *Bird Song Learning*. pp. 315–325; 1.18 Domjan, M. *Adaptive Specializations and Generality of the Laws of Classical and Instrumental Conditioning*. pp. 327–340; 1.19 Cheng, K., and Crystal, J. D. *Learning to Time Intervals*. pp. 341–363; 1.25 De Marco, R. J., and Menzel, R. *Learning and Memory in Communication and Navigation in Insects*. pp. 477–498; 1.28 Heisenberg, M., and Gerber, B. *Behavioral Analysis of Learning and Memory in* Drosophila. pp. 549–559; 1.29 Giurfa, M. *Behavioral and Neural Analysis of Associate Learning in the Honeybee*. pp. 561–585; 1.30 Benjamin, P. R., and Kemenes, G. *Behavioral and Circuit Analysis of Learning and Memory in Mollusks*. pp. 587–604; 1.31 Borrelli, L., and Fiorito, G. *Behavioral Analysis of Learning and Memory in Cephalopods*. pp. 605–627; 1.36 Ostlund, S. B., Winterbauer, N. E., and Balleine, B. W. *Theory of Reward Systems*. pp. 701–720; 2.34 Lee, T. D., and Schmidt, R. A. *Motor Learning and Memory*. pp. 645–662; 3.11 Weinberger, N. M. *Cortical Plasticity in Associative Learning and Memory*. pp. 187–218; 3.14 Ranganath, C., and Blumenfeld, R. S. *Prefrontal Cortex and Memory*. pp. 261–279; 3.15 Chiba, A. A., and Quinn, L. K. *Basal Forebrain and Memory*. pp. 281–301; 3.18 Packard, M. G. *Neurobiology of Procedural Learning in Animals*. pp. 341–356; 3.19 Poulos, A. M., Christian, K. M., and Thompson, R. F. *Procedural Learning: Classical Conditioning*. pp. 357–381; 3.20 Cullen, K. E. *Procedural Learning: VOR*. pp. 383–402; 3.21 Nudo, R. J. *Neurophysiology of Motor Skill Learning*. pp. 403–421; 3.22 Sanes, J. N. *Cerebral Cortex: Motor Learning*. pp. 423–439; 3.23 Mooney, R., Prather, J., and Roberts, T. *Neurophysiology of Birdsong Learning*. pp. 441–474; 3.24 Maren, S. *Emotional Learning: Animals*. pp. 475–502; 4.06 Muller, U. *Molecular Mechanism of Associative Learning in the Bee*. pp. 91–101; 4.07 Isabel, G., and Preat, T. *Molecular and System Analysis of Olfactory Memory in* Drosophila. pp. 103–118; 4.08 Crow, T., Tian, L. -M., and Xue-Bian, J. -J. *Molecular Mechanisms of Associative Learning in* Hermissenda. pp. 119–132; 4.09 Kemenes, G. *Molecular Mechanism of Associative Learning in Lymnaea*. pp. 133–148; 4.10 Lorenzetti, F. D., and Byrne, J. H. *Cellular Mechanisms of Associative Learning in* Aplysia. pp. 149–156; 4.11 Schafe, G. E., and LeDoux, J. E. *Neural and Molecular Mechanisms of Fear Memory*. pp. 157–192; 4.12 Winstanley, C. A., and Nestler, E. J. *The Molecular Mechanisms of Reward*. pp. 193–215; 4.13 Rosenblum, K. *Conditioned Taste Aversion and Taste Learning: Molecular Mechanisms*. pp. 217–234; 4.40 Mozzachiodi, R., and Byrne, J. H. *Plasticity of Intrinsic Excitability as a Mechanism for Memory Storage*. pp. 829–838; 4.41 Jessberger, S., Aimone, J. B., and Gage, F. H. *Neurogenesis*. pp. 839–858.)

References

1. Schafe, G. E., Atkins, C. M., Swank, M. W., Bauer, E. P., Sweatt, J. D., and LeDoux, J. E. (2000). "Activation of ERK/MAP kinase in the amygdala is required for memory consolidation of pavlovian fear conditioning." *J. Neurosci.* 20:8177–8187.

2. McKernan, M. G., and Shinnick-Gallagher, P. (1997). "Fear conditioning induces a lasting potentiation of synaptic currents *in vitro*." *Nature* 390:607–611.

3. Rogan, M. T., Staubli, U. V., and LeDoux, J. E. (1997). "Fear conditioning induces associative long-term potentiation in the amygdala." *Nature* 390:604–607.

4. Blair, H. T., Schafe, G. E., Bauer, E. P., Rodrigues, S. M., and LeDoux, J. E. (2001). "Synaptic plasticity in the lateral amygdala: a cellular hypothesis of fear conditioning." *Learn. Mem.* 8:229–242.

5. Rogan, M. T., and LeDoux, J. E. (1995). "LTP is accompanied by commensurate enhancement of auditory-evoked responses in a fear conditioning circuit." *Neuron* 15:127–136.

6. Ito, M. (2001). "Cerebellar long-term depression: characterization, signal transduction, and functional roles." *Physiol. Rev.* 81:1143–1195.

7. Carey, M., and Lisberger, S. (2002). "Embarrassed, but not depressed: eye opening lessons for cerebellar learning." *Neuron* 35:223–226.

8. Nader, K., Schafe, G. E., and LeDoux, J. E. (2000). "Fear memories require protein synthesis in the amygdala for reconsolidation after retrieval." *Nature* 406:722–726.

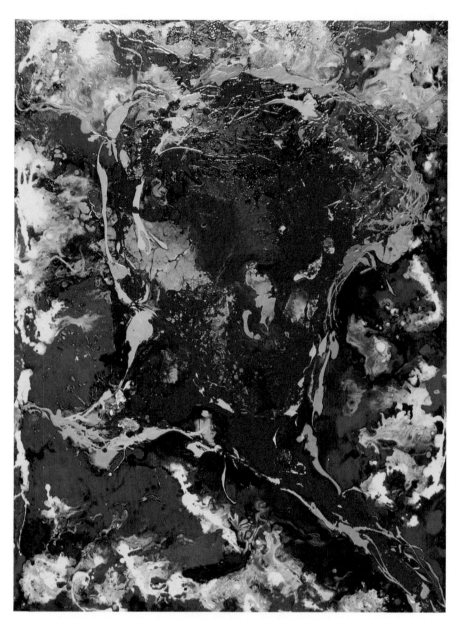

Grid Cell

J. David Sweatt, acrylic on canvas, 2008–2009

Hippocampal Function in Cognition

I. INTRODUCTION

In Chapter 2 we discussed one of the principal functions of the hippocampus, allowing memory consolidation. This is the classic role of the hippocampus—to participate in the formation of long-term memories by helping to convert short-term sensory signals into long-term or permanently encoded memories. It is important to distinguish between memory consolidation and memory storage. The hippocampus generally does not store information for extended periods of time, but rather serves as an intermediate-duration memory buffer that is involved in maintaining memories until they are transferred for more permanent storage in various regions of the cerebral cortex. This is referred to as *consolidation* of memories, that is, consolidation is the process by which memories are converted to very long-lasting forms.

Keep in mind that shorter-term memories also undergo consolidation. The hippocampus is clearly involved in the consolidation of memories lasting from 24 hours to a lifetime, and likely is also involved in the consolidation of memories of even shorter duration. This implies that there may be multiple hippocampus-dependent memory consolidation processes that subserve memories of various durations—this is an open question at this time.

Thus far in the book we have touched on various examples of hippocampus-dependent learning and memory paradigms. For example, in Chapter 4 we discussed a wide variety of rodent learning and memory paradigms that are hippocampus-dependent. In this chapter we will delve into the role of the hippocampus in animal behavior in more detail, drawing specific examples from the literature for each of three categories of function. These three categories involve the role of the hippocampus in information processing and cognition. Specifically we will discuss how the hippocampus is involved in perceptual processing of information regarding space, timing, and relationships among objects. The theme for this chapter, therefore, is that the hippocampus serves a role in multimodal information processing, in addition to its role in memory consolidation (see Figure 1).

Note that these three functions (space, timing, relationships) can conceptually be considered very differently from the classic function of the hippocampus, subserving memory consolidation. The first three functions are related to real-time information processing, perception of environmental stimuli, and cognition in general. This information processing role of the hippocampus can be considered independently of the specific memory-formation aspect of its role in memory consolidation. As a first

**Functions of the
Hippocampus**

• Cognitive processing:
Space
Timing
Relationships

• Memory consolidation

FIGURE 1   Summary of functions of the hippocampus.

approximation it may be useful to think of the first three functions as what is going on *inside* the hippocampus on a minute-to-minute basis, while thinking of the memory consolidation function as what happens to allow the hippocampus to later send its processed messages *outside* to other parts of the brain for long-term storage.

Chapter 2, where we discussed the hippocampus in memory consolidation, plus the overview in this chapter of the three additional general functions of the hippocampus, will prepare us for the next chapter where we will begin to discuss synaptic plasticity in the hippocampal circuit and its attendant cellular physiology. This is in order to begin to explore how the hippocampus achieves its various functions as a signal integrator and as a cellular memory store for subsequent downloading of information to the longer-term storage areas of the cortex. In this chapter we will talk about what the hippocampus does—in the next chapter and for most of the rest of the book we will discuss current ideas about how it does it at the cellular and molecular levels.

II. STUDYING THE HIPPOCAMPUS

If you are interested in studying the roles of the hippocampus in the behaving animal, how do you even begin to go about it? One approach is to remove the hippocampus or inactivate it and assess the cognitive and behavioral consequences of this experimental manipulation. These types of studies were the first to lead to an appreciation of the role of the hippocampus in memory consolidation (reviewed in 1). In fact, studies we discussed in Chapter 2 concerning patient H. M. were breakthrough studies that led to the appreciation of the importance of the hippocampus in converting a short-lived memory into a long-lasting one (2).

A second approach to studying hippocampal function is quite different. If you want to know what is going on in the hippocampus of an animal that is learning, why not stick an electrode in its hippocampus and directly monitor the cellular firing pattern?

This type of approach has been exploited to great effect of late, and in this chapter we will talk about new and important insights into the role of the hippocampus in the behaving animal that have been generated using these techniques.

A. Hippocampal Anatomy

First, a refresher of the basic anatomical structure of the hippocampus will be helpful (see Figure 2). As we have already discussed (see Chapter 2), the hippocampus receives direct or indirect inputs from all the sensory areas of the cortex, including the areas of the cortex involved in late stages of visual information processing, the auditory cortex, and the somatosensory cortex. The hippocampus also receives fairly direct input from the olfactory system via the olfactory bulb. Sensory information of these various sorts is funneled down to the hippocampus via the perirhinal and entorhinal cortices; these are the cortical areas in the immediate anatomical vicinity of the hippocampus near the rhinal fissure in the temporal lobe.

The outputs of the perirhinal and entorhinal cortices then project to the dentate gyrus and the hippocampus proper (these two are referred to jointly as the hippocampal formation). There are four anatomical subdivisions of the hippocampus: areas CA1; CA2; CA3; and CA4. CA1 and CA3 are the largest and most easily identified. The principal neurons in the CA regions are the pyramidal neurons, which comprise about 90% of all the neurons in the CA regions of the hippocampal formation. The output neurons of the hippocampus are the CA1 pyramidal neurons—it is via these axons that information leaves the hippocampus proper. The axons of CA1 neurons project back to the entorhinal cortex, as well as other structures. The hippocampus also receives a number of relatively diffuse modulatory projections from various areas of the brain stem. These projections include axon terminals releasing norepinephrine (NE), acetylcholine (ACh), and 5-hydroxytryptamine (5HT, also known as serotonin).

Via this general circuit, sensory information enters the hippocampus, is processed in the local hippocampal circuit, and then goes out of the hippocampus and ultimately back up into the cortex. As part of this process, information first passes into and subsequently back-tracks its way once again through the entorhinal and perirhinal cortices, as well as the hippocampus (see Figure 3). I emphasize this because it is important to remember that these cortical areas immediately adjacent to the hippocampal formation are functionally an extension of the hippocampus (and *vice versa*). By and large nothing gets into or out of the hippocampus without passing through the neurons

Hippocampal connectivity in the CNS

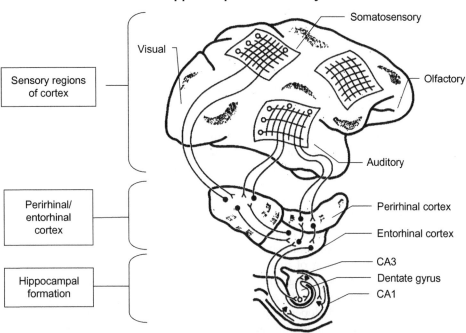

FIGURE 2 Hippocampal connectivity in the CNS. Illustration of the pathway from sensory perceiving regions of the cortex through the perirhinal and entorhinal cortices to the hippocampal formation. Figure adapted from Squire and Zola-Morgan (1). Copyright American Association for the Advancement of Science.

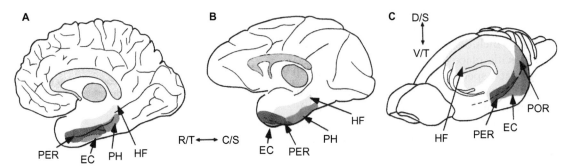

FIGURE 3 Comparative views of the hippocampal system for the human (left), monkey (middle), and rat (right). The upper panel shows the relevant structures in lateral views of the human brain (A), the monkey brain (B), and the rodent brain (C). PER = perirhinal cortex; EC = entorhinal cortex; PH = parahippocampal area; HF = hippocampal formation. Figure adapted from Burwell, R. D., Witter, M. P., and Amaral, D. G. (1995). Copyright Elsevier 2008.

in the entorhinal and perirhinal cortex. Throughout the literature (and this book) there are many references to "hippocampus-dependent" processes. These processes might equally well be described as entorhinal cortex-dependent or perirhinal cortex-dependent. The hippocampal formation and its adjacent cortical regions function in unison in order to execute the sophisticated cognitive and memory processing that is detailed below.

III. HIPPOCAMPAL FUNCTION IN COGNITION

Thus, one major role of the hippocampus and associated cortices is to process a wide variety of sensory information, which we will discuss in this section. The second general function, to download information into the cortex for long-term storage, we will deal with in the final section of this chapter. The types of information that the hippocampus deals with, at least as a first approximation, can be divided into three different categories. First, space—for example the hippocampus is known to be involved in processing spatial information as described in Chapter 4, where we talked about hippocampus-dependent maze learning. The second category is timing—for example, with trace-associative conditioning. Animals can learn associations that have no intervening time period between CS and US just fine without a hippocampus. However, introducing a delay period between the presentation of the CS and the presentation of the US brings the hippocampus into play. Thus, the hippocampus appears to be critical for allowing the animal to make an association between two stimuli separated in time. Finally, complex associations are hippocampus-dependent; the hippocampus is involved in an animal learning complex contingencies. For example, one specific type of learning of this sort that we will return to later is an animal learning how to predict whether or not a container labeled with a specific scent contains a hidden food reward, depending on recent experience. Learning these types of complicated associations and contingencies brings the hippocampus into play. In the following sections we address specific examples for each of these categories, illustrating the categories with specific examples from the literature.

A. Space

When an animal is learning about spatial relationships and positions it utilizes its hippocampus. Specific examples include: learning that a hidden platform is in a specific place (Morris water maze learning); learning that a specific place is a bad place to be (contextual fear conditioning); learning that one place is different from another (context discrimination); and learning the order of left/right turns to take in order to navigate a maze (e.g., the more complicated Lashley mazes).

What happens in the hippocampus when an animal is placed in a novel environment and learns about that environment? This is a question that has intrigued neuroscientists for decades, and many beautiful studies over the years have given us nice insights into a number of specific cellular phenomena that occur in the hippocampus when an animal is exploring and learning about a new environment. Most of these studies have used direct electrical recording of hippocampal electrical activity during exploration of a new environment.

Early studies in this area used electroencephalographic (EEG) recordings. EEG recording techniques allow the monitoring of the electrical activity of fairly large populations of cells, by monitoring the mild electric current that flows between and among active

neurons as they fire, due to the influx and efflux of cellular ions. Because EEG recording monitors populations of neurons, the technique is best at detecting the synchronous firing of groups of neurons.

Pioneering EEG studies identified and defined rhythmic firing in the hippocampus when an animal is exploring a novel environment (3). One pronounced example of this that has received much attention is rhythmic firing at the 4–8 Hz (4–8 per second) rate in rodent hippocampus. This type of rhythmic firing around the 5 Hz range is referred to as theta frequency firing, or more commonly as the "theta rhythm" (see Figure 4). The theta rhythm occurs during locomotion and exploration of a new environment, and many experiments have linked the theta rhythm firing with various spatial learning tasks. These initial studies indicated that specific patterns of neuronal firing in the hippocampus are correlated with spatial and contextual learning in animals.

But what is happening at the level of the firing of individual neurons? For example, suppose you put

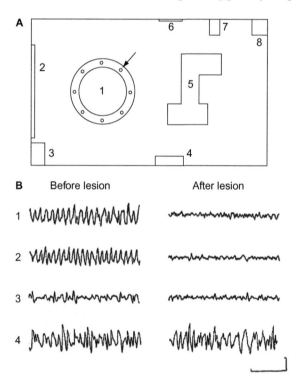

FIGURE 4 Theta pattern in hippocampal EEG. EEG study in which electrodes were implanted to monitor the aggregate electrical activity in a population of neurons during exploration behavior. (A) Plan view of the testing room (5.5 by 9.1 meters). Contents: (1) circular maze; (2) elevated ventilating duct; (3) table; (4) animal cages; (5) test console; (6) door; (7) sink; (8) cabinet. Overhead fluorescent lights provide 330 lumen/m^2 of illumination at the level of the maze. (B) Recordings obtained during: (1) voluntary movement; (2) REM sleep; (3) still-alert; (4) slow-wave sleep. The recordings before and after a medial septal lesion was made which eliminated theta rhythm were from the same electrode. Time and voltage calibration: 1 second and 500 μV. Data and figure reproduced from Winson (3).

an animal in an open round field with visual cues in specific places and allow it to learn about its environment. What happens to the firing patterns of its hippocampal neurons? In classic studies O'Keefe and Dostrovsky identified "place" cells in the hippocampus (4–6). In these experiments the investigators recorded cell firing within the hippocampus by using implanted extracellular electrodes that could monitor the firing of single cells, referred to as single "units." Recording from neurons in the dorsal hippocampus, O'Keefe and Dostrovsky discovered cells in the freely-moving rat that fired only in a specific location within an open field or maze. They referred to these cells as "place cells" and coined the additional nomenclature of "place field" to describe the specific location in the environment where the cell selectively fires (see Figure 5).

Although place cells fire in a way that is highly correlated with the animal's position, these cells fire predominantly when the animal is moving in only one direction (Figure 6). The firing fields are very stable over days and months once established, and place fields are established reasonably quickly (7–8), on the order of a few minutes to 1–2 hours (keep in mind that some consolidation process is likely involved). A given place cell can have more than one place field within an apparatus or in two apparati, in other words, a place cell is not exclusively linked to a specific location but may be called upon in connection with one location in one environment and in connection with another location in another environment.

What are place cells? Place cells are hippocampal pyramidal neurons. The "unit" firing recorded in these early studies was a manifestation of action potential firing in pyramidal neurons in the CA regions of the hippocampus. We will return to these cells and their synaptic and biophysical properties in greater detail in the next two chapters.

The firing pattern is not absolute but relative—for example, place cell firing depends on the animal's perception of visual cues. This can be demonstrated fairly simply by rotating the cues clockwise or counterclockwise between testing trials for a given animal, but keeping their position relative to each other constant. When the cues are rotated the place field for a given place cell stays constant in relation to the cues (see Figure 7), but is independent of the animal's absolute location. This experimental result eliminates the simplest explanation for place fields—the rat is not like a homing pigeon that can reference the earth's magnetic field for navigation.

But the rotated cues experiment has a much greater implication. Place cell firing is an example of cognition. The animal exhibits a specific cellular firing pattern in its hippocampus that depends on its perception of the environment. The place cell firing is in no way dependent on absolute position in space—it is dependent on the animal's perceived position, based on its interpretation of visual and other cues in the environment.

In fact, the place field is somewhat of an abstraction (9–10). Suppose you train an animal in a small circular chamber and allow place fields to develop. If you place the same animal in a much larger round chamber with the same relative visual cues, the place field stays constant relative to the cues, at least for a subset of place cells (see Figure 8). To me this is a mind-boggling example of cognitive processing; it is a direct demonstration that a cellular firing pattern can reflect a generalized construct, an abstract representation of the animal's environment.

Thus, place fields are manifest as a burst of action potential firing in a CA1 pyramidal neuron when an animal enters a *perceived* spatial location. Or, stated more precisely, place fields are manifest as a burst of action potentials when an animal enters what it

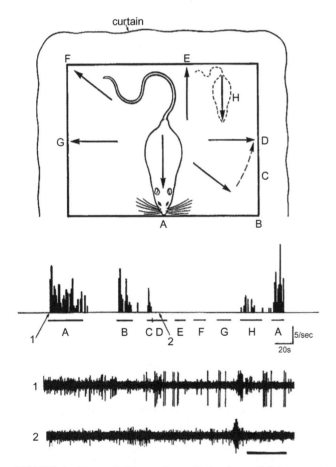

FIGURE 5 Place cell firing patterns. Early place cell firing report from O'Keefe and Dostrovsky (1971). Place cells only fired in position (A), as shown in top diagram. Below, histogram of firing at each location in the diagram and raw firing patterns during periods marked 1 and 2 in the histogram. Figure reproduced from O'Keefe and Dostrovsky (4).

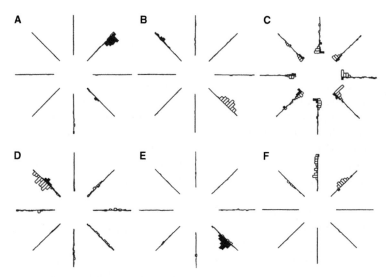

FIGURE 6   Direction selectivity in place cell firing. Typical directional "place fields" exhibited by pyramidal cells while rats move about the radial eight-arm maze. Arms are represented as pulled away from center to facilitate viewing. Spatial firing rates are broken down according to radial direction of motion (open and filled histograms represent outward and inward, respectively). Although, in extremely simplified visual environments, hippocampal cells are much more poorly directionally tuned, in most situations firing in the direction opposite to the preferred one is rarely significantly different from background. Data, figure, and legend reproduced from McNaughton, Chen, and Markus (26).

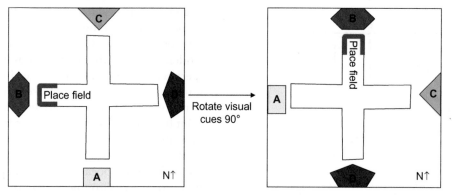

FIGURE 7   Place cells follow rotation of visual cues. Diagram of four-arm radial maze set-up. In this test the maze remains stationary while the visual cues on the walls are rotated 90° clockwise. When the animal is placed in the first set-up the place field is in the arm closest to the cue marked (B) (the western arm before the rotation). When the cues are rotated the place field is again in the arm closest to the cue marked (B) (the northern arm after the rotation). This indicates that the place field is located by the animal's relationship to the distal visual cues, not the animal's absolute location in the room.

perceives to be a particular spatial location. However, it is critically important to keep in mind that the ordering of this sentence may be exactly reversed. It is an equally valid interpretation, because the data are based on correlations, that the burst of action potential firing leads to the animal perceiving itself as being in a certain place. In other words, we might equally well say that an animal perceives itself to be in a particular location whenever a set of hippocampal place cells fires a burst of action potentials. As we learn more about the hippocampus it will hopefully become clearer whether the hippocampus is "upstream" or "downstream" of spatial perception. In the limit we may find that it is exactly in the middle of spatial

perception, that is, that place cell firing is *the* mechanism of spatial perception (see Box 1).

This is the fundamental quandary of the cognitive neurobiologist, and it shows up over and over again in the contemporary literature in experiments involving monitoring of cellular firing (or fMRI signals) in real-time in response to environmental stimulation. Where does sensory processing end and cognition begin? How does cellular firing get translated into an abstract construct in the brain? The real potential of beginning to answer these types of questions, which really are the modern reformulation of the philosophical mind-body problem that has intrigued mankind for millennia, is one of the best reasons I can think of

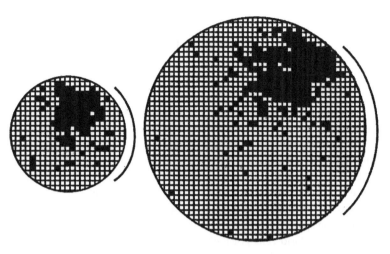

FIGURE 8 Place cells fire in a corresponding location in larger round chamber. Place field in original (left) and larger (right) circular open field is recorded from a hippocampal neuron of a rat searching for food. The larger open field maintains the same orientation in relation to the visual cue (black arc) which is the same size relative to the chamber as in the smaller version. The place field recorded from the rat is shown with black squares and was recorded first in the small chamber then in the large chamber. The place fields are in the same position relative to the visual cue in each chamber, and also the place field is enlarged in the larger chamber. Data and figure reproduced from Muller and Kubie (9).

to be particularly excited about being a neuroscientist in the contemporary era.

B. Timing

The hippocampus is involved not only in the processing of spatial information; it is also involved in what I will refer to, for lack of a better term, as processing temporal information. This does not necessarily mean that the hippocampus is involved in encoding time itself (which could also be true), but rather I am referring to the hippocampus being involved in temporally-dependent learning, such as trace associative conditioning and remembering the order of events, and also that the hippocampus itself exhibits time- and experience-dependent alterations in its cellular firing properties. In this section we will discuss a few examples of timing-dependency of hippocampal function and information processing. We will start with an example of experience-dependent alterations in the behavior of hippocampal place cells, as an example of changes in the hippocampus that occur with repeated environmental signals over time. In the second section we will discuss the important role of the hippocampus in the formation of time-dependent associations, by and large using trace associative conditioning as our example.

In the last section we discussed the impressive, rapid formation of hippocampal place fields when an animal is introduced into a new environment. These place fields are, of course, manifest as a burst of action potential firing in a CA1 pyramidal neuron when an animal enters a particular spatial location (or more

precisely when an animal enters what it perceives to be a particular spatial location). What happens to place cell firing over time when the animal re-enters that same location? Are there time-dependent changes in place cell firing properties?

Work from the laboratories of Matt Wilson, Gyorgi Buzsaki, Bruce McNaughton, and Carol Barnes, along with several others, has given us clear answers to these two questions. There are clearly time-dependent changes in place cell firing properties that depend on the animal's experience. Re-entering the same place field repetitively over time leads to several pronounced effects on cellular firing patterns, at the level of the individual neuron. These changes are a clear example of experience-dependent changes in the firing properties of hippocampal pyramidal neurons, and as described above I use them to illustrate one sort of "time"-dependent information processing by the hippocampus.

Three specific examples of such cellular changes are as follows (see Figure 9). One, with repeated re-entry into the place field of a pyramidal neuron there is an increase in the place cell's firing rate on successive re-exposure (11). Two, with re-entry into a place field there is a decrease in the latency of the time required for firing the first action potential in a place cell's burst of action potentials (11). Three, the extent of dendritic action potential back-propagation increases over time with experience in the place field (12) (we will return to back-propagating action potentials in much more detail in later chapters). Thus, the first entry into a place sets up a hippocampal neuronal place field, but there are subsequent time- and experience-dependent changes in place cell action potential firing properties as well.

BOX 1

GRID CELLS IN THE ENTORHINAL CORTEX

As was emphasized in the main text, sensory input from the sensory cortex converges on the entorhinal cortex and is then passed on to the hippocampus. Thus, the entorhinal cortex is a bridge between the primary sensory cortex and the hippocampus. Recent exciting studies have demonstrated a role for the entorhinal cortex in spatial processing of sensory information (see Further Reading).

The principal cell type encoding spatial information in the entorhinal cortex is the grid cell. Grid cells got their name from the property of firing with peak firing rates occurring at regular intervals when the animal is exploring an open field. Grid cells are somewhat similar to hippocampal place cells, except that instead of firing when the animal is in a single locale, they fire whenever the animal is at any one of a number of points that form a regular grid-like pattern (see Figure). Grid cells appear to encode a repetitive, hexagonally-based representation of space. The selective firing of an individual grid cell has been shown to depend on an animal's perception of its spatial location, based on visual cues. Interestingly, grid cell firing patterns are also stable when the animal is placed in complete darkness, suggesting a stability and constancy to the pattern that may assist the animal with dark navigation and an internal representation of its location.

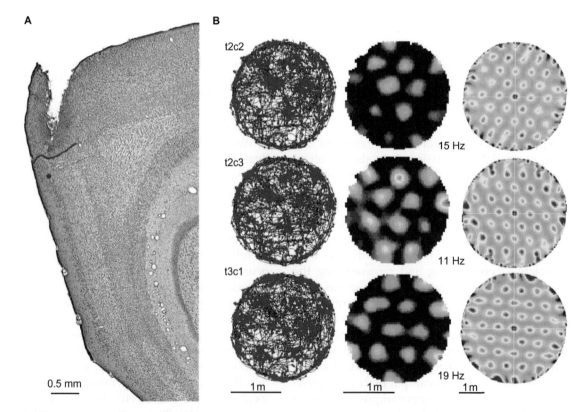

BOX 1   Grid cells in the entorhinal cortex. This figure illustrates the firing properties of a grid cell in the entorhinal cortex. In this experiment the firing of neurons in the entorhinal cortex were monitored *in vivo* in behaving animals using a tetrode (4-unit) recording electrode. In these experiments animals were exploring a circular open field with visual spatial cues corresponding to four spatial directions. (A) Sagittal Nissl-stained section indicating the recording location (red dot) in layer II of the dorsomedial entorhinal cortex (dMEC). Red line indicates border to postrhinal cortex. (B) Firing fields of three simultaneously recorded cells at the dot in **A** during 30 min of running in a large circular enclosure. Cell names refer to tetrode (t) and cell (c). Left, trajectory of the rat (black) with superimposed spike locations (red). Middle, color-coded rate map with the peak rate indicated. Red is maximum, dark blue is zero. Right, spatial autocorrelation for each rate map indicates that a given cell is highly likely to fire at specific points in a hexagonal array pattern in the open field. The color scale is from blue ($r = -1$) through green ($r = 0$) to red ($r = 1$). Figure and legend adapted from (27). Copyright Macmillan Publishers Ltd (2005).

The mechanisms underlying this experience-dependent alteration in hippocampal pyramidal neuron properties is a subject of active investigation. For now, suffice it to say that intriguing mechanisms that could be contributing to these changes include activity-dependent changes in sodium or potassium channels in place cell neurons, changes in neuromodulatory inputs (e.g., acetylcholinergic or noradrenergic inputs) to the hippocampus, or activity-dependent synaptic plasticity within the hippocampus itself (12).

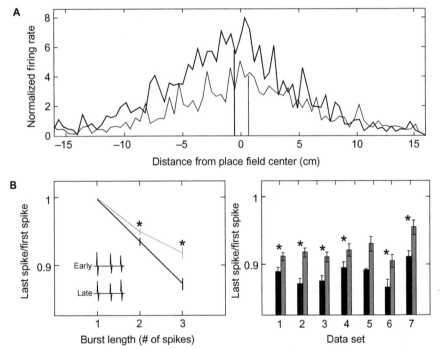

FIGURE 9 Experience-dependent changes in place cell firing. (A) Histogram of the total firing rate at various distances from the place field center during the first and the last visitation to the same place in an environment (light curve, visit 1; solid curve, visit 17. Bin width = 0.41 cm, which corresponds to the resolution of the position tracking camera). Firing rates increase as the animal approaches the place field center. (B) Activity-dependent attenuation in spike amplitude is reduced with experience. The average ($\pm$SE) amplitude attenuation during high-frequency bursts for a population of simultaneously recorded cells is shown on the left. The amplitude of the last spike in a burst is expressed as a fraction of the amplitude of the first spike, and is plotted as a function of the number of spikes in the burst. The black line plots the average attenuation for the animal's first four minutes in the environment, and the gray line plots the attenuation for the animal's last four minutes. The amount of attenuation is reduced with experience. On the right, the average attenuation for bursts of three spikes for the first four minutes of exploration in a familiar environment are shown as black bars, and for the last four minutes are shown as gray bars. A significant (*p <0.05, t test) reduction in amplitude attenuation was seen in all data sets (n = 7). Data and figure from Quirk, Blum, and Wilson (12).

Memory for Real Time—Episodic Memory, Ordering, and the CS-US Interval

Experience-dependent changes in hippocampal place cell firing patterns only begin to scratch the surface of the involvement of the hippocampus in timing-dependent encoding of information and temporal information processing. The hippocampus is necessary for a wide variety of different timing-dependent learning tasks. I will briefly highlight a few examples below, but a common theme that is emerging in modern studies of hippocampal function is that the hippocampus is involved in perceiving and encoding temporal relationships, storing memory traces for brief periods of time in associative learning, and indeed that the hippocampus is involved in "episodic" perception in general. Simply stated, the hippocampus appears to be integral to forming a coherent representation of a temporal series of events, corresponding to what we would refer to as a single episode of personal experience.

Obviously, if the hippocampus is ultimately involved in mediating the storage of a complex set of individual experiences, forming a representation with the appropriate temporal ordering is key. Exciting work by the laboratories of Howard Eichenbaum, Matt Wilson, and John Disterhoft have begun to demonstrate nicely that this type of hippocampal information processing is indeed occurring, and furthermore recent elegant work from these laboratories has begun to explore the cellular and molecular basis for this role.

Early studies in this area asked a simple question: do hippocampal lesions have a greater effect on memory paradigms that involve a time lag during learning? The answer to this question is clearly "Yes." For example, in one pioneering study Chiba et al. investigated memories for temporal ordering in rats that were learning the specific order of presentation of two spatial locations (13). They found that the greater the timelag between visits to the first site and the second site, the more susceptible the memory formation was to hippocampal lesions. Thus, the hippocampus is involved selectively in forming a memory of event orders when there is a longer intervening time between the first event and the second event.

Other work (14) has shown that hippocampal lesions disrupt the ability of rats to learn the ordering of olfactory cues. A rat with a hippocampal lesion, for example, will have a deficit in remembering the specific order: orange; lemon; wintergreen. This is a very nice example of the role of the hippocampus in placing sensory stimuli in the appropriate temporal relationship with each other.

In additional studies, recordings from the hippocampus *in vivo* in behaving animals have suggested that temporal factors can come into play in the firing of "place" cells. For example, place cells can fire selectively depending on the recent history of the animal (15). In one experiment rats are trained to make alternating left-hand and right-hand turns as they repeatedly run a T-maze. An animal in the identical spot in a T-maze can have a given place cell fire selectively, depending on whether it is about to make a left-hand turn or a right-hand turn. These cells may be "intent" cells influencing what the animal will do next. Alternatively, they may be "recent history" cells, because what the animal is *about* to do next depends on what it has just finished doing. Regardless, this cell firing pattern clearly shows that "place" cells are not just place cells but something more complex, influenced by the animal's recent history.

In fact, it is intriguing to consider that a potential clue to this aspect of pyramidal neuron function was there in the very first description of place cells by O'Keefe and Dostrovsky. Place cells don't just fire depending on location, they also only fire when the animal is moving in a specific direction through the place field (as we already discussed). Obviously, an animal moving in one direction in a place field has had a different recent experience than when it crossed the same spot moving in the opposite direction, and this could be the basis for this experimental observation.

The most extensively-studied example of hippocampal involvement in time-dependent information processing is trace-associative conditioning. You will recall from the last chapter that in trace conditioning a time lag is introduced between the CS and the US, typically in the range of a few seconds to a few minutes. The most popular experimental model to study this is trace-eye-blink conditioning, although trace cued fear conditioning has also been utilized. Hippocampal lesions of various sorts (anatomical, pharmacologic, molecular) lead to a loss of trace eye-blink or fear conditioning in animals, up to and including the human (1, 16–17). The time-dependent specificity of the involvement of the hippocampus is illustrated by the observation that delivery of the identical stimuli with no intervening time lag (delay conditioning) is perfectly normal in hippocampally-lesioned animals. Thus, the hippocampus is selectively involved in memory formation that incorporates a timing-dependent component.

What is happening in the hippocampus during trace associative conditioning? This fascinating question is being explored at present, and at least a few answers are available. Hippocampal pyramidal neurons in area CA1 show large increases in their firing rates during the learning period, especially early in training when pyramidal neurons show increased firing in response to both the CS and the US (see Figure 10 and McEchron and Disterhoft (18–19) for more details).

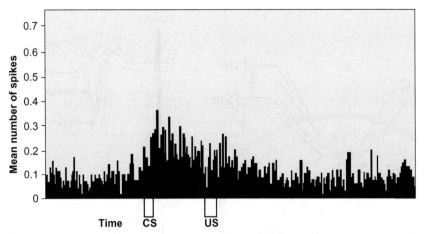

FIGURE 10 Increased hippocampal neuron firing during trace eye-blink conditioning. Average peri-event histograms (10 ms bins) for pyramidal cell response profile recorded from rabbits during trace conditioning. Action potentials (spikes) from each cell were summed across a single training session, then averaged across cells. The duration of the histogram is 3750 ms, and the duration of the baseline period prior to CS onset is 1000 ms. 7.4 percent of all tested pyramidal cells display this type of response profile. Data and figure from McEchron, Weible, and Disterhoft (19).

It is worth noting that many neocortical neurons exhibit this same type of firing pattern, that is, a residual increase in firing after the presentation of an environmental stimulus. This has been most extensively documented in neurons in the visual system. This is important to keep in mind, because clearly the hippocampus is not the only area of the brain encoding temporal information.

Thus, it is possible that pyramidal neurons maintain a representation of the CS over time so that it can be associated with the US. A more sophisticated model has been proposed by Howard Eichenbaum, which he refers to as the episodic encoding model (20–21). In this model the hippocampus forms a temporal representation of a single event, based on the specific order of firing of individual (or groups of) CA1 pyramidal neurons. Thus, the firing of ensembles of cells in a particular order would represent a specific episode in the animal's life, preserving the temporal relationships with fidelity. This type of information could then be used in the storage of a learned relationship between two stimuli separated in time. Overall, while the circuit properties underlying the role of the hippocampus in temporal information processing are still unclear at this time, new insights have been gained and much effort is being devoted to this problem.

If the circuitry is unclear, the cellular and molecular mechanisms are even more mysterious. Tantalizing clues have emerged, however. For example, trace fear conditioning is dependent on NMDA receptor function in CA1 pyramidal neurons, as was demonstrated in a very sophisticated study using genetically-engineered mice (17). Additional studies have also shown that trace eye-blink conditioning results in increases in CA1 pyramidal neuron membrane excitability, and an increase in synaptic efficacy at the connections between neurons in area CA3 and area CA1 (see Figure 11 and reference 22). The contributions of these specific mechanisms to the role of the hippocampus in temporal information processing will hopefully become clearer as work in this area continues.

Overall, these studies directly demonstrating changes in hippocampal pyramidal neuron firing in timing-dependent associative learning are a beautiful example of cognitive processing in real-time. They suggest that hippocampal pyramidal neurons encode the maintenance of a representation of a sensory stimulus, in the absence of any continued presentation of the stimulus itself.[1] This representation functions to allow a subsequent association of that sensory input with a temporally removed, second sensory stimulus (Box 2).

C. Multimodal Associations—The Hippocampus as a Generalized Association Machine and Multimodal Sensory Integrator

Even the earliest reports of place cells noted that they are multimodal sensory integrators. In an early study, where O'Keefe began to investigate "why they fire where they fire", he trained rats in a T-maze using four different external visual cues as the spatial landmarks (6). He then proceeded to query the animal's hippocampus by recording how place cell firing patterns changed with removal of one or several of the spatial cues. He found that some place cells used one or two of the cues as the relevant landmarks, while

---

[1]It is important to note that this may not take place entirely *within* the hippocampus. For example, a larger circuit of which the hippocampus is a part may carry out this function. Particularly appealing in this context is the possibility of reciprocal hippocampal–neocortical projections participating in a short-term memory store, given the variety of evidence demonstrating the maintained firing of cortical neurons *in vivo* after various sensory stimuli.

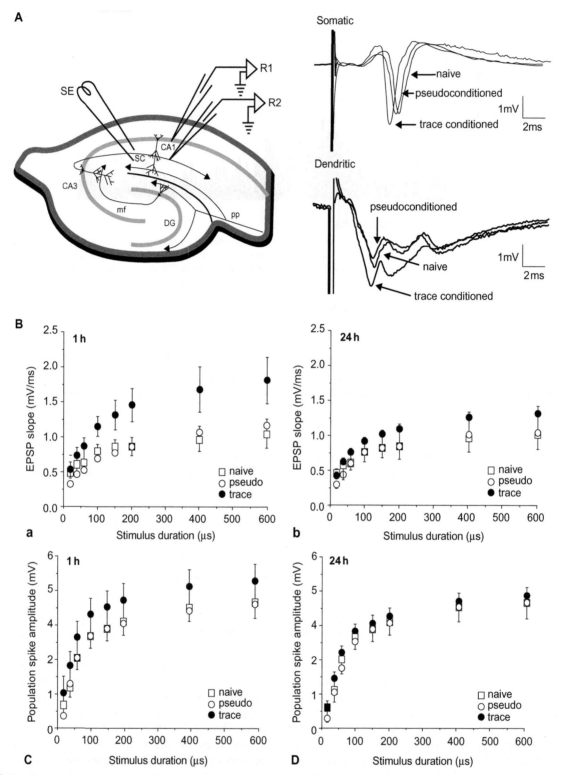

FIGURE 11   Increased connectivity in hippocampal pyramidal neurons with eye-blink conditioning. Hippocampal slices were prepared and physiologic responses monitored *in vitro*, using control animals and trace-conditioned animals. (A) Diagram showing rabbit hippocampal slices *in vitro* with placement of stimulating electrode (SE), and somatic (R1) and dendritic (R2) recording electrodes. To the right are representative field potentials (excitatory post-synaptic responses) from each type of recording one hour after conditioning. The following structures are also labeled: Schaffer collaterals (sc); perforant path (pp); dentate gyrus (DG); mossy fibers (mf); CA1 and CA3. (B) Effects of conditioning on Schaffer collateral evoked field potentials recorded in CA1. Means ± SE are given for trace-conditioned (1 hour, n = 9; 24 hr, n = 13), pseudoconditioned (1 hour, n = 9; 24 hour, n = 8), and naïve (n = 7) animals for each stimulus intensity value. (a) Excitatory postsynaptic potential (EPSP) slope recorded in dendrites was greater in slices prepared from conditioned animals one hour after conditioning.

(Continued on next page)

BOX 2

ARC AND CELLULAR REACTIVATION

"Immediate early genes" (IEGs) is a term that describes a diverse family of genes that have in common rapid regulation at the transcriptional level. Typically in neurons IEGs respond in an activity-dependent fashion within about 5–15 minutes of cellular stimulation. This rapid transcriptional response of a wide variety of genes clearly indicates the presence of signal transduction mechanisms that can quickly carry a signal from the neuronal cell surface to the nucleus.

IEGs code for proteins with a wide variety of cell functions. One major category is transcription factors, and the well-known transcription factors c-fos, c-jun, jun-B, and zif268 are indeed immediate early genes. This category of IEGs indicates that there likely are secondary and tertiary waves of altered transcription in response to increased IEG expression, and implies that activity-dependent alterations in neuronal gene expression are indeed likely to be quite complex and subject to elaborate

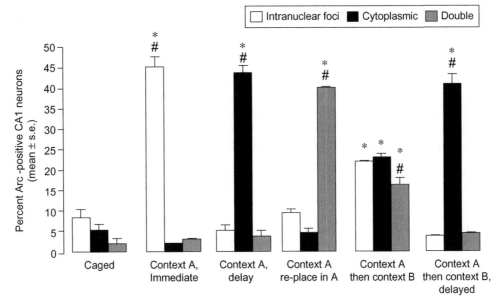

BOX 2 Neuronal activity-dependent arc expression. Arc expression defines CA1 neuronal ensembles that encode distinct environments. Rats explored environments designated A and B. After being placed in context A, some groups of animals were placed back in A or placed in a different context (B). Arc expression in the nucleus □ or cytoplasm ■ was assessed. The time delay in Arc transport from nucleus to cytoplasm allows investigating whether the same cells are activated when an animal is replaced in the same environment. "Double" staining means that Arc is found in both the nucleus and cytoplasm, indicating that the cell has been activated twice by the first and second exposures to environment A. The distinct staining profiles seen in A/A and A/B groups demonstrate that the induction of Arc transcription in CA1 is highly specific to the nature of the behavioral experience. The A/immediate, A/delay and A/B/delay groups define the temporal resolution properties of Arc catfish. From each rat (n=3 rats per group), 97–146 (mean, 120) neurons were counted; the total number of neurons analyzed for this experiment was 2,157. The percentage of positive cells for each staining profile was determined for each individual rat; reported values indicate the group mean (*p <0.002) relative to the other two cell populations for that group by paired t-test. Data, figure, and legend reproduced from Guzowski et al. (28).

Continued

FIGURE 11 (Continued) (b) no significant differences in initial EPSP slope were seen between conditioning groups 24 hours after conditioning. No conditioning effect was seen in population spike amplitude input-output function one hour (c) or 24 hours (d) after conditioning, population spikes indicate action potential firing in the post-synaptic CA1 pyramidal neurons. Diagram and data reproduced from Power, Thompson, Moyer, and Disterhoft (22).

BOX 2—cont'd

ARC AND CELLULAR REACTIVATION

control mechanisms. Along these lines, the term immediate early gene arises from early studies of transcriptional regulation in non-neuronal cells, where temporal waves of altered gene expression were observed and termed immediate early, early, and late.

Another category of IEGs code for cytoskeletal and structural proteins like Homer 1A, actin, and Arc (initially discovered as activity-regulated gene 3.1, or Arg3.1). Work from Paul Worley and his collaborators Ozzie Steward, Carol Barnes, and Bruce McNaughton has demonstrated that Arc regulation is particularly interesting, and we will return to these studies in later chapters. Of course in order to make an active product all genes must be transcribed, processed into mRNA, and then translated into protein. Arc mRNA has the interesting attribute that it is rapidly transported into dendritic processes, and in fact the mRNA is selectively transported and compartmentalized to dendritic regions that have undergone recent excitation. There it undergoes local protein synthesis, the net result of which is selective localization of Arc protein at synapses experiencing recent activity.

Like many other IEGs, Arc transcription is regulated in the brain in response to various types of environmental stimulation. Arc transcription is increased in specific pyramidal neurons in area CA1 within a few minutes of exploration of a novel environment, for example (28). This is most likely a molecular correlate to increased place cell firing and the establishment of place fields in hippocampal pyramidal neurons. In a study that combined molecular biology approaches with behavior, Guzowski et al. (28) capitalized on neuronal activity-dependent Arc expression to demonstrate that the same hippocampal pyramidal neurons that fire initially when place fields are established also fire when the animal is replaced into the same context. In these studies, Guzowski et al. used Arc as an activity-dependent molecular marker to track the activity of specific ensembles of pyramidal neurons over time, an elegant application of molecular approaches in the context of the behaving animal.

---

the remainder of the landmarks were immaterial to their firing—a fairly straightforward result. However, he also observed some place cells that were triggered by any combination of any two landmarks. As far as these cells were concerned, landmarks A + B were equivalent to landmarks C + D were equivalent to A + C, and so on. Thus, two environments that were different from each other visually (A + B versus C + D, for example) were treated as equivalent as long as the animal had had the opportunity to previously learn that A, B, C, and D were always present in a consistent spatial relationship to *each other*. The place cell firing apparently had come to represent an abstraction, an integration of four spatial cues. Apparently, any two cues were sufficient to allow the place cell (or something upstream of it) to reconstruct a representation of the entirety of the space.

More recent work has made clear the role of the hippocampus in general, and "place," i.e., pyramidal, cells in particular, in multimodal sensory integration. Howard Eichenbaum and his collaborators have been leaders in this pursuit and they have made many seminal observations in this area. In this next section I will highlight two of the studies from Eichenbaum and his co-workers that are landmark findings in the field.

The first study used the four-arm radial maze (see Figure 12). The set-up in the basic version of the experiment was quite simple—there were four arms to the plus-shaped maze, and the maze was in a room with one unique visual cue on each wall. The behavioral task was for the animal to learn to use the spatial cues to navigate to food rewards in the maze. In these experiments the firing patterns for hippocampal place cells recapitulated what we described above—they fired depending on the animal's location in space relative to the distal visual cues. In addition, as expected they were direction-dependent, that is they fired selectively when the animal was moving either outward into an arm or inward back toward the center of the maze.

What happens when you have local cues within the arms of the maze? Eichenbaum's group addressed this question by preparing their four-arm maze with distinct visual, olfactory, and tactile cues in each of the four arms, in addition to the four distal visual cues on the wall (23–24). When they trained their animals in this maze they found cells that fired selectively depending on the texture of the floor and the olfactory cues that were present (see Figure 12). If there are cells in the hippocampus which fire in response to distal visual cues and also cells that fire in response to local

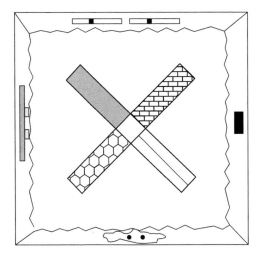

FIGURE 12 Four-arm radial maze with local and distal cues. Diagram of the four-arm radial maze set-up used in the experiments such as those performed by Tanila et al. (1997, 1998) (see text and Figure 13). This maze is used to assess effects of manipulation of local and distal cues. Local cues are coverings of the arms that give a set of visual, tactile, and olfactory cues distinct form the other arms. The distal cues are objects on each wall surrounding the maze. Reproduced from Tanila, Sipila, Shapiro, and Eichenbaum (7).

hippocampal pyramidal neuron firing can track local cues, can track distal cues, or can track both independently. In the latter case the cell appears to encode an A + B + C + D representation like we talked about above, where either A + B or C + D is sufficient to trigger firing. In this case it is even more complex, because the different cues are non-equivalent, i.e., some are distal visual cues and some are local tactile and olfactory cues.

Thus we have seen our first example of the fact that "place cell" is really a misnomer. Hippocampal pyramidal neurons are place cells, but they also can be texture cells and olfactory cells, and they also can be place plus texture plus olfactory cells. In the next experiment I will describe, Eichenbaum's laboratory went on to show that the world of the hippocampal pyramidal neuron is even more complex than that. Hippocampal pyramidal neurons are multimodal association cells that are involved in encoding a wide variety of contingencies and relationships.

In this experiment Eichenbaum and his colleagues first trained rats in a contingency task—a task with the accurate but cumbersome descriptor "continuous odor-guided non-matching to sample" (25). One aspect of the task is that rats learn that small cups filled with sand sometimes have food rewards in them. Moreover, each sand cup has one of nine odor cues mixed in with it, spicy smells such as thyme or paprika. How does a rat know if a specific sand cup has food buried in it or not? The sand cups are presented sequentially, and if the smell of the cup presented is different from the previous one, then the rat knows there is food buried in the new cup. Thus: "continuous" (presented sequentially) "odor-guided" (smell of the cup) "non-matching" (different) "to sample" (from the previous one). In presenting many odors in a row the investigators were also careful to vary the order of presentation so that sequences of odors could not be used to predict the food—in other words, only the odor presented immediately before could be used to predict the food reward.

After rats learned this fundamental contingency, an additional layer of complexity was added that was irrelevant to the rats, but of fundamental importance to the rat-testers (see Figure 14). The food cups were presented to the rats randomly at one of nine different locations in an open field surrounded by spatial cues (can you say place cell?). The positions of placement in the matrix were carefully controlled so that this variable did not allow prediction of the presence or absence of the food reward.

In considering the entirety of the task, then, a number of different individual components can be identified. The rats at any given time will be in a particular *place*. At some times they will be *approaching*

cues, are they mutually exclusive? The answer is no—in fact, there were individual cells that fired in response to both local cues and distal cues when they were presented separately. Moreover, there were some cells that fired only when all the cues are presented together. Their firing depended on the simultaneous presence of all the various cues. This latter finding suggests that these cells are firing in response to (or in order to produce) an aggregate representation of all the cues!

Finally, we come to the *piece de resistance*—what happens to these multimodal cells, cells which respond to both local cues and distal cues, if you change the relationship of the local cues to the distal cues? Eichenbaum and his colleagues did a clever manipulation where they asked that question, the "double rotation" experiment (Figure 13). They trained animals in a multi-cue maze that contained both local cues and distal visual cues and then rotated the visual cues 90° counter-clockwise and the local cues 90° clockwise. When the animal was placed back in the manipulated maze what happens to the firing of the cells? The firing of some cells tracked the visual cues, as expected of place cells. The firing of other cells tracked the local olfactory, tactile, and visual cues—a sort of variant of the classic place cell. However, there were some single cells that tracked both the local and distal cues. They continued to fire when the animal was in a particular arm of the maze with specific local cues, and fired in a different arm of the maze that was in the original orientation relative to the distal visual cues. Thus,

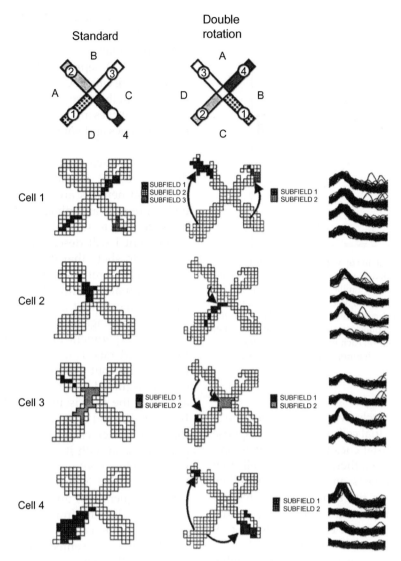

FIGURE 13   Double rotation four-arm maze experiment. In this experiment the four local cues were rotated 90° to the left as the distal cues were rotated 90° to the right. The responses of four simultaneously recorded cells (cells 1–4) are shown here before and after the double rotation of the cues. Data and figure reproduced from Tanila, Shapiro, and Eichenbaum (24). Copyright John Wiley and Sons, Inc.

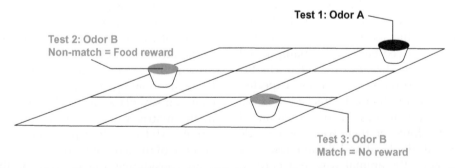

FIGURE 14   Continuous odor-guided non-matching to sample. This diagram outlines an experiment to assess the ability of the animal to distinguish between a matching or non-matching stimulus. The animal must determine if the second smell that they experience is the same or different than the first, if the third is the same or different than the second and so on. In this example test one has Odor A; test two has Odor B, a non-match. Test three also has Odor B, so the third is a match to the second. Only non-matches contain a food reward.

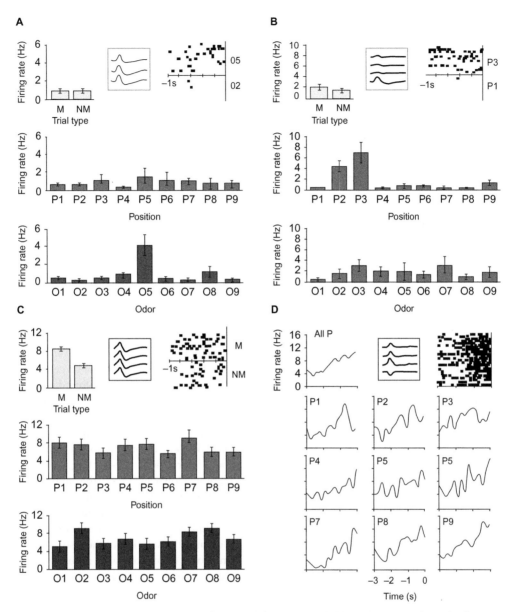

FIGURE 15 Task-related firing patterns of hippocampal pyramidal neurons. (A)–(C) in this figure show the firing rate in one second analysis period for each trial type (M = match; NM = non-match); cup location (P1–P9); and odor (O1–O9) for three different types of cells: (A) an odor cell (odor, $F_{(8,74)}$ = 8.59, P <0.0001; trial type, $F_{(1,74)}$ = 0.04, not significant (NS); cup location $F_{(8,74)}$ = 1.03, NS; odor × trial type, $F_{(8,74)}$ = 1.74, NS); (B) a location cell (cup location, $F_{(8,74)}$ = 8.60; P <0.0001; odor, $F_{(8,74)}$ = 0.84, NS; trial type $F_{(1,74)}$ = 2.76, NS; odor × trial type $F_{(8,74)}$ = 1.14, NS; cup location × trial type, $F_{(8,74)}$ = 1.58, NS); (C) a match cell (trial type, $F_{(1,74)}$ = 22.95, P <0.0001; odor, $F_{(8,74)}$ = 1.42, NS; location, $F_{(8, 74)}$ = 1.17, NS; odor × trial type, $F_{(8,74)}$ = 0.68, NS; location × trial type, $F_{(8, 74)}$ = 1.20, NS). (D) shows firing rates (200 ms bins) for a three second period when the rat approached each cup position (P1–P9), and averaged across all positions (all P) for an approach cell (trial period, $t_{(1,107)}$ = 10.77, P <0.001; trial type, $F_{(1,74)}$ = 0.06, NS; odor $F_{(8,74)}$ = 0.47, NS; location $F_{(8,74)}$ = 1.42, NS; odor × trial type, $F_{(8,74)}$ = 0.96, NS; location × trial type, $F_{(8,74)}$ = 1.00, NS). Each panel also shows the waveform of the cell recorded on each tetrode channel, and a raster display of firing patterns time-locked to the end of the odor sample period. Data, figure, and figure legend reproduced from Wood, Dudchenko, and Eichenbaum (25).

the location of the new food cup, as they move from one place to the next. When they smell the new cup they will be sensing the *odor*. After sensing the new odor they will ascertain whether it is a *match/non-match* to the previous odor.

What happened when Eichenbaum and colleagues recorded pyramidal neuron firing in the rat

hippocampus while animals performed this task? They found that hippocampal pyramidal neurons exhibit an amazing array of sophisticated firing patterns (Figure 15). Some cells fire selectively only when the animal is approaching a food cup, regardless of where it is (Figure 15D). Perhaps these cells are encoding that the animal is about to have to make a decision

BOX 3

SLEEP AND MEMORY CONSOLIDATION

One of the most interesting areas of current investigation into memory formation in general, and hippocampus-dependent memory formation specifically, are studies asking whether sleep is involved in memory formation (29–33). Specifically, current hypotheses from several groups posit that hippocampus-dependent memory consolidation *requires* sleep, or at least sleep-associated processes.

Sleep is, of course, a mysterious process, so testing the role of sleep specifically is quite difficult (33). It is not sufficient to define sleep as a lack of consciousness, and indeed it is clear from monitoring of CNS activity patterns that being unconscious is different from being asleep. In the modern era, sleep is specifically defined in the context of EEG patterns: several different specific stages of sleep have been defined including four progressive stages of "slow-wave" sleep, and rapid eye movement (REM) sleep. Intriguingly, REM sleep is associated with the same synchronized theta-frequency discharges in the hippocampus as are observed in exploring animals (see text). Thus, while "sleep" seems a fairly intuitive term, in fact the phenomenon is a very complex CNS circuit phenomenon, involving almost all areas of the brain, which is quite inconstant over the course of a single sleep episode. Thus, testing the hypothesis that sleep is required for memory is not straightforward. Moreover, sleep disruption obviously has a great number of secondary effects on disposition, attention, and motivation—further complicating attempts to approach the problem experimentally.

Nevertheless, there are a number of intriguing observations consistent with a role for sleep-associated neuronal activity in memory consolidation. Work in this area has come primarily from Bruce McNaughton, Carol Barnes, Matt Wilson, Gyorgi Buzsaki, and their respective colleagues. These investigators have shown sleep-associated reproduction of specific patterns of hippocampal pyramidal neuron firing: firing patterns that mimic firing patterns that the animal had established while awake and learning. In other words, it appears that the hippocampus and cortex are "replaying" episodic events while asleep as part of a process of consolidation of memory. In addition, there are a number of correlative studies suggesting that loss of these types of replay episodes causes memory dysfunction.

On the other hand, in the human literature there is not as much support for the idea of a necessity for sleep *per se* in memory consolidation. For example, patients with specific types of brain lesions or on certain types of medication never sleep or have profound disruptions of their sleep pattern (34). There are also a few examples of individuals who spontaneously lose the desire to sleep and are essentially insomniac for their entire remaining lifetime. These phenomena do not lead to any profound memory disruption, dissociating sleep from memory formation. However, given the ambiguity in defining sleep, it is certainly possible that insomniac individuals may have certain sleep-like patterns of CNS activity that functionally substitute for the lack of sleep.

Obviously, resolution of the issue of the role of sleep in memory formation will require much additional study. At this point, however, the answer looks as if it could be fascinating.

---

about the content of the cup. Or perhaps they encode some abstract representation of the food cup itself. Some cells responded selectively to specific odors only (Figure 15A). Some cells fired selectively depending on whether the odor matched or didn't match the previous odor, regardless of the odor being presented or where it was (Figure 15C). Perhaps they are reward/no reward cells, or perhaps they are contingency cells. Thus, specific hippocampal pyramidal neurons can be considered odor cells, or approach cells, or match/non-match cells—an amazing array of possibilities.

Not surprisingly, some cells are simply place cells (Figure 15B). However, some cells were specific place plus odor cells, firing at only one place in the matrix and only on the presentation of a specific odor. Some cells were place plus match/non-match cells. Finally, a few cells were even so specialized as to be place plus odor plus match/non-match cells. Imagine—these cells will fire only in a specific place in response to a specific odor, and only if it does not match the previous odor. These cells appear to encode complex, multimodal associations among locations, sensory stimuli, and recent history—a significant step up from "place" cells.

These findings from Eichenbaum's laboratory fundamentally change the way we should think about the hippocampus. Pyramidal neurons are sensory integration cells. They are involved in making sophisticated associations and correlations of sensory stimuli with specific places, in the context of the animal's prior history.

Overall, the wide variety of studies we discussed in this section, which used *in vivo* recording techniques in the behaving animal, suggest an amazingly complex involvement of the hippocampus in sensory processing—suggesting its involvement in cognitive processing of space, time, and relationships.

D. The Hippocampus is also Required for Memory Consolidation

As we discussed in Chapter 2, a quite wide variety of studies using many different approaches have demonstrated that involvement in memory consolidation is a central attribute of hippocampal function. We will spend much of the rest of the book discussing the cellular and molecular particulars of this process. In brief, the hippocampus, in addition to its information processing role that we discussed above, serves as a short-term memory store that ultimately downloads information to the cortex for longer-term storage. The basis for this process is still somewhat mysterious, but one thing that is clear is that the hippocampus must be able to hold a memory trace for some appreciable period of time—hours to days or weeks at least.

In the next chapter we will talk about cellular mechanisms likely to be critical to allowing the hippocampus to serve as this sort of memory buffer, for example—long-term potentiation (LTP). Long-lasting synaptic potentiation is also likely involved in the precise formation and maintenance of hippocampal place cell firing patterns. We also will touch on shorter-lasting forms of synaptic plasticity that may be involved in short-term storage of information and information processing in the hippocampus; phenomena such as post-tetanic potentiation (PTP) and short-term potentiation (STP) that may be involved in the "timing" aspect of hippocampal processing of CS-US contingencies over the period of a few seconds.

In the next chapter we also will talk about complex mechanisms regulating the induction of LTP, specifically ending up with examples of how lasting plastic change in hippocampal neurons can be triggered depending on three-way or four-way contingencies. These latter examples are the types of cellular mechanisms that are likely to allow the multimodal sensory integration examined in the studies by Eichenbaum's group that we have discussed in this chapter.

IV. SUMMARY

In this chapter we explored hippocampal function in more detail, drawing specific examples from the literature for each of the four broad categories of cognition in which the hippocampus participates:

1. *Space*—The hippocampus is involved in spatial cognition and spatial memory formation. One intriguing type of cell that is heavily represented among the hippocampal neurons are place cells, which fire very selectively when an animal perceives itself to be in a particular spatial location. Place cells are quite likely to be involved in the actual representation of space in the CNS.

2. *Timing*—The hippocampus participates in the encoding of episodic memory, that is, memory for sequences of events and particular episodes in an individual's life. What defines a particular sensory sequence or episode is a particular timing and temporal relationship of a series of occurrences, and the hippocampus helps encode sequencing of this sort. In addition, in the case of ordered contingencies that are separated by a time period, for example with trace associative conditioning, firing of cells in the hippocampus may participate in storing a representation of the first stimulus so that it can be associated with the second stimulus when it arrives. Alternatively, the hippocampus could be involved in encoding the time delay interval itself, so that the timing of the association of the two stimuli can be represented.

3. *Multimodal associations*—The hippocampus serves to integrate diverse sensory inputs to help encode relationships among those inputs. For example, a given hippocampal neuron may be involved in encoding a complex relationship for a given stimulus that includes its place, its smell, its reward salience, and its contingency relationship to other recent sensory stimuli.

4. *Memory consolidation*—This was the first function clearly linked to the hippocampus, and in many ways its classic role.

This outline of the complexities and diversity of hippocampal function prepare us for the next chapter, where we will begin to dissect the hippocampal synaptic circuit and its cellular physiology. This will allow us to begin to understand how the hippocampus achieves its various functions as a signal integrator and as a transient cellular memory store for subsequent downloading of information to the longer-term storage areas of the cortex.

Further Reading

Eichenbaum, H., Yonelinas, A. P., and Ranganath, C. (2007). The medial temporal lobe and recognition memory. *Annu. Rev. Neurosci.* 30:123–152.

Eichenbaum, H. (2000). A cortical-hippocampal system for declarative memory. *Nat. Rev. Neurosci.* 1:41–50.

Eichenbaum, H., Dudchenko, P., Wood, E., Shapiro, M., and Tanila, H. (1999). The hippocampus, memory, and place cells: is it spatial memory or a memory space? *Neuron* 23:209–226.

Eichenbaum, H., and Cohen, N. J. (2004). *From Conditioning to Conscious Recollection: Memory Systems of the Brain*. Upper Saddle River, NJ: Oxford University Press.

Fyhn, M., Molden, S., Witter, M. P., Moser, E. I., and Moser, M. B. (2004). Spatial representation in the entorhinal cortex. *Science* 305(5688):1258–1264.

Hafting, T., Fyhn, M., Molden, S., Moser, M. B., and Moser, E. I. (2005). Microstructure of a spatial map in the entorhinal cortex. *Nature* 436(7052):801–806.

Leutgeb, S., Leutgeb, J. K., Barnes, C. A., Moser, E. I., McNaughton, B. L., and Moser, M. B. (2005). Independent codes for spatial and episodic memory in hippocampal neuronal ensembles. *Science* 309(5734):619–623.

Louie, K., and Wilson, M. A. (2001). Temporally structured replay of awake hippocampal ensemble activity during rapid eye movement sleep. *Neuron* 29:145–156.

Moser, E. I., Kropff, E., and Moser, M. B. (2008). Place cells, grid cells, and the brain's spatial representation system. *Annu. Rev. Neurosci.* 31:69–89.

Journal Club Articles

Guzowski, J. F., McNaughton, B. L., Barnes, C. A., and Worley, P. F. (1999). Environment-specific expression of the immediate-early gene Arc in hippocampal neuronal ensembles. *Nat. Neurosci.* 2:1120–1124.

O'Keefe, J., and Dostrovsky, J. (1971). The hippocampus as a spatial map. Preliminary evidence from unit activity in the freely-moving rat. *Brain Res.* 34:171–175.

Wood, E. R., Dudchenko, P. A., and Eichenbaum, H. (1999). The global record of memory in hippocampal neuronal activity. *Nature* 397:613–616.

For more information—relevant topic chapters from: John H. Byrne (Editor-in-Chief) (2008). *Learning and Memory: A Comprehensive Reference*. Oxford: Academic Press (ISBN 978-0-12-370509-9). (1.21 Fortin, N. *Navigation and Episodic-Like Memory in Mammals*. pp. 385–417; 1.33 Rolls, E. T. *Computational Models of Hippocampal Functions*. pp. 641–665; 1.35 Koene, R. A., and Hasselmo, M. E. *Connectionist Memory Models of Hippocampal Function*. pp. 681–700; 1.37 Singer, W. *Synchronous Oscillations and Memory Formation*. pp. 721–728; 3.03 Burwell, R. D., and Agster, K. L. *Anatomy of the Hippocampus and the Declarative Memory System*. pp. 47–66; 3.05 Voss, J. L., and Paller, K. A. *Neural Substrates of Remembering—Electroencephalographic Studies*. pp. 79–97; 3.06 Nyberg, L. *Structural Basis of Episodic Memory*. pp. 99–112; 3.07 Martin, A., and Simmons, W. K. *Structural Basis of Semantic Memory*. pp. 113–130; 4.29 Dynes, J. L., and Steward, O. *Dendritic Transport of mRNA, the IEG Arc, and Synaptic Modifications Involved in Memory Consolidation*. pp. 587–610.)

References

1. Squire, L. R., and Zola-Morgan, S. (1971). The medial temporal lobe memory system. *Science* 253:1380–1386.

2. Scoville, W. B., and Milner, B. (2000). Loss of recent memory after bilateral hippocampal lesions, 1957. *J. Neuropsychiatry Clin. Neurosci.* 12:103–113.

3. Winson, J. (1978). Loss of hippocampal theta rhythm results in spatial memory deficit in the rat. *Science* 201:160–163.

4. O'Keefe, J., and Dostrovsky, J. (1971). The hippocampus as a spatial map. Preliminary evidence from unit activity in the freely-moving rat. *Brain Res.* 34:171–175.

5. O'Keefe, J. (1976). Place units in the hippocampus of the freely moving rat. *Exp. Neurol.* 51:78–109.

6. O'Keefe, J., and Conway, D. H. (1978). Hippocampal place units in the freely moving rat: why they fire where they fire. *Exp. Brain Res.* 31:573–590.

7. Tanila, H., Sipila, P., Shapiro, M., and Eichenbaum, H. (1997). Brain aging: impaired coding of novel environmental cues. *J. Neurosci.* 17:5167–5174.

8. Lever, C., Wills, T., Cacucci, F., Burgess, N., and O'Keefe, J. (2002). Long-term plasticity in hippocampal place-cell representation of environmental geometry. *Nature* 416:90–94.

9. Muller, R. U., and Kubie, J. L. (1987). The effects of changes in the environment on the spatial firing of hippocampal complex-spike cells. *J. Neurosci.* 7:1951–1968.

10. Muller, R. U., Kubie, J. L., and Ranck, J. B., Jr. (1987). Spatial firing patterns of hippocampal complex-spike cells in a fixed environment. *J. Neurosci.* 7:1935–1950.

11. Mehta, M. R., Barnes, C. A., and McNaughton, B. L. (1997). Experience-dependent, asymmetric expansion of hippocampal place fields. *Proc. Natl. Acad. Sci. USA* 94:8918–8921.

12. Quirk, M. C., Blum, K. I., and Wilson, M. A. (2001). Experience-dependent changes in extracellular spike amplitude may reflect regulation of dendritic action potential back-propagation in rat hippocampal pyramidal cells. *J. Neurosci.* 21:240–248.

13. Chiba, A. A., Kesner, R. P., and Reynolds, A. M. (1994). Memory for spatial location as a function of temporal lag in rats: role of hippocampus and medial prefrontal cortex. *Behav. Neural Biol.* 61:123–131.

14. Fortin, N. J., Agster, K. L., and Eichenbaum, H. B. (2002). Critical role of the hippocampus in memory for sequences of events. *Nat. Neurosci.* 5:458–462.

15. Wood, E. R., Dudchenko, P. A., Robitsek, R. J., and Eichenbaum, H. (2000). Hippocampal neurons encode information about different types of memory episodes occurring in the same location. *Neuron* 27:623–633.

16. Clark, R. E., and Squire, L. R. (1998). Classical conditioning and brain systems: the role of awareness. *Science* 280:77–81.

17. Huerta, P. T., Sun, L. D., Wilson, M. A., and Tonegawa, S. (2000). Formation of temporal memory requires NMDA receptors within CA1 pyramidal neurons. *Neuron* 25:473–480.

18. McEchron, M. D., and Disterhoft, J. F. (1997). Sequence of single neuron changes in CA1 hippocampus of rabbits during acquisition of trace eyeblink conditioned responses. *J. Neurophysiol.* 78:1030–1044.

19. McEchron, M. D., Weible, A. P., and Disterhoft, J. F. (2001). Aging and learning-specific changes in single-neuron activity in CA1 hippocampus during rabbit trace eyeblink conditioning. *J. Neurophysiol.* 86:1839–1857.

20. Eichenbaum, H., Dudchenko, P., Wood, E., Shapiro, M., and Tanila, H. (1999). The hippocampus, memory, and place cells: is it spatial memory or a memory space? *Neuron* 23:209–226.

21. Eichenbaum, H. (2000). A cortical-hippocampal system for declarative memory. *Nat. Rev. Neurosci.* 1:41–50.

22. Power, J. M., Thompson, L. T., Moyer, J. R., Jr., and Disterhof, J. F. (1997). Enhanced synaptic transmission in CA1 hippocampus after eyeblink conditioning. *J. Neurophysiol.* 78:1184–1187.

23. Shapiro, M. L., Tanila, H., and Eichenbaum, H. (1999). Cues that hippocampal place cells encode: dynamic and hierarchical representation of local and distal stimuli. *Hippocampus* 7:624–642.

24. Tanila, H., Shapiro, M. L., and Eichenbaum, H. (1997). Discordance of spatial representation in ensembles of hippocampal place cells. *Hippocampus* 7:613–623.

25. Wood, E. R., Dudchenko, P. A., and Eichenbaum, H. (1999). The global record of memory in hippocampal neuronal activity. *Nature* 397:613–616.

26. McNaughton, B. L., Chen, L. L., and Markus, E. J. (1991). Dead reckoning, landmark learning, and the sense of direction: A

neurophysiological and computational hypothesis. *J. Cognitive Neurosci.* 3:190–202.

27. Hafting, T., Fyhn, M., Molden, S., Moser, M. B., and Moser, E. I. (2005). Microstructure of a spatial map in the entorhinal cortex. *Nature* 436(7052):801–806.

28. Guzowski, J. F., McNaughton, B. L., Barnes, C. A., and Worley, P. F. (1999). Environment-specific expression of the immediate-early gene Arc in hippocampal neuronal ensembles. *Nat. Neurosci.* 2:1120–1124.

29. Wilson, M. A., and McNaughton, B. L. (1994). Reactivation of hippocampal ensemble memories during sleep. *Science* 265:676–679.

30. Graves, L., Pack, A., and Abel, T. (2001). Sleep and memory: a molecular perspective. *Trends Neurosci.* 24:237–243.

31. Kudrimoti, H. S., Barnes, C. A., and McNaughton, B. L. (1999). Reactivation of hippocampal cell assemblies: effects of behavioral state, experience, and EEG dynamics. *J. Neurosci.* 19:4090–4101.

32. Louie, K., and Wilson, M. A. (2001). Temporally structured replay of awake hippocampal ensemble activity during rapid eye movement sleep. *Neuron* 29:145–156.

33. Maquet, P. (2001). The role of sleep in learning and memory. *Science* 294:1048–1052.

34. Lavie, P., Pratt, H., Scharf, B., Peled, R., and Brown, J. (1984). Localized pontine lesion: nearly total absence of REM sleep. *Neurology* 34:118–120.

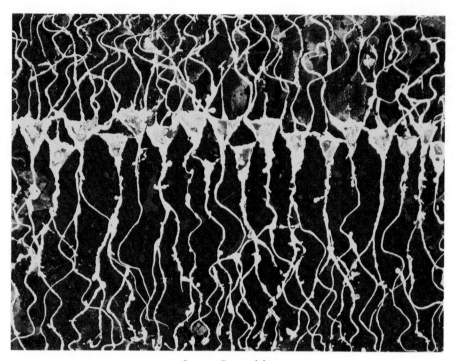

Stratum Pyramidale
J. David Sweatt, acrylic on canvas, 2008–2009

Long-Term Potentiation—A Candidate Cellular Mechanism for Information Storage in the Central Nervous System

This chapter reviews long-term potentiation (LTP) of synaptic transmission, currently one of the most widely-studied and popular candidate mechanisms for a cellular phenomenon underlying long-term storage of information in the nervous system. This chapter will briefly describe the overall phenomenon and basic attributes of LTP. This background is important because an understanding of LTP is a prerequisite

to understanding most of the rest of this book. This chapter also is a transition point for this volume; we transition from analyzing behavior, cognition, and anatomy to investigating cellular and molecular mechanisms underlying memory.

The particular circuits and neuronal connections that underlie hippocampus-dependent forms of mammalian learning and memory are mysterious at present.

There is little understanding of the means by which complex episodic and declarative memories are stored and recalled at the neural circuit level. In many ways the study of LTP serves only as a surrogate for studying hippocampus-dependent memory directly. Nevertheless, this chapter will focus on LTP. We will focus on it for three main reasons. First, it has been extensively studied and is the form of synaptic plasticity best-understood at the molecular level. Second, it is a robust form of synaptic plasticity and worthy of investigation in its own right. Finally, it is a specific candidate cellular mechanism for mediating certain forms of associative learning, spatial learning, and adaptive change in the central nervous system (CNS), in particular in the amygdala, hippocampus, and cerebral cortex respectively.

I. HEBB'S POSTULATE

Despite the various caveats concerning the specific role of LTP in hippocampus-dependent memory formation, there is a general hypothesis for memory storage that is available and broadly accepted. This hypothesis is that:

Memories are stored as alterations in the strength of synaptic connections between neurons in the CNS.

The significance of this general hypothesis should be emphasized—this is one of the few areas of contemporary cognitive research for which there is a unifying hypothesis. This general hypothesis has a solid underlying rationale. Learning and memory manifest themselves as a change in an animal's behavior, and scientists capitalize on this in order to study these phenomena by observing and measuring changes in an animal's behavior in the wild or in experimental situations. However, all of the behavior exhibited by an animal is a result of activity in the animal's nervous system. The nervous system comprises many kinds of cells, but the primary functional units of the nervous system are neurons. As neurons are cells, an animal's entire behavioral repertoire is a manifestation of an underlying cellular phenomenon. By extension, changes in an animal's behavior such as occurs with learning, must also be subserved by an underlying cellular change.

By and large, the vast majority of the communication between neurons in the nervous system occurs at synapses. As synapses mediate the neuron–neuron communication that underlies an animal's behavior, changes in behavior are ultimately subserved by alterations in the nature, strength, or number of interneuronal synaptic contacts in the animal's nervous system.

The capacity for alterations of synaptic connections between neurons is referred to as "synaptic plasticity." One of the great unifying theories to emerge out of neuroscience research in the last century was that synaptic plasticity subserves learning and memory. LTP (of some sort at least) is the specific form of synaptic plasticity that is the leading candidate as a mechanism subserving behavior-modifying changes in synaptic strength that mediate higher-order learning and memory in mammals.

One of the pioneers in advancing the idea that changes in neuronal connectivity are a mechanism for memory was the Canadian psychologist Donald Hebb, who published his seminal formulation as what is now generally known as "Hebb's Postulate:"

When an axon of cell A … excites cell B and repeatedly or persistently takes part in firing it, some growth process or metabolic change takes place in one or both cells so that A's efficiency as one of the cells firing B is increased.

Hebb, D. O. (1949). The Organization of Behavior.

Note the important contrast between Hebb's Postulate and its popular contemporary formulation—one (Hebb's) specifies cell firing and the other (the modern formulation) specifies synaptic change. These two phenomena are clearly different and the current, exclusively synaptic, variant is incomplete. Changes in synapses are certainly important in information storage in the CNS, but we need to consider that the post-synaptic receptors sit in a membrane whose biophysical properties are carefully controlled. Regulation of membrane sodium channels, chloride channels, and potassium channels also contribute significantly to the net effect in the cell that any neurotransmitter-operated process can achieve (see Boxes 1 and 2).

II. A BREAKTHROUGH DISCOVERY— LONG-TERM POTENTIATION IN THE HIPPOCAMPUS

As a young post-doctoral researcher, Tim Bliss (Figure 1) set out to find a long-lasting form of synaptic plasticity in the hippocampus, and by teaming up with Terje Lomo in Per Anderson's laboratory in Oslo, he did just that. The seminal report by Bliss and Lomo in 1973, describing a phenomenon they termed "long-term potentiation" of synaptic transmission, set the stage for what is now over three decades of progress in understanding the basics of long-term synaptic alteration in the CNS.

BOX 1

TYPES OF RECEPTORS AND POTENTIAL SITES OF PLASTICITY

Neurotransmitters can be broadly categorized into two types, based on the types of receptors they bind to and their effects on the post-synaptic cell. Some neurotransmitters directly mediate neuron–neuron communication by binding to and opening ligand (neurotransmitter)-gated ion channels. A second major category generally serves a more subtle role—modulating neuronal function through eliciting intracellular second-messenger generation.

The first types of receptors form neurotransmitter-regulated pores which can open on binding of neurotransmitter, which allows ions to flux across the cell membrane, and results in an electrical change (generally depolarizing or hyperpolarizing) in the cellular membrane. Neurotransmission of this sort is typically how one neuron excites (or inhibits) another follower neuron within a neuronal circuit. The two predominant types of ligand-gated ion channels found in the hippocampus, and elsewhere in the CNS, bind glutamate (excitatory) or gamma-amino-butyric acid (GABA, inhibitory). The major glutamate receptor subtype is named for a selective agonist at this receptor, alpha-amino-3-hydroxy-5-methyl-4-isoxazolepropionic acid; mercifully abbreviated to AMPA. The AMPA subtype of receptors are glutamate-gated cation channels that when opened lead to membrane depolarization. Another subtype of glutamate receptor that is very similar is activated by kainic acid (KA, kainate), and this subtype is referred to as the kainate receptor. The typical EPSP in a hippocampal neuron is mediated by ion flux through the AMPA subtype of glutamate receptor. Inhibitory post-synaptic potentials (IPSPs) are mostly mediated by the GABA-A subtype of GABA receptors. GABA-A receptors are GABA-gated chloride channels. Opening these channels moves the membrane potential in a negative direction, toward the hyperpolarized chloride ion equilibrium potential. This tends to hyperpolarize the membrane and clamp it there.

The second major category of neurotransmitter receptor doesn't produce electrical changes in the post-synaptic neuron directly, but rather elicits biochemical changes within the post-synaptic neuron. Typically these types of neurotransmitters couple to second-messenger generating enzymes that can lead to alterations in a wide variety of cellular chemical processes. These types of neurotransmitters are referred to as modulatory neurotransmitters, because their effects typically (but by no means exclusively) sculpt and fine-tune the electrical and cellular responses to the neurotransmitters that open ligand-gated ion channels. Almost all neurotransmitters have specific subtypes of receptors that act in this fashion, including specific receptors for glutamate, GABA, norepinephrine, dopamine, serotonin, acetylcholine, and for a large number of different neuropeptides.

The second messenger-generating enzymes that these modulatory neurotransmitter receptors couple to are also quite diverse. A partial listing includes: adenylyl cyclase, which makes cyclic AMP (cAMP) and activates the cAMP-dependent protein kinase (PKA); phospholipase C (PLC), which makes diacylglycerol (DAG) and activates protein kinase C (PKC); PLC also makes inositol tris-phosphate (IP3) which mobilizes intracellular calcium and can activate the calcium/calmodulin-dependent protein kinase type II (CaMKII); and phospholipase A2 (PLA2), which liberates free arachidonic acid that can be converted into a wide variety of active metabolites. We will explore these systems and others in detail later in this book.

Finally, it is important to note that the targets of these various signaling pathways are as diverse as the genome itself. In terms of neuronal function particularly important targets are: pre-synaptic proteins associated with neurotransmitter release, membrane K^+ channels, Ca^{++} channels and Na^+ channels, nuclear transcription factors regulating gene expression, the protein synthesis machinery, and the cytoskeleton.

In their experiments Bliss and Lomo recorded synaptic responses in the dentate gyrus, stimulating the perforant path inputs from the entorhinal cortex (1). They used extracellular stimulating and recording electrodes implanted into the animal, and the basic experiment was begun by recording baseline synaptic transmission in this pathway. They discovered that

a brief period of high frequency (100 Hz "tetanic") stimulation, led to a robust increase in the strength of synaptic connections between the perforant path inputs from the entorhinal cortex onto the dentate granule neurons in the dentate gyrus (Figure 2). They also observed an increased likelihood of the cells firing action potentials in response to a constant synaptic

---

BOX 2

GLOBAL CELL-WIDE CHANGES AS MECHANISMS CONTRIBUTING TO MEMORY

As mentioned in the main text, limitations arise from ignoring potential long-term regulation of membrane biophysical properties. We need to consider that local changes in dendritic membrane excitability may be involved in cellular information processing, and also that global changes in cellular excitability that alter the likelihood of the cell firing an action potential may also be a mechanism for information storage.

Another potential mechanism involved in memory that involves the entire cell and not specific synapses is adult *neurogenesis*, the growth and functional integration of new neurons in the adult CNS. Finally, one can think of inhibition (e.g., GABAergic modulation) as operating above the level of the single synapse, because it can control the likelihood of the cell firing an action potential. The role of inhibition in plasticity, and the plasticity of inhibition *per se*, are also potential mechanisms contributing to memory.

The possibility that global or cell-wide alterations might be involved in memory is also relevant when considering global genomic (transcriptional) and epigenomic changes, which affect the nucleus, and potentially the entire cell. One solution to the "problem" of global changes due to altered transcription is specific trafficking of the products of global changes in transcription. Various aspects of this are dealt with in later chapters.

The idea of processes such as excitability being involved in memory, processes that encompass the entire cell, has been criticized as too limiting, because with global changes in excitability one loses the computational power of selectively altering the response at a single synaptic input, i.e., synapse specificity. However, we don't know how the neuron or the CNS computes a memory output. The fundamental unit of information storage may not be the synapse, but the neuron. Future experiments will be necessary to resolve this issue, but it is nevertheless worthwhile to keep in mind the possibility that regulation of excitability and regulation of neuronal properties cell-wide, as well as the more typically-considered alterations in synaptic connections, may play a role in memory storage.

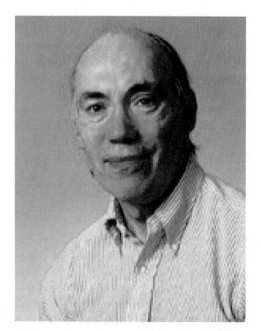

FIGURE 1   T. V. P. Bliss, *FRS*. Photo courtesy of Tim Bliss.

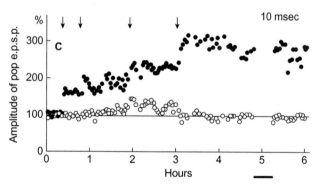

FIGURE 2   Bliss and Lomo's first published LTP experiment. As described in more detail in the text, in this pioneering work Tim Bliss and Terje Lomo demonstrated long-term potentiation of synaptic transmission. This specific experiment investigated synaptic transmission at perforant path inputs into the dentate gyrus. Arrows indicate the delivery of high-frequency synaptic stimulation, resulting in LTP. Filled circles are responses from the tetanized pathways; open circles are a control pathway that did not receive tetanic stimulation. The bar, where no data points are available, indicates a period of time where Tim Bliss fell asleep. Data acquisition in this era involved the investigator directly measuring synaptic responses by hand from an oscilloscope screen. Moreover, it was not unusual for experiments to extend overnight due to the long time involved in preparing the rabbit for the experiment, implanting the electrodes into the brain, and establishing a stable recording configuration. From Bliss and Lomo, (1).

input, a phenomenon they termed E-S (EPSP-to-Spike) potentiation. These two phenomena, synaptic potentiation and increased action potential firing, together were termed LTP. LTP lasted many, many hours in this intact rabbit preparation. The appeal of LTP as an analog of memory was immediately apparent—it is a long-lasting change in neuronal function that is produced by a brief period of unique stimulus, exactly the sort of mechanism that had long been postulated to be involved in memory formation. This pioneering work of Bliss and Lomo set in motion a several-decade-long pursuit by numerous investigators geared toward understanding the attributes and mechanisms of LTP.

A. The Hippocampal Circuit and Measuring Synaptic Transmission in the Hippocampal Slice

Bliss and Lomo did their experiment using the intact rabbit, stimulating and recording in the anesthetized animal using implanted electrodes. In recent times this preparation has been largely supplanted by the use of recordings from hippocampal slices maintained *in vitro* (see Figure 3). As most of the LTP experiments that will be described in the rest of the book come from this type of preparation, the next section will describe the hippocampal neuronal and synaptic circuit, and give an overview of extracellular recording in a typical LTP experiment.

As we have already discussed in earlier chapters, the main information processing circuit in the hippocampus is the relatively simple tri-synaptic pathway, and much of this basic circuit is preserved in transverse slices across the long axis of the hippocampus (Figure 4).

Various types of LTP can be induced at all three of these synaptic sites, and we will discuss below some mechanistic differences between these. Most experiments on the basic attributes and mechanisms of LTP have been studies of the synaptic connections between axons from area CA3 pyramidal neurons that extend into area CA1. These are the synapses onto CA1 pyramidal neurons that are known as the Schaffer collateral inputs.

The main excitatory (i.e., glutamatergic) synaptic circuitry in the hippocampus, in overview, consists of three modules (see Figure 4) (2–4). Information enters the dentate gyrus of the hippocampal formation from cortical and subcortical structures via the perforant path inputs from the entorhinal cortex (Figure 4). These inputs make synaptic connections with the dentate granule cells of the dentate gyrus. After synapsing in the dentate gyrus, information is moved to area CA3 via the mossy fiber pathway, which consists of the axonal outputs of the dentate granule cells and their connections with pyramidal neurons in area CA3. After synapsing in area CA3, information is moved to area CA1 via the Schaffer collateral path, which consists largely of the axons of area CA3 pyramidal neurons along with other projections from area CA3 of the contralateral hippocampus. After synapsing in CA1, information exits the hippocampus via projections from CA1 pyramidal neurons and returns to subcortical and cortical structures.

The connections in this synaptic circuit are retained in a fairly impressive manner if one makes transverse slices of the hippocampus, as the inputs, "tri-synaptic circuit," and outputs are laid out in a generally laminar fashion along the long axis of the hippocampal formation. This is a great advantage for *in vitro* electrophysiological experiments.

It is important to emphasize that the tri-synaptic circuit outlined above is a great oversimplification,

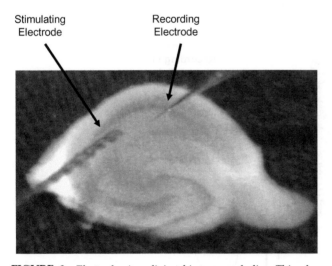

Stimulating Electrode

Recording Electrode

FIGURE 3 Electrodes in a living hippocampal slice. This photograph illustrates the appearance of a mouse hippocampal slice, maintained in a recording chamber. Responses in area CA1 are recorded using a saline-filled glass micropipette electrode (right) and a bipolar platinum stimulating electrode (left). See text and Figure 4 for additional details. Image courtesy of Susan Campbell.

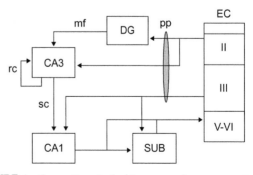

FIGURE 4 Connections in the hippocampal memory system. The excitatory pathways in the hippocampal formation. EC, entorhinal cortex; DG, dentate gyrus: mf, mossy fibers; pp, perforant path; rc, recurrent collateral axons of the CA3 pyramidal neurons; sc, Schaffer collateral/commissural axons; SUB, submiculum. Figure and legend from (48). Copyright Elsevier 1996.

as there are a great many additional synaptic components of the hippocampus. For example, there are inhibitory GABAergic interneurons that make synaptic connections with all of the principal excitatory neurons outlined above. These GABAergic inputs serve in both a feedforward and feedback fashion to control excitability. There are also many recurrent and collateral excitatory connections between the excitatory pyramidal neurons, particularly in the area CA3 region. There is a direct projection from the entorhinal cortex to the distal regions of CA1 pyramidal neuron dendrites, a pathway known as the stratum lacunosum moleculare.

Finally, as we discussed in Chapter 2, there are many modulatory projections into the hippocampus that make synaptic connections with the principal neurons. These inputs are via long projection fibers from various anatomical nuclei in the brainstem region, and they are, by and large, not directly excitatory or inhibitory, but rather serve to modulate synaptic connectivity in a fairly subtle way. There are four predominant extrinsic modulatory projections into the hippocampus. First, there are inputs of norepinephrine (NE)-containing fibers that project from the locus ceruleus. Second, there are dopamine (DA)-containing fibers that arise from the substantia nigra. There also are inputs using acetylcholine (ACh) from

the medial septal nucleus, and 5-hydroxytryptamine (5HT, serotonin) from the raphe nuclei.

B. Long-Term Potentiation of Synaptic Responses

In a popular variation of the basic LTP experiment, extracellular field potential recordings in the dendritic regions of area CA1 are utilized to monitor synaptic transmission at Schaffer collateral synapses (see Figure 5). A bipolar stimulating electrode is placed in the stratum radiatum subfield of area CA1 and stimuli (typically constant current pulses ranging from 1–30 μA) are delivered. Stimuli delivered in this fashion stimulate the output axons of CA3 neurons that pass nearby, causing action potentials to propagate down these axons. Cellular responses to this stimulation are recorded using extracellular or intracellular electrophysiologic recording techniques.

The typical waveform in an extra cellular recording consists of a "fiber volley," which is an indication of the pre-synaptic action potential arriving at the recording site, and the excitatory post-synaptic potential (EPSP) itself. The EPSP responses are a manifestation of synaptic activation (depolarization) in the CA1 pyramidal neurons. For measuring "field" i.e., extracellularly recorded EPSPs, the parameter typically measured is the initial slope of the EPSP waveform (see Figure 5).

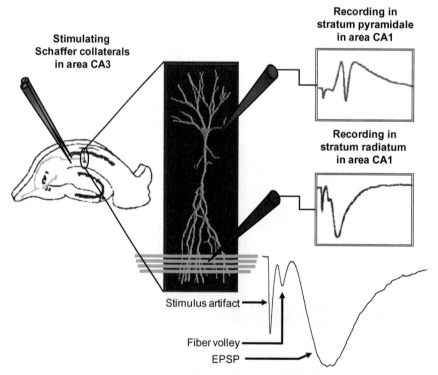

FIGURE 5   Recording configuration and typical physiologic responses in a hippocampal slice recording experiment. Electrode placements and responses from stratum pyramidale (cell body layer) and stratum oriens (dendritic regions) are shown. In addition, the typical waveform of a population EPSP is illustrated, showing the stimulus artifact, fiber volley, and population EPSP.

Absolute peak amplitude of EPSPs can also be measured, but the initial slope is the preferred index. This is because the initial slope is less subject to contamination from other sources of current flow in the slice. For example, currents are generated by feedforward inhibition due to GABA-ergic neuron activation. Also, if the cells fire action potentials this can contaminate later stages of the EPSP, even when one is recording from the dendritic region.

Extracellular field recordings measure responses from a population of neurons, so EPSPs recorded in this fashion are referred to as population EPSPs (pEPSPs). Note that pEPSPs are downward-deflecting for stratum radiatum recordings (see Figure 5). If one is recording from the cell body layer (stratum pyramidale) the EPSP is an upward deflection, and if the cells fire action potentials the EPSP has superimposed on it a downward deflecting "spike," the population spike.

As a prelude to starting an LTP experiment, input–output (I–O) functions for stimulus intensity versus EPSP magnitude are recorded in response to increasing intensities of stimulation (see Figure 6). For the remainder of the experiment, the test stimulus intensity is set to elicit an EPSP that is approximately 35–50% of the maximum response recorded during the I–O measurements. Baseline synaptic transmission at this constant test stimulus intensity is usually monitored for a period of 15–20 minutes to ensure a stable response.

Once the health of the hippocampal slice is confirmed, as indicated by a stable baseline synaptic response, LTP can be induced using any one of a wide variety of different LTP induction protocols. Many popular variations include a single or repeated period of one second 100 Hz stimulation (with delivery of the 100 Hz trains separated by 20 seconds or more) where stimulus intensity is at a level necessary for approximately half-maximal stimulation (see Figure 6 and Box 3). A variation is a "strong" induction protocol where LTP is induced with three pairs of 100 Hz, one-second stimuli, where stimulus intensity is near that necessary for a maximal EPSP. This latter protocol gives robust LTP that lasts for essentially as long as one can keep the hippocampal slice alive. A final major variation is high-frequency stimulation patterned after the endogenous hippocampal theta rhythm; this will be described in more detail in a later section of this chapter.

C. Short-Term Plasticity—Paired-Pulse Facilitation and Post-Tetanic Potentiation

There are two types of short-term plasticity exhibited at hippocampal Schaffer collateral synapses and elsewhere that are just as activity-dependent as LTP. These are paired-pulse facilitation (PPF) and post-tetanic potentiation (PTP). PPF is a form of short-term synaptic plasticity that is commonly held to be due to residual

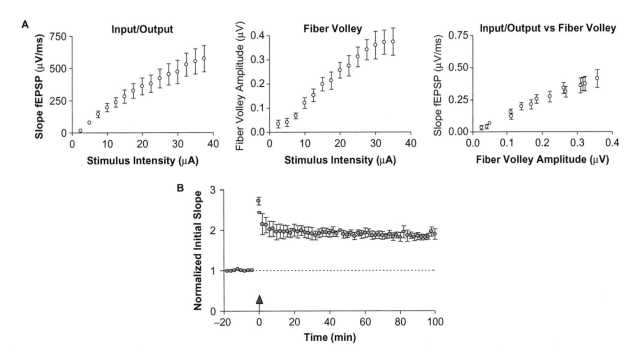

FIGURE 6 An input–output curve and typical LTP experiment. The top panel shows the relationship of EPSP magnitude versus stimulus intensity (in microAmps), and the same data converted to an input–output relationship for EPSP versus fiber volley magnitude in order to allow an evaluation of post-synaptic response versus pre-synaptic response in the same hippocampal slice. The lower panel illustrates a typical high-frequency stimulation induced potentiation of synaptic transmission in area CA1 of a rat hippocampal slice *in vitro*. The arrow indicates the delivery of 100 Hz (100 pulses per second) synaptic stimulation. Data courtesy of Ed Weeber and Coleen Atkins.

BOX 3

MONITORING BASELINE SYNAPTIC TRANSMISSION

In most pharmacologic experiments using physiologic recordings in hippocampal slice preparations, effects of drug application on baseline synaptic transmission can be evaluated by simply monitoring EPSPs before and after drug application using constant stimulus intensity. A more elaborate alternative is to produce input–output curves for EPSP initial slope (or magnitude) versus stimulus intensity for the pre-synaptic stimulus (see Figure 6). These types of within-slice experiments are very straightforward, but in some experimental comparisons this type of within-preparation design is not possible. For example, if one is comparing a wildtype with a knockout animal, of necessity, there must be a comparison across preparations. How does one evaluate if there is a difference in basal synaptic transmission in this situation? The principal confound is that while one has control over the magnitude of the stimulus one delivers to the pre-synaptic fibers, differences in electrode placement, slice thickness, etc., from preparation to preparation cause variability in

the magnitude of the synaptic response elicited by a constant stimulus amplitude. One commonly used approach in order to compare from one preparation (or animal strain) to the next is to quantitate the EPSP relative to the amplitude of the fiber volley in that same hippocampal slice (see Figure 6A). The rationale is that the fiber volley, which represents the action potentials firing in the pre-synaptic fibers, is a pre-synaptic physiologic response from within the same slice, and that one can at least normalize the EPSP to a within-slice parameter. The underlying assumption is that the magnitude of the fiber volley is representative of the number of axons firing an action potential. While not a perfect control, evaluating input–output relationships for fiber volley magnitude versus EPSP is a great improvement when making comparisons between different types of animals. If differences are observed, an increase in the fiber volley amplitude-EPSP slope relationship suggests an augmentation of synaptic transmission.

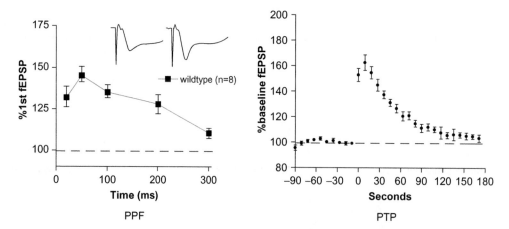

FIGURE 7 Paired-pulse facilitation (left panel) and post-tetanic potentiation (right panel). See text for details. Data for both panels courtesy of Michael Levy.

---

calcium augmenting neurotransmitter release pre-synaptically. When two single stimulus pulses are applied with interpulse intervals ranging from 20–300 milliseconds, the second EPSP produced is larger than the first (see Figure 7). This effect is referred to as PPF. The role of this type of synaptic plasticity in the behaving animal is unknown at this time; however, it is clearly a robust form of temporal integration of synaptic transmission and could be used in information processing behaviorally.

The second form of short-term plasticity, PTP, is a large enhancement of synaptic efficacy observed after brief periods of high-frequency synaptic activity. For example, in experiments where LTP is induced with one or two one-second, 100 Hz tetani, a large and transient increase in synaptic efficacy is produced immediately after high-frequency tetanus (see Figure 7). This is PTP. The mechanisms for PTP are unknown, but both PTP and PPF are NMDA receptor-independent phenomena.

III. NMDA RECEPTOR-DEPENDENCE OF LONG-TERM POTENTIATION

In 1983 Graham Collingridge made the breakthrough discovery that induction of tetanus-induced forms of LTP is blocked by blockade of the NMDA subtype of glutamate receptor (5). Collingridge's fascinating discovery was that the glutamate analog aminophosphono-valeric acid (APV), an agent that selectively blocks the NMDA subtype of glutamate receptor, could block LTP induction while leaving baseline synaptic transmission entirely intact (Figure 8).

This was the first experiment to give a specific molecular insight into the mechanisms of LTP induction. The properties of the NMDA receptor that allow it to function in this unique role of triggering LTP are important, and we will return to a detailed analysis of regulation of the NMDA receptor later in this book. For our purposes right now, suffice it to say that pharmacologic blockers of NMDA receptor function have allowed the definition of different types of LTP that can be selectively induced with various physiologic stimulation protocols. For example, subsequent work has shown that an NMDA receptor-independent type of LTP can be induced in area CA1, and elsewhere in the hippocampus (mossy fibers, to be precise), as well as other parts of the CNS. We will return to a brief description of these types of LTP at the end of this chapter, but for now will continue to focus on NMDA receptor-dependent types of LTP.

Early studies of LTP used mostly high-frequency (100 Hz) stimulation, in repeated one-second-long trains, as the LTP-inducing stimulation protocol. While these protocols are still widely used to good effect, it is clear that such prolonged periods of high-frequency firing do not occur physiologically in the behaving animal. However, LTP can also be induced by stimulation protocols that are much more like naturally occurring neuronal firing patterns in the hippocampus. To date the forms of LTP induced by these types of stimulation have all been found to be NMDA receptor-dependent in area CA1. Two popular variations of these protocols are based on the natural occurrence of an increased rate of hippocampal pyramidal neuron firing while a rat or mouse is exploring and learning about a new environment. Under these circumstances, hippocampal pyramidal neurons fire bursts of action potentials at about five bursts per second, i.e., 5 Hz. This is the hippocampal "theta" rhythm that has been described in the literature. One variation of LTP-inducing stimulation that mimics this pattern of firing is referred to as Theta-Frequency Stimulation (TFS), which consists of 30 seconds of single stimuli delivered at 5 Hz. Another variation, Theta-Burst Stimulation (TBS) consists of three trains of stimuli delivered at 20-second intervals, each train composed of ten stimulus bursts delivered at 5 Hz, with each burst consisting of four pulses at 100 Hz (see Figure 9). These patterns of stimulation, which are based on naturally-occurring firing patterns *in vivo*, lead to LTP in hippocampal slice preparations.

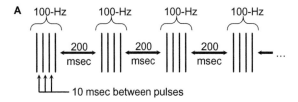

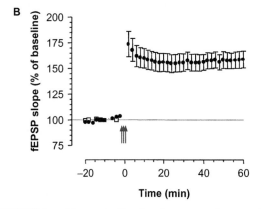

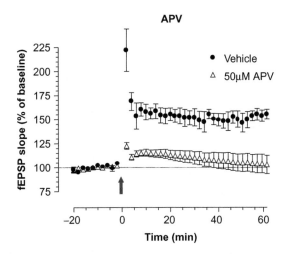

FIGURE 8 APV block of LTP. These data are from recordings *in vitro* from mouse hippocampal slices, demonstrating the NMDA receptor-dependence of tetanus-induced LTP. Identical high-frequency synaptic stimulation was delivered in control (filled circles) and NMDA receptor antagonist (APV, open triangles) treated slices. Data courtesy of Joel Selcher.

FIGURE 9 LTP triggered by theta burst stimulation in the mouse hippocampus. (A) Schematic depicting theta burst stimulation. This LTP induction paradigm consists of three trains of 10 high-frequency bursts delivered at 5 Hz. (B) LTP induced with theta burst stimulation (TBS-LTP) in hippocampal area CA1. The three red arrows represent the three TBS trains.

A. Pairing Long-Term Potentiation

Of course, there are much more sophisticated electrophysiologic techniques than extracellular recording that one can use to monitor synaptic function. Intracellular recording and patch-clamp techniques that measure electrophysiologic responses in single neurons have also been used widely in studies of LTP (see Box 4). These types of recording techniques perturb the cell that is being recorded from, and lead to "run-down" of the post-synaptic response in the cell impaled by the electrode. This limits the duration of the LTP experiment to however long the cell stays alive—somewhere in the range of 60 to 90 minutes for an accomplished physiologist. Regardless, in these recording configurations one can induce synaptic potentiation using tetanic stimulation or theta-pattern stimulation and measure LTP as an increase in post-synaptic currents through glutamate-gated ion channels, or as an increase in post-synaptic depolarization when monitoring the membrane potential.

Control of the post-synaptic neuron's membrane potential with cellular recording techniques also allows for some sophisticated variations of the LTP induction paradigm. In one particularly important series of experiments it was discovered that LTP can be induced by pairing repeated single pre-synaptic stimuli with post-synaptic membrane depolarization, so-called "pairing" LTP (see Figure 10) (6).

The basis for pairing LTP comes from one of the fundamental properties of the NMDA receptor (see Figure 11). The NMDA receptor is both a glutamate-gated channel and a voltage-dependent one. The simultaneous presence of glutamate and a depolarized membrane is necessary and sufficient (when the co-agonist glycine is present) to open the channel. Pairing synaptic stimulation with membrane depolarization provided via the recording electrode (plus the low levels of glycine always normally present) opens the NMDA receptor channel and leads to the induction of LTP.

How does the NMDA receptor trigger LTP? The NMDA receptor is a calcium channel and its opening leads to elevated intracellular calcium in the post-synaptic neuron. It is this calcium influx that triggers LTP, and indeed many subsequent chapters in this volume deal with the various processes this calcium influx triggers. It is important to remember that it is not necessarily the case that every calcium molecule involved in LTP induction actually comes through the

---

BOX 4

RECORDING FROM INDIVIDUAL NEURONS

While most of the data under discussion in this chapter were generated using extracellular recording techniques, there are a number of much more sophisticated electrophysiologic techniques that have been used to great effect in studies of LTP. These types of techniques fall into two broad categories generally referred to as sharp electrode recording and patch-clamp recording. The basic difference in the two techniques is that sharp electrode recording impales the neuron with the recording electrode, while patch-clamping involves forming a tight seal between the recording electrode and the cell membrane. In general, sharp electrode recording is used for current clamp experiments or experiments where one monitors the membrane potential passively. Patch-clamp experiments, in general, involve voltage clamp of the membrane potential. In these experiments one can hold the membrane potential constant while measuring current flow through membrane channels. Alternatively, one can use the electrode to manipulate the membrane potential directly. This latter type of experiment was the sort used to discover pairing LTP as described in the text, and also in key experiments demonstrating that depolarization of the post-synaptic cell is required for LTP induction. More recent applications of patch-clamping approaches have allowed the direct recording of dendritic membrane potential (prior studies had all recorded from the much larger cell body region), and this dendritic patch recording technique allowed the seminal finding of back-propagating action potentials in dendrites.

A great strength that single-cell recording techniques have in common is that they allow access to the cytoplasm of a single post-synaptic neuron. This allows the introduction of pharmacologic agents, including large proteins, specifically into the single post-synaptic cell. Application of this approach has led to a number of landmark findings in investigations of LTP, including the discovery of a necessity for post-synaptic calcium for LTP induction, and the necessity for post-synaptic protein kinase activity for LTP induction.

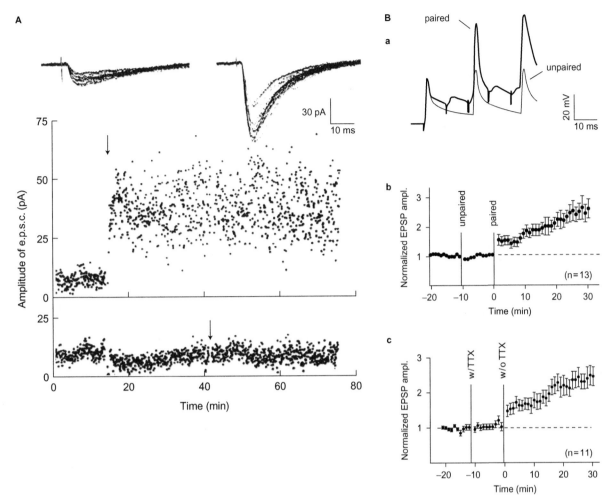

FIGURE 10 Pairing LTP. (A) LTP of synaptic transmission induced by pairing post-synaptic depolarization with synaptic activity. The upper panels illustrate post-synaptic currents recorded directly from the post-synaptic neuron using voltage-clamp techniques (see Box 2). The lower panels are a pairing TLP experiment (upper), and control, non-paired pathway (lower). In the pairing LTP experiment hippocampal CA1 pyramidal neurons were depolarized from −70 mV to 0 mV while the paired pathway was stimulated at 2 Hz 40 times. Control received no stimulation during depolarization. From Malinow and Tsien (7). (B) Pairing small EPSPs with back-propagating dendritic action potentials induces LTP. Inset (a) subthreshold EPSPs paired with back-propagating action potentials increase dendritic action potential amplitude. Voltage-clamp recording at approximately 240 μm from soma, that is, in the dendritic tree of the neuron (see Figure 10). Action potentials were evoked by 2 ms current injections through a somatic whole-cell electrode at 20 ms intervals. Alone, action potential amplitude was small (unpaired). Paired with EPSPs (5 stimuli at 100 Hz), the action potential amplitude increased greatly (paired). Inset (b) grouped data showing normalized EPSP amplitude after unpaired and paired stimulation. The pairing protocol shown in (a) was repeated five times at 5 Hz at 15 second intervals twice. (C) A similar pairing protocol was given with and without applying the sodium channel blocker tetrodotoxin (TTX, to block action potential propagation) to the proximal apical dendrites to prevent back-propagating action potentials from reaching the synaptic input sites. LTP was induced only when action potentials fully back-propagated into the dendrites. Reproduced with permission from Magee and Johnston, (8).

NMDA receptor. Calcium influx through membrane calcium channels and calcium released from intracellular stores may also be involved.

The gating of the NMDA receptor/channel involves a voltage-dependent Mg^{++} block of the channel pore. Depolarization of the membrane in which the NMDA receptor resides is necessary to drive the divalent Mg^{++} cation out of the pore, which then allows calcium ions to flow through. Thus, the simultaneous occurrence of both glutamate in the synapse and a depolarized post-synaptic membrane is necessary to

open the channel and allow LTP-triggering calcium into the post-synaptic cell.

These properties, glutamate dependence *and* voltage-dependence, of the NMDA receptor allow it to function as a coincidence detector. This is a critical aspect of NMDA receptor regulation, and this allows for a unique contribution of the NMDA receptor to information processing at the molecular level. Using the NMDA receptor the neuron can trigger a unique event, calcium influx, specifically when a particular synapse is both active pre-synaptically (glutamate is present in the

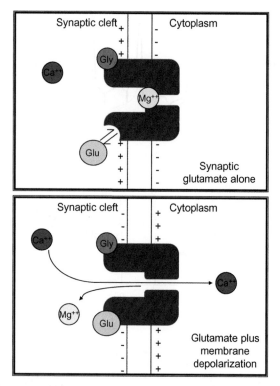

FIGURE 11   Coincidence detection by the NMDA receptor. The simultaneous presence of glutamate and membrane depolarization is necessary for relieving Mg^{++} blockade and allowing calcium influx.

synapse) and post-synaptically (when the membrane is depolarized).

This confers a computational property of associativity on the synapse. This attribute is nicely illustrated by "pairing" LTP, as described above, where low-frequency synaptic activity paired with post-synaptic depolarization can lead to LTP. The associative property of the NMDA receptor allows for many other types of sophisticated information processing as well. For example, activation of a weak input to a neuron can induce potentiation, provided a strong input to the same neuron is activated at the same time (9). These particular features of LTP induction have stimulated a great deal of interest, as they are reminiscent of classical conditioning with depolarization and synaptic input roughly corresponding to unconditioned and conditioned stimuli, respectively.

The associative nature of NMDA receptor activation also allows for synapse specificity of LTP induction, which has been shown to occur experimentally. If one pairs post-synaptic depolarization with activity at one set of synaptic inputs to a cell, while leaving a second input silent or active only during periods at which the post-synaptic membrane is near the resting potential, then selective potentiation of the paired input pathway occurs.

Similarly, in field stimulation experiments LTP is restricted to tetanized pathways—even inputs convergent on the same dendritic region of the post-synaptic neuron are not potentiated if they receive only baseline synaptic transmission in the absence of synaptic activity sufficient to adequately depolarize the post-synaptic neuron (10). This last point illustrates the basis for LTP "cooperativity." LTP induction in extracellular stimulation experiments requires cooperative interaction of afferent fibers, which in essence means there is an intensity threshold for triggering LTP induction. Sufficient total synaptic activation by the input fibers must be achieved such that the post-synaptic membrane is adequately depolarized to allow opening of the NMDA receptor (11).

B. Dendritic Action Potentials

In the context of the functioning hippocampal neuron *in vivo*, the associative nature of NMDA receptor activation means that a given neuron must reach a critical level of depolarization in order for LTP to occur at any of its synapses. Specifically, in the physiologic context, the hippocampal pyramidal neuron generally must reach the threshold for firing an action potential. While action potentials are, of course, triggered in the active zone of the cell body, hippocampal pyramidal neurons along with many other types of CNS neurons can actively propagate action potentials into the dendritic regions: the so-called back-propagating action potential (see Figure 12)(8). These dendritic action potentials are just like action potentials propagated down axons, in that they are carried predominantly by voltage-dependent ion channels such as sodium channels. The penetration of the back-propagating action potential into the dendritic region provides a wave of membrane depolarization that allows for the opening of the voltage-dependent NMDA receptor/ion channels. As a generalization, in many instances in the intact cell back-propagating action potentials are what allow sufficient depolarization to reach hippocampal pyramidal neuron synapses in order to open NMDA receptors. In an ironic twist, this has brought us back to a more literal reading of Hebb's postulate where, as we discussed in the introduction to this chapter, Hebb actually specified firing of the post-synaptic neuron as being necessary for the strengthening of its connections.

In fact, the timing of the arrival of a dendritic action potential with synaptic glutamate input appears to play an important part in precise, timing-dependent triggering of synaptic plasticity in the hippocampus (see Figures 10 and 13)(8). It has been observed that a critical timing window is involved *vis-à-vis* back-propagating action potentials: glutamate arrival in

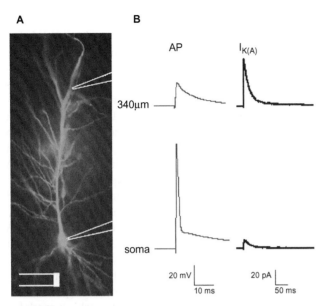

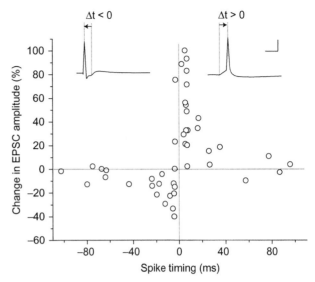

FIGURE 12 Back-propagating action potentials in dendrites of CA1 pyramidal neurons. (A) The recording set-up, with a bipolar stimulating electrode used to trigger action potentials at the cell body region (lower left), a recording electrode in the cell soma to monitor firing of an action potential, and a recording electrode in the dendrites (upper right) to monitor propagation of the action potential into the distal dendritic region. (B) Traces indicate the data recorded from the soma (lower) and dendritic (upper) electrodes. The left-hand traces from (B) (labeled AP) indicate the membrane depolarization achieved at the soma and dendrite when an action potential is triggered and propagates into the dendritic region. Note that the dendritic action potential is of lower magnitude and broader due to the effects of dendritic membrane biophysical properties as the action potential propagates down the dendrite. The right half of (B) shows current flow through "A-type" voltage-dependent potassium currents observed in the soma and dendrites. The density of A-type potassium currents increases dramatically as one progresses outward from the soma into the dendritic regions, as illustrated by the much larger potassium current observed in the distal dendritic electrode. These voltage-dependent potassium channels are key regulators of the likelihood of back-propagating action potentials reaching various parts of the dendritic tree. Data and figure reproduced from Yuan et al. (12).

FIGURE 13 The timing of back-propagating action potentials with synaptic activity determines whether synaptic strength is altered, and in which direction. Precise timing of the arrival of a back-propagating action potential (a "spike") with synaptic glutamate determines the effect of paired depolarization and synaptic activity. A narrow window when the arrival of the synaptic EPSP immediately precedes or follows the arrival of the back-propagating action potential determines whether synaptic strength is increased,

the synaptic cleft must slightly precede the back-propagating action potential in order for the NMDA receptor to be effectively opened. This timing dependence arises in part due to the time required for glutamate to bind to and open the NMDA receptor. The duration of an action potential is, of course, quite short so in essence the glutamate must be there first and already bound to the receptor in order for full activation to occur. (Additional factors are involved, see references 13–16.)

This order-of-pairing specificity allows for a precision of information processing—not only must the membrane be depolarized, but also as a practical matter the cell must fire an action potential. Moreover, the timing of the back-propagating action potential

arriving at a synapse must be appropriate. It is easy to imagine how the nervous system could capitalize on these properties to allow for forming precise timing-dependent associations between two events.

One twist to the order-of-pairing specificity is that if the order is reversed and the action potential arrives before the EPSP, then synaptic depression is produced (see Figure 13). The mechanisms for this attribute are under investigation at present—one hypothesis is that the backward pairing by various potential mechanisms leads to a lower level of calcium influx, which produces synaptic depression (see below).

In later chapters we will discuss in more detail the molecular mechanisms by which local effects regulating membrane depolarization within specific dendritic branches or dendritic subregions may be achieved. Moreover, we will discuss the signal transduction mechanisms by which modulatory neurotransmitter systems can regulate the likelihood of action potential back-propagation through controlling dendritic potassium channels, and we will discuss how this might allow for sophisticated information processing through the interplay of action potential propagation, glutamate release, and neuromodulation. All of these things become possible because the dendritic membrane in which the NMDA receptors reside is not passive, but contains voltage-dependent ion channels. Thus, controlling the post-synaptic membrane biophysical properties can be a critical determinant for regulating the triggering of synaptic change.

IV. NMDA RECEPTOR-INDEPENDENT LONG-TERM POTENTIATION

While the vast majority of studies of LTP and its molecular mechanisms have investigated NMDA receptor-dependent processes, as mentioned above there are also several types of NMDA receptor-independent LTP. The next section will briefly describe a few different types of NMDA receptor-independent LTP (see Figure 14).

A. 200 Hz Long-Term Potentiation

NMDA receptor-independent LTP can be induced at the Schaffer collateral synapses in area CA1, the same synapses discussed thus far. This allows for somewhat of a compare-and-contrast of two different types of LTP at the same synapse. A protocol that elicits NMDA receptor-independent LTP in area CA1 is the use of four half-second, 200 Hz stimuli separated by five seconds (18). LTP induced with this stimulation protocol is insensitive to NMDA receptor-selective antagonists such as APV. It is interesting that simply doubling the rate of tetanic stimulation from 100 Hz to 200 Hz appears to shift activity-dependent mechanisms for synaptic potentiation into NMDA receptor independence. At the simplest level of thinking, this indicates that there is some unique type of temporal integration going on at the higher frequency stimulation that allows the necessity for NMDA receptor activation to be superseded. What might the 200 Hz stimulation be uniquely stimulating? One appealing hypothesis arises from the observation that 200 Hz LTP is blocked by blockers of voltage-sensitive calcium channels. Thus, the current working model is that 200 Hz stimulation elicits sufficiently large and sufficiently prolonged membrane depolarization, resulting in the opening of voltage-dependent calcium channels, to trigger elevation of post-synaptic calcium

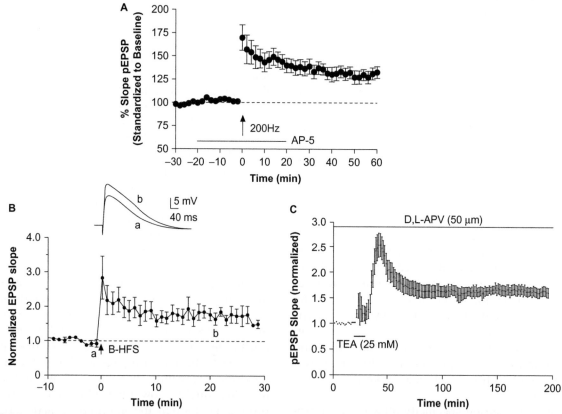

FIGURE 14 Examples of NMDA receptor-independent LTP. (A) 200 Hz stimulation in area CA1 elicits LTP, even in the presence of the NMDA receptor antagonist APV. Data courtesy of Ed Weeber. (B) LTP at mossy fiber inputs into area CA3 is also NMDA receptor-independent—the potentiation shown occurred in the presence of blockers of the NMDA receptor. Data courtesy of Rick Gray. From Kapur et al. (17). (C) Application of the K channel blocker tetra-ethyl ammonium (TEA) also elicits NMDA receptor-independent LTP in area CA1. Data courtesy of Craig Powell (Ph.D. thesis, Baylor College of Medicine, pg 50).

sufficient to trigger LTP synaptic potentiation. One observation consistent with this hypothesis is that injection of post-synaptic calcium chelators blocks 200 Hz stimulation-induced LTP.

B. Tetra-Ethyl Ammonium Long-Term Potentiation

NMDA receptor-independent LTP in area CA1 can also be induced using tetra-ethyl ammonium (TEA$^+$) ion application, a form of LTP which is referred to as LTP$_k$ (19, 20). TEA$^+$ is a non-specific potassium channel blocker, the application of which greatly increases membrane excitability. Like 200 Hz LTP, LTP$_k$ is insensitive to NMDA receptor antagonists, and is blocked by blockade of voltage-sensitive calcium channels. Moreover, LTP$_k$ is also blocked by post-synaptic calcium chelator injection. The induction of LTP$_k$ is dependent on synaptic activity, as its induction is blocked by AMPA receptor antagonists. Similar to 200 Hz LTP, the current model for TEA LTP is that synaptic depolarization via glutamate receptor activation, augmented by the hyperexcitable membrane due to K$^+$ channel blockade, leads to a relatively large and prolonged membrane depolarization. This leads to the triggering of LTP through post-synaptic calcium influx.

C. Mossy Fiber Long-Term Potentiation in Area CA3

The predominant model system for studying NMDA receptor-independent LTP is not the Schaffer collateral synapses, but rather the mossy fiber inputs into area CA3 pyramidal neurons. Considerable excitement accompanied the discovery of NMDA receptor-independent LTP at these synapses by Harris and Cotman (21). The mossy fiber synapses are unique, large synapses with unusual pre-synaptic specializations, and there has been much interest in comparing the attributes and mechanisms of induction of mossy fiber LTP (MF-LTP) with those of NMDA receptor-dependent LTP in area CA1 (17, 22, 23).

V. A ROLE FOR CALCIUM INFLUX IN NMDA RECEPTOR-DEPENDENT LONG-TERM POTENTIATION

NMDA receptor-dependent LTP at Schaffer collateral synapses has achieved a broad consensus of a necessity for elevations of post-synaptic calcium for triggering LTP (24). In fact, this is one of the few areas of LTP research where there is almost universal agreement.

The case for a role for elevated post-synaptic calcium in triggering LTP is quite clear-cut and solid (25–27). A principal line of evidence is that injection of calcium chelators post-synaptically blocks the induction of LTP. Also, inhibitors of a variety of calcium-activated enzymes also block LTP induction, including specifically when they are introduced into the post-synaptic neuron. Fluorescent imaging experiments using calcium-sensitive indicators have clearly demonstrated that post-synaptic calcium is elevated with LTP-inducing stimulation. Finally, elevating post-synaptic calcium is sufficient to cause synaptic potentiation (although there has been some controversy on this point). Thus, the hypothesis of a role for post-synaptic calcium elevation in triggering LTP has met the three classic criteria (block, measure, mimic) necessary for "proving" a hypothesis, and this idea is on a solid experimental footing.

VI. PRE-SYNAPTIC VERSUS POST-SYNAPTIC MECHANISMS

One of the most intensely studied and least satisfactorily resolved aspects of LTP concerns the locus of LTP maintenance and expression. One component of LTP is an increase in the EPSP, which could arise from increasing glutamate concentrations in the synapse or by increasing the responsiveness to glutamate by the post-synaptic cell (see Figure 15). The "pre-" versus "post-" debate is whether the relevant changes reside pre-synaptically, manifest as an increase in neurotransmitter release or similar phenomenon, or post-synaptically, as a change in glutamate receptor responsiveness, etc. Over the last fifteen years or so numerous experiments have been performed to try to address this question, and as of yet there is no clear consensus answer. Popularity of the "pre-" hypothesis versus the "post-" hypothesis has waxed and waned, and this oscillation may continue for some time yet. In the next few paragraphs I will summarize a few representative findings to provide background on these issues.

In some of the earliest studies to begin to get at LTP mechanistically, it became clear that infusing compounds into the post-synaptic cell led to a block of LTP. A few of these studies involving calcium chelators were described in the last section, and some studies investigating protein kinases are described in later chapters of this book (see Box 5). If compounds that are limited in their distribution to the post-synaptic compartment block LTP, the most parsimonious hypothesis is that LTP resides post-synaptically.

However, shortly thereafter evidence began to accumulate suggesting that there were also pre-synaptic changes involved in LTP expression. For example,

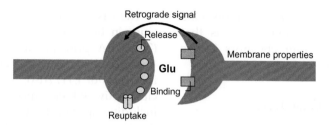

Pre-synaptic = Altered
• Neurotransmitter amount in vesicles
• Number of vesicles released
• Kinetics of release
• Glutamate reuptake
• Probability of vesicle fusion

Post-synaptic = Altered
• Number of AMPA receptors
• Insertion of AMPA receptors
• Ion flow through AMPA channels
• Membrane electrical properties

Additional possibilities include changes in number of total synaptic connections between two cells

FIGURE 15   Potential sites of synaptic modification in LTP.

BOX 5

A NEED FOR POST-SYNAPTIC PROTEIN KINASE ACTIVITY IN LONG-TERM POTENTIATION INDUCTION

Experiments using intracellular electrodes to perfuse membrane-impermeant peptides directly and selectively into the post-synaptic cell have been instrumental in clarifying a necessity for post-synaptic events in LTP induction. Based on many studies of this sort, it is clear that LTP induction is blocked by infusion of compounds whose permeation is restricted to the intracellular compartment of the post-synaptic cell. Some of the pioneering studies of this sort utilized injection of protein kinase inhibitors post-synaptically, which not only illustrated a need for post-synaptic events generally, but also clarified a need for post-synaptic signal transduction events specifically for the induction of LTP.

In some of the earliest studies, involvement of Ca^{2+}-dependent protein kinases was tested by intracellular injection of peptides that inhibited either PKC or CaMKII. As we will discuss later, many second messenger-regulated protein kinases have auto-inhibitory domains within their amino acid sequence. Synthetic peptides that inhibit these domains are some of the most selective pharmacologic tools available. In one early experiment, peptides corresponding to the protein kinase C autoinhibitory domain were infused post-synaptically and found to block LTP induction. While a variety of other earlier studies had shown that less-selective kinase inhibitors could block LTP induction,

these early studies were landmark findings, because of the specificity of the experimental manipulation.

In other early studies a role for post-synaptic CaMKII was also investigated, using a similar approach. Two different types of peptides were used to inhibit CaMKII activation in these studies. In one series of studies the investigators used the pseudosubstrate peptide CaMKII(273–302), which inhibits CaMKII by mimicking the autoinhibitory domain. In a separate series of experiments a different type of approach was used—the infusion of calmodulin-binding peptides. These peptides bind to the calcium signal-transducing protein calmodulin and inhibit its activation of downstream targets including CaMKII. The results from both these experiments are consistent with a role for post-synaptic signal transduction events in LTP induction in general, and suggest a role for CaMKII specifically. It turns out that subsequent work has shown that both these manipulations are doing more than just blocking CaMKII activation, because both types of peptides can affect other relevant signal transduction cascades. Nevertheless, these were key findings at the time, motivating pursuit of the CaMKII system as a player in LTP induction, and a wide variety of subsequent work has supported a role for CaMKII activation in LTP.

various types of "quantal" analysis that had been successfully applied at the neuromuscular junction to dissect pre-synaptic changes from post-synaptic changes suggested that LTP is associated with changes pre-synaptically. In a series of investigations, several laboratories used whole-cell recordings of synaptic transmission in hippocampal slices, and found an increase in the probability of release, a strong indicator of pre-synaptic changes in classic quantal analysis (7, 28–32). These findings fit nicely with earlier studies from Tim Bliss's laboratory suggesting an increase in glutamate release in LTP as well (30). Given findings supporting post-synaptic locus on the one hand and pre-synaptic locus on the other, why not just hypothesize that there are changes both pre-synaptically and post-synaptically? The rub came in that some of the quantal analysis results seemed to exclude post-synaptic changes occurring.

These findings in the early 1990s ushered in an exciting phase of LTP research that was important independent of the pre-versus-post debate *per se*. If there are changes pre-synaptically but these changes are triggered by events originating in the post-synaptic cell, as the earlier inhibitor-perfusion experiments had indicated, then the existence of a retrograde messenger is implied. A retrograde messenger is a compound generated in the post-synaptic compartment that diffuses back to, and signals changes in, the pre-synaptic compartment—the opposite (retrograde) direction from normal synaptic transmission. Moreover, if the compound is generated intracellularly in the post-synaptic neuron, then the compound must somehow be able to traverse the post-synaptic membrane. The data supporting pre-synaptic changes in LTP implied the existence of such a signaling system, and this hypothesis launched a number of interesting and important experiments to determine what types of molecules might serve such a role—some of these are highlighted in Figure 16.

However, in the mid-1990s the pre- versus post-pendulum began to swing back in the opposite direction, toward the post-synaptic side. Several groups found evidence for post-synaptic changes that could account for the apparently pre-synaptic changes identified by quantal analysis studies. Specifically, evidence was generated for what are termed "silent synapses" (see Figure 17). These are synapses that contain NMDA receptors but no alpha-amino-3-hydroxy-5-methyl-4-isoxazole propionic acid (AMPA) receptors—they are capable of synaptic plasticity mediated by NMDA receptor activation, but are physiologically silent in terms of baseline synaptic transmission. Silent synapses are rendered active by NMDA receptor-triggered activation of latent AMPA receptors post-synaptically. Such uncovering of silent

AMPA receptors could involve membrane insertion or post-translational activation of already-inserted receptors. Activation of silent synapses is a post-synaptic mechanism that could explain the effects (decreased failure rate, for example) in quantal analysis experiments that implied pre-synaptic changes. Thus, there is now an argument that all LTP physiology and biochemistry could be post-synaptic. For example, this model for conversion of silent synapses into active synapses by AMPA receptor insertion is an entirely post-synaptic phenomenon.

Given the variety of evidence described so far, should one conclude that LTP resides pre-synaptically, post-synaptically, or both? While there is not yet an unambiguous consensus in the pre- versus post- debate, overall the available literature indicates that changes are occurring in both the pre-synaptic and post-synaptic compartments. There are two

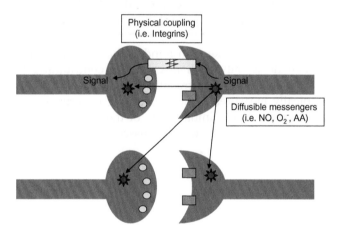

FIGURE 16   Potential mechanisms for retrograde signaling.

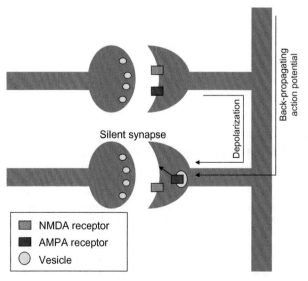

FIGURE 17   A simplified model of silent synapses.

different types of approaches I will briefly mention here. First, a number of experiments using sophisticated imaging techniques have found LTP to be associated with pre-synaptic changes such as increased vesicle recycling and increased pre-synaptic membrane turnover (see, for example, references 31–32). Also, direct biochemical measurements of the phosphorylation of proteins selectively localized to the pre-synaptic compartment have shown LTP-associated changes. Conceptually similar experiments looking at phosphorylation of post-synaptic proteins have found the same thing. Thus, imaging and biochemistry studies have fairly clearly illustrated that sustained biochemical changes are happening in both the pre-synaptic and post-synaptic cell.

VII. LONG-TERM POTENTIATION CAN INCLUDE AN INCREASED ACTION POTENTIAL FIRING COMPONENT

One caveat to keep in mind is that the discussion above deals only with mechanisms contributing to increases in synaptic strength. The increased EPSP is typically measured in field recording experiments as an increase in the initial slope of the EPSP (or EPSP magnitude), and as was discussed above a second

component of LTP is referred to as EPSP-spike (E-S) potentiation. As I have already mentioned, E-S potentiation was identified by Bliss and Lomo in the first published report of LTP (1), and is defined as an increase in population spike amplitude that cannot be attributed to an increase in synaptic transmission (i.e., initial EPSP slope in field recordings). Thus, E-S potentiation is a term used to refer to the post-synaptic cell having an increased probability of firing an action potential at a constant strength of synaptic input.

E-S potentiation at Schaffer collateral synapses can be observed using recordings in stratum pyramidale, as illustrated in Figure 18. In this example input–output curves for the initial slope of the EPSP and the population spike amplitude were generated using various stimulus intensities, before and after LTP induction. E-S potentiation is manifest as an increase in population spike amplitude even when responses are normalized to EPSP slope.

What is the mechanism for this long-term increase in the likelihood of firing an action potential? One possibility is that there are changes in the intrinsic excitability of the post-synaptic neuron. Particularly appealing is the idea that long-term down-regulation of dendritic potassium channel function could cause a persistent increase in cellular excitability and action potential firing. While investigations of this hypothesis are still at an early stage, some recent work has

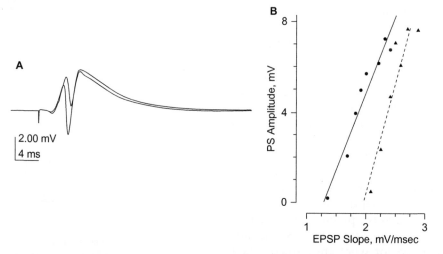

FIGURE 18 E-S potentiation in area CA1. Extracellular recordings were made in the cell body layer of area CA1 (using stimulation of the Schaffer collateral inputs), and input–output curves were performed using a range of 5–45 μA constant current stimulation. Initial slopes of the EPSP and population spike (PS) amplitude were then determined from the tracings, and the data plotted as population spike amplitude versus EPSP slope. Right panel: Plots are shown for pre-tetanus (triangles) and 75 minutes post-tetanus (circles). Left panel: Superimposed representative tracings for before and 75 minutes after tetanic stimulation, showing the increased population spike amplitude after tetanic stimulation. In this experiment, five 100 Hz tetani were delivered. EPSP to spike (E-S) coupling was assayed in hippocampal slices by taking a second set of input–output measurements after the induction of LTP. The baseline I–O curve and the post-stimulation I–O curve were then compared to assess whether a change in excitability had occurred over the course of the experiment. Although in the illustration I have presented we measured both EPSP slope and population spike amplitude from the same waveform, recording from the cell body layer, the preferred approach is to record EPSPs in the dendritic region and simultaneously record spikes independently from the cell body layer. This minimizes cross-contamination of the pop spike changes in the EPSP measurements, and *vice versa*.

suggested that E-S potentiation has a component due to intrinsic changes in the post-synaptic neuron.

Progress in testing this hypothesis has been slow, due to the technically difficult nature of the experiments. Most patch-clamp physiologic studies of LTP have utilized recordings from the cell body which are not capable of detecting changes in channels localized to the dendrites due to technical limitations. Thus, testing the idea of changes in dendritic excitability as a mechanism contributing to E-S potentiation requires dendritic patch-clamp recording, which at present only a few laboratories do routinely.

However, a more thoroughly investigated mechanism for E-S potentiation is based on alterations in feedforward inhibitory connections onto pyramidal neurons in area CA1 (see Figure 19). The next few paragraphs present an overview of this area.

There are a number of different types of neurons in the hippocampus that are called interneurons (or intrinsic neurons) because their inputs and outputs are restricted to local areas of the hippocampus. In other words, they only communicate with other neurons nearby in the hippocampus. Most of these neurons in area CA1 use the inhibitory neurotransmitter GABA, and their actions are to inhibit firing of CA1 pyramidal neurons. Different GABA-ergic interneurons make connections in all the dendritic regions of CA1 pyramidal neurons, as well as the initial segment of the axon where the action potential originates. A single GABA-ergic interneuron may contact a thousand pyramidal neurons, thus the effects of altered interneuron function are not generally limited to a single follower cell.

Interneurons in area CA1 receive glutamatergic Schaffer collateral projections, just as the pyramidal neurons do—in fact the inputs to the interneurons are branches of the same axons impinging the pyramidal neurons. Glutamate release at these interneuron synapses activates the interneurons and causes downstream release of GABA onto the pyramidal neurons. This inhibitory action is, of course, slightly delayed at the level of the single cell that receives input from the same Schaffer collateral axon that is activating the GABA-ergic interneuron, because there is an extra synaptic connection involved.

How does this local circuit contribute to E-S potentiation? Two different groups have shown that the same stimulation that produces LTP at the Schaffer collateral–pyramidal neuron synapses simultaneously produces a decreased efficacy of coupling (long-term depression, LTD) of the Schaffer collateral–interneuron synapses (33–34). Thus, while the excitatory input to the pyramidal neuron is being enhanced, the feedforward inhibitory GABA input is diminished. This causes a net increase in excitability and increased likelihood of firing an action potential, added on to the increased EPSP due to the normal LTP mechanisms. This is, of course, the definition of E-S potentiation.

There are a couple of interesting properties for this LTD at the Schaffer collateral–interneuron synapse. First, it is NMDA receptor-dependent, just like LTP. This explains why one does not see E-S potentiation independent of synaptic potentiation in experiments where APV is infused onto the slice. Second, and more interesting, the LTD is not specific to the activated synapse—other Schaffer collateral inputs onto the same interneuron are also depressed (33). Therefore, there is decreased feedforward inhibition across all the inputs (and outputs of course) for the whole interneuron. The interneuron has a diminished response to all its inputs, and therefore decreased feedforward inhibition to all its outputs. Thus, the interneuron LTD appears to be serving to modulate the behavior of an entire small local circuit of neuronal connections.

VIII. LONG-TERM POTENTIATION CAN BE DIVIDED INTO PHASES

Contemporary models divide very long-lasting LTP, i.e., LTP lasting in the range of 5–6 hours, into at least three phases. LTP comprising all three phases can be induced with repeated trains of high-frequency stimulation in area CA1 (see Figure 20), and the phases are expressed sequentially over time to constitute what we call "LTP." Late LTP (L-LTP) is hypothesized to be dependent for its induction on changes in gene expression, and this phase of LTP lasts many

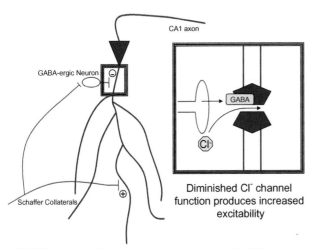

FIGURE 19 The GABA-ergic interneuron model of E-S potentiation. One potential mechanism for E-S potentiation is diminution of inhibitory feedforward inhibition through GABA-ergic interneurons in area CA1. Specific possible sites for this effect include LTD of the Schaffer collateral inputs onto GABA-ergic neurons, or synaptic depression of the interneuron-CA1 pyramidal neuron synapse.

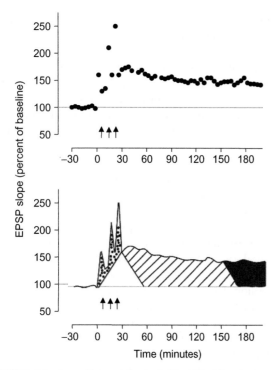

FIGURE 20 Immediate, early, and late LTP. The upper panel is real data from a late-phase LTP experiment, courtesy of Erik Roberson. The lower panel is a cartoon adaptation of the same data approximating the initial, early, and late stages of LTP. Adapted from *A Biochemists View of LTP* (35).

hours (see also 35). Early LTP (E-LTP) is likely subserved by persistently activated protein kinases, as we will discuss in the next chapter, and starts at around 30 minutes or less post-tetanus and is over by about 2–3 hours. The first stage of LTP, generally referred to as short-term potentiation (STP), is independent of protein kinase activity for its induction, and lasts about 30 minutes. The mechanisms for STP are essentially a complete mystery at present.

Readers may note some degree of ambiguity in the times specified for each phase of LTP. This is in part because the phases are very descriptive and different laboratories often use slightly different conditions for their LTP experiments.

A. Early-Long-Term Potentiation and Late-Long-Term Potentiation—Types Versus Phases

E-LTP and L-LTP refer to different temporal phases of LTP. These phases are subserved by different maintenance mechanisms of different time-courses and durations. These two phases of LTP, E-LTP and L-LTP, are not exclusive of each other. In fact, depending on the LTP induction protocol used, E-LTP can be ongoing while L-LTP is developing, and one supplants the other over time (35). These definitions contain an underlying assumption about the biochemistry of LTP

that is an organizing principle for the rest of this book, which is that different phases of LTP are subserved by distinct molecular mechanisms.

However, the terms E-LTP and L-LTP have also been used in a slightly different fashion, in particular as popularized by the Kandel laboratory (36). The Kandel laboratory and others use a terminology that divides the NMDA receptor-dependent form of LTP in area CA1 into E-LTP and L-LTP as well. E-LTP and L-LTP in this terminology refer to what one can characterize as two subtypes of LTP; a transient form (typically lasting 1–2 hours) and a long-lasting form (lasting at least five hours or more). The latter form of LTP is characterized by its dependence on intact protein synthesis, and the induction of this form of LTP requires delivery of multiple tetanic stimuli. E-LTP in this alternative nomenclature is induced by fewer tetanic stimuli, and is protein synthesis independent. In this usage, E-LTP and L-LTP are defined as different *types* of LTP, not as temporal phases of LTP. Thus, one must keep in mind that two slightly different variations in the use of E-LTP and L-LTP exist in the literature.

Before turning to a discussion of some implications of LTP having phases, there is one final set of three terms I must introduce—three terms widely used in the LTP literature. These terms arose from pharmacological inhibitor studies of LTP and I will go through these types of studies in a moment. However, first I will simply introduce the terms.

Induction refers to the transient events serving to trigger the formation of LTP. *Maintenance*, or more specifically a maintenance mechanism, refers to the persisting biochemical signal that lasts in the cell. This persisting biochemical signal acts on an effector, for example a glutamate receptor or the pre-synaptic release machinery, resulting in the *expression* of LTP.

It is important to keep in mind that, depending on the design of the experiment, induction, maintenance, and expression could be differentially inhibited (see Figure 21). The simplest type of experiment

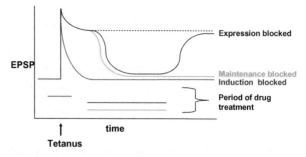

FIGURE 21 Induction, maintenance, and expression of LTP. This schematic illustrates the different experimental approaches to dissecting effects on the biochemical mechanisms subserving LTP induction, maintenance, or expression. See text for additional details.

does not do this—for example imagine if one applies an enzyme inhibitor (or knocks out a gene) before, during, and after the period of LTP-inducing high-frequency stimulation, this manipulation may block LTP. However, this does not distinguish whether the missing activity is required for the induction, the expression, or the maintenance of LTP. To distinguish between these possibilities, imagine instead applying the inhibitor selectively at different time points during the experiment. If inhibitor is applied only during the tetanus and then washed out and it blocks the generation of LTP, one can conclude that the enzyme is necessary for LTP induction. If the inhibitor is applied after the tetanus and it reverses the potentiation, it may be blocking either the maintenance or expression of LTP, as was nicely illustrated in an early experiment by Malinow, Madison, and Tsien (37) where they applied a protein kinase inhibitor after LTP induction. In this experiment, transient application of a kinase inhibitor after tetanus blocked synaptic potentiation, but the potentiation recovered after removal of the inhibitor. This is a blockade of LTP *expression*. However, if the kinase inhibitor had caused the potentiation to be lost irreversibly, the inhibitor would then, by definition, have blocked the *maintenance* of LTP.

Finally, it is important to synthesize the concepts of induction, maintenance, and expression with the concept of phases. Simply stated, three phases of LTP (STP, E-LTP, and L-LTP) times three distinct underlying mechanisms for each phase (induction, maintenance, and expression) gives nine separate categories into which any particular molecular mechanism contributing to LTP may fit (see Figure 22).

IX. MODULATION OF LONG-TERM POTENTIATION INDUCTION

In one sense the hippocampal slice is a denervated preparation. In the intact animal the hippocampus receives numerous input fibers that provide modulatory inputs of the neurotransmitters dopamine (DA), norepinephrine (NE), serotonin (5HT), and acetylcholine (ACh). Functionally these inputs are largely lost in physically preparing the hippocampal slice for the

experiment. However, these lost modulatory inputs can be partially reconstituted by directly applying the neurotransmitters (or more commonly pharmacologic substitutes) to the slice preparation *in vitro*. This approach has been used quite successfully to gain insights into the physiologic mechanisms and functional roles of these inputs in the intact brain.

Norepinephrine, DA, and ACh-mimicking compounds can all modulate the induction of LTP at Schaffer collateral synapses (see Figure 23). Specifically, agents acting at various subtypes of receptors for these compounds can increase the likelihood of LTP induction and the magnitude of LTP that is induced. Several examples of this type of modulation experiment are shown in Figure 23. In one example (Figure 23A) 5 Hz stimulation of Schaffer collateral synapses for three minutes essentially gives no potentiation. Coapplication of isoproterenol, a beta-adrenergic receptor agonist that mimics endogenous NE, converts a non-potentiating signal into a potentiating one (38). Under other conditions beta-adrenergic agonists can also augment the magnitude of LTP induced, if different physiologic stimulation protocols are used that evoke modest LTP. Similar types of effects can be observed for activation of various subtypes of receptors for ACh and DA (12).

One known site of action of neuromodulators is regulation of back-propagating action potentials in pyramidal neuron dendrites. All of these agents which modulate LTP induction can modulate the magnitude of back-propagating action potentials (see Figure 23B). The augmentation of back-propagating action potentials is a means by which these neurotransmitters can enhance membrane depolarization and thereby enhance NMDA receptor opening (Box 6).

The growth factor brain-derived neurotrophic factor (BDNF) can also modulate the induction of LTP by a number of mechanisms, at least one of which is pre-synaptic (see Figure 23C, and references 40–42). BDNF, acting through its cell-surface receptor TrkB, acts on pre-synaptic terminals to selectively facilitate neurotransmitter release during high-frequency stimulation. This is an interesting example of modulation of LTP induction that is activity-dependent but localized to the pre-synaptic compartment. The mechanisms controlling the levels of BDNF in the adult

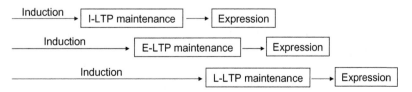

FIGURE 22 Mechanisms of induction, maintenance, and expression. This diagram highlights the importance of considering that each different phase of LTP may have separate and parallel induction, maintenance, and expression mechanisms.

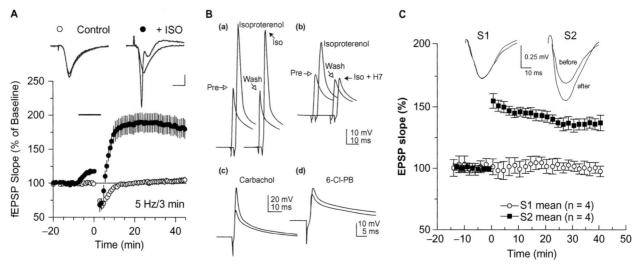

FIGURE 23 Neuromodulation of LTP induction. (A) Modulation of LTP induction by the beta-adrenergic agonist Isoproterenol. Activity-dependent β-adrenergic modulation of low frequency stimulation induced LTP in the hippocampus CA1 region. In control experiments (no ISO), 3 minutes of 5 Hz stimulation (delivered at time 5 0, open symbols, n 5 26) had no lasting effect on synaptic transmission (45 minutes after 5 Hz stimulation, fEPSPs were not significantly different from pre-5 Hz baseline, t(25) 5 1.01). However, 3 minutes of 5 Hz stimulation delivered at the end of a 10 minute application of 1.0 mM ISO (indicated by the bar) induced LTP (closed symbols, p <0.01 compared with baseline). The traces are fEPSPs recorded during baseline and 45 minutes after 5 Hz stimulation in the presence and absence (control) of ISO. Calibration bars are 2.0 mV and 5.0 ms. Reproduced from Thomas et al. (38). (B) One potential mechanism for neuromodulation is regulation of back-propagating action potentials in CA1 dendrites. The data shown illustrate amplification of dendritic action potentials by isoproterenol (a) and its susceptibility to inhibition by the protein kinase inhibitor H7 (b). The traces shown are from dendritic patch-clamp recordings from hippocampal pyramidal neurons. Muscarinic agonist (carbachol, c) and the dopamine receptor agonist 8-Cl-PB can also give various degrees of action-potential modulation. (a) Bath application of 1 μM isoproterenol resulted in a 104% increase in amplitude, from 41 mV("Pre") to 84 mV, of an antidromically initiated action potential recorded 220 μm from the soma. Wash-out of isoproterenol amplitude (38 mV; "wash"). With a second application of isoproterenol (dark arrow labeled "Iso"), the amplitude again increased twofold to 80 mV. (b) In a different recording 300 μM H-7, a generic kinase inhibitor, was included in the control saline during the wash-out of isoproterenol. The subsequent second application of isoproterenol failed to lead to a second increase in amplitude (dark arrow labeled "Iso + H7"). (c) In a distal recording (300 μM), 1 μM carbachol increased the action potential amplitude by 81%, from 27–60 mV. In the carbachol experiments, cells were held hyperpolarized to −80 mV to remove Na$^+$ channel inactivation (d) one of the 6 out of 10 recordings where 6-Cl-PB led to an increase in amplitude. In a recording 220 μm from the soma, 10 μM 6-Cl-PB increased dendritic action potential amplitude by 26%, from 21 to 26.5 mV. The cells were held at −70 mV in all 6-Cl-PB experiments. Adapted from Johnston et al. (39). (C) BDNF also modulates LTP induction in response to theta-frequency type stimulation. Two stimulating electrodes were positioned on either side of a single recording electrode to stimulate two different groups of afferents converging in the same dendritic field in CA1. Stimulation was applied to Schaffer collaterals alternately at low frequency (1 per minute). After a period of baseline recording, LTP was induced with a theta burst stimulation applied at time 0 only to one pathway (S1, filled squares). Simultaneous recording of an independent pathway (S2, open circles) showed no change in its synaptic strength after the theta burst was delivered to S1. BDNF (closed squares) selectively facilitates the induction of LTP in the tetanized pathway without affecting the synaptic efficacy of the untetanized pathway. EPSPs were recorded in the CA1 area of BDNF-treated slices. Synaptic efficacy (initial slope of field EPSPs) is expressed as a percentage of baseline value recorded during the 20 min before the tetanus. Representative traces of field EPSPs from S1 and S2 pathways were taken 10 minutes before and 40 minutes after the theta burst stimulation. Adapted from Gottschalk et al. (40).

hippocampus are not entirely clear at this point, but it is well-established that hippocampal BDNF levels can be regulated by a variety of neuronal activity-dependent processes, and indeed in response to environmental signals impinging on the behaving animal.

X. DEPOTENTIATION AND LONG-TERM DEPRESSION

If synapses can be potentiated and this potentiation is very long-lasting, over time the synapses will be driven to their maximum synaptic strength. In this condition there is no longer synaptic plasticity and no further capacity for that synapse to participate in synaptic-plasticity-dependent processes. Worse still, over the lifetime of an animal synapses will, by random chance, experience LTP-inducing conditions (pre-synaptic activity coincident with a post-synaptic action potential, for example) many times. If LTP is irreversible, ultimately every synapse will be maximally potentiated—obviously not a desirable condition *vis-à-vis* memory storage.

Consideration of this conundrum raises two implications. First, synapses that are involved in lifelong memory storage must be rendered essentially aplastic. In order to have good fidelity of memory storage over

BOX 6

TEMPORAL INTEGRATION IN LONG-TERM POTENTIATION INDUCTION

At one level it is a statement of the obvious to say that LTP induction depends on temporal integration. After all, the characteristic that distinguishes LTP induction protocols from baseline stimulation is that during an LTP induction protocol, stimulation is delivered at a higher rate. It is obviously the case that if the only attribute that is different is that the synapse is seeing activity at 100 pulses per second rather than once every 20 seconds then LTP is being triggered by unique timing-dependent processes, which is simply a restatement of one definition of temporal integration. But what are the unique events that are happening physiologically with high-frequency stimulation? Stated briefly, the answer to this question is that temporal integration is occurring such that the cell is reaching a threshold of depolarization in order to fire an action potential. This action potential firing then leads to membrane depolarization to allow opening of NMDA receptors. Below I will describe two different ways in which this can happen.

The first mechanism can be illustrated by considering what happens during the 1-second period of 100 Hz tetanus (see Figure A). Such closely-spaced stimulation means that post-synaptic depolarization from the first EPSP carries over into the second stimulation, and so on, and so on, including 96 more times. Stated more precisely, the post-synaptic membrane potential does not recover to the original resting potential before an additional depolarizing EPSP is triggered, and temporal summation of post-synaptic depolarization occurs. The summed depolarization eventually reaches threshold for the cell to fire an action potential. This is one of the classic examples of neuronal temporal integration, and of course such a process is not limited to hippocampal pyramidal neurons. One unique aspect of this in hippocampal neurons and probably other cortical neurons as well, is that triggering of the action potential is used to generate a back-propagating action potential into the dendrites, which is involved in depolarizing the NMDA receptor and triggering synaptic plasticity.

A second example comes from considering LTP induced by theta-pattern stimulation. With this type of LTP induction protocol, delivered at the slower 5 Hz (once per 200 milliseconds) rate, temporal integration is similarly involved, but occurs via a different route. After all, 200 milliseconds is long enough for the post-synaptic membrane potential to recover completely before the next wave of depolarization, so temporal integration of the sort described above is inadequate as an explanation. One can investigate this question by examining the physiologic events occurring during the period of theta-frequency stimulation. For illustrative purposes, results with theta-frequency stimulation will be discussed, although similar effects are also observed with theta-burst stimulation.

The experiments I will describe used theta-frequency stimulation (TFS) consisting of 30 seconds of 5 Hz stimulation. This stimulation paradigm evokes stable LTP as illustrated in Figure B. Population spikes were assessed during the theta-frequency stimulation period, utilizing a dual recording electrode technique. The stimulating electrode remained in hippocampal area CA3, and activated Schaffer collateral fibers innervating area CA1. One recording electrode was positioned in stratum radiatum of area CA1 in order to record synaptic responses, field EPSPs (Figure B, (B)). Another electrode was placed in stratum pyramidale, the cell body layer, in order to record action potential firing in response to the same input. For each single stimulus, the initial slope of the EPSP recorded in stratum radiatum and the amplitude of the population spike recorded in stratum pyramidale were measured, throughout the period of 5 Hz stimulation.

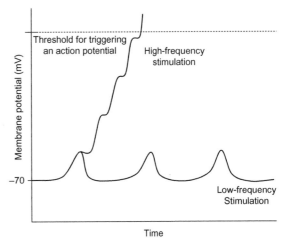

BOX 6 FIGURE A Temporal integration in LTP induction. Temporal summation of EPSPs is one mechanism contributing to bringing the post-synaptic neuron to threshold for firing an action potential, one contribution to the selective ability of high-frequency stimulation to produce LTP.

Continued

BOX 6—cont'd

TEMPORAL INTEGRATION IN LONG-TERM POTENTIATION INDUCTION

Theta-frequency stimulation resulted in a short-lived increase in action potential firing during the 30 seconds of 5 Hz stimulation (see Figure B, (C) and (D)). For roughly the first 20 seconds of the stimulation, the amplitude of the population spike increased dramatically. Meanwhile, over this same time period, the EPSP slope recorded in stratum radiatum gradually declined. Therefore, the ratio of the population spike amplitude

to the EPSP slope increased over time, indicating an increased likelihood of action potential firing over the short time-course of the theta-frequency stimulation (Figure D). Once again, for theta-frequency stimulation as for 100 Hz tetanic stimulation, some temporal integration process is taking place to cause action potential firing during the period of LTP-inducing stimulation.

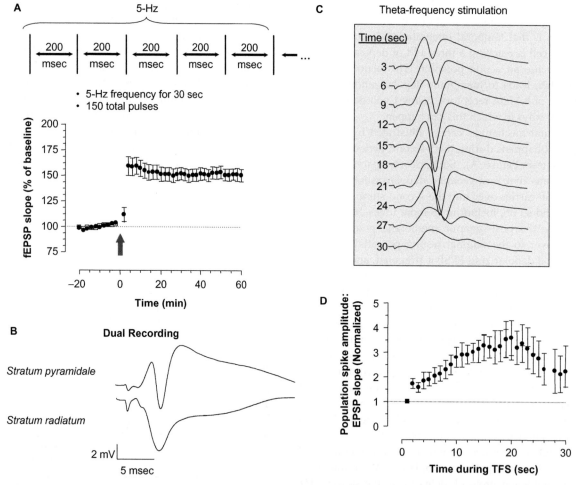

BOX 6   FIGURE B Increased action potential firing over the course of theta-frequency stimulation. (A) The TFS protocol and TFS-induced LTP in mouse hippocampal slices. (B) Electrode placement configuration for recording EPSP and Population spikes simultaneously during TFS. (C) Representative traces in response to TFS from a hippocampal slice. Note the difference in the population spike between the first and 18th stimulation of the stimulation paradigm. (D) Quantitation of increased spike amplitude during TFS. Population spike counts recorded in stratum pyramidale of hippocampal area CA1 during theta burst stimulation is plotted versus burst number during TFS. Slices showed a progressive increase in spike generation during the first two-thirds of TFS.

BOX 6—cont'd

TEMPORAL INTEGRATION IN LONG-TERM POTENTIATION INDUCTION

The mechanism for this temporal integration is not completely clear at present. A variety of previous studies have suggested that for LTP induced by theta-frequency stimulation there is an important role for attenuation of feedforward GABA-ergic inhibition onto pyramidal neurons (Figure C) (72–74). One current hypothesis is that short-term synaptic depression in the GABA-ergic local circuit during theta-frequency stimulation, due to stimulation of pre-synaptic GABA-b autoreceptors, leads to a loss of GABA-mediated inhibition, increased excitability, and increased firing of action potentials during the period of theta-frequency stimulation.

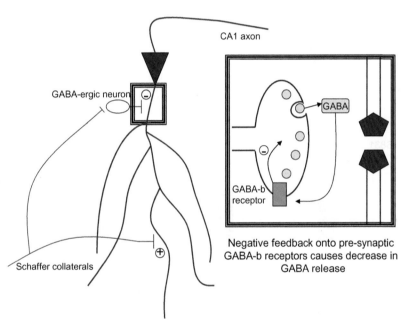

BOX 6 FIGURE C 100 GABA-b receptors in temporal integration with TBS. This figure presents one model for the increased excitability that occurs during TBS, based on auto-inhibition at GABA-ergic inputs onto CA1 pyramidal neurons during the period of stimulation.

the lifetime of an animal, a synapse involved in permanent memory storage must be rendered immutable to a change in synaptic strength due to the random occurrence of what would normally be LTP-inducing stimulation.

But what about synapses like those in the hippocampus that are not sites of memory storage, but whose plasticity is part of the active processing in forming new long-term memories? In order to retain their plasticity, and hence their capacity to contribute to memory formation, their potentiation must be reversible. Schaffer collateral synapses can undergo activity-dependent reversal of LTP; a phenomenon termed *depotentiation* (see Figure 24). Another activity-dependent way to decrease synaptic strength is long-term depression (LTD), the mirror image of LTP. As we discussed in previous chapters, LTD is a long-lasting decrease of synaptic strength below baseline. Using logic similar to that of the first paragraph of this section, the phenomenon of de-depression of synaptic transmission is implied, although this has not been widely studied at this point.

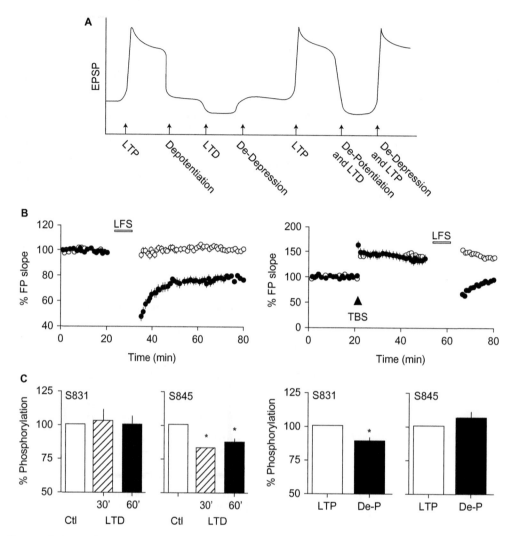

FIGURE 24 Depotentiation and LTD. (A) Schematic illustrating LTP, depotentiation, LTD, de-depression, and combinations of them. (B) LTD and depotentiation in hippocampal neurons. Simultaneous recording of slices receiving baseline stimulation (control, open circles) and 1 Hz stimulation (closed circles). FP, field potential. Regulation of distinct AMPA receptor phosphorylation sites during bidirectional synaptic plasticity. (C) Homosynaptic LTD in CA1 is associated with dephosphorylation of GluR1 at a PKA site (ser845). Depotentiation gives dephosphorylation at a CaMKII/PKC site (ser 831). Adapted from Lee et al. (43).

As a practical matter, it is often difficult to separate depotentiation from LTD experimentally. For example, a "baseline" response in hippocampal slices or *in vivo* likely is a mixture of basal synaptic activity and activity at previously potentiated synapses. Moreover, for the most part, the stimulation protocols used to induce depotentiation are variations of the protocols used to induce LTD. Nevertheless, mechanistic investigations have made clear that depotentiation and LTD use different mechanisms (43–44), and thus must be considered as distinct processes.

In the hippocampus and neocortex, physiologic LTD (and depotentiation) induction protocols generally involve variations of repetitive 1 Hz stimulation (43, 45). A common protocol is to deliver 900 stimuli at 1 Hz, but there also are LTD protocols that use random small variations in frequency in the 1 Hz region, and variations that use paired-pulse stimuli delivered at 1 Hz. Synaptic depression appears to be fairly robust *in vivo*, but is quite difficult to induce in hippocampal slices from adult animals. LTD *in vitro* is almost always studied using slices from immature animals, or cultured immature neurons, and it is possible that LTD as it is currently studied *in vitro* is largely a manifestation of what is normally a developmental mechanism.

One ironic aspect of the LTP/LTD story is that both phenomena at Schaffer collateral synapses can be blocked by NMDA receptor antagonists. This suggests that calcium influx triggers both processes, and indeed current models of LTD induction hypothesize that LTD is caused by an influx of calcium that achieves a lower level than that needed for LTP induction. This lower level of calcium is hypothesized to selectively activate protein phosphatases, and by this mechanism lower synaptic efficacy.

Another very different type of LTD is cerebellar LTD. As we discussed in Chapter 5, cerebellar LTD occurs at synapses onto Purkinje neurons in the cerebellar cortex. Cerebellar LTD is a very interesting phenomenon, because its behavioral role is much better understood than the hippocampal plasticity phenomena we are discussing in this chapter. As we have already discussed, cerebellar LTD is involved in associative eye-blink conditioning, a cerebellum-dependent classical conditioning paradigm.

XI. A ROLE FOR LONG-TERM POTENTIATION IN HIPPOCAMPAL INFORMATION PROCESSING, HIPPOCAMPUS-DEPENDENT TIMING, AND CONSOLIDATION OF LONG-TERM MEMORY

In this final section we will address a few simple illustrative examples of how LTP might contribute to the principal roles of the hippocampus that we discussed in the last chapter. Thus, we will discuss how LTP might be involved in spatial learning, timing and sequencing, and memory consolidation. Before beginning it is important to emphasize that current thinking among workers in the area is that LTP is obligatorily involved in hippocampus-dependent memory formation; however, LTP does not equate to memory. LTP is one of those processes contributing in an essential way to memory formation. Think of LTP as a component mechanism utilized by the hippocampus to allow it to perform its multitudinous functions. It is a physiologic and molecular tool that allows the hippocampus to do what it needs to do.

In the next section I will review several key studies that support a role for LTP in the various hippocampus-dependent processes mentioned above. Please note the important caveat that I am going to focus mostly on studies manipulating hippocampal NMDA receptor function as a means of blocking LTP. Blocking NMDA receptors is not the same thing as selectively blocking LTP, but it is probably as close as we can get right now in terms of practicable experiments. For example, despite decades of investigation, no one has observed that NMDA receptors function in baseline synaptic transmission in the hippocampus. Thus, manipulations that selectively block the NMDA receptor appear to be selective for blocking LTP induction, but not background neuronal activity

in the hippocampus. Loss of NMDA receptor function by various manipulations in general does not appear to cause derangement of overall activity in the hippocampal circuit, but rather a selective loss of the capacity to trigger changes in synaptic strength. Nevertheless, loss of NMDA receptor function may cause additional effects besides loss of LTP: loss of LTD and derangement of the post-synaptic molecular infrastructure are two prominent possibilities. Thus, blockade of NMDA receptors may be doing other things besides blocking LTP induction.

One other thing to keep in mind is that while I will focus on NMDA receptor-related studies, these are by no means the only relevant data. Many other manipulations that block LTP also affect memory formation, consolidation, and hippocampal information processing. The NMDA receptor manipulation is simply the one I will use for our present purposes, to give an example of the types of experiments that have formed current thinking in this area.

A. Long-Term Potentiation in Hippocampal Information Processing

This potential role for LTP harkens back to the extensive discussion we had in Chapter 6 concerning the formation of pyramidal neuron place fields. It is clear that LTP is not necessary for hippocampal place field formation (46–49). However, molecular disruptions that block LTP formation do have consistent effects on place fields. Specifically, loss of LTP is associated with a decreased stability of place fields (49). There also are effects on the spatial specificity of place fields and the coordinated firing of pyramidal neurons that have the same place fields (46). Overall, these data provide one explanation for the loss of hippocampus-dependent spatial learning in animals deficient in LTP. The effects on place fields specifically are consistent with the idea that NMDA receptor-dependent LTP is necessary in forming an accurate and lasting representation of complex visuo-spatial environments.

NMDA receptor-dependent LTP in area CA1 of the hippocampus also appears to be necessary for multimodal associative learning (50). Mice can learn to form complex associations among three different odor cues in order to make predictions about food rewards. In one type of task, mice must learn that odor A + B is different from odor B + C, is different from odor C + A. Mice deficient in NMDA receptor-dependent LTP in area CA1 are deficient in making the types of complex multiple associations necessary to execute this task efficiently (34). Thus, LTP appears to be necessary for the formation of relational memories involving complex associative information processing.

A final and fascinating recent example illustrates that NMDA receptor-dependent processes are necessary for reconstituting spatial locations using partial visual cues (51). In these experiments, NMDA receptors were selectively eliminated in hippocampal area CA3 using genetic engineering approaches. Mice deficient in NMDA receptor-dependent LTP in area CA3 can learn the Morris water maze normally, but exhibit a deficiency in being able to recall the hidden platform location when they are primed for recollection using a partial set of visual cues. In other words, animals are selectively deficient in recalling a spatial location when some of the training-associated visual stimuli are removed. These deficits are associated with a similar derangement of place cell activity in a partial-cue environment. These findings indicate that hippocampal LTP is involved in the animal forming a complete and unified representation of a complex set of visual stimuli.

Two important experiments using infusion of the NMDA receptor antagonist APV into the CNS also bear directly on this idea—in fact, these two papers from Richard Morris's laboratory are seminal findings that both shaped general thinking in the area and served as a foundation for much of the later work in this area. In a pioneering study Morris and his colleagues found that intraventricular infusions of APV, at concentrations that block LTP induction, block spatial learning in the water maze (see Figure 25, reference 52). A few years later, Morris demonstrated that this effect was not due to a loss of the capacity of the animal to learn the spatial relationship of the hidden platform to the visual cues (55), but rather NMDA receptor blockade appears to block the capacity of the animal to learn the task, which is to learn that there is a consistent relationship between the spatial cues and the hidden platform, and that they can use spatial cues to predict where the platform will be located. The NMDA receptor (and by inference LTP) is not necessary for spatial learning *per se*—it is necessary for learning more complex relationships about

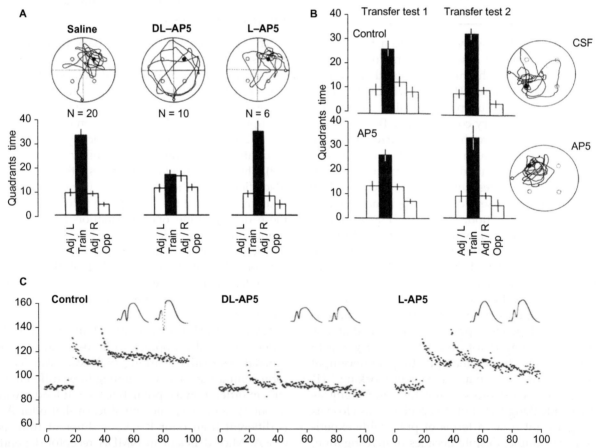

FIGURE 25 The NMDA receptor antagonist D-AP5 (i.e., APV) blocks learning in the Morris water maze. These data are from the landmark paper by Richard Morris and his colleagues (53), demonstrating that infusion into the CNS of d,l-AP5 (an active mixture) but not the control, inactive enantiomer l-AP5 blocks learning in the water maze task. The upper panel illustrates that pre-training infusion of d,l-AP5 blocks learning of a spatially selective search strategy for locating the hidden platform. The middle panel illustrates that post-training blockade of NMDA receptors does not affect memory recall. The lower panel illustrates that the same infusion protocol leads to effective blockade of NMDA receptor-dependent LTP in the dentate gyrus. See text for additional discussion.

spatial information. These pioneering data are in nice agreement with the more recent work described above indicating that NMDA receptor-dependent processes are necessary for an animal to reconstitute a special representation from partial visual stimuli (51).

How might NMDA receptor-dependent LTP contribute to these types of multimodal information processing in the hippocampus? One can imagine a couple of ways in which the cellular and molecular properties of LTP induction might contribute to the processing of complex associations and the establishment of a lasting representation of the association. Please keep in mind that these examples are markedly oversimplified. They are not based on realistic circuits, nor are they sufficient to account for the entirety of the observations. They simply serve to provide a frame of reference for how the molecular and cellular processes we have been discussing might enter into our thinking

about unique roles for hippocampal LTP in forming complex associations.

Two possibilities are shown in Figure 26. In the first example, imagine that initially a pyramidal neuron receives one strong input (input 1) and two weak inputs (inputs 2 and 3). Either input 1 by itself or inputs 2 and 3 firing simultaneously can trigger an action potential in their follower neuron. Now imagine that one produces paired activity in input 1 plus input 2, causing LTP at input 2. Similarly, one produces paired activity of input 1 and input 3, and gets LTP at input 3. Now inputs 1, 2, and 3 are all "strong" inputs and capable of firing an action potential. This means that input 2 alone or input 3 alone can reconstitute the response that previously required both 2 and 3. In essence, a partial representation of a single stimulus can reproduce what previously required two simultaneous, separate stimuli.

LTP in multimodal information processing

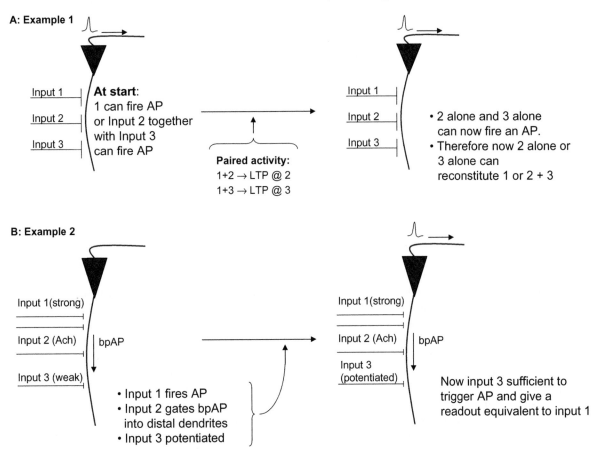

FIGURE 26   LTP in multimodal information processing. Example 1 illustrates how pairing synaptic activity of strong plus weak activity can allow a single input to achieve the same effect that formerly required its activity plus another input. Associative activity allows a single input to subsequently represent either an entirely different input from its original meaning, or can allow a partial representation of an original stimulus to reconstitute the entire original effect. Example 2 illustrates how an excitatory input (Input 1) coupled with a modulatory input (ACh in this example) allows a different input (Input 3) to trigger a new response. The new response to Input 3 is now functionally equivalent to the original response to Input 1. See text for additional discussion.

A second example is conceptually similar. Imagine that a pyramidal neuron receives a strong input (input 1), a modulatory input such as ACh (input 2), and a weak input (input 3). Input 1 triggers a back-propagating action potential, which ACh modulation of dendritic K channels allows propagation into the distal dendrites. This back-propagating action potential is paired with input 3, causing LTP at this site. Input 3 is now sufficient to cause an action potential on its own and give a read-out equivalent to input 1. Thus, input 3, by virtue of its association with a salience signal (ACh in this example), is now uniquely able to trigger the same response as input 1.

As I emphasized above, these examples are not realistic models to try to account for the complex behavioral changes described in the last chapter. They are merely simple examples to give an idea of how multiple coincidence detection mechanisms that result in LTP, which we know occur in hippocampal pyramidal neurons, might play a part in representing complex associations.

B. Timing-Dependent Information Storage in the Hippocampus

A second and distinct role for LTP that we will touch on briefly is its participation as a mechanism for storing timing- and sequencing-dependent information in the hippocampus.

One experimental observation that specifically prompts the conclusion that LTP is involved in timing-dependent information storage in the hippocampus is the finding that NMDA receptor activation is necessary for trace fear conditioning. Huerta et al. (56) used a sophisticated engineered mouse lacking NMDA receptors in area CA1 in order to probe the role of the

---

BOX 7

SPINE ANATOMY AND BIOCHEMICAL COMPARTMENTALIZATION

So far we have discussed the synapse in largely abstract terms, related largely to its function. However, the synapse is also a physical entity and the structural attributes of this entity confer some interesting properties. This brief section will describe certain physical aspects of the synapse that will be important to consider before moving on to later chapters of this book, which discuss details about the molecular mechanisms for LTP. In brief, there are three points highlighted in this section. First, most synapses in the CNS and almost all excitatory synapses in the hippocampus are at specialized structures called *dendritic spines*. Second, spines are small, well-circumscribed biochemical compartments that localize proteins and signaling molecules to a specific post-synaptic compartment. Third, spines are of course contiguous with dendrites, and thus continuously sense the local dendritic membrane potential.

A picture of part of the dendritic region of an area CA1 pyramidal neuron is shown in the Figure. The fuzzy appearance of the CA1 dendritic tree in this picture is due to the abundance of small dendritic spines protruding at right angles to the dendritic shaft. Almost all (about 95%) of the Schaffer collateral synapses we have been discussing in the abstract are actually physically present at spines. Most spines have a fairly simple elongated mushroom-like (i.e., chicken drumstick) shape, although there is clearly great diversity of their

morphology. For example, a low percentage (about 2%) of CA1 pyramidal neuron spines are bifurcated and actually have two synapses on them. Spines have an actin-based cytoskeleton and most have both smooth endoplasmic reticulum which can contribute to local calcium release and polyribosomes where local protein synthesis occurs. In hippocampal pyramidal neurons microtubules and mitochondria are limited to the dendritic shaft.

A distinguishing feature of the area of synaptic contact at the spine is the post-synaptic density, or PSD. This is a highly compact biochemical structure containing scaffolding proteins, receptors, and signal transduction components. The calcium/calmodulin sensitive protein kinase CaMKII is particularly enriched at the PSD, as is a structural protein called PSD-95, a name which is based on its molecular weight.

The dendritic spine membrane surrounds the PSD and the area immediately below it, and thus circumscribes a discrete biochemical compartment. The spine neck, however, is open to the dendritic shaft so there is still considerable diffusion of soluble spine contents (such as calcium and second messengers) into the local dendritic region. Nevertheless, on short time-scales the spine compartment may serve to effectively localize signaling molecules to a specific synapse. Moreover, molecules tethered to the PSD by scaffolding proteins and

BOX 7—cont'd

SPINE ANATOMY AND BIOCHEMICAL COMPARTMENTALIZATION

the like probably have fairly limited diffusion, because the spine compartment will make them tend to rebind at the same PSD as they unbind and rebind. Thus, this spine morphology is likely to be an important component for achieving synaptic specificity in LTP and other forms of synaptic plasticity.

The compartmentalization of molecules by the dendritic spine is not paralleled by an electrical compartmentalization, by and large. As a first approximation we can assume that the spine membrane potential reflects the local dendritic shaft membrane potential. However, it is likely that electrical compartmentalization does occur in dendrites, but this is at the level of the various dendritic branches, as well as a component contributed by their overall distance from the soma. This introduces the fascinating possibility that local generation and restricted propagation of action potentials within a specific dendritic subregion might be used as a mechanism for generating dendritic branch-specific plasticity.

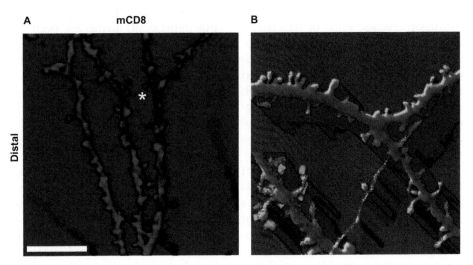

BOX 7   Dendrites with spines in a hippocampal pyramidal neuron. This figure illustrates the presence and shapes of dendritic spines on pyramidal neurons in the hippocampus. The spines are the small mushroom-shaped lateral projections containing synaptic contacts. (A) Courtesy of Liqun Lou, Stanford University. (B) Courtesy of E Korkotian, The Weizmann Institute.

hippocampus and NMDA receptor-dependent processes in timing-dependent learning. The specific paradigm that they used was trace fear conditioning. They found that the introduction of even a brief 30 second delay between CS and US presentation rendered the learning dependent on hippocampal NMDA receptors. These data strongly suggest that one role for LTP in area CA1 is the temporary storage of information so that events can be associated over time.

In earlier work, Richard Morris made a conceptually similar observation indicating a role for NMDA receptor-dependent processes in short-term information storage. Morris trained animals in a delayed match-to-place task and found that the extent of NMDA receptor dependency varied based on the length of the delay period between stimulus and match (55). Again, these data indicate a role for LTP or similar processes in temporary information storage.

The general idea coming out of studies of this sort is that LTP or a similar process in the hippocampus is involved in the storage of episodes of experience for brief periods of time (56–59). This allows the episode to be processed into the appropriate temporal context (i.e., what came before, what came after) so that associations can be made between one event, or sequence of events, and another. As with the other roles for LTP that we have been discussing, the precise function that LTP might play in contributing to this phenomenon is not clear. However, knowing that LTP is an activity-dependent phenomenon that results in a persisting change, it certainly seems reasonable that LTP could be participating in buffering time-dependent information locally in the hippocampus.

C. Consolidation—Storage of Information within the Hippocampus for Down-Loading to the Cortex

In this final section we will discuss the possible role of LTP in the classic function of the hippocampus—memory consolidation. As we have already discussed in several sections of the book, a wide variety of evidence has already shown that the hippocampus is involved in consolidation of long-term memories. For example, lesion studies including studies of human patients have shown this to be the case. Also, numerous drug infusion studies, some of which will be described below, have shown a role for the hippocampus in memory consolidation. A key point with the drug infusion studies is that drugs can be infused into the hippocampus post-training and interfere with long-term memory formation. Appreciation of the significance of this was what led to the distinction of hippocampal memory consolidation as a distinct process from the initial events triggering memory formation.

A number of different experiments have shown that hippocampal protein synthesis and mRNA synthesis is necessary for the consolidation of long-term memories (60, 61). In fact, these same studies make it clear that multiple stages of protein-synthesis-dependent cellular processes are required for memory consolidation, as injection of protein synthesis inhibitors at different time points after training can lead to disruption of memory consolidation. Moreover, specific molecular processes such as ERK activation, CREB activation, Arc induction, and C/EBP induction are necessary for hippocampus-dependent memory consolidation (62–64). The NMDA receptor is also necessary for hippocampus-dependent memory consolidation (65–68). The necessity of these specific molecular events for memory consolidation, mechanisms which are also known to be necessary for LTP induction, strongly implicate LTP as a component of memory consolidation.

More direct evidence for a role for LTP in hippocampal memory consolidation was obtained in an additional study by Brun et al. (69). These investigators showed that delivering LTP-inducing stimulation to the dentate gyrus after training led to disruption of memory consolidation. This effect was blocked by NMDA receptor blockade, demonstrating that the triggering of LTP or a related phenomenon, as opposed to network firing, is what is disrupting the consolidation.

Thus, taken together there is a substantial body of direct and indirect findings that indicate that LTP is participating in the consolidation of hippocampus-dependent memory formation. The model is that the relevant LTP is occurring in the hippocampus, and it is triggering changes downstream in cortical targets of the hippocampus that store the memory. We will discuss a broad-brush-stroke model of how this might happen in the next few paragraphs.

D. A Model for Long-Term Potentiation in Consolidation of Long-Term Memory

The upshot of the hypothesized role of LTP in memory consolidation is that hippocampal LTP is not a long-term memory storage mechanism—it is a memory buffer. The long-term storage of hippocampus-dependent memories occur downsteam of the hippocampus in various regions of the cortex. In these final few paragraphs I will present a thumbnail sketch of how hippocampal LTP might participate in cortical memory consolidation. Once again, I emphasize that this is not a sophisticated or realistic model—it is an illustrative example of how LTP in the hippocampus could lead to long-term changes downstream in the cortex.

The basics of the model are based on what we have seen thus far: that LTP serves to maintain information in the hippocampus, represented as a pattern of synaptic weights, during the process of memory consolidation. The output of the potentiated circuit, manifest as a result of these altered synaptic strengths, triggers long-lasting changes in the cortex and the formation of long-term memory. The "model" will simply be an elaboration of this basic idea, but with a few more specifics added.

Figure 27 shows a simplified diagram of the hippocampus—only area CA1 is specified to any extent. The hippocampus receives "sensory input" and neuromodulatory "arousal/attention/emotion" signals. These are simply a lumping together of the various inputs to the hippocampus and area CA1 that we have discussed extensively in previous chapters. The "consolidation signal" designates activity that is triggered externally or internally as part of the consolidation process—it basically represents the baseline neuronal activity that is known to be necessary for memory consolidation.

The output from area CA1 goes to the entorhinal cortex and perirhinal cortex, and these are treated in block fashion as a way-station to the cerebral cortex. The entirety of the cerebral cortex is reduced to two neurons in the model, which is about how many

BOX 8

SATURATING LONG-TERM POTENTIATION BLOCKS MEMORY FORMATION

An interesting series of "occlusion" experiments have strongly supported a role for hippocampal LTP in memory formation *in vivo*. The rationale in these types of experiments is that if one goes in and saturates LTP in the hippocampus, further naturally-occurring LTP is not possible; thus, learning deficits should arise because of the lost capacity of the hippocampus to trigger its necessary synaptic plasticity.

Pioneering studies using this approach were executed by Bruce McNaughton and Carol Barnes' groups, which indicated that saturating hippocampal LTP produced learning deficits (75–76). A more recent collaborative study by the Moser and Morris laboratories has confirmed and solidified the original conclusions (77). The studies from both groups used a similar rationale and approach, although there were appreciable and significant differences in the technical execution of the studies and the types of data analysis brought to bear. Regardless, the overall conclusions were the same—saturating LTP at the perforant path inputs to the dentate gyrus leads to a loss of the capacity for hippocampus-dependent memory formation (see Figure). These data strongly support the hypothesis that synaptic changes of a sort similar or identical to LTP are necessary for memory formation *in vivo*.

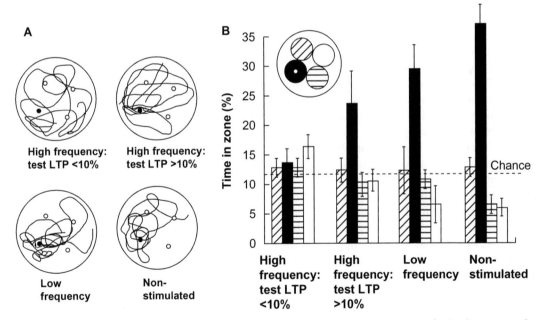

BOX 8 Saturating hippocampal LTP occludes Morris water maze learning. Four groups of animals were tested. Two groups were controls that received no LTP-inducing stimulation (non-stimulated and low frequency). Another group received LTP-inducing stimulation, but that did not saturate LTP (high frequency test LTP >10%). The final group, which exhibited saturated LTP (test LTP <10%) had learning deficits. (A) Records of the search pattern of a representative animal from each group during the final spatial probe test (60 seconds). (B) Time spent inside a circle (radius of 35 cm) around the platform position (black bar) and in corresponding, equally large zones in the three other pool quadrants (diagonally striped, horizontally striped, and white bars) during the final spatial probe test (60 seconds). The dotted line indicates the chance level. Error bars indicate SEM. Reproduced from Moser et al. (77).

BOX 9

HIPPOCAMPAL LONG-TERM POTENTIATION HAPPENS WHEN AN ANIMAL LEARNS

The hypothesis that hippocampal LTP is involved in memory makes the prediction that when an animal learns LTP should be induced at hippocampal synapses. In the ideal "measure" experiment of this sort we would be able to put stimulating and recording electrodes into the hippocampus, have the animal learn, and then directly measure an increased strength of synaptic connections *in situ* attendant with the memory formation. This would demonstrate that LTP is indeed occurring with memory formation in the behaving animal.

In vivo recordings from the hippocampus have revealed a number of important and relevant findings that are consistent with the prediction that LTP is indeed occurring in the hippocampus during learning. For example, the basic observation that hippocampal neurons form of place field firing patterns implies altered hippocampal connectivity when an animal is learning about a new environment. Physiologic changes such as altered excitability occur with spatial learning that is consistent with the induction and maintenance of LTP-like phenomena. Endogenous learning-related firing patterns are consistent with the occurrence of LTP-triggering high-frequency synaptic activity. Moser et al. have also directly observed synaptic potentiation in the dentate gyrus with learning (78–79), although the observable potentiation is fairly short-lived. Finally, and most recently, Bear and colleagues have observed long-lasting potentiation of synaptic transmission in the hippocampus when an animal learns a spatially dependent task, the most clear demonstration of learning-associated LTP in the hippocampus so far (80).

---

functioning cortical neurons I have left after a long day of writing. When memory is to be assessed, the cortex receives a "recall signal"—you might imagine this as an environmental signal, such as being asked the question "What is the capital of Alabama?" Before training your "behavioral output" is the answer "Birmingham." After training and the ministrations of your hippocampus, your behavior output is altered—it becomes "Montgomery."

How might the hippocampus bring about this change, utilizing its capacity for LTP? You receive sensory input in the form of new information, such as the preceding sentence, manifest as firing of hippocampal neurons. The importance of the information is clear, so your hippocampal synapses receive a blast of neuromodulatory neurotransmitter (i.e., your professor just told you that the question will be on the exam). The simultaneous activity of neuronal projections into area CA1 and the neuromodulatory signal leads to the formation of LTP at one (for our purposes) of your Schaffer collateral synapses. These events are shown in Figure 27A and B.

If you are going to store this new information long enough to make it to the test next week, your hippocampus has to receive the "consolidation signal" (Figure 27C). This relays neuronal activity through the hippocampus, including your newly-potentiated CA1 synapse. This heightened firing of one of your CA1 pyramidal neurons is manifest as a potentiation of synapses downstream in the entorhinal/perirhinal cortices, and ultimately potentiation of a synapse downstream of there in one of your two functioning cortical neurons (Figure 27D).

The potentiated synapse in your cerebral cortex is the result of a very long-lasting variety of LTP.[1] The potentiated cortical synapse participates in a network of neurons storing information. Its potentiated state leads to an altered behavioral output when its circuit receives a recall signal (Figure 27E). Your cortical circuit stays altered long past the duration of the potentiation in the hippocampus (Figure 27F). Hippocampal synapses are free to relax back to their original state—the hippocampus, after all, is not storing the memory long-term, just participating in consolidating the memory in the cortex. Thus, your hippocampal synapses return to an unpotentiated state, but their potentiation was an absolute requirement for storing the memory in the cortex.

Please keep in mind that the model is deliberately oversimplified. I made it up using the absolute

---

[1]This aspect of the model is probably accurate. Long-lasting memory storage in the cortex may well involve LTP or LTP-like processes (70–71). Ultra-long-term LTP may be the mechanism for cortical information storage, triggered by the potentiated outputs of the hippocampus and entorhinal cortex.

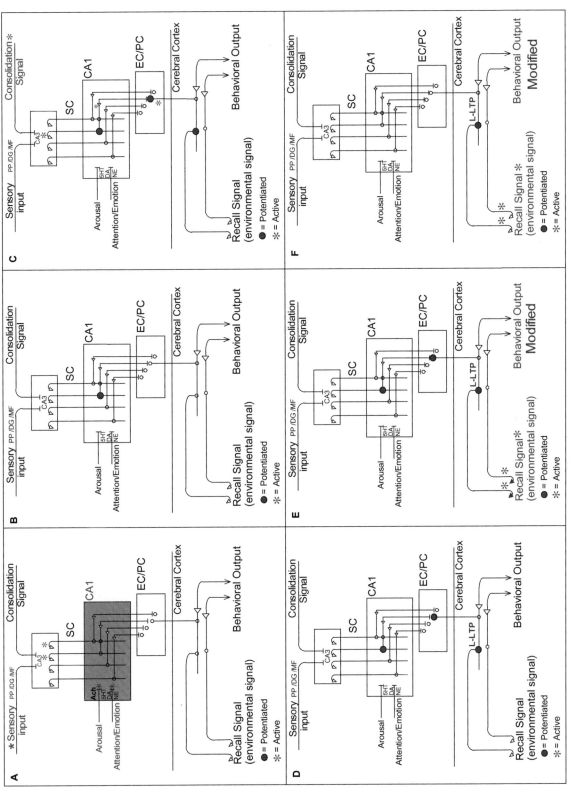

FIGURE 27 A simple model of how LTP might participate in memory consolidation. See text for discussion. (A) Activity in a sensory input plus activation of an ACh input into area CA1 (54). PP/DG/MF = inputs via the perforant path, dentate gyrus, and mossy fiber pathway. EC/PC = entorhinal cortex/perirhinal cortex. Note also that a recall signal routed through the cerebral cortex elicits a given pre-training behavioral output. (B) LTP at a set of synapses in Area CA1. (C) A consolidation signal played through the potentiated pathway results in synaptic potentiation in downstream synapses, including in the cerebral cortex. (D) L-LTP is now established at specific synapses in the cortex. (E) Sending a recall signal through the modified cortical synapses elicits a modified behavioral output. It is important to note that part of the recall signal will likely involve the original "sensory input" specified in (A). (F) Even when synaptic potentiation is lost in the hippocampus and its immediate targets the modified behavior persists.

minimum number of components that I could, simply to illustrate the basic idea of a role for the hippocampus in cortical memory consolidation. It highlights several important points to keep in mind. First, hippocampal LTP does not participate in long-term storage. Second, defined cognitive phenomena like consolidation and recall must somehow impact on LTP after it is generated. Hippocampal LTP doesn't just happen and then there is memory—LTP is a tool that is used as part of a much more complicated cognitive circuit in order to allow memory storage and recall. Finally, associative sensory stimuli that impinge on the hippocampus can use the associative properties of LTP to encode their relationship.

All these considerations illustrate that LTP does not equal memory. Rather, it is a critical component of the complicated process of memory formation.

XII. SUMMARY

Like learning, LTP can be defined as a long-lasting change in output in response to a transient input. The persistence of this effect has been demonstrated to extend many hours *in vitro* and several weeks *in vivo*. We do not know exactly how LTP relates to memory although there is considerable evidence for the hypothesis that hippocampal LTP is involved in memory. Regardless, it is the best understood example of long-lasting synaptic plasticity in the mammalian CNS, and it is a model for how long-lasting memory-associated changes are likely to occur in the CNS. Understanding LTP will yield valid insights into the mechanisms of plasticity that underlie learning and memory in the brain. The *bona fide* changes in neuronal connections that occur *in vivo* may or may not be identical to LTP as it is presently studied in the laboratory, but this does not diminish its utility as a cellular model system for studying lasting neuronal change in the mammalian CNS.

There are several specific themes and concepts that we introduced in this chapter:

1. LTP is a striking example of a "Hebbian," activity-dependent change in synaptic strength.
2. There are different forms and phases of LTP that are subserved by different molecular mechanisms.
3. The second messenger calcium is nearly universally involved in triggering LTP.
4. Regulation of neuronal excitability is an important contributor to controlling synaptic plasticity.
5. The induction of LTP is subject to a wide variety of modulatory influences due to neurotransmitters such as dopamine, norepinephrine, and acetylcholine.

6. Hippocampal LTP does not equal long-term memory; rather, LTP is a cellular process contributing to hippocampus-dependent cognitive function and long-term memory consolidation.

Further Reading

Barrionuevo, G., and Brown, T. H. (1983). "Associative long-term potentiation in hippocampal slices." *Proc. Natl. Acad. Sci. U S A* 80:7347–7351.

Chittajallu, R., Alford, S., and Collingridge, G. L. (1998). "Ca^{2+} and synaptic plasticity." *Cell Calcium* 24:377–385.

Grover, L. M., and Teyler, T. J. (1990). "Two components of long-term potentiation induced by different patterns of afferent activation." *Nature* 347:477–479.

Harris, E. W., and Cotman, C. W. (1986). "Long-term potentiation of guinea pig mossy fiber responses is not blocked by N-methyl D-aspartate antagonists". *Neurosci. Lett.* 70:132–137.

Johnston, D., and Amaral, D. G. (1983). "Hippocampus". In *The Synaptic Organization of the Brain*, Shepherd, G. M. (Ed.), 4th ed. New York: Oxford University Press, pp. 417–458.

Johnston, D., Hoffman, D. A., Colbert, C. M., and Magee, J. C. (1999). "Regulation of back-propagating action potentials in hippocampal neurons." *Curr. Opin. Neurobiol.* 9:288–292.

Johnston, D., and Wu, S. M-S. (1995). *Foundations of Cellular Neurophysiology*. Cambridge, MA: MIT Press.

Linden, D. J. (1999). "The return of the spike: postsynaptic action potentials and the induction of LTP and LTD." *Neuron* 22:661–666.

Lynch, G., Larson, J., Kelso, S., Barrionuevo, G., and Schottler, F. (1983). "Intracellular injections of EGTA block induction of hippocampal long-term potentiation." *Nature* 305:719–721.

Malinow, R., Madison, D. V., and Tsien, R. W. (1988). "Persistent protein kinase activity underlying long-term potentiation." *Nature* 335:820–824.

Maren, S. (1999). "Long-term potentiation in the amygdala: a mechanism for emotional learning and memory." *Trends Neurosci.* 22:561–567.

Martin, S. J., Grimwood, P. D., and Morris, R. G. (2000). "Synaptic plasticity and memory: an evaluation of the hypothesis." *Annu. Rev. Neurosci.* 23:649–711.

Rioult-Pedotti, M. S., Friedman, D., and Donoghue, J. P. (2000). "Learning-induced LTP in neocortex." *Science* 290:533–536.

Stevens, C. F. (1998). "A million dollar question: does LTP = memory?." *Neuron* 20:1–2.

Thomas, M. J., Moody, T. D., Makhinson, M., and O'Dell, T. J. (1996). "Activity-dependent beta-adrenergic modulation of low frequency stimulation induced LTP in the hippocampal CA1 region." *Neuron* 17:475–482.

Wigstrom, H., and Gustafsson, B. (1986). "Postsynaptic control of hippocampal long-term potentiation." *J. Physiol.* (Paris) 81:228–236.

Journal Club Articles

Bliss, T. V., and Lomo, T. (1973). "Long-lasting potentiation of synaptic transmission in the dentate area of the anaesthetized rabbit following stimulation of the perforant path." *J. Physiol.* 232:331–356.

Collingridge, G. L., Kehl, S. J., and McLennan, H. (1983). "Excitatory amino acids in synaptic transmission in the Schaffer collateral-commissural pathway of the rat hippocampus." *J. Physiol.* 334:33–46.

Lee, H. K., Barbarosie, M., Kameyama, K., Bear, M. F., and Huganir, R. L. (2000). "Regulation of distinct AMPA receptor phosphorylation sites during bidirectional synaptic plasticity." *Nature* 405:955–959.

Magee, J. C., and Johnston, D. (1997). "A synaptically controlled, associative signal for Hebbian plasticity in hippocampal neurons." *Science* 275:209–213.

Whitlock, J. R., Heynen, A. J., Shuler, M. G., and Bear, M. F. (2006). "Learning induces long-term potentiation in the hippocampus." *Science* 313:1093–1097.

For more information—relevant topic chapters from: John H. Byrne (Editor-in-Chief) (2008). *Learning and Memory: A Comprehensive Reference*. Oxford: Academic Press (ISBN 978-0-12-370509-9). (4.02 Bailey, C. H., Barco, A., Hawkins, R. D., and Kandel, E. R. *Molecular Studies of Learning and Memory in* Aplysia *and the* Hippocampus: *A Comparative Analysis of Implicit and Explicit Memory Storage.* pp. 11–29; 4.17 Giles, A. C., and Rankin, C. H. *Behavioral Analysis of Learning and Memory in* C. elegans. pp. 629–640; 4.18 Maccaferri, G., and McBain, C. J. *GABAergic Interneurons in Synaptic Plasticity and Information Storage.* pp. 367–385; 4.19 Shilyansky, C., Wiltgen, B. J., and Silva, A. J. *Neurofibromatosis Type I Learning Disabilities.* pp. 387–407; 4.24 Banko, J. L., and Weeber, E. J. *Angelman Syndrome.* pp. 489–500; 4.30 Alvestad, R. M., Goebel, S. M., Coultrap, S. J., and Browning, M. D. *Glutamate Receptor Trafficking in LTP.* pp. 611–632; 4.31 Lee, H. -K., and Huganir, R. L. *AMPA Receptor Regulation and the Reversal of Synaptic Plasticity—LTP, LTD, Depotentiation, and Dedepression.* pp. 633–648; 4.37 Lovinger, D. M. *Regulation of Synaptic Function by Endocannabinoids.* pp. 771–792; 4.38 Hawkins, R. D. *Transsynaptic Signaling by NO during Learning-Related Synaptic Plasticity.* pp. 793–802; 4.39 Waters, J. Nevian, T. Sakmann, B. and Helmchen, F. *Action Potentials in Dendrites and Spike-Timing-Dependent Plasticity.* pp. 803–828; 4.40 Mozzachiodi, R., and Byrne, J. H. *Plasticity of Intrinsic Excitability as a Mechanism for Memory Storage.* pp. 829–838.)

References

1. Bliss, T. V., and Lomo, T. (1973). "Long-lasting potentiation of synaptic transmission in the dentate area of the anaesthetized rabbit following stimulation of the perforant path." *J. Physiol.* 232:331–356.

2. van Groen, T., and Wyss, J. M. (1990). "Extrinsic projections from area CA1 of the rat hippocampus: olfactory, cortical, subcortical, and bilateral hippocampal formation projections." *J. Comp. Neurol.* 302:515–528.

3. Johnston, D., and Amaral, D. G. (1983). "Hippocampus". In *The Synaptic Organization of the Brain*, Shepherd, G. M. (Ed.), 4th ed. New York: Oxford University Press, pp. 417–458.

4. Naber, P. A., and Witter, M. P. (1998). "Subicular efferents are organized mostly as parallel projections: a double-labeling, retrograde-tracing study in the rat." *J. Comp. Neurol.* 393:284–297.

5. Collingridge, G. L., Kehl, S. J., and McLennan, H. (1998). "Excitatory amino acids in synaptic transmission in the Schaffer collateral-commissural pathway of the rat hippocampus". *J. Physiol.* 334:33–46.

6. Wigstrom, H., and Gustafsson, B. (1986). Postsynaptic control of hippocampal long-term potentiation. *J. Physiol. (Paris)* 81:228–236.

7. Malinow, R., and Tsien, R. W. (1990). "Presynaptic enhancement shown by whole-cell recordings of long-term potentiation in hippocampal slices". *Nature* 346:177–180.

8. Magee, J. C., and Johnston, D. (1997). "A synaptically controlled, associative signal for Hebbian plasticity in hippocampal neurons". *Science* 275:209–213.

9. Barrionuevo, G., and Brown, T. H. (1983). "Associative long-term potentiation in hippocampal slices". *Proc. Natl. Acad. Sci. U S A* 80:7347–7351.

10. Andersen, P., Sundberg, S. H., Sveen, O., and Wigstrom, H. (1977). "Specific long-lasting potentiation of synaptic transmission in hippocampal slices". *Nature* 266:736–737.

11. McNaughton, B. L., Douglas, R. M., and Goddard, G. V. (1978). "Synaptic enhancement in fascia dentata: cooperativity among coactive afferents". *Brain Res.* 157:277–293.

12. Yuan, L. L., Adams, J. P., Swank, M., Sweatt, J. D., and Johnston, D. (2002). "Protein kinase modulation of dendritic K^+ channels in hippocampus involves a mitogen-activated protein kinase pathway". *J. Neurosci.* 22:4860–4868.

13. Johnston, D., Hoffman, D. A., Magee, J. C., Poolos, N. P., Watanabe, S., Colbert, C. M., and Migliore, M. (2000). "Dendritic potassium channels in hippocampal pyramidal neurons." *J. Physiol.* 525 Pt 1:75–81.

14. Bi, G. Q., and Poo, M. M. (1998). "Synaptic modifications in cultured hippocampal neurons: dependence on spike timing, synaptic strength, and postsynaptic cell type". *J. Neurosci.* 18:10464–10472.

15. Linden, D. J. (1999). "The return of the spike: postsynaptic action potentials and the induction of LTP and LTD". *Neuron* 22:661–666.

16. Kamondi, A., Acsady, L., and Buzsaki, G. (1998). "Dendritic spikes are enhanced by cooperative network activity in the intact hippocampus". *J. Neurosci.* 18:3919–3928.

17. Kapur, A., Yeckel, M. F., Gray, R., and Johnston, D. (1998). "L-type calcium channels are required for one form of hippocampal mossy fiber LTP". *J. Neurophysiol.* 79:2181–2190.

18. Grover, L. M., and Teyler, T. J. (1990). "Two components of long-term potentiation induced by different patterns of afferent activation". *Nature* 347:477–479.

19. Aniksztejn, L., and Ben-Ari, Y. (1991). "Novel form of long-term potentiation produced by a K^+ channel blocker in the hippocampus". *Nature* 349:67–69.

20. Powell, C. M., Johnston, D., and Sweatt, J. D. (1994). "Autonomously active protein kinase C in the maintenance phase of N-methyl-D-aspartate receptor-independent long term potentiation". *J. Biol. Chem.* 269:27958–27963.

21. Harris, E. W., and Cotman, C. W. (1986). "Long-term potentiation of guinea pig mossy fiber responses is not blocked by N-methyl-D-aspartate antagonists". *Neurosci.Lett.* 70:132–137.

22. Zalutsky, R. A., and Nicoll, R. A. (1990). "Comparison of two forms of long-term potentiation in single hippocampal neurons". *Science* 248:1619–1624.

23. Yeckel, M. F., Kapur, A., and Johnston, D. (1999). "Multiple forms of LTP in hippocampal CA3 neurons use a common postsynaptic mechanism". *Nat. Neurosci.* 2:625–633.

24. Lynch, G., Larson, J., Kelso, S., Barrionuevo, G., and Schottler, F. (1983). "Intracellular injections of EGTA block induction of hippocampal long-term potentiation". *Nature* 305:719–721.

25. Nicoll, R. A., and Malenka, R. C. (1995). "Contrasting properties of two forms of long-term potentiation in the hippocampus". *Nature* 377:115–118.

26. Chittajallu, R., Alford, S., and Collingridge, G. L. (1998). "Ca^{2+} and synaptic plasticity". *Cell Calcium* 24:377–385.

27. Johnston, D., Williams, S., Jaffe, D., and Gray, R. (1992). "NMDA-receptor-independent long-term potentiation". *Annu. Rev. Physiol.* 54:489–505.

28. Bekkers, J. M., and Stevens, C. F. (1990). "Presynaptic mechanism for long-term potentiation in the hippocampus". *Nature* 346:724–729.

29. Malinow, R. (1991). "Transmission between pairs of hippocampal slice neurons: quantal levels, oscillations, and LTP". *Science* 252:722–724.

30. Dolphin, A. C., Errington, M. L., and Bliss, T. V. (1982). "Long-term potentiation of the perforant path *in vivo* is associated with increased glutamate release". *Nature* 297:496–498.

31. Zakharenko, S. S., Zablow, L., and Siegelbaum, S. A. (2001). "Visualization of changes in presynaptic function during long-term synaptic plasticity". *Nat. Neurosci.* 4:711–717.

32. Malgaroli, A., Ting, A. E., Wendland, B., Bergamaschi, A., Villa, A., Tsien, R. W., and Scheller, R. H. (1995). "Presynaptic component of long-term potentiation visualized at individual hippocampal synapses". *Science* 268:1624–1628.

33. McMahon, L. L., and Kauer, J. A. (1997). "Hippocampal interneurons express a novel form of synaptic plasticity". *Neuron* 18:295–305.

34. Lu, Y. M., Mansuy, I. M., Kandel, E. R., and Roder, J. (2000). "Calcineurin-mediated LTD of GABAergic inhibition underlies the increased excitability of CA1 neurons associated with LTP". *Neuron* 26:197–205.

35. Roberson, E. D., English, J. D., and Sweatt, J. D. (1996). "A biochemist's view of long-term potentiation". *Learn. Mem.* 3:1–24.

36. Winder, D. G., Mansuy, I. M., Osman, M., Moallem, T. M., and Kandel, E. R. (1998). "Genetic and pharmacological evidence for a novel, intermediate phase of long-term potentiation suppressed by calcineurin". *Cell* 92:25–37.

37. Malinow, R., Madison, D. V., and Tsien, R. W. (1988). "Persistent protein kinase activity underlying long-term potentiation". *Nature* 335:820–824.

38. Thomas, M. J., Moody, T. D., Makhinson, M., and O'Dell, T. J. (1996). "Activity-dependent beta-adrenergic modulation of low frequency stimulation induced LTP in the hippocampal CA1 region". *Neuron* 17:475–482.

39. Johnston, D., Hoffman, D. A., Colbert, C. M., and Magee, J. C. (1999). "Regulation of back-propagating action potentials in hippocampal neurons". *Curr. Opin. Neurobiol.* 9:288–292.

40. Gottschalk, W., Pozzo-Miller, L. D., Figurov, A., and Lu, B. (1998). "Presynaptic modulation of synaptic transmission and plasticity by brain-derived neurotrophic factor in the developing hippocampus". *J. Neurosci.* 18:6830–6839.

41. Xu, B., Gottschalk, W., Chow, A., Wilson, R. I., Schnell, E., Zang, K., Wang, D., Nicoll, R. A., Lu, B., and Reichardt, L. F. (2000). "The role of brain-derived neurotrophic factor receptors in the mature hippocampus: modulation of long-term potentiation through a presynaptic mechanism involving TrkB". *J. Neurosci.* 20:6888–6897.

42. Lu, B., and Chow, A. (1999). "Neurotrophins and hippocampal synaptic transmission and plasticity". *J. Neurosci. Res.* 58:76–87.

43. Lee, H. K., Barbarosie, M., Kameyama, K., Bear, M. F., and Huganir, R. L. (2000). "Regulation of distinct AMPA receptor phosphorylation sites during bidirectional synaptic plasticity". *Nature* 405:955–959.

44. Lee, H. K., Kameyama, K., Huganir, R. L., and Bear, M. F. (1998). "NMDA induces long-term synaptic depression and dephosphorylation of the GluR1 subunit of AMPA receptors in hippocampus". *Neuron* 21:1151–1162.

45. Kemp, N., McQueen, J., Faulkes, S., and Bashir, Z. I. (2000). "Different forms of LTD in the CA1 region of the hippocampus: role of age and stimulus protocol". *Eur. J. Neurosci.* 12:360–366.

46. McHugh, T. J., Blum, K. I., Tsien, J. Z., Tonegawa, S., and Wilson, M. A. (1996). "Impaired hippocampal representation of space in CA1-specific NMDAR1 knockout mice". *Cell* 87:1339–1349.

47. Tsien, J. Z., Chen, D. F., Gerber, D., Tom, C., Mercer, E. H., Anderson, D. J., Mayford, M., Kandel, E. R., and Tonegawa, S. (1996). "Subregion- and cell type-restricted gene knockout in mouse brain". *Cell* 87:1317–1326.

48. Tsien, J. Z., Huerta, P. T., and Tonegawa, S. (1996). "The essential role of hippocampal CA1 NMDA receptor-dependent synaptic plasticity in spatial memory". *Cell* 87:1327–1338.

49. Kentros, C., Hargreaves, E., Hawkins, R. D., Kandel, E. R., Shapiro, M., and Muller, R. V. (1998). "Abolition of long-term stability of new hippocampal place cell maps by NMDA receptor blockade". *Science* 280:2121–2126.

50. Rondi-Reig, L., Libbey, M., Eichenbaum, H., and Tonegawa, S. (2001). "CA1-specific N-methyl-D-aspartate receptor knockout mice are deficient in solving a nonspatial transverse patterning task". *Proc. Natl. Acad. Sci. USA* 98:3543–3548.

51. Nakazawa, K., Quirk, M. C., Chitwood, R. A., Watanabe, M., Yeckel, M. F., Sun, L. D., Kato, A., Carr, C. A., Johnston, D., Wilson, M. A., and Tonegawa, S. (2002). "Requirement for hippocampal CA3 NMDA receptors in associative memory recall". *Science* 297:211–218.

52. Davis, S., Butcher, S. P., and Morris, R. G. (1992). "The NMDA receptor antagonist D-2-amino-5-phosphonopentanoate (D-AP5) impairs spatial learning and LTP in vivo at intracerebral concentrations comparable to those that block LTP in vitro". *J. Neurosci.* 12:21–34.

53. Morris, R. G. (1989). "Synaptic plasticity and learning: selective impairment of learning rats and blockade of long-term potentiation in vivo by the N-methyl-D-aspartate receptor antagonist AP5". *J. Neurosci.* 9:3040–3057.

54. Cobb, S. R., Bulters, D. O., Suchak, S., Riedel, G., Morris, R. G., and Davies, C. H. (1999). "Activation of nicotinic acetylcholine receptors patterns network activity in the rodent hippocampus". *J. Physiol.* 518(Pt 1):131–140.

55. Bannerman, D. M., Good, M. A., Butcher, S. P., Ramsay, M., and Morris, R. G. (1995). "Distinct components of spatial learning revealed by prior training and NMDA receptor blockade". *Nature* 378:182–186.

56. Huerta, P. T., Sun, L. D., Wilson, M. A., and Tonegawa, S. (2000). "Formation of temporal memory requires NMDA receptors within CA1 pyramidal neurons". *Neuron* 25:473–480.

57. Morris, R. G. (1996). "Further studies of the role of hippocampal synaptic plasticity in spatial learning: is hippocampal LTP a mechanism for automatically recording attended experience?" *J. Physiol.* (Paris) 90:333–334.

58. Morris, R. G., and Frey, U. (1997). "Hippocampal synaptic plasticity: role in spatial learning or the automatic recording of attended experience?" *Philos. Trans. R. Soc. Lond. B. Biol. Sci.* 352:1489–1503.

59. Shapiro, M. L., and Eichenbaum, H. (1999). "Hippocampus as a memory map: synaptic plasticity and memory encoding by hippocampal neurons". *Hippocampus* 9:365–384.

60. Igaz, L. M., Vianna, M. R., Medina, J. H., and Izquierdo, I. (2002). "Two time periods of hippocampal mRNA synthesis are required for memory consolidation of fear-motivated learning". *J. Neurosci.* 22:6781–6789.

61. Grecksch, G., and Matthies, H. (1980). "Two sensitive periods for the amnesic effect of anisomycin". *Pharmacol. Biochem. Behav.* 12:663–665.

62. Guzowski, J. F., Lyford, G. L., Stevenson, G. D., Houston, F. P., McGaugh, J. L., Worley, P. F., and Barnes, C. A. (2000). "Inhibition of activity-dependent Arc protein expression in the rat hippocampus impairs the maintenance of long-term potentiation and the consolidation of long-term memory". *J. Neurosci.* 20:3993–4001.

63. Guzowski, J. F., and McGaugh, J. L. (1997). "Antisense oligodeoxynucleotide-mediated disruption of hippocampal cAMP response element binding protein levels impairs consolidation of memory for water maze training". *Proc. Natl. Acad. Sci. U S A* 94:2693–2698.

64. Taubenfeld, S. M., Milekic, M. H., Monti, B., and Alberini, C. M. (2001). "The consolidation of new but not reactivated memory requires hippocampal C/EBPbeta". *Nat. Neurosci.* 4:813–818.

65. Kim, J. J., Fanselow, M. S., DeCola, J. P., and Landeira-Fernandez, J. (1992). "Selective impairment of long-term but not short-term conditional fear by the N-methyl-D-aspartate antagonist APV". *Behav. Neurosci.* 106:591–596.

66. Steele, R. J., and Morris, R. G. (1999). "Delay-dependent impairment of a matching-to-place task with chronic and intrahippocampal infusion of the NMDA-antagonist D-AP5". *Hippocampus* 9:118–136.

67. Day, M., and Morris, R. G. (2001). "Memory consolidation and NMDA receptors: discrepancy between genetic and pharmacological approaches". *Science* 293:755.

68. Shimizu, E., Tang, Y. P., Rampon, C., and Tsien, J. Z. (2000). "NMDA receptor-dependent synaptic reinforcement as a crucial process for memory consolidation". *Science* 290:1170–1174.

69. Brun, V. H., Ytterbo, K., Morris, R. G., Moser, M. B., and Moser, E. I. (2001). "Retrograde amnesia for spatial memory induced by NMDA receptor-mediated long-term potentiation". *J. Neurosci.* 21:356–362.

70. Rioult-Pedotti, M. S., Friedman, D., and Donoghue, J. P. (2000). "Learning-induced LTP in neocortex". *Science* 290:533–536.

71. Rioult-Pedotti, M. S., Friedman, D., Hess, G., and Donoghue, J. P. (1998). "Strengthening of horizontal cortical connections following skill learning". *Nat. Neurosci.* 1:230–234.

72. Chapman, C. A., Perez, Y., and Lacaille, J. C. (1998). "Effects of GABA(A) inhibition on the expression of long-term potentiation in CA1 pyramidal cells are dependent on tetanization parameters". *Hippocampus* 8:289–298.

73. Mott, D. D., and Lewis, D. V. (1991). "Facilitation of the induction of long-term potentiation by GABAB receptors". *Science* 252:1718–1720.

74. Davies, C. H., Starkey, S. J., Pozza, M. F., and Collingridge, G. L. (1991). "GABA autoreceptors regulate the induction of LTP". *Nature* 349:609–611.

75. Castro, C. A., Silbert, L. H., McNaughton, B. L., and Barnes, C. A. (1989). "Recovery of spatial learning deficits after decay of electrically induced synaptic enhancement in the hippocampus". *Nature* 342:545–548.

76. McNaughton, B. L., Barnes, C. A., Rao, G., Baldwin, J., and Rasmussen, M. (1986). "Long-term enhancement of hippocampal synaptic transmission and the acquisition of spatial information". *J. Neurosci.* 6:563–571.

77. Moser, E. I., Krobert, K. A., Moser, M. B., and Morris, R. G. (1998). "Impaired spatial learning after saturation of long-term potentiation". *Science* 281:2038–2042.

78. Moser, E., Moser, M. B., and Andersen, P. (1993). "Synaptic potentiation in the rat dentate gyrus during exploratory learning". *Neuroreport* 5:317–320.

79. Andersen, P., Moser, E., Moser, M. B., and Trommald, M. (1996). "Cellular correlates to spatial learning in the rat hippocampus." *J. Physiol.* (Paris) 90:349.

80. Whitlock, J. R., Heynen, A. J., Shuler, M. G., and Bear, M. F. (2006). "Learning induces long-term potentiation in the hippocampus". *Science* 313(5790):1093–1097.

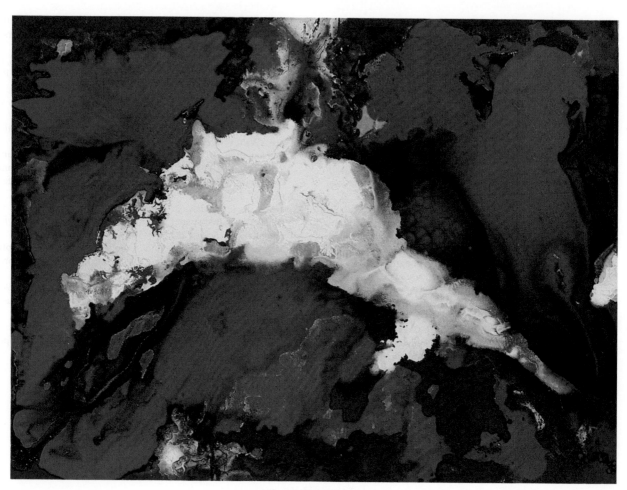

The NMDA Receptor
J. David Sweatt, acrylic on canvas, 2008–2009

8

The NMDA Receptor

I. INTRODUCTION

As we discussed in the last chapter, many forms of LTP are blocked by antagonists of the N-methyl-D-aspartate (NMDA) subtype of glutamate receptor (1). For example, the glutamate analog amino-phosphono-valeric acid (APV, also known as AP-5) selectively blocks the NMDA receptor, and blocks LTP induction while leaving baseline synaptic transmission intact. Furthermore, seminal studies by Richard Morris also demonstrated that NMDA receptor blockade also blocks hippocampus-dependent long-term memory formation (2). More recently, genetically-engineered mice lacking the NMDA receptor gene, selectively in area CA1 of the hippocampus, have been shown to be deficient in LTP and spatial memory (see Figures 1 and 2).

The properties of the NMDA receptor that allow it to function in this unique role of selectively triggering long-term synaptic potentiation, and indeed memory, are important, and in this chapter we will discuss regulation of the NMDA receptor.

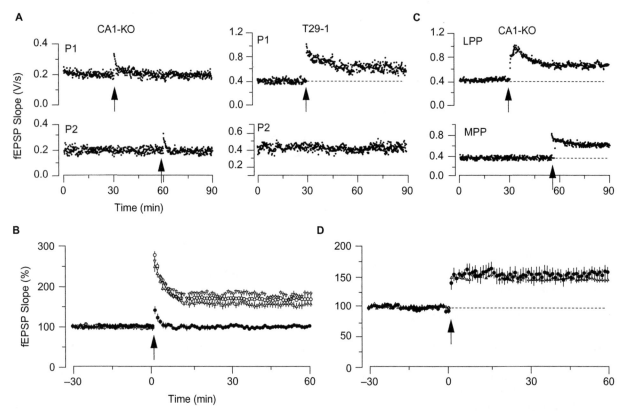

FIGURE 1 Loss of the NMDA receptor selectively in hippocampal area CA1 leads to selective deficits in LTP in this area of the hippocampus. Lack of LTP in CA1 and normal LTP in dentate gyrus from area CA1 selective NMDA receptor knockout mice. (A) Representative experiments in a CA1-KO slice (left) and a T29–1 control slice (right). Field EPSPs were recorded in the stratum radiatum in CA1 by stimulating two independent inputs (labeled P1 and P2). After a period of baseline recording (30 minutes), a tetanic train (100 Hz for 1 second) was given to P1 (arrow). This pathway remained unchanged in the CA1-KO slice, whereas it became potentiated in the T29–1 slice. Picrotoxin (100 mM) was present throughout the experiments. (B) The mean (6 SEM) field EPSPs in the four groups tested for LTP induction in CA1. The CA1-KO (closed circles, n = 5, 21) did not show LTP, whereas the other groups, which are controls for the genetic manipulations in the CA1-KO mouse, presented clear LTP (T29–1, open circles, n = 5, 12; fNR1, upward triangles, n = 5, 4; wt, downward triangles, n = 5, 5). (C) A single experiment in which dentate field EPSPs were recorded on stimulation of two pathways, the lateral perforant path (LPP) and the medial perforant path (MPP), recording from the dentate gyrus. A tetanus-induced (40 shocks at 100 Hz, arrow) clear LTP in both pathways. Picrotoxin (100 mM) was present throughout the experiment. (D) The mean (±SEM) field EPSPs in the CA1-KO (closed circles, n = 5, 10) and fNR1 (open triangles, n = 5, 6) dentate gyrus. Significant dentate gyrus LTP was elicited in both groups after the tetanus. Figure and legend from Tsien et al. (1996). *Cell* 87:1327–1338. Copyright Elsevier 1996.

As we discussed in the last chapter, the NMDA receptor is both a glutamate-gated channel and a voltage-dependent one. The simultaneous presence of glutamate and a depolarized membrane is necessary and sufficient (when the co-agonist glycine is present) to gate the channel (Figure 3). Pairing synaptic stimulation with membrane depolarization provided via either AMPA-subtype glutamate receptors or neuronal action potential firing (plus the low levels of glycine always normally present) opens the NMDA receptor channel. Channel gating in this fashion leads to the induction of long-term changes in synaptic strength and contributes to long-term memory formation *in vivo*.

The NMDA receptor is a calcium channel and its gating leads to elevated intracellular calcium in the post-synaptic neuron. It is this calcium influx that triggers lasting changes in synaptic function, and indeed

the next two chapters of this book deal with the various processes this calcium influx triggers.

The gating of the NMDA receptor/channel involves a voltage-dependent Mg^{++} block of the channel pore. Depolarization of the membrane in which the NMDA receptor resides is necessary to drive the divalent Mg^{++} cation out of the pore, which then allows calcium ions to flow through (Figure 3). Thus, the simultaneous occurrence of both glutamate in the synapse and a depolarized post-synaptic membrane is necessary to open the channel and allow LTP-triggering calcium into the post-synaptic cell. These properties of the NMDA receptor, glutamate dependence and voltage-dependence, allow it to function as a coincidence detector.

Thus, the NMDA receptor is a critical molecular locus for triggering lasting changes that has unique biophysical properties allowing it to perform a coincidence

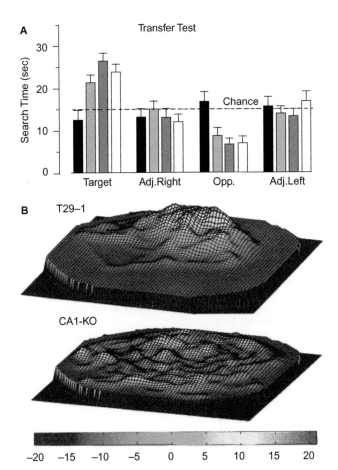

FIGURE 2 Loss of the NMDA receptor in area CA1 blocks learning in the Morris water maze. CA1-KO mice show a deficient performance during the transfer test component of the Morris water maze. (A) Average time (±SEM) in each quadrant during a transfer test in the Morris water maze for the four groups of genetically-engineered mice: the area CA1-selective knockout and three genetic controls (closed bars, CA1-KO; hatched bars, T29-1; shaded bars, fNR1; open bars, wt). The CA1-KO mice spent equal amounts of time in each quadrant, whereas the control groups spent significantly more time than chance in the target quadrant. (B) Three-dimensional graphs representing the total occupancy by six T29-1 mice and six CA1-KO mice during the last transfer test. The control mice focused their search in the trained location (where the platform was during training), whereas the mutant mice visited the whole maze area equivalently. Figure and legend from Tsien et al. (2006). *Cell* 87:1327–1338. Copyright Elsevier 1996.

detection role in the neuron. For these intriguing reasons the most-studied molecule in the short history of molecular studies of learning and memory is the NMDA subtype of glutamate receptor.

A. STRUCTURE OF THE NMDA RECEPTOR

The NMDA receptor is a glutamate-gated cation channel, and as such is a multisubunit transmembrane protein. Current models hypothesize that it is a tetrameric hetero-oligomeric protein with more than one glutamate binding site. It is, of course, voltage-dependent and this arises from the voltage-dependent Mg block of the pore that we discussed above. The protein has binding sites for zinc, polyamines, and glycine (a co-agonist necessary for activity).

Abundantly expressed individual subunits of the receptor are named NR1, NR2A, NR2B, NR2C, and NR2D (the somewhat unusual nomenclature arose for historical reasons related to the cloning of the first NMDA receptor subunits). One functional NMDA receptor is comprised of one or more NR1 subunits plus one or more NR2-type subunits. The NR2 subunits determine the calcium permeability of the channel and can influence the voltage-dependence of its activation, kinetics of opening, and other biophysical properties. NR1 and NR2A and 2B are phosphorylated at a number of different sites—NR1 by PKC and PKA, NR2A by cyclin-dependent kinase 5, and NR2A and NR2B by various tyrosine kinases such as src and fyn.

Indeed, the NMDA receptor is subject to a wide variety of direct modulatory influences, some of which are shown in Figure 4 and listed in Table 1. Moreover, recent work by Seth Grant and his colleagues has shown that the NMDA receptor is in fact a large multiprotein complex (3–4). This complex includes a striking representation of many different types of scaffolding proteins and signal transduction molecules (see Figure 5). In fact, the NMDA receptor supramolecular complex includes a number of proteins whose function has been directly implicated in human learning, including: neurofibromatosis type 1 protein (NF1); PKA; raf-1; Mitogen- and extracellular signal-regulated kinase (MEK); ERK; and ribosomal S-6 kinase 2 (RSK-2). These gene products have all directly or indirectly been implicated in human learning, as they are associated with various human mental retardation syndromes. The presence of gene products linked to human mental retardation within the NMDA receptor complex is intriguing and consistent with a role for this complex in human cognition.

Given the dozens of individual molecular events that have been reported as being involved in NMDA receptor regulation in the literature, how can one begin to organize this immense molecular system into a coherent picture? In order to do this, in this chapter, regulation of the NMDA receptor will be broken down into the following three basic components:

1. Mechanisms upstream of the NMDA receptor that directly regulate NMDA receptor function.
2. Mechanisms upstream of the NMDA receptor that control membrane depolarization.
3. The components of the synaptic infrastructure which are necessary for the NMDA receptor, and the associated synaptic signal transduction machinery, to function normally.

NMDA Receptor Activation and Calcium Influx

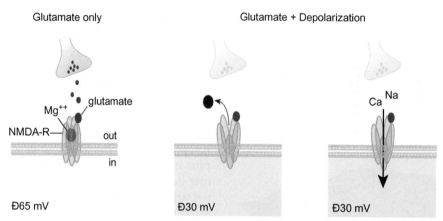

FIGURE 3   NMDA receptors are involved in synaptic plasticity. The simultaneous presence of glutamate and membrane depolarization is necessary for relieving Mg^{++} blockade and allowing calcium influx. The NMDA receptor is activated by a combination of glutamate binding and membrane depolarization. A positively charged magnesium ion blocks the NMDA receptor channel at rest. Depolarization causes the magnesium ion to be ejected, and this permits sodium and calcium ions to flow in. Figure and legend adapted from Cline et al. (1987); Cline and Constantine-Paton (1990). *Development of the Nervous System*, 2nd ed. Copyright Elsevier, 2006.

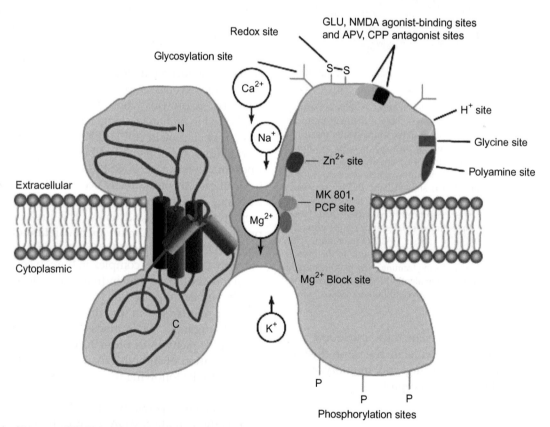

FIGURE 4   Diagram of NMDA receptor highlighting binding sites for numerous agonists, antagonists, and other regulatory molecules. The location of these sites is a crude approximation for the purpose of discussion. Adapted from Hollmann and Heinemann (1994). Copyright Elsevier 2004.

TABLE 1   Direct Modulators of the NMDA Receptor

Modulator	Mechanism	Effect
Src family tyrosine kinases (src, fyn)	tyrosine phosphorylation loss of Zn inhibition	enhancement
Scaffolding proteins		
RACK1	binding	inhibitory
PSD-95	scaffolding	modulatory
PKC	ser/thr phosphoryation (direct)	enhancement
	src activation (indirect)	enhancement
PKA/PP1/Yotiao	phosphorylation	enhancement
	dephosphorylation	inhibition
Cyclin dependent kinase 5	ser/thr phosphorylation	enhancement
Nitric oxide/reactive oxygen species	sulfhydryl nitrosylation or oxidation	inhibition
Polyamines (e.g., spermine, spermidine)	direct binding to a modulatory site	augmentation
Caseine kinase II	ser/thr phosphorylation modulation of polyamine effects	enhancement

Molecule	Mr(kD)
Glutamate receptors	
NR1	120
NR2A	180
NR2B	180
GluR6 + 7	117
mGluR1a	200
Scaffolding and adaptors	
PSD-95	95
ChapSyn110/PSD-93	110
Sap102	115
GKAP/SAPAP	95–140
Shank	200
Homer	28/45
Yotiao	200
AKAP150	150
NSF	83
PKA	
PKA catalytic subunit	40
PKA-R2β	53
PKC	
PKCβ	80
PKCγ	80
PKCε	90
CaM kinase	
CaM kinase II β	60
phosph-CaM kinase	60

Molecule	Mr(kD)
Phosphatases	
PP1	36
PP2A	36
PP2B(calcineurin)	61
PPs	50
PTPID/SHP2	72
Tyrosine kinases	
Src	60
PYK2	116
MAP Kinase pathway	
ERK (pan ERK)	42/44
ERK1	42/44
ERK2	42
MEK1	45
MEK2	46
MKP2	43
Rsk	90
Rsk-2	90
c-Raf1	74
Small G-proteins and modulators	
Rac1	21
Rap2	21
SynGAP	10,12,35,60
NF1	60,101

Molecule	Mr(kD)
Other signaling molecules	
Calmodulin	15
nNOS	155
PI3 Kinase	85
PLCγ	130
cPLA2	110
Citron	183
Arg3.1	55
Cell adhesion and cytoskeletal proteins	
N-Cadherin	150
Desmoglein	165
β-Caternin	92
LI	200
pp120cas	120
MAP2B	280
Actin	45
α-actinin 2	110
Spectrin	240/280
Myosin (brain)	205
Tubulin	50
Coractin	80/85
CortBP-1	180/200
Clathryn heavy chain	180
Dynamin	100
Hsp-70	70

FIGURE 5   Summary of molecular composition of the NMDAR supramolecular complex. The component molecules and their molecular weights are listed. Adapted from Husi et al. (3–4).

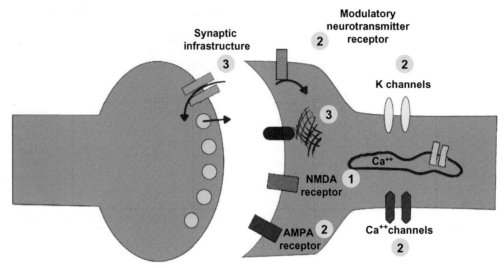

FIGURE 6 LTP induction machinery. Schematic diagram summarizing examples of the three different components of NMDA receptor regulation discussed in this chapter. See text and Tables 1–3 for explanation.

TABLE 2   Mechanisms Upstream of the NMDA Receptor Involved in Membrane Depolarization

Ionic Current	Molecules Involved	Role	Mechanisms of Modulation
K currents			
Voltage-dependent "A" currents	Kv4.2 (and Kv4.3)	limit bpAPs	ERK, PKA, CaMKII
		limit EPSP magnitude	
"H" currents	NCN channels (HCN)	regulate excitability	cyclic nucleotides (direct)
Na currents			
AMPA receptors	GluR1, GluR2 Aka GluR-A,B	depolarize membrane	PKA, CaMKII, PKC
Voltage-dependent Na$^+$ currents	Na(v)1.6, 1.1,1.2	AP propagation	PKC (decreased inactivation)
Ca currents	?—likely many	AP propagation (hypothetical)	PKA
Cl currents			
GABA receptors	all GABA-A receptor subunits	AP firing excitability	numerous

These various components of the NMDA receptor regulatory machinery are schematized in Figure 6 and listed in more detail in, Tables 1–3. The remainder of this chapter will fill in the molecular details necessary to flesh out this general model.

II. NMDA RECEPTOR REGULATORY COMPONENT 1—MECHANISMS UPSTREAM OF THE NMDA RECEPTOR THAT DIRECTLY REGULATE NMDA RECEPTOR FUNCTION

The NMDA receptor is a biochemical signal integrator. Its capacity for signal integration and coincidence detection is not limited to determining the simultaneous presence of glutamate and depolarization. It also senses biochemical signals that are used in computing the degree of calcium influx. This section will describe many of the biochemical mechanisms known to regulate the NMDA receptor directly. In general, the discussion will be limited to those processes which have been directly implicated in LTP induction, memory formation, or both.

These biochemical processes generally are not all-or-none such as the glutamate/depolarization mechanism, but rather serve to modulate the magnitude of post-synaptic calcium influx. Section III below will describe biochemical processes that are used to control the NMDA receptor in an all-or-none fashion indirectly through controlling the membrane potential.

As described above, the NMDA receptor is a coincidence detector, but in addition the NMDA receptor is also a temporal integrator. These temporal integration mechanisms operate on a longer time-frame and are limited to biochemical, as opposed to biophysical,

TABLE 3   Components of the Synaptic Infrastructure Necessary for NMDA Receptor Function

Component	Targets	Role
Cell Adhesion Molecules		
Integrins	src, rho, rac, ras/MAPKs	transmembrane signaling, interactions with extracellular matrix, NMDAR regulation
Syndecan-3	MLCK, FAK?	spine morphology?
	fyn, NMDAR	signaling from matrix heparan sulfates to the NMDA receptor
N-Cadherin	other Cadherins,	spine morphology?
	cytoskeleton	pre-/post-adhesion?
Actin Cytoskeleton/Associated Proteins		
Rho	membrane/cytoskeleton interactions	regulate synaptic structure
Cdk5	NMDA receptor	increase NMDA receptor function
Filamin	K channels	K channel localization
Pre-synaptic processes		
Glutamate release	synaptic glutamate	NMDA receptor activation
Glutamate reuptake	synaptic glutamate	limiting NMDA receptor desensitization
Anchoring/Interacting Proteins		
PSD-95	receptors, signal transduction mechanisms nNOS, SynGAP, GKAP	post-synaptic organization
Rack1/fyn	NMDA receptor	direct regulation of NMDA receptor
Shank/HOMER	metabotropic receptors	effector localization, cytoskeleton
GRIP	AMPA receptors, PICK-1/PKC	post-synaptic organization
AKAP	PKA, PP2B	kinase and phosphatase localization
CaMKII	signal transduction	regulate likelihood of LTP induction

processes. The time-frame in which the NMDA receptor can detect the simultaneous presence of depolarization and glutamate is, of course, quite limited because the membrane depolarization is so brief. In contrast, a biochemical signal, such as elevation of a second messenger or increased protein kinase activity, has a much longer half-life. Thus, a temporal integration mechanism of seconds (or longer) time-scale must use these types of processes. The capacity of the NMDA receptor to be modulated by protein kinases and other messenger molecules allows for this sort of temporal integration.

In the following three sections I will provide a few specific examples of these types of regulatory mechanisms that operate on the NMDA receptor. Please note that this is not a comprehensive description—instead, I will present a few examples to illustrate the concepts. It is important to bear in mind that there are a number of different mechanisms that can cause increased current flow through a ligand-gated ion channel:

1. The probability that the channel will open can be increased, which is referred to as increased "channel open probability."
2. The conductance, i.e., the rate at which ions flow through the channel can be increased.
3. The number of channels in the membrane can increase.

4. The affinity of the channel for its ligand can increase—a mechanism that, of course, can only operate at sub-saturating ligand concentrations.

This chapter will not go into detail about which of these mechanisms is involved in channel modulation, except where the mechanism is directly relevant to the molecular mechanisms that are involved (for example, increased membrane insertion of a channel implies the involvement of specific molecular processes). In addition, in many cases the specifics are not known or the channel modulation involves multiple mechanisms.

A. Kinase Regulation of the NMDA Receptor

One of the oncogene products produced by the Rous sarcoma virus, which also has a homolog in the mammalian genome, is the tyrosine kinase src. Src family tyrosine kinases like src and fyn directly phosphorylate the NMDA receptor (5–6), increasing calcium flux through the receptor. Tyrosine phosphorylation of the NMDA receptor increases current flow through the ion channel by reducing a tonic, zinc-dependent inhibition (7). Src modulation of the NMDA receptor at a minimum involves increased channel open probability. Protein tyrosine kinase phosphorylation of the NMDA receptor may be required for LTP induction, and at a minimum this mechanism serves an important modulatory role controlling the likelihood of LTP induction (8).

Protein kinase C (PKC) can not only act indirectly through Src to modulate the NMDAR, but PKC can also directly phosphorylate the receptor on serine/threonine residues and affect its function (9–10). Phosphorylation of the NMDAR by PKC causes increased calcium flow through the receptor (11). The potential importance of this is quite straightforward—any cell surface receptor coupled to a phospholipase C cascade can modulate the likelihood of LTP induction through direct regulation of the NMDA receptor complex (see Figure 7).

The cAMP-dependent protein kinase (PKA) can also augment NMDA receptor function, although the mechanism is complex and not entirely understood (12). PKA binds to the NMDA receptor via an associated protein, Yotiao (Yotiao is a specific isoform of a kinase anchoring protein, which we will discuss again in a later section of this chapter). Yotiao binds both PKA and protein phosphatase 1 (PP1) to the NMDA receptor, and when all three are bound together the PP1 activity predominates and keeps the NMDA receptor phosphorylation (and activation) low. PKA activation by cAMP leads to enhancement of NMDA currents, although it is not entirely clear if this is due to PKA phosphorylation of the NMDA receptor, loss of tonic dephosphorylation by PP1, or both. Again, in the context of the hippocampal pyramidal neuron this mechanism represents a basis for any neurotransmitter receptor coupled to adenylyl cyclase to be able to modulate NMDA receptor function and the induction of LTP.

B. Redox Regulation of the NMDA Receptor

Modulation of the NMDA receptor is, of course, not restricted to post-translational modifications involving phosphorylation. An interesting and novel type of regulation that is gaining increased attention is redox modulation of protein function. In the context of NMDA receptor function there are two specific examples of this type of regulation, both of which elicit inhibition of NMDA receptor function. The reactive nitrogen species nitric oxide (NO), a free radical, can react with sulfhydryl moieties in cysteine side-chains, a reaction leading to S-nitrosylation of the side-chain. This reaction occurs in NR2A subunits at reasonably low levels of free NO, and leads to decreased channel opening (24). A second example of redox regulation of NMDA receptors involves reactive oxygen species (ROS) such as superoxide and peroxynitrite, the product of the reaction of superoxide plus NO (25). ROS inhibition of the NMDA receptor likely occurs via cysteine oxidation in a fashion reminiscent of the effects of NO, although the mechanisms of this effect are not clear at present.

The physiologic role of NO and ROS inhibition of NMDA receptor function is not clear. One interesting speculation is that oxidative inhibition of NMDA receptors might serve to "lock" the synapse in a particular state after plasticity has been triggered, or the mechanism might serve as a basis for inhibitory crosstalk limiting the capacity of a synapse to undergo LTP.

C. Polyamine Regulation of the NMDA Receptor

Finally, polyamine compounds such as spermine, spermidine, and putrescine can modulate NMDA receptor function. Polyamines are synthesized normally in cells and are essentially long aliphatic chains with several amino moieties covalently attached. Polyamines have diverse modulatory effects on NMDA receptors *in vitro* and *in vivo*, but one effect that they have is augmentation of NMDA receptor function. This effect is through the unusual mechanism of relief of tonic proton inhibition of the channel (26–27). Polyamine co-application with NMDA leads to an enhancement of NMDA-induced synaptic potentiation in area CA1. Evidence exists which suggests activity-dependent increased polyamine synthesis in the hippocampus (28), so these mechanisms might serve a role in temporal integration with repeated stimulation or in setting a baseline likelihood of LTP induction.

III. NMDA RECEPTOR REGULATORY COMPONENT 2—MECHANISMS UPSTREAM OF THE NMDA RECEPTOR THAT CONTROL MEMBRANE DEPOLARIZATION

As we discussed in the last chapter, recent discoveries have highlighted the importance of mechanisms for controlling membrane depolarization in LTP induction. In particular, recent emphasis was catalyzed by the discovery of back-propagating action potentials and of their involvement in providing the depolarization of the synaptic membrane necessary for LTP induction (29–31). A second important development was the emergence of the "silent synapse" model of LTP induction, wherein there are synapses that contain NMDA receptors but no AMPA receptors. Obviously, in the silent synapse model the membrane depolarization necessary for NMDA receptor activation cannot come from local AMPA receptors, but must be propagated via the membrane from a distal site. Taken together, these two considerations bring into focus the necessity for understanding the mechanisms that control the electrical properties of the dendrite and dendritic spines, and their role in regulating

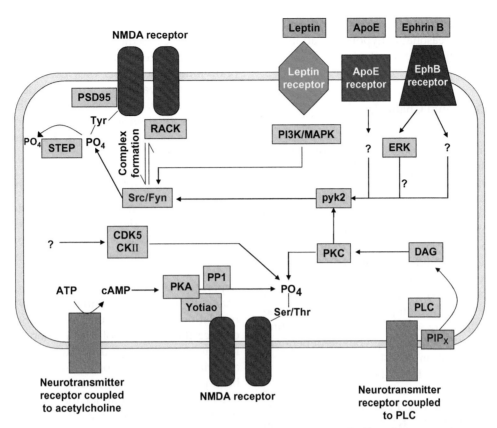

FIGURE 7 Receptor modulation of the NMDA receptor by the src, PKA, and PKC cascade. These kinase cascades are represented here in relation to modulation of NMDA receptors, which could potentially lead to regulating LTP induction. See text for discussion of the PKA- and PKC-dependent regulation of the NMDA receptor. Concerning src family tyrosine kinases, the activities of Src and Fyn in neurons are controlled by a number of upstream signal transduction cascades. One important regulator of Src is the focal adhesion kinase (FAK) CAKbeta, also known as pyk2, and this cascade has been shown to be involved, through Src, in regulating LTP induction (13). In addition, the ERK MAP kinase cascade and the PKC cascades, which will be discussed below, can also activate Src-family kinases and these pathways may also modulate NMDA receptor function and LTP induction via Src (14). Dephosphorylation of the src/fyn sites on NMDA receptors likely occurs through the action of the tyrosine phosphatase STEP.

A number of interesting cell surface receptors modulate NMDA receptor function, and thus potentially LTP induction, acting through the src cascade. The Ephrins, which have mostly been studied in the context of nervous system development, modulate NMDA receptors in cultured neurons (15). EphrinB2, acting through its receptor EphB2, activates src and modulates NMDA receptors via this mechanism. Genetic deletion of EphB2 leads to an attenuation of LTP in area CA1 (16–17). Apolipoprotein E receptors in hippocampus also modulate LTP induction via a src/NMDA receptor pathway (18). Finally, the obese gene product leptin acts through its cell surface receptor and a PI3-Kinase/MAPK/src pathway to modulate NMDA receptors and LTP induction in the hippocampus (19). Thus, the Src/Fyn pathways serve an important role in funneling cell surface signals to the NMDA receptor itself, modulating its activity and regulating LTP induction.

Src tyrosine kinase potentiation of NMDA receptors is also subject to a variety of other influences. RACK1 (Receptor for Activated C Kinase 1) promotes formation of a Fyn/RACK1/NR2B complex that actually inhibits fyn phosphorylation of the NMDA receptor and diminishes current through the receptor (20). Also, the post-synaptic density core protein PDS-95 modulates src phosphorylation of NMDARs, and src potentiation of NMDAR currents appears to require the presence of PSD-95 (21).

The cyclin-dependent kinases (CDKs) are key regulators of cell division, controlling progression through the cell cycle. However, this role is, of course, not germane to understanding the function of non-dividing neurons in the adult CNS. However, one cdk isoform, cdk-5, is selectively expressed in post-mitotic neurons and functions in regulating neuronal migration and neurite outgrowth in development. Moreover, recent work has shown that this kinase is involved in synaptic plasticity and learning in adult animals (22). Specifically, inhibition of cdk-5 blocks NMDA receptor-dependent LTP in area CA1 and blocks contextual fear conditioning. One possible mechanism for this effect is cdk-5 regulation of NMDA receptor function, as cdk-5 phosphorylates the NR2A subunit and cdk-5 inhibitors reduce NMDA-induced currents in hippocampal neurons (23). Thus, cdk-5 may modulate NMDA receptor function in a manner reminiscent of src, PKC, etc. The mechanisms controlling cdk-5 regulation in hippocampal pyramidal neurons have yet to be explained.

the NMDA receptor through controlling the depolarization envelope that the receptor experiences.

Table 2 lists a number of the important molecules contributing to regulation of membrane depolarization in neuronal dendrites. Progress in this area has

been greatly facilitated by relatively recent technical advances that allow direct cell-attached patch recording from the distal dendritic regions of CA1 pyramidal neurons. These studies have identified a number of relevant membrane currents that control dendritic membrane depolarization and excitability, and in most cases there are reasonable hypotheses about the molecules underlying these currents.

A. Dendritic Potassium Channels—A-type Currents

"A-type," or voltage-dependent, rapidly inactivating K^+ channels localized in the dendrites of hippocampal pyramidal neurons play a critical role in shaping the local electrical responses of the dendritic membrane and dendritic tree. The functions of A-type channels in general are to: repolarize the membrane after an action potential; contribute to the resting membrane potential (modestly); and regulate firing frequency. Dan Johnston and his co-workers have proposed a model in which A-type channels in distal dendrites of the hippocampus are critical regulators of back-propagating action potentials, regulating LTP induction through controlling voltage-dependent NMDA receptor activation (32–34).

Moreover, this type of regulatory mechanism is subject to modulation by cellular signal transduction cascades. Activation of PKA or PKC shifts the activation curve of A-type K^+ currents recorded in hippocampal area CA1 dendrites (32). The voltage-dependence of their activation is shifted in the depolarizing direction, leading to increases in dendritic excitability and increased back-propagating action potentials in dendrites. More recent work has shown that the alterations in A-current voltage-dependence caused by application of PKA, PKC or β-adrenergic receptor activators are secondary to activation of ERK MAP kinase (33–34). Overall, these observations indicate that K^+ channel regulation of dendritic membrane properties is regulated by cell surface neurotransmitter receptors coupled to ERK activation. The implication of this, as will be discussed in more detail below, is that neuromodulation of K^+ channel function could serve a critical role in controlling action potential back-propagation and local membrane electrical properties. This mechanism would then allow indirect but critical control over the membrane depolarization necessary for NMDA receptor activation.

What is the molecular basis for this regulation of voltage-dependent K^+ channel function? The A-type potassium channel pore-forming subunit Kv4.2 is localized to sub-synaptic compartments of dendrites in CA1 pyramidal neurons, and is likely the pore-forming subunit of dendritic A-type channels in these regions. Thus, one contemporary hypothesis is that ERK phosphorylation of Kv4.2, the K^+ channel pore-forming subunits likely to mediate A-currents in hippocampal dendrites, decreases the probability of channel opening or the number of channels in the membrane. Once these channels in a particular region of a dendrite are rendered nonfunctional due to phosphorylation, the ability of a back-propagating action potential to invade that particular dendrite increases. This will allow, or increase the likelihood of, NMDA receptor activation and Ca^{2+} influx locally, and thus control the induction of LTP at that synapse.

B. Voltage-Dependent Sodium Channels

Just like in axons, propagation of action potentials along dendrites depends on voltage-gated sodium channels. In situations where back-propagating action potentials provide the depolarization necessary for NMDA receptor activation, this effect is, of course, dependent on the function of voltage-gated sodium channels. This is a potential site of plasticity for the regulation of LTP induction (35). Specifically, PKC can regulate the rate of inactivation of sodium channels in pyramidal neuron dendrites, a mechanism allowing PKC control of the extent of action potential back-propagation. Mechanistically, PKC decreases the extent of sodium channel inactivation, allowing for repetitive action potentials (where Na channel inactivation is relevant) to more effectively penetrate the dendrites (30, 36). By this mechanism, PKC activation can promote the induction of LTP.

C. AMPA Receptor Function

The next chapter will cover in detail a variety of mechanisms by which protein kinases augment AMPA receptor function. This is one of the principal mechanisms by which synaptic strength is enhanced during the expression of E-LTP. However, it should not escape our attention that these mechanisms could also play a critical role in the induction of LTP. In this context it is important to note that CaMKII, PKC, and PKA all enhance AMPA receptor function—any cell surface receptor or calcium influx process that leads to activation of these kinases could influence the likelihood of LTP induction through augmenting AMPA receptor membrane depolarization.

This amplification of AMPA receptor function could be important in several contexts. First, AMPA receptors provide the initial depolarization of the membrane that brings the cell to threshold for firing an action potential. An augmentation of AMPA receptor function means that for any given level of glutamate at the synapse there is greater depolarization, at least until the concentration of glutamate reaches a saturating level. Thus, the cell is more likely to reach threshold for firing an action potential, and therefore be more likely to trigger NMDA receptor activation. In "non-silent" synapses where AMPA receptors and NMDA receptors are both present, AMPA receptor augmentation will lead directly to greater local membrane depolarization and enhanced NMDA receptor function. This is an appealing model in the context of second messenger-coupled neurotransmitter receptors modulating LTP induction.

D. GABA Receptors

As described in Chapter 7, GABA-gated chloride ion channels (GABA-A receptors) control numerous processes relevant to the triggering of LTP. As these processes were described already in the context of hippocampal circuit information processing mechanisms, they will not be covered here. Suffice it to say that dendritic GABA-A receptor activation could play a powerful role in controlling NMDA receptor activation locally, and regulate plasticity and memory formation via this mechanism.

IV. NMDA RECEPTOR REGULATORY COMPONENT 3—THE COMPONENTS OF THE SYNAPTIC INFRASTRUCTURE THAT ARE NECESSARY FOR THE NMDA RECEPTOR AND THE SYNAPTIC SIGNAL TRANSDUCTION MACHINERY TO FUNCTION NORMALLY

The components of the synaptic infrastructure, such as scaffolding proteins, cytoskeletal proteins, and cell surface adhesion molecules, are now coming to be appreciated as important signaling components in the cell that respond rapidly and with great variety to extracellular and intracellular signals. However, placing them into a scheme for NMDA receptor regulation is fairly speculative at this point, and in some cases the most that can be said is that they are known to interact with other proteins known to be involved in NMDA receptor regulation. With these caveats in mind, what follows is a brief listing of the more notable components of the synaptic infrastructure that have been implicated as potentially contributing to NMDA receptor regulation. While this section will delve into several specific categories of molecules, it is important to keep in mind that the overall take-home message of this section is that the NMDA receptor does not function in isolation. It is a component of a richly-complicated physical structure that is itself subject to regulation.

A. Cell Adhesion Molecules and the Actin Matrix

A prominent category of synaptic adhesion molecules are the integrins (37). Integrins are cell surface molecules that transduce signals from the extracellular matrix to the inside of the cell. They are single-transmembrane-domain proteins that usually function as heterodimers of alpha and beta subunits. Knockout mice deficient in alpha5 and beta3 integrin exhibit hippocampus-dependent learning deficits, and deficits in NMDA receptor-dependent LTP in area CA1.

Integrins interact with a wide variety of intracellular effectors; three categories of these are clearly important to keep in mind in terms of LTP induction in general and regulating NMDA receptor function specifically (see Figure 8). First, integrins couple to src activation in many cells, and as we discussed in the first section of this chapter this is a mechanism for directly augmenting NMDA receptor function. Second, integrins couple to ras and via this mechanism can lead to ERK activation—this might play a role in K channel regulation (and regulating other effectors) as was discussed in the second section of this chapter. Finally, the prototype function of integrins is in regulating the actin cytoskeleton. This potential role of integrins has taken on special significance given findings by a number of laboratories that normal dynamic regulation of the actin cytoskeleton is necessary for LTP induction. Exactly how the actin cytoskeleton regulates LTP induction is unclear at present, but one model is presented in Figure 8.

B. Pre-Synaptic Processes

It is a statement of the obvious that any pre-synaptic process that regulates glutamate release can impinge on NMDA receptor function through controlling the level of synaptic glutamate that is attained. For our purposes here, I simply note that these are potentially relevant mechanisms for regulating NMDA receptor function indirectly.

C. Anchoring and Interacting Proteins of the Post-Synaptic Compartment—Post-Synaptic Density Proteins

The post-synaptic density (PSD) is a multiprotein assembly that is the organizing center for many receptors and effectors, and the cytoskeleton, in the post-synaptic compartment (43–44). PSD-95 is a protein enriched in the post-synaptic density and a prominent player in this context (45). Understanding its role in the organization of the complex post-synaptic infrastructure is important, so we will discuss this in some detail.

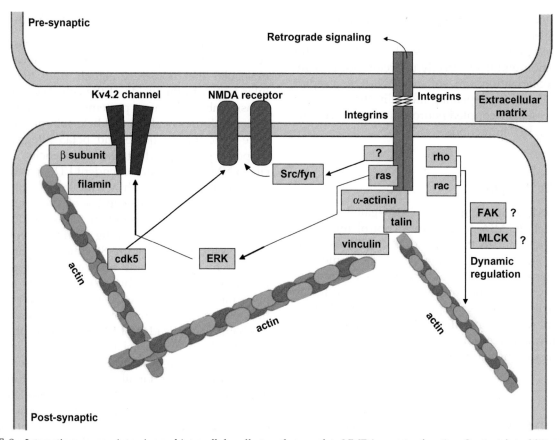

FIGURE 8 Interactions among integrins and intracellular effectors that regulate NMDA receptor function. See text for additional discussion and definitions. Integrin regulation of the actin cytoskeletal matrix is complex. One principal role is linking the extracellular matrix to sites of actin matrix adhesion on the cytoplasmic side of the membrane. Integrin cytoplasmic tails bind to alpha-actinin and talin, which in turn recruit actin-binding proteins such as vinculin to the complex. This complex serves to anchor the cytoskeleton to the peri-synaptic plasma membrane and synaptic zone.

Integrins also regulate the small G proteins rho (ras homolog, first identified in *Aplysia*) and rac, which regulate actin dynamics—this dynamic regulation of the actin matrix may contribute to activity-dependent changes in spine morphology. Consideration of integrin regulation of rho activity is especially appealing in this context because the classic role of rho is in regulating actin–myosin based movement through activating myosin light-chain kinase. Another potential integrin effector in this context is the focal adhesion kinase (FAK), which also serves to control cell morphology via the actin cytoskeletal matrix in many cells.

The actin cytoskeletal matrix may also contribute to NMDA receptor regulation in fairly direct ways. For example, actin microfilaments can serve as anchors for signaling components that affect the NMDA receptor directly. One example of this is actin filaments serving as the anchor for cdk5, which as was discussed above can phosphorylate and activate the NMDA receptor. Also, A-type potassium channels interact with the actin-binding protein filamin via their cytoplasmic c-terminal domain, and potassium channel beta subunits couple these channels to the actin cytoskeleton. These interactions certainly help localize A-channels appropriately in the dendritic spine. Perhaps more importantly, disruption of these interactions can cause attenuation of potassium channel function, and as we discussed above A-channel inhibition promotes increased membrane excitability and enhanced NMDA receptor function.

An additional transmembrane, extracellular-matrix-binding protein that has been directly implicated in LTP induction is Syndecan-3. Inhibition of this molecule using various approaches leads to deficits in LTP (38). Syndecan-3 binds heparan sulfates in the extracellular space, which are components of the glycosaminoglycan family of molecules present there. Syndecan-3 associates with the tyrosine kinase fyn, which might regulate NMDA receptor activity through direct tyrosine phosphorylation. The cell adhesion molecules L1 and N-CAM have also been implicated in the expression of LTP in some studies, however, recent results from knockout mice have suggested that loss of these molecules does not lead to LTP deficits (39–41). Finally, the N-cadherin subtype of cell adhesion molecule has been implicated in LTP induction and maintenance (42). A likely role for the cadherins is in stabilizing strong connections between the pre-synaptic and post-synaptic membranes, although like other cell adhesion molecules the cadherins also interact with and can regulate the actin cytoskeleton.

PSD-95 binds to NMDA receptors (specifically the NR2 subunit) post-synaptically, and serves as a multi-domain anchoring protein for a large number of scaffolding and structural proteins post-synaptically (see Figure 9). PSD-95 helps anchor nitric oxide synthase (NOS), localizing this source of the reactive nitrogen species NO. PSD-95 also binds the ras GTPase activating protein synGAP, whose function is still under investigation but which may regulate the ras/ERK cascade locally at the synapse. PSD-95 also anchors the cytoskeleton through its interations with a protein termed SPAR, which is a GTPase activating protein

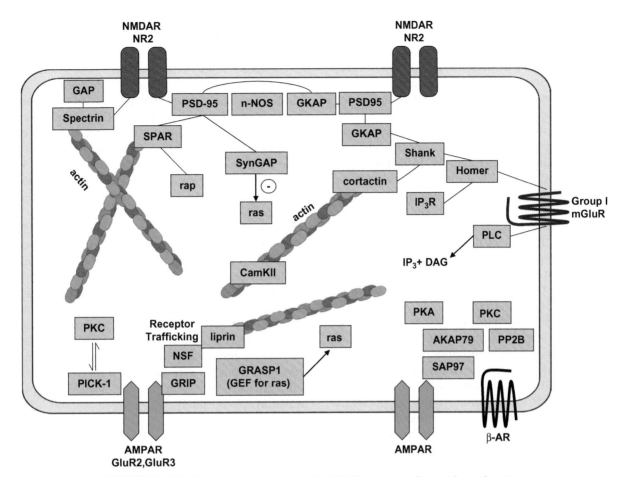

FIGURE 9   PSD-95 as an anchoring protein for NMDA receptors. See text for explanation.

(GAP) for rap, and also an actin-interacting protein in its own right. Rap helps control the cytoskeleton indirectly through its target signal transduction processes, such as the MAP kinase cascades.

PSD-95 also binds to proteins that seem to be more explicitly structural, such as the scaffolding protein Shank. Shank is another multi-domain molecule that links the PSD-95 binding protein GKAP to the actin skeleton through cortactin. Shank also binds to HOMER, a metabotropic receptor binding protein. Thus, via shank and HOMER, group I metabotropic receptors coupled to PLC can be localized near the NMDA receptor. HOMER also binds the IP3 receptor, which may help localize the endoplasmic reticulum close to the NMDA receptor, allowing for proximity of intracellular calcium release mechanisms to the principal pathway for extracellular calcium influx, the NMDA receptor.

Genetic deletion of PSD-95 leads to striking alterations in LTP in area CA1—LTP is enhanced (45). This is associated with learning deficits. It is unclear how the loss of PSD-95 leads to the augmentation of

LTP—interpretation of the result is difficult because of the many complex roles of PSD-95 at the synapse, as outlined above. Overall, the data suggest that PSD-95 is somehow altering the threshold for LTP induction, a result consistent with the idea that PSD-95 and its associated proteins serve as dynamic modulators of NMDA receptor function.

Finally, the NMDA receptor NR1 and NR2 subunits also bind spectrin, the actin-binding protein. This may serve as an additional cytoskeleton anchoring site postsynaptically. Consideration of the complicated structure and regulation of the post-synaptic density complex highlights the importance of thinking of the entire postsynaptic domain as a large functional unit. The NMDA receptor is embedded in a dynamic multiprotein complex that it regulates, and that in turn regulates it. While many details of the structural components of the PSD complex are still being worked out, and their roles in LTP induction and memory formation are being actively investigated, it is clear that disrupting one or more of the cogs in this machine can lead to disruption of the proper function of the NMDA receptor.

D. AMPA Receptors

AMPA receptors, of course, provide the initial depolarization that ultimately results in NMDA receptor activation. However, in this section we will focus on the AMPA receptor as a structural component of the synapse.

AMPA receptors, like the NMDA receptor, also reside post-synaptically, but are in much more of a state of flux than NMDA receptors. In fact, the average half-life for an AMPA receptor in the post-synaptic membrane is 15 minutes. Also, AMPA receptor membrane insertion can be activity-dependent. Thus, in terms of its structural role, the AMPA receptor should not be thought of like the NMDA receptor—the NMDA receptor likely serves a frankly structural role in addition to its function as a ligand-gated ion channel, while the AMPA receptor is more peripherally associated with the PSD (46).

The AMPA receptor binds at least two "structural" proteins—PICK-1, which binds PKC, and GRIP (43). GRIP is a multi-domain scaffolding protein that likely functions in AMPA receptor trafficking. GRIP also binds to GRASP1, a GEF for ras (47–48)—the functional role of GRASP1 at the synapse is unclear at present. AMPA receptors can also bind NSF, a vesicle-associated protein that may also be involved in receptor membrane insertion in a fashion reminiscent of its role pre-synaptically in neurotransmitter vesicle fusion.

AMPA receptors also bind the A kinase anchoring protein AKAP79, an interaction that appears to be mediated by the PSD-95 homolog SAP-97 (49–51). As the name implies, AKAPs bind and localize PKA through interacting with the regulatory subunits of the kinase. The general role of AKAPs is to help localize PKA near relevant targets, such as the AMPA receptor, post-synaptically. The story is actually more complicated than that, as AKAP79 in the hippocampus also binds and localizes a protein phosphatase, PP2B (or Calcineurin). As a first approximation it is useful to think of proteins such as AKAPs serving a role to increase the signal-to-noise ratio for signal transduction—localizing kinases close to their substrates to increase the efficacy of phosphorylation, but also localizing phosphatases to those same substrates in order to keep their basal phosphorylation low and to allow for rapid reversal of phosphorylation events once the kinase activation is over (51). AKAP79 may also serve specifically to localize the calcium-sensitive phosphatase PP2B to the AMPA receptor in order to facilitate calcium-dependent AMPA receptor dephosphorylation and down-regulation (52).

E. CaMKII—the Calcium/Calmodulin-Dependent Protein Kinase II

CaMKII is highly enriched at the post-synaptic density complex. This enrichment occurs through CaMKII binding to the actin cytoskeleton, and the anchor for the cytoskeleton is the NMDA receptor, as we have discussed extensively. Thus, one purpose of the NMDA receptor/PSD-95/cytoskeleton complex is to help localize CaMKII to the PSD domain. This keeps a critical effector of the NMDA receptor, CaMKII, tightly bound and localized for effective responsiveness to NMDA receptor activation.

While the various scaffolding proteins, PSD-95, etc., that are discussed above are involved upstream of the NMDA receptor, regulating its function, CaMKII is downstream of the NMDA receptor. However, it is listed as a component of the synaptic infrastructure necessary for proper NMDA receptor function because it is such an important and direct target of the NMDA receptor. In addition, CaMKII binding to the PSD complex may play a structural role in concert with the actin cytoskeleton to serve as part of the infrastructure necessary for the NMDA receptor to function appropriately.

V. SUMMARY

The above discussion makes it clear that the NMDA receptor does not reside in isolation in the membrane. In fact, the NMDA receptor is the anchor for a large multiprotein complex of structural proteins and signal transduction components (see Figure 3). In fact, experiments using various deletion mutants missing the cytoplasmic anchoring domains of the NMDA receptor have allowed dissection of the role of the NMDA receptor as a scaffolding protein versus its role as a ligand-gated ion channel (53). Deletion of the intracellular domain of the NMDA receptor appears to be sufficient to account for many, if not all, of the physiologic and behavioral deficits observed in NMDA receptor knockout mice. An important message from this finding is that the role of the NMDA receptor as a component of the PSD infrastructure is just as important as its role as a ligand-gated ion channel.

In this chapter we have discussed three major categories of molecular components and processes that are involved in NMDA receptor regulation:

1. Molecular mechanisms upstream of the NMDA receptor that directly regulate its function, processes like phosphorylation, redox regulation,

and modulatory ligand binding. These processes can serve to integrate signals over a longer time-span than the relatively short-lived glutamate binding and membrane depolarization. These mechanisms also greatly increase the number of discrete molecular signals that the NMDA receptor is able to integrate or use for coincidence detection.

2. Mechanisms upstream of the NMDA receptor that control membrane depolarization. These mechanisms localized in the post-synaptic cell serve to fine-tune and regulate the depolarization envelope that the NMDA receptor senses. Again, these mechanisms provide a powerful system for increasing the integrative capacity of the NMDA receptor.

3. Components of the synaptic infrastructure that control its function. The NMDA receptor is embedded in the post-synaptic density, a rich milieu of molecules many of which are able to directly or indirectly affect NMDA receptor function. In addition, many components of the PSD serve as targets of the NMDA receptor in terms of its triggering downstream molecular consequences.

It is very important not to think of these in isolation from each other—they are functional categories to help organize the complex biochemical machinery of NMDA receptor regulation, not compartmentalized biochemical processes in the cell. Thus, we need to begin to think of the NMDA receptor as an immensely complicated information processing machine. It integrates a plethora of biochemical signals and computes, based on a number of molecular inputs, whether to trigger a lasting molecular change. The interactions of these various processes are what allow the NMDA receptor to serve in its role as a molecular decision-maker, and allows for at least part of the necessary sophistication required for deciding when to trigger memory formation in the animal *in vivo*.

Further Reading

Bannerman, D. M., Good, M. A., Butcher, S. P., Ramsay, M., and Morris, R. G. (1995). "Distinct components of spatial learning revealed by prior training and NMDA receptor blockade". *Nature* 378:182–186.

Davis, S., Butcher, S. P., and Morris, R. G. (1992). "The NMDA receptor antagonist D-2-amino-5-phosphonopentanoate (D-AP5) impairs spatial learning and LTP *in vivo* at intracerebral concentrations comparable to those that block LTP *in vitro*". *J. Neurosci.* 12:21–34.

Day, M., and Morris, R. G. (2001). "Memory consolidation and NMDA receptors: discrepancy between genetic and pharmacological approaches". *Science* 293:755.

Husi, H., and Grant, S. G. (2001). "Proteomics of the nervous system". *Trends Neurosci.* 24:259–266.

Kentros, C., Hargreaves, E., Hawkins, R. D., Kandel, E. R., Shapiro, M., and Muller, R. V. (1998). "Abolition of long-term stability of new hippocampal place cell maps by NMDA receptor blockade". *Science* 280:2121–2126.

Kim, J. J., Fanselow, M. S., DeCola, J. P., and Landeira-Fernandez, J. (1992). "Selective impairment of long-term but not short-term conditional fear by the N-methyl-D-aspartate antagonist APV". *Behav. Neurosci.* 106:591–596.

Konnerth, A., Li, J., McNamara, J. O., and Seeburg, P. H. (1998). "Importance of the intracellular domain of NR2 subunits for NMDA receptor function *in vivo*". *Cell* 92:279–289.

McHugh, T. J., Blum, K. I., Tsien, J. Z., Tonegawa, S., and Wilson, M. A. (1996). "Impaired hippocampal representation of space in CA1-specific NMDAR1 knockout mice". *Cell* 87:1339–1349.

Nakazawa, K., Quirk, M. C., Chitwood, R. A., Watanabe, M., Yeckel, M. F., Sun, L. D., Kato, A., Carr, C. A., Johnston, D., Wilson, M. A., and Tonegawa, S. (2002). "Requirement for hippocampal CA3 NMDA receptors in associative memory recall". *Science* 297:211–218.

Roberts, A. C., and Glanzman, D. L. (2003). "Learning in *Aplysia*: looking at synaptic plasticity from both sides". *Trends Neurosci.* 26(12):662–670.

Rondi-Reig, L., Libbey, M., Eichenbaum, H., and Tonegawa, S. (2001). "CA1-specific N-methyl-D-aspartate receptor knockout mice are deficient in solving a nonspatial transverse patterning task". *Proc. Natl. Acad. Sci. U S A* 98:3543–3548.

Sheng, M. (2001). "Molecular organization of the postsynaptic specialization". *Proc. Natl. Acad. Sci. U S A* 98:7058–7061.

Tang, Y. P., Shimizu, E., Dube, G. R., Rampon, C., Kerchner, G. A., Zhuo, M., Liu, G., and Tsien, J. Z. (1999). "Genetic enhancement of learning and memory in mice". *Nature* 401:63–69.

Tsien, J. Z., Huerta, P. T., and Tonegawa, S. (1996). "The essential role of hippocampal CA1 NMDA receptor-dependent synaptic plasticity in spatial memory". *Cell* 87:1327–1338.

Journal Club Articles

Hoffman, D. A., Magee, J. C., Colbert, C. M., and Johnston, D. (1997). "K+ channel regulation of signal propagation in dendrites of hippocampal pyramidal neurons". *Nature* 387:869–875.

Husi, H., Ward, M. A., Choudhary, J. S., Blackstock, W. P., and Grant, S. G. (2000). "Proteomic analysis of NMDA receptor-adhesion protein signaling complexes". *Nat. Neurosci.* 3:661–669.

Mayer, M. L., Westbrook, G. L., and Guthrie, P. B. (1984). "Voltage-dependent block by Mg^{2+} of NMDA responses in spinal cord neurones". *Nature* 309:261–263.

Morris, R. G. (1989). "Synaptic plasticity and learning: selective impairment of learning rats and blockade of long-term potentiation *in vivo* by the N-methyl-D-aspartate receptor antagonist AP5". *J. Neurosci.* 9:3040–3057.

Nowak, L., Bregestovski, P., Ascher, P., Herbet, A., and Prochiantz, A. (1984). "Magnesium gates glutamate-activated channels in mouse central neurones". *Nature* 307:462–465.

For more information—relevant topic chapters from: John H. Byrne (Editor-in-Chief) (2008). *Learning and Memory: A Comprehensive Reference*. Oxford: Academic Press (ISBN 978-0-12-370509-9). (4.10 Lorenzetti, F. D., and Byrne, J. H. *Cellular Mechanisms of Associative Learning in Aplysia*. pp. 149–156; 4.11 Schafe, G. E., and LeDoux, J. E. *Neural and Molecular Mechanisms of Fear Memory*. pp. 157–192; 4.13 Rosenblum, K. *Conditioned Taste Aversion and Taste Learning: Molecular Mechanisms*. pp. 217–234; 4.30 Alvestad, R. M., Goebel, S. M., Coultrap, S. J., and Browning, M. D. *Glutamate Receptor Trafficking in LTP*. pp. 611–632; 4.32 Marcora, E., Carlisle, H. J., and Kennedy, M. B. *The Role of the Postsynaptic Density and the Spine Cytoskeleton in Synaptic Plasticity.* pp. 649–673; 4.33 Costa-Mattioli, M., Sonenberg, N., and Klann, E. *Translational Control Mechanisms in Synaptic Plasticity and Memory.* pp. 675–694; 4.35 Chan, C.-S., and Davis, R. L. *Integrins and Cadherins—Extracellular Matrix in Memory Formation.* pp. 721–740; 4.39 Waters, J. Nevian, T., Sakmann, B., and Helmchen, F. *Action Potentials in Dendrites and Spike-Timing-Dependent Plasticity.* pp. 803–828.)

References

1. Collingridge, G. L., Kehl, S. J., and McLennan, H. (1983). "Excitatory amino acids in synaptic transmission in the Schaffer collateral-commissural pathway of the rat hippocampus". *J. Physiol.* 334:33–46.

2. Morris, R. G. (1989). "Synaptic plasticity and learning: selective impairment of learning rats and blockade of long-term potentiation *in vivo* by the N-methyl-D-aspartate receptor antagonist AP5". *J. Neurosci.* 9:3040–3057.

3. Husi, H., and Grant, S. G. (2001). "Proteomics of the nervous system". *Trends Neurosci.* 24:259–266.

4. Husi, H., Ward, M. A., Choudhary, J. S., Blackstock, W. P., and Grant, S. G. (2000). "Proteomic analysis of NMDA receptor-adhesion protein signaling complexes". *Nat. Neurosci.* 3:661–669.

5. Raymond, L. A., Tingley, W. G., Blackstone, C. D., Roche, K. W., and Huganir, R. L. (1994). "Glutamate receptor modulation by protein phosphorylation." *J. Physiol.* (Paris) 88:181–192.

6. Suzuki, T., and Okumura-Noji, K. (1995). "NMDA receptor subunits epsilon 1 (NR2A) and epsilon 2 (NR2B) are substrates for Fyn in the postsynaptic density fraction isolated from the rat brain". *Biochem. Biophys. Res. Commun.* 216:582–588.

7. Zheng, F., Gingrich, M. B., Traynelis, S. F., and Conn, P. J. (1998). "Tyrosine kinase potentiates NMDA receptor currents by reducing tonic zinc inhibition". *Nat. Neurosci.* 1:185–191.

8. Lu, Y. M., Roder, J. C., Davidow, J., and Salter, M. W. (1998). "Src activation in the induction of long-term potentiation in CA1 hippocampal neurons". *Science* 279:1363–1367.

9. Logan, S. M., Rivera, F. E., and Leonard, J. P. (1999). "Protein kinase C modulation of recombinant NMDA receptor currents: roles for the C-terminal C1 exon and calcium ions". *J. Neurosci.* 19:974–986.

10. Liao, G. Y., Kreitzer, M. A., Sweetman, B. J., and Leonard, J. P. (2000). "The postsynaptic density protein PSD-95 differentially regulates insulin- and Src-mediated current modulation of mouse NMDA receptors expressed in Xenopus oocytes". *J. Neurochem.* 75:282–287.

11. Ben-Ari, Y., Aniksztejn, L., and Bregestovski, P. (1992). "Protein kinase C modulation of NMDA currents: an important link for LTP induction". *Trends Neurosci.* 15:333–339.

12. Westphal, R. S., Tavalin, S. J., Lin, J. W., Alto, N. M., Fraser, I. D., Langeberg, L. K., Sheng, M., and Scott, J. D. (1999). "Regulation of NMDA receptors by an associated phosphatase-kinase signaling complex". *Science* 285:93–96.

13. Huang, Y., Lu, W., Ali, D. W., Pelkey, K. A., Pitcher, G. M., Lu, Y. M., Aoto, H., Roder, J. C., Sasaki, T., Salter, M. W., and MacDonald, J. F. (2001). "CAKbeta/Pyk2 kinase is a signaling link for induction of long-term potentiation in CA1 hippocampus". *Neuron* 29:485–496.

14. Grosshans, D. R., and Browning, M. D. (2001). "Protein kinase C activation induces tyrosine phosphorylation of the NR2A and NR2B subunits of the NMDA receptor". *J. Neurochem.* 76:737–744.

15. Takasu, M. A., Dalva, M. B., Zigmond, R. E., and Greenberg, M. E. (2002). "Modulation of NMDA receptor-dependent calcium influx and gene expression through EphB receptors". *Science* 295:491–495.

16. Grunwald, I. C., Korte, M., Wolfer, D., Wilkinson, G. A., Unsicker, K., Lipp, H. P., Bonhoeffer, T., and Klein, R. (2001). "Kinase-independent requirement of EphB2 receptors in hippocampal synaptic plasticity". *Neuron* 32:1027–1040.

17. Henderson, J. T., Georgiou, J., Jia, Z., Robertson, J., Elowe, S., Roder, J. C., and Pawson, T. (2001). "The receptor tyrosine kinase EphB2 regulates NMDA-dependent synaptic function". *Neuron* 32:1041–1056.

18. Weeber, E. F., Beffert, U., Jones, C., Christian, J. M., Forster, E., Sweatt, J. D., and Herz, J. (2002). "Reelin and ApoE receptors cooperate to enhance hippocampal synaptic plasticity and learning". *J. Biol. Chem.* 51:49958–49964.

19. Shanley, L. J., Irving, A. J., and Harvey, J. (2001). "Leptin enhances NMDA receptor function and modulates hippocampal synaptic plasticity". *J. Neurosci.* 21:RC186.

20. Yaka, R., Thornton, C., Vagts, A. J., Phamluong, K., Bonci, A., and Ron, D. (2002). "NMDA receptor function is regulated by the inhibitory scaffolding protein, RACK1". *Proc. Natl. Acad. Sci. USA* 9:5710–5715.

21. Liao, G. Y., Wagner, D. A., Hsu, M. H., and Leonard, J. P. (2001). "Evidence for direct protein kinase-C mediated modulation of N-methyl-D-aspartate receptor current". *Mol. Pharmacol.* 59:960–964.

22. Fischer, A., Sananbenesi, F., Schrick, C., Spiess, J., and Radulovic, J. (2002). "Cyclin-dependent kinase 5 is required for associative learning". *J. Neurosci.* 22:3700–3707.

23. Li, B. S., Sun, M. K., Zhang, L., Takahashi, S., Ma, W., Vinade, L., Kulkarni, A. B., Brady, R. O., and Pant, H. C. (2001). "Regulation of NMDA receptors by cyclin-dependent kinase-5". *Proc. Natl. Acad. Sci. USA* 98:12742–12747.

24. Choi, Y. B., Tenneti, L., Le, D. A., Ortiz, J., Bai, G., Chen, H. S., and Lipton, S. A. (2000). "Molecular basis of NMDA receptor-coupled ion channel modulation by S-nitrosylation". *Nat. Neurosci.* 3:15–21.

25. Choi, Y. B., and Lipton, S. A. (2000). "Redox modulation of the NMDA receptor". *Cell Mol. Life Sci.* 57:1535–1541.

26. Traynelis, S. F., Hartley, M., and Heinemann, S. F. (1995). "Control of proton sensitivity of the NMDA receptor by RNA splicing and polyamines". *Science* 268:873–876.

27. Gallagher, M. J., Huang, H., Grant, E. R., and Lynch, D. R. (1997). "The NR2B-specific interactions of polyamines and protons with the N-methyl-D-aspartate receptor". *J. Biol. Chem.* 272:24971–24979.

28. Ingi, T., Worley, P. F., and Lanahan, A. A. (2001). "Regulation of SSAT expression by synaptic activity". *Eur. J. Neurosci.* 13:1459–1463.

29. Stuart, G. J., and Sakmann, B. (1994). "Active propagation of somatic action potentials into neocortical pyramidal cell dendrites". *Nature* 367:69–72.

30. Spruston, N., Schiller, Y., Stuart, G., and Sakmann, B. (1995). "Activity-dependent action potential invasion and calcium influx into hippocampal CA1 dendrites". *Science* 268:297–300.

31. Magee, J. C., and Johnston, D. (1995). "Synaptic activation of voltage-gated channels in the dendrites of hippocampal pyramidal neurons". *Science* 268:301–304.

32. Hoffman, D. A., Magee, J. C., Colbert, C. M., and Johnston, D. (1997). "K^+ channel regulation of signal propagation in dendrites of hippocampal pyramidal neurons". *Nature* 387:869–875.

33. Yuan, L. L., Adams, J. P., Swank, M., Sweatt, J. D., and Johnston, D. (2002). "Protein kinase modulation of dendritic K^+ channels in hippocampus involves a mitogen-activated protein kinase pathway". *J. Neurosci.* 22:4860–4868.

34. Watanabe, S., Hoffman, D. A., Migliore, M., and Johnston, D. (2002). "Dendritic K^+ channels contribute to spike-timing dependent long-term potentiation in hippocampal pyramidal neurons". *Proc. Natl. Acad. Sci. USA* 99:8366–8371.

35. Colbert, C. M., and Johnston, D. (1998). "Protein kinase C activation decreases activity-dependent attenuation of dendritic

Na$^+$ current in hippocampal CA1 pyramidal neurons". *J. Neurophysiol.* 79:491–495.

36. Tsubokawa, H. (2000). "Control of Na$^+$ spike backpropagation by intracellular signaling in the pyramidal neuron dendrites". *Mol. Neurobiol.* 22:129–141.

37. Martin, K. H., Slack, J. K., Boerner, S. A., Martin, C. C., and Parsons, J. T. (2002). "Integrin connections map: to infinity and beyond". *Science* 296:1652–1653.

38. Lauri, S. E., Kaukinen, S., Kinnunen, T., Ylinen, A., Imai, S., Kaila, K., Taira, T., and Rauvala, H. (1999). "Regulatory role and molecular interactions of a cell-surface heparan sulfate proteoglycan (N-syndecan) in hippocampal long-term potentiation". *J. Neurosci.* 19:1226–1235.

39. Bliss, T., Errington, M., Fransen, E., Godfraind, J. M., Kauer, J. A., Kooy, R. F., Maness, P. F., and Furley, A. J. (2000). "Long-term potentiation in mice lacking the neural cell adhesion molecule L1". *Curr. Biol.* 10:1607–1610.

40. Holst, B. D., Vanderklish, P. W., Krushel, L. A., Zhou, W., Langdon, R. B., McWhirter, J. R., Edelman, G. M., and Crossin, K. L. (1998). "Allosteric modulation of AMPA-type glutamate receptors increases activity of the promoter for the neural cell adhesion molecule, N-CAM". *Proc. Natl. Acad. Sci. USA* 95:2597–2602.

41. Luthl, A., Laurent, J. P., Figurov, A., Muller, D., and Schachner, M. (1994). "Hippocampal long-term potentiation and neural cell adhesion molecules L1 and NCAM". *Nature* 372:777–779.

42. Huntley, G. W., Gil, O., and Bozdagi, O. (2002). "The cadherin family of cell adhesion molecules: multiple roles in synaptic plasticity". *Neuroscientist* 8:221–233.

43. Sheng, M., and Pak, D. T. (2000). "Ligand-gated ion channel interactions with cytoskeletal and signaling proteins". *Annu. Rev. Physiol.* 62:755–778.

44. Sheng, M. (2001). "Molecular organization of the postsynaptic specialization". *Proc. Natl. Acad. Sci. USA* 98:7058–7061.

45. Migaud, M., Charlesworth, P., Dempster, M., Webster, L. C., Watabe, A. M., Makhinson, M., He, Y., Ramsay, M. F., Morris, R. G., Morrison, J. H., O'Dell, T. J., and Grant, S. G. (1998). "Enhanced long-term potentiation and impaired learning in mice with mutant postsynaptic density-95 protein". *Nature* 396:433–439.

46. Passafaro, M., Piech, V., and Sheng, M. (2001). "Subunit-specific temporal and spatial patterns of AMPA receptor exocytosis in hippocampal neurons". *Nat. Neurosci.* 4:917–926.

47. Sweatt, J. D. (2001). "Protooncogenes subserve memory formation in the adult CNS". *Neuron* 31:671–674.

48. Vetter, I. R., and Wittinghofer, A. (2001). "The guanine nucleotide-binding switch in three dimensions". *Science* 294:1299–1304.

49. Colledge, M., Dean, R. A., Scott, G. K., Langeberg, L. K., Huganir, R. L., and Scott, J. D. (2000). "Targeting of PKA to glutamate receptors through a MAGUK-AKAP complex". *Neuron* 27:107–119.

50. Coghlan, V. M., Perrino, B. A., Howard, M., Langeberg, L. K., Hicks, J. B., Gallatin, W. M., and Scott, J. D. (1995). "Association of protein kinase A and protein phosphatase 2B with a common anchoring protein". *Science* 267:108–111.

51. Dodge, K., and Scott, J. D. (2000). "AKAP79 and the evolution of the AKAP model". *FEBS Lett.* 476:58–61.

52. Tavalin, S. J., Colledge, M., Hell, J. W., Langeberg, L. K., Huganir, R. L., and Scott, J. D. (2002). "Regulation of GluR1 by the A-kinase anchoring protein 79 (AKAP79) signaling complex shares properties with long-term depression". *J. Neurosci.* 22:3044–3051.

53. Sprengel, R., Suchanek, B., Amico, C., Brusa, R., Burnashev, N., Rozov, A., Hvalby, O., Jensen, V., Paulsen, O., Andersen, P., Kim, J. J., Thompson, R. F., Sun, W., Webster, L. C., Grant, S. G., Eilers, J., Konnerth, A., Li, J., McNamara, J. O., and Seeburg, P. H. (1998). "Importance of the intracellular domain of NR2 subunits for NMDA receptor function *in vivo*". *Cell* 92:279–289.

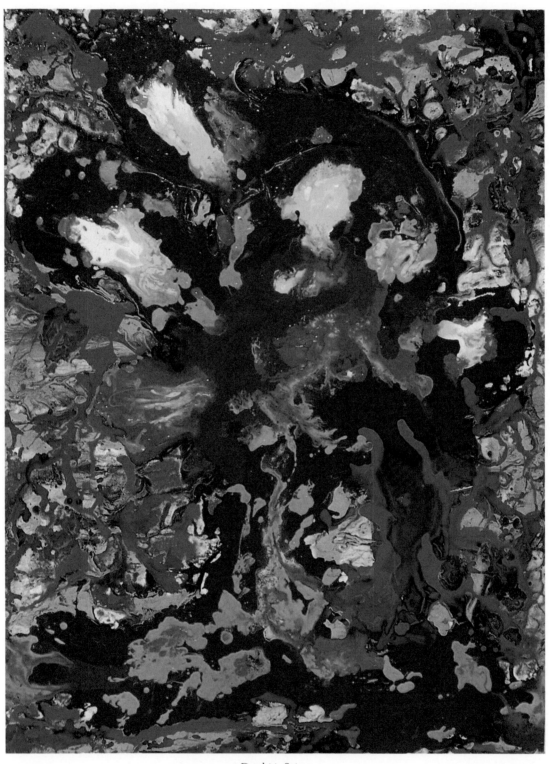

Dendritic Spine

J. David Sweatt, acrylic on canvas, 2008–2009

Biochemical Mechanisms for Information Storage at the Cellular Level

Chapter Overview

In the last chapter we discussed the complex mechanisms and biochemical "computations" involved in NMDA receptor regulation. Overall these mechanisms determine whether an LTP- and memory-inducing level of calcium will be reached post-synaptically in response to synaptic activity. In this chapter we will deal with the first stages of those processes that are actually triggered by that calcium signal when it is attained. In essence, this chapter deals with the transition of synaptic plasticity induction mechanisms into the maintenance and expression of plasticity and memory.

In this chapter we begin to deal with the fundamental biochemical problem that has to be solved in order for memory to exist—the generation of a persisting biochemical signal by a transient inducing stimulus. In many ways, this is the heart of the matter

for memory at the molecular level, the reduction of the problem to its smallest finite components. We will deal specifically in this chapter with the issue of how a transient calcium signal gets converted to a persisting biochemical trace in a CA1 pyramidal neuron. Almost all of the mechanisms we will discuss have been studied in the context of NMDA receptor-dependent early LTP (E-LTP). We will focus on E-LTP, because the vast majority of detailed molecular studies of synaptic plasticity have focused on this phenomenon, so it is the area richest in available information. In addition, as discussed in earlier chapters, there is a strong correlation between LTP mechanisms and mechanisms known to be relevant to memory *in vivo*.

A second issue we will deal with in this chapter is how the biochemical traces involved in maintaining synaptic potentiation get converted into actual potentiation of synaptic transmission. These are the mechanisms of E-LTP expression. For the most part this means discussing mechanisms of augmenting AMPA receptor function, although we also will touch briefly on facilitation of pre-synaptic glutamate release and potential alterations in post-synaptic excitability.

CHAPTER OVERVIEW

The chapter will be broken down into three broad sections (see Figure 1). The first section will deal with two well-established targets of the calcium that triggers LTP and other memory-associated forms of synaptic plasticity: CaMKII and PKC. In this section I will focus principally on the known mechanisms for generation of persistently activated forms of these kinases; forms of the molecules that are capable of serving as molecular memory traces in LTP and memory in general.

This section, then, deals with maintenance mechanisms for plasticity. The second section of this chapter will deal with potential effectors of the persistently activated kinases: post-synaptic glutamate receptors; the pre-synaptic release mechanism; and the cytoskeleton. This section therefore deals with mechanisms of expression of synaptic potentiation. The final section deals with dendritic protein synthesis in perpetuating lasting functional changes, and the notion that there are synaptic "tags" that are generated in response to plasticity-inducing stimulation.

I. TARGETS OF THE CALCIUM TRIGGER

We discussed the elaborate mechanisms involved in generating a level of post-synaptic calcium sufficient to trigger LTP in the last chapter. What is it that

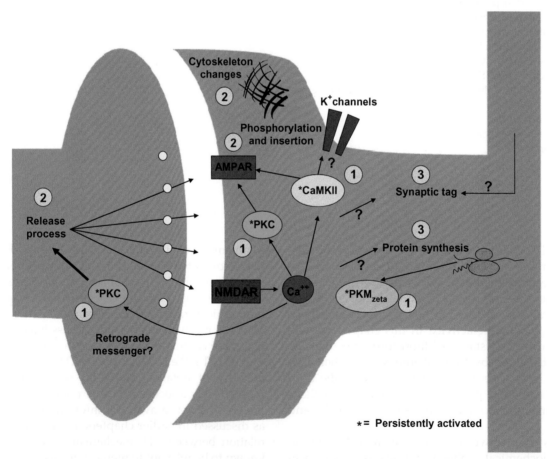

FIGURE 1   Chapter summary. This chapter deals with three primary issues related to mechanisms for E-LTP. First, describing mechanisms for generating and maintaining persisting signals at the synapse, (1). Second, discussing molecular sites of action of these persisting signals which operate in the expression of E-LTP, (2). Third, reviewing some of the mechanisms involved in the regulation of local dendritic protein synthesis and synaptic tagging, mechanisms involved in the E-LTP to L-LTP transition (3).

this calcium signal does? Obviously any direct target of the calcium signal has to be a calcium-binding protein. While there are a number of calcium-binding proteins in cells, based on the known functional categories of calcium-binding proteins and those that have been implicated in LTP, there are two proteins we need to pay particular attention to: calmodulin (CaM); and PKC(s). In this section of the chapter we will discuss these two proteins and their targets, focusing mostly on CaM-regulated kinases, CaM-dependent adenylyl cyclases (ACs), and PKC, because these have been by far the most extensively studied in the context of LTP and memory.

Interestingly, CaM and the calcium-binding isoforms of PKC are the prototype molecules for the two major categories of calcium-binding proteins (see Figure 2). Each of these molecules has calcium binding domains in their structure that define whole families of calcium-binding proteins. CaM is the prototype molecule for the "E-F hand" family of calcium-binding

proteins. The "E-F hand" terminology derives from esoteric naming of the calcium-binding domain based on a lettered alpha-helix nomenclature (the E-F part), coupled with the fact that the domain could be modeled to look like a human hand in a specific configuration. (OK, since you asked, the hand configuration is the classic "six-shooter" configuration that boys use when they want to pretend to shoot each other.) As a first approximation you can think of the E-F hand structure as the generic calcium-binding domain in proteins. A wide variety of proteins, including CaM, troponin C, the S100s, and the calcium-binding subunits of the protease calpain and protein phosphatase 2B all contain E-F hand calcium-binding domains.

PKC is the prototype for the "C2 domain" family of calcium-binding proteins. As we will discuss later, the PKC superfamily is a heterogeneous group of proteins with variable ("V") and conserved ("C") domains. The second conserved domain ("C2") is a calcium-binding domain. The C2 domain family of calcium-binding

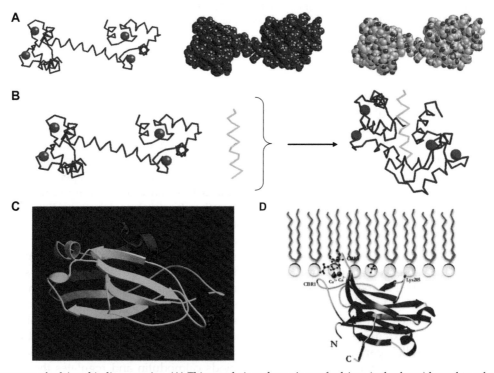

FIGURE 2   Structures of calcium-binding proteins. (A) This panel gives three views of calcium (red spheres) bound to calmodulin, illustrating the structure of the "E-F hand" subtype of calcium-binding protein. The first rendering shows the peptide backbone of calmodulin in dark blue. The second rendering is identical to the first except that the calmodulin structure is illustrated in space-filling spheres. The third rendering is identical to the second except that amino acids are rendered in the CPK convention (red = oxygen, blue = nitrogen, gray = carbon, yellow = sulphur. (B) This panel illustrates the interaction of Ca/calmodulin with a target effector. An alpha-helical domain of CaMKII is illustrated in light green to the right of the calmodulin molecule. As part of achieving its effects on target effectors calmodulin changes the structure of its own inter-domain alpha helix, wrapping itself around the target. (C) and (D) Illustrations of the "C2 domain" subtype of calcium-binding domain. These figures illustrate two different conformations of this type of calcium-binding domain, typified by the C2 domain of PKC alpha. (D) Structural changes induced by calcium (shown as red spheres) binding to the calcium-binding domain and adjacent regions of the molecule typically cause allosteric changes, promoting binding to phospholipid membranes. Structures based on data in Verdaguer et al. (1).

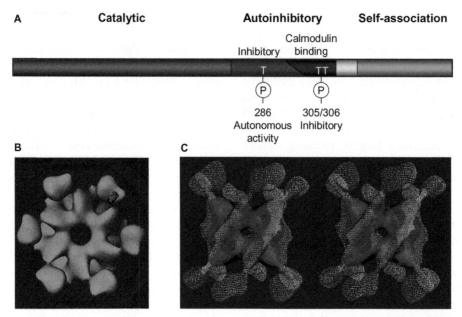

FIGURE 3   Structure of CAMKII. (A) Line diagram illustrating the catalytic, autoinhibitory, and association domains of CaMKII, as well as two sites of autophosphorylation. Reproduced from Lisman et al. (6). (B) and (C) illustrate a detailed and realistic model of CaMKII based on sophisticated high-resolution electron microscopy and X-ray diffraction techniques. (B) is a "top-down" view of CaMKII showing 6 of the 12 individual subunits comprising the holoenzyme. Adapted from Lisman et al. (6). (C) is a stereo rendering of a "side view" of the same structure. This model shows that the core comprises an aggregate of 12 association domains (residues 315–478) and that the 12 "foot" regions extending from the core are the functional domains (residues 1–314). The ATP- and calmodulin-binding sites are near the middle of the foot (as indicated by the shaded region on one foot in (B)). (C) is reproduced from Kolodziej et al. (2).

proteins typically binds both calcium and phospholipids, and calcium regulation of protein-membrane interactions is typical of this group (see Figure 2). Specific examples of C2 domain-containing proteins include the PKCs, the synaptic vesicle-associated protein synaptotagmin, and various phospholipases.

A. CaMKII

Calmodulin-Sensitive Enzymes

Calmodulin, in the absence of calcium (apo-calmodulin), has a dumbbell-shaped structure with four E-F hand calcium-binding domains (see Figure 2). On binding of calcium, which is a cooperative interaction, CaM undergoes an extensive conformational change in which the "handle" part of the dumbbell twists itself around a target molecule alpha helix (see Figure 2). This calcium-dependent interaction leads to a conformational change in the target, and typically triggers enzyme activation.

One of the most widely studied and important targets of CaM are the calcium/calmodulin-dependent protein kinases (the CaMK's). There are two CaMK isoforms of particular significance in neurons: CaMKII and CaMKIV. CaMKIV is most likely involved in regulating neuronal gene expression, and we will return to this molecule in the next chapter. CaMKII has achieved special notoriety for its importance in the induction, maintenance, and expression of LTP, as we will discuss in the next section (6).

The Ca^{2+}/calmodulin-dependent protein kinase II (CaMKII) is enriched in the brain and exhibits multi-functional roles in calcium-mediated signal transduction processes. CaMKII is composed of homologous alpha and beta subunits with a size of 52 and 60 kDa, respectively. The CaMKII holoenzyme, i.e., the functional structure, is a dodecamer (12 subunits) and is a mixture of both alpha and beta subunits. The individual subunit structure and the structure of the holoenzyme are shown in Figure 3. Each subunit comprises three domains: an interaction domain that allows formation of the holoenzyme complex; a regulatory domain that binds calmodulin and regulates the enzyme's activity; and a catalytic domain that executes the phosphotransfer reaction from Mg^{++}/ATP to the substrate protein.

The activity of CaMKII is highly sensitive to calcium influx, and the calcium-dependency of activation has an absolute requirement for calmodulin. In the simplest mode of regulation of CaMKII activity, calcium binds to calmodulin, the complex activates CaMKII, and enzymatic activity returns to baseline after calcium

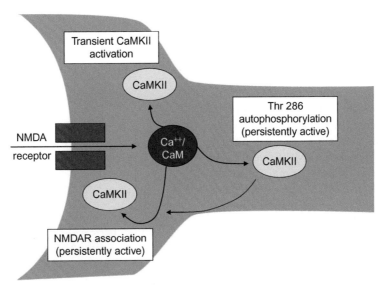

FIGURE 4 Three different effects of Ca/CaM onAMKII. Calcium and calmodulin can produce CaMKII activation by various mechanisms, with the duration of the activation differing among the mechanisms. CaMKII can be transiently activated by direct binding of Ca/CaM—the activation terminates when calcium levels return to baseline. CaMKII can also be translocated to the NMDA receptor, independent of autophosphorylation, which leads to a calcium-independent activation lasting seconds to minutes. CaMKII, which undergoes autophosphorylation at Thr 286, can be rendered active independent of Ca/CaM, which is a mechanism for persistent activation. This persistently-activated, autophosphosphorylated CaMKII can also associate with the NMDA receptor. See text for additional discussion.

levels diminish (see Figure 4). This obviously can be relevant to LTP induction, but is not a mechanism for generating a persistently activated enzyme that can serve as an LTP maintenance molecule.

However, the activity of the enzyme and its sensitivity to successive increases in calcium concentrations are altered following CaMKII autophosphorylation. Autophosphorylation, the act of a kinase phosphorylating itself, occurs in CaMKII in response to calcium/calmodulin stimulation. Changes in the phosphorylation state of the alpha or beta subunits of CaMKII alter the kinetic properties of the holoenzyme—the enzyme becomes active independent of any need for calcium/calmodulin. Thus, autophosphorylation of CaMKII can generate a persistently active (or autonomously active) enzyme—a persisting biochemical signal in response to a transient intitiating event.

The principal autophosphorylation site, which renders the enzyme autonomously active, is Thr 286 in CaMKII alpha (and the homologous Thr 287 site in the beta subunit). Autophosphorylation at this site occurs via an intraholoenzyme but intersubunit reaction. In other words, individual CaMKII subunits phosphorylate their neighbors, but not themselves. Thus, CaMKII autophosphorylation is self-delimited to a single 12-subunit holoenzyme. Activation of CaMKII by Ca^{2+}/Calmodulin causes the alpha and beta subunits to undergo autophosphorylation at Thr 286/287, rendering the enzyme autonomously active and partially

insensitive to further increases in Ca^{2+}/CaM concentrations. An additional consequence of autophosphorylation is that activated CaMKII associates with NMDA receptors (7–8), a process that can also lead to persistent activation of the enzyme (see Figure 4). Thus, autophosphorylation at the Thr 286 site leads to a persistently activated CaMKII enzyme, localized post-synaptically at its site of activation—an ideal molecular memory trace.

How is it that the autophosphorylation of CaMKII is maintained in the face of protein phosphatases that can reverse the autophosphorylation? Current models (9) capitalize on data indicating that protein phosphatase activity is low in the PSD, where the autophosphorylated CaMKII is located. Thus, all that needs to occur is that the rate of intersubunit autophosphorylation is greater than the net rate of CaMKII dephosphorylation in order for the phosphorylation to persist for the life of the enzyme. Thus, the capacity for intersubunit transphosphorylation synergizes with a low level of phosphatase activity to give a persisting signal in the cell.

In the mid-1980s there was much excitement about the idea that autophosphorylated CaMKII might serve as a self-perpetuating signal that could subserve permanent memory storage. However, a variety of experimental results generated since then suggests that perpetual activation of CaMKII does not occur with LTP-inducing stimulation or memory formation.

BOX 1

CAMKII AS A TEMPORAL INTEGRATOR

It is interesting to note that while CaMKII can serve as an information storage molecule in E-LTP maintenance, a role for this mechanism is not limited to longer-term information storage. CaMKII can, by similar mechanisms, serve to allow temporal integration between spaced periods of NMDA receptor activation. That CaMKII can by itself serve as a temporal integrator was elegantly demonstrated in a series of studies by DeKoninck and Schulman (16). When CaMKII sees repeated, spaced pulses of calcium and calmodulin it integrates these signals and gives a read-out of calcium spike frequency in terms of autonomous CaMKII activity (see Figure). Thus, increasing frequencies and levels of calcium give increased autonomous CaMKII activity. In this amazing example all that is needed for temporal integration is a single molecular complex sensing the ambient level of free calcium. This is likely a means by which multiple, spaced tetanic stimuli are able to selectively produce unique long-lasting effects on CaMKII activity post-synaptically.

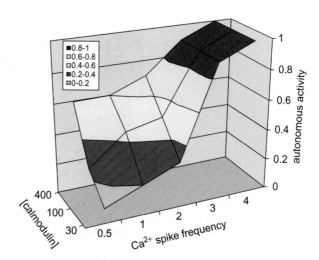

BOX 1 Temporal integration of a calcium signal by CAMKII as a function of availability of calmodulin. Graphical representation of autonomous CaMKII activity, illustrating the dependence on the frequency of calcium concentration spikes and the concentration of calmodulin. Adapted from data in De Koninck and Schulman, (16). Reproduced with permission from Dineley et al. (74).

Direct assays for autonomously activated CaMKII indicate that the autophosphorylated enzyme only persists for 1–2 hours. Thus, CaMKII autophosphorylation does not appear to be a mechanism for permanent memory storage.

The necessity of CaMKII autophosphorylation for LTP is reasonably well-established. The induction of NMDA receptor-dependent LTP requires CaMKII activation in the post-synaptic neuron (10–11), and mice deficient for alpha CaMKII show deficits in hippocampal LTP (12–14). The sites of CaMKII autophosphorylation are also important in LTP induction. Mutations of the Thr 286 site to prevent autophosphorylation, or conversely to produce a calcium-independent form of CaMKII result in LTP deficits for some types of LTP-inducing stimulation (15). Persistently activated CaMKII, and indeed increased CaMKII autophosphorylation at Thr 286, have been demonstrated in LTP (15).

Moreover, activation of NMDA receptors results in translocation of CaMKII from the cytosol to the post-synaptic density regions, and LTP-inducing stimulation triggers a transient translocation of CaMKII from the cytosol to the PSD that is largely dependent on the autophosphorylation state of the CaMKII at Thr 286. Finally, injection or transfection of autonomously active CaMKII into neurons likewise leads to enhancement of synaptic strength and an occlusion of LTP induced by tetanic stimulation, further data consistent with a role of autonomously active CaMKII in E-LTP maintenance.

Inhibitory Autophosphorylation of CaMKII

Further *in vitro* experiments indicate that autophosphorylation of CaMKII at additional sites can also occur. Specifically, autophosphorylation of Thr 305/306 sites on alpha and beta CaMKII occurs following Thr 286 autophosphorylation under circumstances of prolonged or robust stimulation. This can inhibit both the calcium/CaM-independent activity, and the calcium/CaM-dependent activity. Thr 305/306 autophosphorylation also leads to dissociation of the enzyme from the PSD. We will return to a possible role for this event in a human mental retardation syndrome, Angelman Syndrome, in a later chapter.

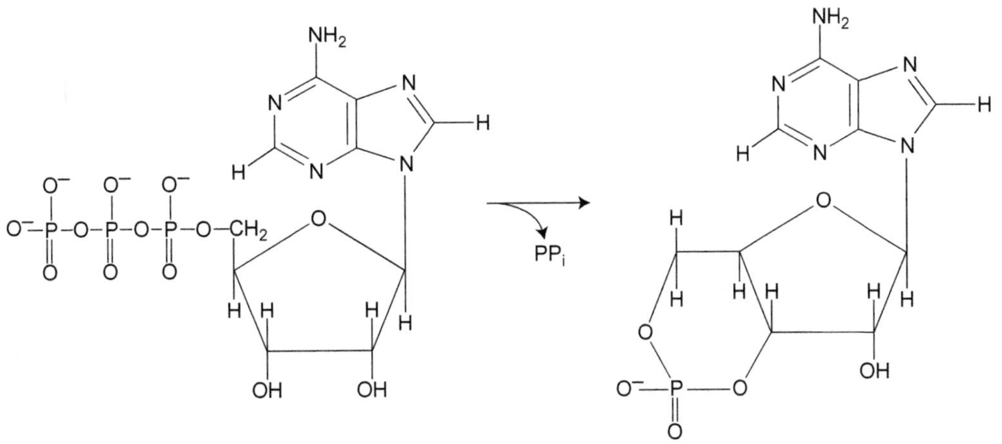

FIGURE 5 Catalysis of cAMP by adenylyl cyclases. Adenylyl cyclases catalyze the conversion of adenosine triphosphate (ATP) on the left, to cyclic adenosine monophosphate (cAMP) on the right. Adenylyl cyclases catalyze this conversion by attacking the 3′ hydroxyl group on the ribose of the nucleoside triphosphate, ATP. Figure and legend from D. Storm and K. L. Eckel-Mahan, *Learning and Memory: A Comprehensive Reference*, Volume 4: Molecular Mechanisms of Memory. Copyright Elsevier 2008.

B. Two Additional Targets of CaM—Adenylyl Cyclase and Nitric Oxide Synthase

Adenylyl cyclase (AC), the enzyme that converts ATP to the second messenger cAMP (see Figure 5), is also a target of CaM in neurons. The CaM-sensitive AC isoforms are AC1 and AC8, and simultaneous knockout of these two genes gives a pronounced LTP and memory deficit (see Figure 6, reviewed in reference 17). Calcium/calmodulin stimulation of AC likely contributes to regulating the responsiveness of the post-synaptic cell to intracellular calcium, and this is likely a mechanism of attenuation of LTP in the AC knockout mice. However, there is no evidence that there is any persisting activation of AC that contributes to LTP maintenance (18), so AC likely serves only in the induction phase of LTP.

Nitric oxide synthase (NOS) is also CaM-sensitive. When NOS is activated by CaM it converts arginine to citrulline plus the free radical species NO (nitric oxide). It is clear that generation of NO through NOS activation modulates LTP induction, but the precise mechanisms by which this happens are still being investigated (19). As we discussed in the last chapter, NMDA receptors are modulated by NO, and NO-sensitive guanylyl cyclase has also been implicated as a target of NO in LTP induction (20–22). The ras/ERK cascade is also a potential target of NO. These are all relevant mechanisms for NO in modulating LTP induction, but as with AC it seems unlikely that there is any role for ongoing NOS activation in E-LTP maintenance.

One of the most interesting potential roles for NO derives from its capacity to cross cell membranes directly. Thus, NO, like other membrane-permeant species, could be a "retrograde messenger" that carries a signal from the post-synaptic compartment to the pre-synaptic compartment (23). One specific retrograde messenger role that has been proposed for NO is activation of pre-synaptic guanylyl cyclase and the cyclic GMP-dependent protein kinase (PKG) (24). This proposed role is also limited to LTP induction, and has not been proposed to serve an LTP maintenance function. However, pre-synaptic NO and NO-derived reactive species might also be particularly important in generating persisting signals pre-synaptically. The possible role of oxidatively modified PKC in E-LTP maintenance is discussed in Box 2.

In summary, then, both AC and NOS are additional targets of CaM in E-LTP induction. They serve as important triggering mechanisms, involved in the induction of persisting signals. They are not, however, persistently activated, and do not directly participate in LTP maintenance.

C. Another Major Target of Calcium—PKC

The calcium/phospholipid-dependent protein kinases (PKCs) are pluripotent regulators of synaptic transmission and neuronal function. PKC has not been as extensively studied as its cousin CaMKII in the context of LTP; nevertheless, there is a fairly broad literature implicating PKC as a molecule contributing to the maintenance of E-LTP. PKC inhibitors can block the expression of E-LTP (25–28), PKC is persistently activated in E-LTP (29–36), and activation of PKC or injection of the enzyme into the post-synaptic cell elicits synaptic potentiation (37–40). Thus, the molecule

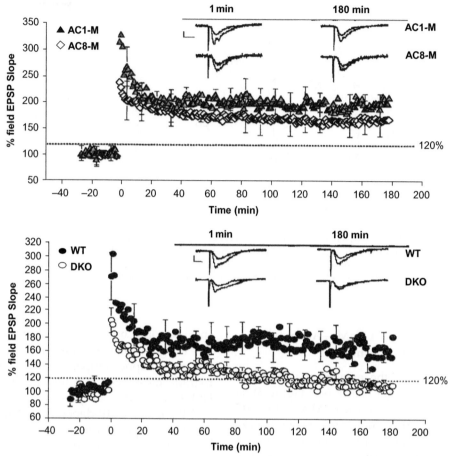

FIGURE 6   LTP in adenylyl cyclase-deficient mice. "DKO" mice lacking both the AC1 and AC8 calmodulin-sensitive isoforms of adenylyl cyclase have a defect in LTP. Upper panel: LTP was induced in AC1 mutant (AC1-M, shaded triangles; n >9 mice, 17 slices) and AC8 mutant mice (AC8-M, open diamonds; n >13 mice, 25 slices) slices by four tetanic trains of 100Hz (200ms, 6s apart) stimulus. There was no statistically significant difference between the mean fEPSP of AC1-M and AC8-M mutant mice 180 minutes after tetanization (p = 0.28). Representative fEPSP traces taken from area CA1 in AC1-M and AC8-M slices at 1 minute and 180 minutes after tetani are shown in the insets. Each trace is superimposed over a baseline trace taken 2 minutes before tetani for ease of comparison. Scale bar, 1mV, 10ms. Lower panel: LTP was diminished in DKO mice. Wildtype mice (closed circles; n = 13 mice, 26 slices) preparations gave an L-LTP lasting up to 180 minutes, whereas potentiation in the DKO (open circles; n = 8 mice, 19 slices) preparations declined to near baseline values within 80 minutes. Representative fEPSP traces taken from area CA1 in wildtype and DKO brain slices at 1 minute and 180 minutes after tetani are shown in insets. The dashed lines (C and D) represent an arbitrary cutoff (120%), below which potentiation was considered to be near baseline. Scale bar, 1mV, 10ms. Figure and legend reproduced from Wong et al. (3).

BOX 2

OXIDATION OF PKC

Eric Klann and his colleagues have discovered a quite novel route for persistent PKC activation in LTP, and indeed a novel signal transduction mechanism in its own right. In oxidative activation of PKC (and other proteins regulated by oxidation) a reactive oxygen species directly reacts chemically with its target. Thus, instead of binding reversibly to an allosteric site, in this case the second messenger causes a direct and persistent modification of an amino acid side-chain of its effector enzyme. This reaction is probably not readily reversible—thus the modification has a built-in persistence, lasting until the PKC molecule is broken down completely.

In the case of oxidative PKC activation in LTP the reactive species is a superoxide or a superoxide-derived reactive oxygen species such as peroxynitrite or hydrogen peroxide (see Figure and reference 44). PKC is

BOX 2—cont'd

OXIDATION OF PKC

activated by reactive oxygen species in a complex manner. Hydrogen peroxide and superoxide increase both autonomous (i.e., calcium-independent) and calcium/phospholipid-dependent PKC activity. The α, βII, ε, and ζ isoforms of PKC are autonomously activated by reactive oxygen species through thiol side-chain oxidation and release of zinc from the cysteine-rich "zinc finger" regions of PKC (see Figure). In a biochemical *tour de force* Lauren Knapp and Eric Klann showed that the generation of this persistently activated form of PKC occurs concomitantly with induction of NMDA receptor-dependent E-LTP (45).

Several lines of evidence show that the source of the reactive oxygen species in LTP is secondary to NMDA receptor activation (44). For example, NMDA receptor activation in area CA1 of hippocampal slices results in superoxide free radical production, providing a source of reactive oxygen species. This finding is nicely complemented by the observation that superoxide scavengers inhibit E-LTP induction in area CA1. Finally, NMDA receptor blockade blocks the generation of the persistently activated oxidized form of PKC in E-LTP. However, the precise source of the superoxide-derived

messenger is not known at this time, and this is an area of active investigation. Possibilities include NOS (which can produce superoxide as well as nitric oxide), NADPH oxidases, mitochondrial electron transport, and lipid peroxidases.

One additional interesting aspect of this model is that superoxide and other reactive oxygen species, such as NO, can cross cell membranes by mechanisms that are still under investigation. Thus, oxidative activation of PKC may not be limited to the post-synaptic compartment. This mechanism presents an intriguing possibility for a retrograde signaling mechanism in E-LTP, especially given that pre-synaptic PKC activation apparently is sufficient to give increased neurotransmitter release.

Finally, I should note that not just PKC but several protein kinases and phosphatases are regulated by reactive oxygen species, as are a variety of transcription factors. Typically, protein kinases are activated by reactive oxygen species, whereas protein phosphatases are inhibited, potentially enabling a concerted modulation of protein phosphorylation levels within the cell. Persistent phosphatase inhibition in E-LTP is also a potential mechanism contributing to E-LTP maintenance (see 6, reviewed in 44).

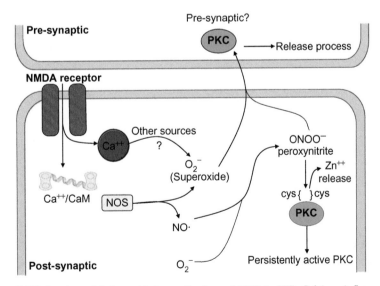

BOX 2 A model for oxidative activation of PKC in LTP. Calcium influx through the NMDA receptor triggers production of reactive oxygen species (NO, superoxide, and peroxynitrite), which directly act on cysteine side-chains in PKC. This oxidation results in Zn release and autonomously active PKC. Reactive oxygen species can also cross the synapse as retrograde messengers to activate PKC pre-synaptically.

meets the three principal criteria establishing it as a candidate E-LTP maintenance molecule.

In mammals, the PKC enzyme family is quite heterogeneous and comprises 11 known isozymes that have been divided into three major subsets: conventional (α, βI, βII, and γ); novel (δ, ε, η, θ and μ); and atypical (λ and ζ) (see Figure 7). Each isoform is encoded by a separate gene with the exception of the βI and βII isoforms, which are splice variants from a single gene. Each subfamily of PKC isoforms is subject to distinct control mechanisms. The conventional isoforms are regulated by calcium in concert with diacylglycerol and membrane phospholipid (see Box 3). The novel and atypical classes are structurally homologous, but can be regulated independent of calcium. Brain subregion-specific and neuronal subtype-specific expression is the rule rather than the exception for the various isoforms. Almost all the various subtypes are expressed to varying degrees in the hippocampus.

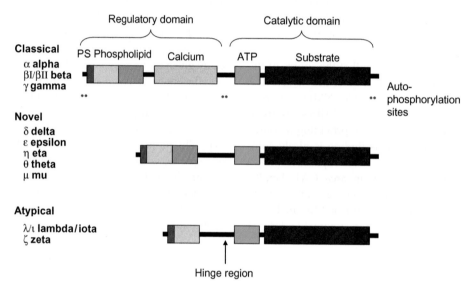

FIGURE 7   Domain structures of isoforms of PKC. The regulatory and catalytic domains of various PKC isoforms are illustrated, illustrating regions of structural conservation. Autophosphorylation sites in the classical isoforms are indicated by red dots. Figure courtesy of Coleen Atkins.

BOX 3

ANOTHER POTENTIAL TARGET OF CALCIUM—PHOSPOHOLIPASES

There are a number of calcium-activated phospholipases in neurons that are potential targets of the LTP-inducing calcium signal. These include phospholipases C, D, and A2, which cleave off various parts of membrane phospholipids (see Figure). Phospholipase C (PLC) is important in the context of PKC activation in LTP induction, because PKCs are sensitive to the PLC product diacylglycerol (DAG).

Phospholipases also are noteworthy in this context because they can generate membrane-permeant compounds such as arachidonic acid (AA) and DAG, which if persistently produced could serve as retrograde signaling compounds in order to trigger changes in the presynaptic compartment.

One specific mechanism that has been proposed in this context is the persistent generation of AA by post-synaptic

BOX 3—cont'd

ANOTHER POTENTIAL TARGET OF CALCIUM—PHOSPOHOLIPASES

BOX 3 Sites of cleavage of membrane phospholipids by phospholipases. The left-hand panel illustrates bonds that are hydrolyzed by phospholipases A1, A2, C, and D. Note that each cleavage is a hydrolysis reaction, leaving free hydroxyl (OH) groups at the cleavage site for each of the two products. PLA1 and PLA2 liberate a free fatty acid (FA, see lower right panel) and a lyso-phospholipid. PLC liberates diacyl-glycerol (DAG) and a phosphorylated head group (see upper right panel). PLD liberates phosphatidic acid (PA) and the free, hydroxylated head group.

PLA2 (49–50). Tim Bliss's group has published evidence that there is a persisting increase in AA after LTP-inducing stimulation *in vivo*, and proposed that this might serve as a persisting potentiating signal in E-LTP. Potential targets of AA are numerous. For example, AA can activate PKC and this could serve as a presynaptic facilitation mechanism. However, AA can also be converted to a wide variety of active metabolic products by the cyclo-oxygenase pathway (which produces prostaglandins and associated compounds) and the lipoxygenase pathway (which produces active "HPETE" metabolites). Any of a number of these compounds could serve as potentiating signals by binding to cell surface receptors pre- or post-synaptically. I should note, however, that at present this mechanism remains more in the category of interesting possibility versus established mechanism.

Good evidence exists that a wide variety of PKC isoforms are activated in response to LTP-inducing stimulation (34). The first isoform-specific investigation of a role for PKC in LTP involved characterization of a knockout of the brain-specific, gamma isoform of PKC (41). In fact, this was one of the very first knockout animal studies ever published. In these studies modest effects on hippocampus-dependent memory were observed due to the loss of PKCγ. In addition, the PKCγ knockout animal has a very pronounced but idiosyncratic LTP deficit. Tetanus-induced LTP in area CA1 is completely lost in gamma knockout

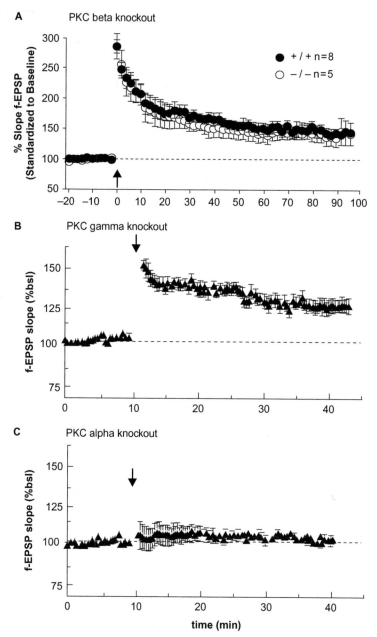

FIGURE 8 Hippocampal LTP in PKC isoform-specific knockout mice. Hippocampal slices obtained from PKC beta (upper), gamma (middle), or alpha (lower)-deficient mice or wildtype mice (+/+ in upper panel) were given an LTP-inducing stimulus (arrows) delivered after stable baseline responses were recorded for 20 minutes. Each set of tetani consisted of a single train of 100 Hz stimulation for 1 second, while maintaining slices at 25°C. Reproduced with permission from Weeber et al. (42) and unpublished data.

animals (see Figure 8). However, LTP can be recovered in PKCγ-deficient mice by delivery of an LTD-inducing stimulus prior to LTP-inducing tetanic stimulation (41). These data suggest that the role of PKCγ is limited to the induction of LTP, and that the gamma isoform of PKC is not necessary for LTP maintenance. Overall, these studies suggest the hypothesis that while PKCγ is involved in regulating LTP induction, other isoforms of PKC are involved in LTP maintenance. Studies of the

PKCβ knockout mouse gave a set of results that were in some ways the mirror image of the PKCγ knockout (42–43). Deletion of the PKCβ gene resulted in pronounced memory defects: strong attenuation of cued and contextual fear conditioning. However, the beta knockout animal had no discernible LTP phenotype in area CA1 of hippocampus (see Figure 8). Based on these studies it seems clear that the beta isoforms of PKC are not necessary for tetanus-induced, NMDA receptor-dependent

LTP induction or early maintenance in area CA1 of hippocampus.

Calpain and PKMζ

PKC was originally discovered not as second messenger-regulated enzyme, but rather as a kinase activated secondary to proteolytic cleavage. Various proteases like trypsin and the calcium-activated protease calpain can clip PKC in its central "hinge" region (see Figure 7), releasing the N-terminal inhibitory domain and liberating the free, active C-terminal catalytic domain. This active fragment of PKC is referred to as "PKM."

Of course, this mechanism of proteolytic activation of PKC has great appeal as a potential mechanism for generating a long-lasting signal in LTP. Making a long story short, it turns out that this acute proteolysis of PKC is not a dominant mechanism in NMDA receptor-dependent LTP in area CA1, although it does appear to be involved in NMDA receptor-independent LTP in this same region (34, 36). An additional mechanism for persistent activation of PKC is discussed in Box 2. However, there is a role for a constitutively active PKM as a persisting signal in E-LTP; it is just that the mechanism of its generation is not proteolysis. Todd Sacktor's research group has spent many years tracking down the basis for generation of this persistent signal in LTP, and I will briefly summarize their findings (4, 5).

Sacktor's group has shown that a constitutively active PKC isoform, the *PKM zeta* (PKMζ) isoform, is synthesized *de novo* after LTP induction (see Figure 1 and reference 46). PKMζ is a second messenger-independent, constitutively active fragment of PKCζ which lacks the regulatory domain. This fragment is synthesized from a unique mRNA that codes for the truncated form of the enzyme (see Figure 9). An LTP-associated increase in the amount of PKMζ protein lasts at least two hours after LTP-inducing tetanus, an effect which is NMDA receptor-dependent (34, 46). Also, inhibitors of PKMζ applied after LTP-inducing stimulation reverse the expression of LTP (see Figure 10 and reference 47). Interestingly, a decrease of PKMζ is seen after LTD induction in area CA1, which suggests that bidirectional regulation of PKMζ may contribute to potentiation and depression of synaptic transmission in area CA1 (48).

Thus, increased synthesis of a constitutively active PKC fragment represents a major category of persisting signal in LTP. It is interesting that the seemingly more straightforward mechanism of direct proteolysis of pre-existing PKCζ is not used. Rather, the formation of PKMζ in LTP is protein synthesis-dependent, a mechanism for generating an autonomously active kinase

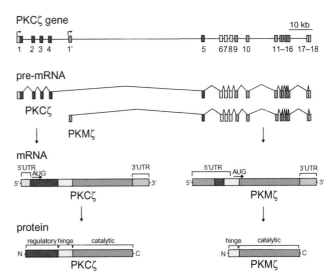

FIGURE 9 PKMζ mRNA formation from an internal promoter within the PKCζ gene. (Top) The intron-exon structure of the human PKCζ gene shows two exon clusters separated by a large intron: exons 1–4, encoding the PKCζ 5'UTR (light blue) and regulatory domain (red), and exons 5–18, encoding the remaining regulatory domain, hinge (yellow), catalytic domain (green), and 3'UTR (gray). The unique 5' PKMζ mRNA sequence is in a single exon (exon 1', dark blue) within the large intron. PKCζ mRNA transcription begins at exon 1, resulting in full length PKCζ (bottom left). Transcription from exon 1' and splicing to exon 5 generates PKMζ mRNA, translation of which begins in the hinge to generate PKMζ (bottom right). From Hernandez, Al., Blace, N., Cary, J. F., et al. (2003). "Protein kinase Mζ synthesis from a brain mRNA encoding an independent protein kinase Cζ catalytic domain. Implications for the molecular mechanism of memory." *J. Biol. Chem.* 278:40305–40316. Figure courtesy of Todd Sacktor, adapted from *Learning and Memory: A Comprehensive Reference*, Volume 4: Molecular Mechanics of Memory. Copyright Elsevier 2008.

distinct from other post-translational mechanisms we have discussed (e.g., CaMKII autophosphorylation).

D. Section Summary—Mechanisms for Generating Persisting Signals in Long-Term Potentiation and Memory

As was emphasized at the beginning of the chapter, the capacity to generate a persisting signal in response to a transient stimulus is the biochemical *sine qua non* of memory formation. In this section we have seen several examples of these types of processes that have been proposed to be involved in the maintenance of early stages of LTP (see Table 1). These are the best-characterized solutions to the problem of making a lasting signal in E-LTP, and these reactions serve as general prototypes for solutions to the problem of neuronal activity-dependent generation of molecular memory traces.

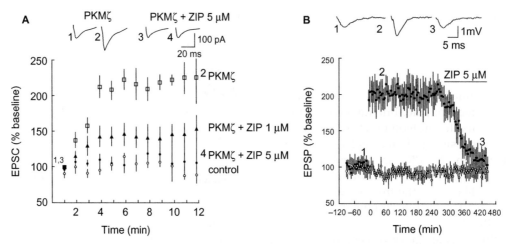

FIGURE 10 PKMζ is necessary and sufficient for LTP maintenance. (A) Whole-cell perfusion of PKMζ into a CA1 pyramidal cell potentiates AMPAR-mediated synaptic transmission. A total of $1\,\mu mol\,l^{-1}$ ZIP applied to the bath partially blocks and $5\,\mu mol\,l^{-1}$ ZIP fully blocks the PKMζ-mediated potentiation of AMPAR responses. (B) A total of $5\,\mu mol\,l^{-1}$ ZIP applied to the bath five hours after tetanization reverses LTP maintenance, but does not affect synaptic transmission of a control pathway simultaneously recorded within the hippocampal slice. EPSC, excitatory post-synaptic current; EPSP, excitatory post-synaptic potential. From Serrano, P., Yao, Y., and Sacktor, T. C. (2005). "Persistent phosphorylation by protein kinase Mζ maintains late-phase long-term potentiation." *J. Neurosci.* 25:1979–1984. Figure courtesy of Todd Sacktor, adapted from *Learning and Memory: A Comprehensive Reference*, Volume 4: Molecular Mechanics of Memory. Copyright Elsevier 2008.

TABLE 1   Proposed Mechanisms for Generating Persisting Signals in E-LTP

Molecule	Mechanism	Role
CaMKII	Self-perpetuating autophosphorylation coupled with low phosphatase activity	Effector phosphorylation, structural changes
Various PKCs	Direct, irreversible covalent modification by reactive oxygen species	Effector phosphorylation
PKMζ	*De novo* synthesis of a constitutively active kinase	Effector phosphorylation

It is a useful exercise to perform a compare-and-contrast concerning these three documented mechanisms for molecular information storage (see Table 1). In the case of CaMKII, current models propose that Ca/CaM stimulation of the enzyme results in self-perpetuating intersubunit autophosphorylation which, coupled with low phosphatase activity, leads to a persisting level of active enzyme in the PSD. The read-out of this persisting signal potentially includes structural changes in the PSD and increased phosphorylation of target effectors. A second example is that various PKCs can undergo direct, irreversible covalent modification by reactive oxygen species. Oxidation of zinc finger domains in

the enzyme leads to essentially irreversible activation of the enzyme, which is then free to phosphorylate target effectors. Finally, in the case of PKMζ, *de novo* synthesis of a constitutively active kinase lacking the normal autoinhibitory domain leads to the presence of a persistently activated kinase in the cell. Overall, these are three unique and elegant biochemical solutions to the problem of making a lasting signal in response to a transient signal. In the next section we will discuss the targets of these persisting signals that lead to enhanced synaptic transmission—the translation of the persisting signal into persisting effects at the synapse.

II. TARGETS OF THE PERSISTING SIGNALS

How is it that a persistently activated kinase or other persisting biochemical signal is converted to an enhancement of the coupling between two neurons? This is the essential question concerning the mechanism of expression of synaptic potentiation. Maintenance can be served by an autonomously active kinase, for example, but that persisting signal must be converted to some functional consequence at the synapse in order for synaptic potentiation to occur.

This is the issue we will focus on in this section. In considering the possible mechanisms for enhanced neuronal coupling, it is useful to think about the basics of synaptic transmission and post-synaptic responsiveness. There are three basic components of synaptic transmission: release of neurotransmitter; post-synaptic depolarization due to activation of ligand-gated ion channels; and the biophysical response of the post-synaptic membrane to that depolarization. Thus, potential sites for the expression of LTP and other forms of potentiation include:

1. The machinery of the pre-synaptic terminal involved in pre-synaptic calcium influx and the neurotransmitter release process;
2. Post-synaptic glutamate receptors plus their associated proteins, specifically receptors of the AMPA subtype involved in glutamatergic responses; and
3. Potassium and sodium channels that shape the post-synaptic response to glutamatergic receptor-mediated depolarization.

I will discuss each of these three categories of effectors separately as a means of organizing the following discussion, but it is important to remember that they do not operate in isolation, nor are the mechanisms mutually exclusive. In fact, evidence exists that each of these three mechanisms participates in E-LTP expression, as we discussed in the chapter on LTP physiology. However, there is a much greater abundance and variety of results implicating glutamate receptor regulation in LTP, and much more is known about the mechanisms relevant to this category than the other two categories. Thus we will direct more attention to this effector system than to the other two.

A. AMPA Receptors in E-LTP

The E-LTP-associated increase in synaptic strength, i.e., the increase in the EPSP, clearly results in part from increased levels of post-synaptic glutamate receptor activation (reviewed in reference 51). One set of mechanisms contributing to this phenomenon is fairly well-understood: enhancement of AMPA receptor function. As both PKC and CaMKII are persistently activated in E-LTP and can affect AMPA receptor function, a parsimonious explanation for the increased synaptic response post-synaptically in LTP is increased phosphorylation of AMPA receptors and their associated proteins by these kinases.

Three specific mechanisms for augmenting AMPA receptor function, mediated by CaMKII or PKC, have been implicated as playing a part in E-LTP (see Table 2). One mechanism is that the level of AMPA receptor phosphorylation is increased during E-LTP, phosphorylation at a site that can be phosphorylated by either CaMKII or PKC. Increased phosphorylation at this site results in increased receptor current (52–54). A second

TABLE 2   Proposed Mechanisms for Augmenting AMPA Receptor Function in E-LTP

Mechanism	Likely molecular basis
Increased single-channel conductance	Direct phosphorylation of AMPA receptor alpha subunits by CaMKII or PKC
Increased steady-state levels of AMPAR	CaMKII (+ PKC?) phosphorylation of AMPAR-associated trafficking and scaffolding proteins
Insertion of AMPAR into silent synapses	CaMKII phosphorylation of GluR1-associated trafficking proteins

proposed mechanism is that the steady-state level of membrane AMPA receptor protein is increased in a dynamic fashion by CaMKII through regulation of AMPA receptor trafficking and stabilization (9, 55). Finally, AMPA receptors can be inserted into previously "silent" synapses, increasing the strength of connections between two neurons in an essentially all-or-none fashion (reviewed in reference 56), and this mechanism has been proposed as contributing to E-LTP. In the next section I will briefly review some of the mechanisms underlying these three processes.

B. Direct Phosphorylation of the AMPA Receptor

AMPA (α-amino-3-hydroxy-5-methylisoxazole-4-propionic acid) receptors mediate the majority of fast synaptic transmission throughout the nervous system, including at Schaffer collateral synapses in area CA1. There are four homologous alpha subunits (GluR1–GluR4) that combine in a mix-and-match fashion into a multiunit complex (likely tetrameric) which forms a functional AMPA receptor. The GluR1 alpha subunit can be phosphorylated at Ser831 by CaMKII or PKC *in vitro* and *in vivo*. Phosphorylation of GluR1 at this site increases the receptor's ionic conductance, providing a direct route for CaMKII or PKC to enhance synaptic efficacy during LTP (57). In fact, phosphorylation of GluR1 at this site is known to be increased in LTP and memory (54). In addition, LTP induction is associated with increased conductance of AMPA receptors (53), which is consistent with increased phosphorylation at the Ser831 site. Thus, phosphorylation of GluR1 at Ser831 has been shown to occur in LTP and memory, and this mechanism is sufficient to enhance synaptic transmission. Although most models for E-LTP posit the phosphorylation of Ser831 to be mediated by CaMKII, of course persistently active PKC could also perform this role. An interesting variation on this idea is that CaMKII and PKC might be functionally redundant in E-LTP, each phosphorylating

AMPA receptors and serving as a fail-safe mechanism for maintaining synaptic potentiation.

The AMPA receptor is also a substrate for PKA, and PKA phosphorylation likewise increases AMPA channel activity. In a fascinating series of studies regulation of AMPA receptors by PKA was found to predominantly be involved in de-depression of synaptic strength in area CA1 (58). These studies showed that potentiation and depotentiation revolved around the CaMKII/PKC phosphorylation site, while LTD and de-depression revolved around the PKA site. This important study separated mechanisms for synaptic potentiation from mechanisms for synaptic de-depression by demonstrating that one process is not simply the reversal of the other.

C. Regulation of Steady-State Levels of AMPA Receptors

Active CaMKII can also lead to an increase in the level of post-synaptic AMPA receptor density in hippocampal pyramidal neurons in culture. A wide variety of sophisticated studies have shown that transfection of active CaMKII into pyramidal neurons leads to increased trafficking of AMPA receptors into the dendritic spine and into active synapses (56). Thus, one target for CaMKII in E-LTP and memory is regulation of steady-state levels of AMPA receptors post-synaptically.

The mechanism for this increased trafficking and membrane insertion is under active investigation, and is summarized in Figure 11. The initial insertion of

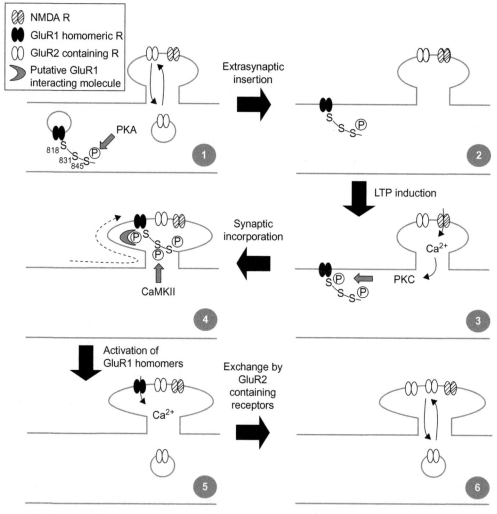

FIGURE 11   A model of AMPA receptor regulation during LTP. PKA phosphorylation of GluR1-S845 primes AMPA receptors for LTP by trafficking the receptors to extrasynaptic sites. Activation of NMDA receptors by LTP-inducing stimuli causes calcium influx and results in phosphorylation of GluR1-S818, which is likely mediated by PKC. Phosphorylation of GluR1-S818 is thought to bind a putative GluR1 binding protein, which ultimately incorporates AMPA receptors to synapses. GluR1 homomeric receptors inserted into synapses then may be activated to allow calcium influx that exchanges them with GluR2-containing receptors. This process may resemble calcium-permeable AMPA receptor plasticity (CARP) observed in cerebellar granule cells. Phosphorylation of synaptic GluR1 homomeric receptors at S831 by constitutively active CaMKII at synapses may facilitate the exchange process by perhaps allowing a large influx of calcium. Figure and legend from Richard Huganir, *Learning and Memory: A Comprehensive Reference*, Volume 4: Molecular Mechanisms of Memory. Copyright Elsevier 2008.

new AMPA receptors is known to be independent of Ser831 phosphorylation, clearly rendering this mechanism as distinct and separable from the mechanism described above for increasing current flow through the AMPA channel (59). Current models posit that one component of E-LTP is activity-dependent delivery of GluR1/2-containing AMPA receptors into the spine and post-synaptic density, possibly mediated by Ser818 phosphorylation. This insertion of new receptors is a process distinct from a second constitutive pathway that delivers GluR2/3-containing receptors and maintains baseline synaptic transmission.

It is important to note that insertion of AMPA receptors into the post-synaptic membrane is not a mechanism for the maintenance of E-LTP. Post-synaptic membrane AMPA receptors turn over with a lifetime of about 15 minutes (60–61). Thus, regulation of AMPA receptor insertion is an active process maintained by some other persisting signal. As mentioned above, one relevant persisting signal is autophosphorylated, autonomously active CaMKII.

How is it that CaMKII increases steady-state levels of AMPA receptors? The mechanisms are currently under investigation and are complex, but Figure 12 summarizes one current model. In this model calcium influx through the NMDA receptor leads to activation of CaMKII and triggers membrane insertion of AMPA receptors. The calcium signal also causes CaMKII autophosphorylation, which as we discussed earlier leads to a self-perpetuating increase in autophosphorylated CaMKII. Autophosphorylated CaMKII binds with high affinity to the cytoplasmic domain of the NMDA receptor, and also to the actin-binding protein alpha-actinin. The actinin linkage couples the CaMKII/NMDA receptor complex to actin, and as we discussed in the last chapter actin filaments cross-link to AMPA receptors via a number of mechanisms, including by binding through the 4.1protein and SAP97. Thus, by this mechanism autophosphorylated CaMKII stabilizes AMPA receptors in the PSD, through linking them to the more stable NMDA receptor complex.

An additional component of the model is that the calcium signal acting through persistently activated PKC and src leads to increased insertion of NMDA receptors in the post-synaptic membrane (62). This second signal increases the number of NMDA receptor "anchors" in the PSD, and thus by this mechanism contributes to elevating the steady-state level of AMPA receptors post-synaptically. As was shown in Figure 11, one additional possible mechanism for perpetuating the increased AMPA receptor levels is a positive reinforcement loop whereby Ser831-phosphorylated receptors maintain the recruitment of new AMPA receptors to potentiated synapses.

Several components of the model are worth noting. First, minimally it does not require CaMKII phosphorylation of AMPA receptors, or indeed any other CaMKII substrate beside CaMKII itself—autophosphorylated CaMKII might serve a purely structural and not a catalytic role. Second, it involves a number of receptor-interacting proteins in the PSD that stabilize the presence of AMPA receptors. Third, it involves the cytoskeleton and thus could serve as a signaling system beyond simply regulating AMPA receptor function. Fourth, it involves the NMDA receptor as well as the AMPA receptor, with the NMDA receptor serving as a PSD-organizing molecule.

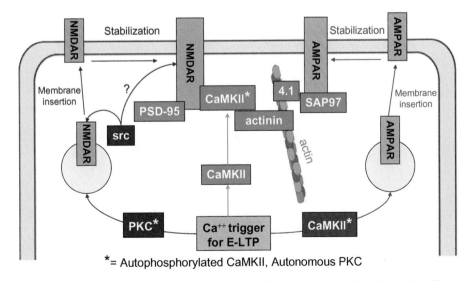

FIGURE 12   A model for glutamate receptor insertion and stabilization in E-LTP. See text for details. Adapted from Lisman and Zhabotinsky (9).

Finally, it involves parallel actions of PKC and CaMKII, as opposed to the two kinases converging on the same target phosphorylation site.

D. Silent Synapses

As we discussed in the earlier chapter on LTP physiology, *de novo* insertion of AMPA receptors is an additional potential mechanism for enhanced synaptic strength in LTP. "Silent" synapses containing NMDA receptors but not functional AMPA receptors occur with reasonable frequency in prenatal and neonatal brain. NMDA receptor-dependent triggering of AMPA receptor insertion into silent synapses occurs in an activity-dependent fashion in neurons, likely by mechanisms quite similar to those described above for elevating AMPA receptor levels in the PSD. Thus, activation of silent synapses through AMPA receptor insertion is clearly a potential mechanism for E-LTP, and "AMPA-fication" of synapses occurs under a number of experimental conditions (reviewed in reference 56).

However, the quantitative contribution of silent synapse activation in LTP in the adult hippocampus is unclear. At our present level of understanding, it appears that increasing AMPA receptor ionic conductance and regulating the steady-state levels of AMPA receptors at the synapse may be the predominant mechanisms for E-LTP at adult synapses, while activation of silent synapses may be more important in the context of developmental synaptic plasticity.

E. Pre-Synaptic Changes—Increased Release

LTP is typically measured as an increase in the initial slope of the EPSP (or EPSP magnitude), and this effect can be subserved by an increase in post-synaptic receptor number or efficacy as described above, or by an increase in pre-synaptic neurotransmitter release, or both of these mechanisms together. The locus of LTP expression (pre- versus post-synaptic) has been widely debated and is a source of continuing controversy, as was described in a previous chapter. The evidence for post-synaptic changes in LTP seems quite convincing at this point and not much argument about this aspect of LTP exists. However, there is much evidence indicative of a change in release pre-synaptically in E-LTP, and convincing biochemical evidence exists that pre-synaptic changes do indeed occur in LTP. One mechanism that could account for lasting changes in the pre-synaptic compartment is discussed in Box 2 and shown in Figure 13. In this model, calcium-induced generation of reactive oxygen species post-synaptically allows retrograde signaling to PKC pre-synaptically. Persistently activated PKC pre-synaptically phosphorylates GAP43 and other targets, leading to increased neurotransmitter release and synaptic potentiation.

F. Post-Synaptic Changes in Excitability?

As we have already discussed, LTP, as originally defined by Bliss and Lomo, is manifest as two physiologic components. The first component is an increase in synaptic strength, and the second component of LTP is referred to as EPSP-slope (E-S) potentiation. E-S potentiation is a general term used to refer to the post-synaptic cell having an increased probability of firing an action potential at a constant strength of synaptic input. E-S potentiation can be explained based on alterations in recurrent inhibitory connections in area CA1. The other possibility is that E-S potentiation is a manifestation of increased excitability in the post-synaptic neuron, but the molecular mechanisms that could account for this aspect of LTP are completely mysterious at present. In an extension of

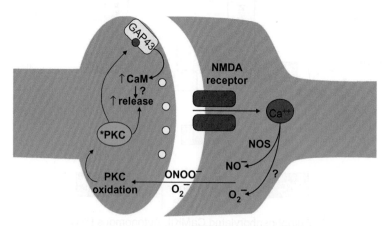

FIGURE 13 Retrograde signaling in E-LTP. Two potential pre-synaptic sites of PKC action are illustrated—direct effects on the release process and the calmodulin binding protein GAP43.

the variety of mechanisms that we have been talking about in the context of AMPA receptor regulation, one can hypothesize that persistently-activated CaMKII or PKC could regulate potassium or sodium channels in order to increase excitability. Investigations to test whether such phenomena occur are currently under way, although these experiments are quite difficult due to the need for recording directly from CA1 pyramidal neuron dendrites after LTP induction.

III. DENDRITIC PROTEIN SYNTHESIS

In this final section we will discuss a complex but critical additional mechanism for generating a persisting biochemical effect in neurons—alterations in protein synthesis. You will likely recall that some of the original experiments that demonstrated a necessity for memory consolidation arose from studies of the effects of inhibiting protein synthesis on memory formation. Thus, from the earliest era of molecular studies of memory there was an interest in proteins synthesis in memory.

There was a resurgence of interest in this area when Eric Kandel's laboratory published a seminal finding demonstrating that localized dendritic protein synthesis is involved in synapse-specific potentiation of synaptic transmission in *Aplysia* sensory neurons (63). This discovery, along with a variety of earlier findings, led to the formulation of the model that local dendritic protein synthesis could provide a solution to the vexing problem of synapse-specificity for protein synthesis-dependent long-term synaptic plasticity and memory.

The conundrum was that LTP and memory are dependent on protein synthesis, but dogma had it that protein synthesis happened exclusively in the rough ER in the cell body. The synapse specificity problem can be solved simply if there is activity-regulated protein synthesis limited to specific dendritic or synaptic regions, as had been suggested by earlier groundbreaking work that indicated the existence of *dendritically* localized protein synthesis machinery (polyribosomes).

Work from a wide variety of laboratories has supported the relevance of local protein synthesis to explaining synapse specificity of protein-synthesis-dependent LTP, and indeed to activity-dependent synaptic plasticity in the CNS in general. It is clear that there is activity-dependent regulation of protein synthesis for a variety of proteins, notably among them CaMKII (64), PKMζ (as described above) and Arc (see Box 2 in Chapter 6). It is also now quite clear that local, regulated protein synthesis occurs in dendrites (reviewed in references 65–66). Of course, the oft-replicated finding that protein synthesis inhibitors can block L-LTP is what first precipitated the local protein synthesis model (67–68).

How is local protein synthesis regulated in LTP and memory? The mechanisms for regulating protein synthesis are themselves horrendously complicated, even without the added complexity of trying to understand how neuronal activity-dependent mechanisms might impinge upon them. Figure 14 and the following discussion summarize some of the signal transduction mechanisms that are hypothesized to operate in the LTP-associated regulation of local protein synthesis in CA1 pyramidal neurons (65–67).

Protein synthesis must, of course, begin with the recognition of an mRNA by the ribosomal complex, which

---

BOX 4

SYNAPTIC TAGGING AND THE E-LTP/L-LTP TRANSITION

In 1997 Uwe Frey and Richard Morris published an interesting series of studies where they formulated the "synaptic tag" hypothesis of L-LTP induction (see Figure and reference 72). Without repeating the entirety of the details of their seminal paper and a variety of subsequent work in this area, the basic idea is as follows. L-LTP is dependent on protein synthesis and presumably on altered gene expression as well. How is it that one can have synapse specificity, which is known to occur with L-LTP, in the face of certainly a central (nuclear) source of mRNA and potentially a central (rough ER)

source of newly-synthesized proteins? Frey and Morris proposed that local activity-regulated generation of persisting signals establishes a "synaptic tag" that marks synapses for potentiation when the synapse experiences an L-LTP-inducing stimulation.

The synaptic tag allows the capture of new gene products (mRNAs or proteins) sent out from the nucleus and cell body (also triggered by LTP-inducing stimulation), localizing these potentiating products at the appropriate synapses. Frey and Morris also showed in their original paper that the generation of the synaptic tag

Continued

BOX 4—cont'd

SYNAPTIC TAGGING AND THE E-LTP/L-LTP TRANSITION

could be pharmacologically isolated from the more generalized induction of L-LTP. In other words, they could generate the tag in the absence of protein synthesis by giving E-LTP-inducing stimulation. Then, subsequent L-LTP inducing stimulation at another set of synapses allowed the original group of synapses to capture the potentiating gene products. While the biochemical identity of the synaptic tag is unknown at present, any one of the variety of persisting post-translational modifications that we are discussing in this chapter are viable candidate mechanisms for contributing to the synaptic tag.

The synaptic tagging work of Frey and Morris also has another very important implication as a mechanism for generating long-lasting synaptic plasticity. Their findings imply that after a cell has received an L-LTP-inducing strong stimulation, subsequent weaker stimuli can capture the L-LTP-inducing products at their synapses. Thus, a weaker stimulation, when following a strong stimulation, could produce L-LTP. This is a powerful mechanism for temporal integration of signals across time (72–73). Depending on the timing of the signals, at any particular time a signal of a given strength may or may not trigger LTP depending on the prior recent "experience" of the cell.

I find this a fascinating finding, in part because this and similar mechanisms of temporal integration have

the potential to explain one of the long-standing mysteries in learning and memory. As described in Chapter 4, a highly reproducible feature of learning across species and learning paradigms is the improved efficacy of "spaced" versus "massed" training. Ten training sessions separated by 15 minutes are much more effective in producing long-lasting and robust memory than ten training sessions back-to-back, for example. Synaptic tagging and other temporal integration mechanisms of this sort have the capacity to explain this phenomenon. Subsequent stimuli, when timed appropriately, can have stronger effects than they would otherwise. A weak signal, that normally might not cross the threshold for triggering change, can be converted to a long-lasting signal if it follows a previous training session. If the subsequent training trials come too soon after the initial stimulus, the synaptic tag generated by the weak stimulus may have nothing to capture, because the nuclear products have not diffused far enough to be captured. If the weak stimulus comes too late (i.e., the training is too spaced out), the genomic products will have been generated but not captured before they decayed. Thus, temporal integration mechanisms of this sort involving synaptic tagging and the generation of other persisting but transient signals allow for the cell to build an optimal time window for the efficacy of repeated stimuli.

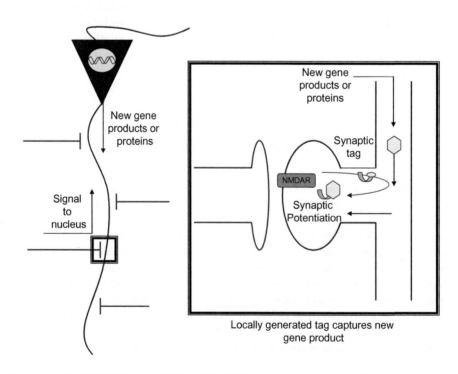

Locally generated tag captures new gene product

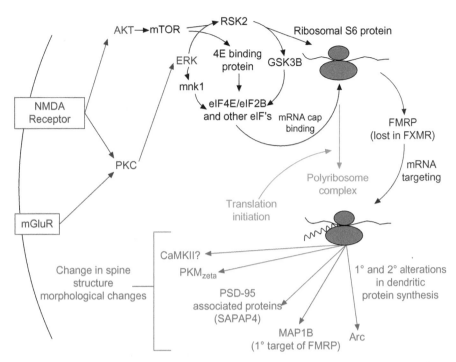

FIGURE 14 A model for activity-dependent regulation of local protein synthesis and spine morphological changes in LTP. See text for details and discussion.

allows the initiation of peptide chain elongation starting from the 5′ end of the message. One mechanism for translational initiation involves the eukaryotic translation initiation factor 4e (eIF4e). Activated eIF4e associates with a number of co-activating proteins and this complex recruits the ribosome to the mRNA, which initiates the process of scanning for the AUG start codon. Activation of eIF4e is regulated by phosphorylation at one major site, Ser 209. The kinase likely to mediate this phosphorylation is MNK1. MNK1 is Mitogen-activated protein kinase-iNteracting-kinase 1 (MNK1). MNK1 is regulated by ERK MAPK, which as we have already discussed is involved in the induction of LTP and memory.

Another target of ERK that may transduce a signal to the protein synthesis machinery is ribosomal S6 kinase 2 (RSK2). ERK directly phosphorylates and activates RSK2, which can then act on the ribosome complex. Both RSK2 and its target glycogen synthase kinase 3β (GSK3b) have been proposed to regulate protein synthesis through phosphorylation of ribosome-associated initiation factors (see Figure 15)—one specific candidate in this context is eIF2B (68). Thus, the ERK pathway has been proposed to regulate protein synthesis in plasticity and memory.

Another player implicated in regulating dendritic protein synthesis is PKC (69). Metabotropic glutamate receptors linked to PLC lead directly to PKC activation (see Box 3) and indirectly to ERK activation.

Metabotropic glutamate receptors via this pathway affect phosphorylation of ribosome-associated proteins (68). A parsimonious model integrating these findings is given in Figure 15, which shows one possible means of coupling glutamate receptors to protein synthesis in dendrites.

What are the messenger RNAs regulated by this mechanism? One of the most interesting possibilities is FMRP. FMRP is the protein encoded by the fragile X mental retardation type 1 gene (70). FMRP is an mRNA binding protein that has both a nuclear localization signal and a nuclear export signal—it is hypothesized to be involved in trafficking of mRNAs. Moreover, FMRP co-localizes with polyribosomes in neuronal cell bodies and dendrites. FMRP knockout mice have altered dendritic spine morphology (in cortical neurons at least), which is consistent with a role for FMRP in regulating localized protein synthesis in dendrites. In addition, FMRP knockout animals exhibit alterations in mGluR-induced LTD at CA1 synapses (71). mGluR agonists can also regulate the synthesis of FMRP itself (69). Thus, one clear candidate as a target of local protein synthesis is FMRP, a protein involved in a human mental retardation syndrome.

While FMRP is a target of the local synthesis machinery, as an mRNA binding protein localized to dendrites, it also likely contributes to regulating local protein synthesis. Two known targets of FMRP regulation are microtubule-associated protein 1B (MAP1B)

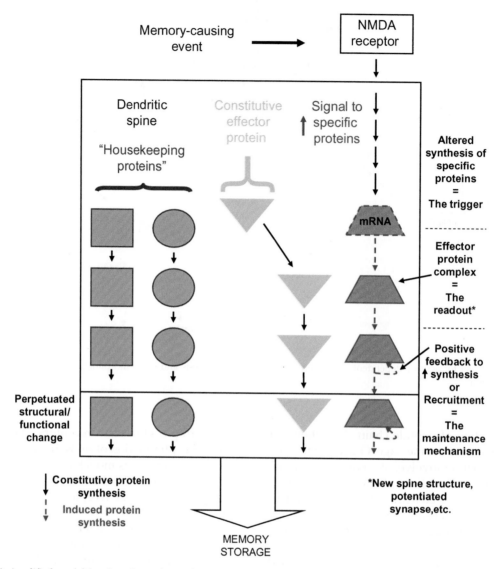

FIGURE 15   A simplified model for altered protein synthesis as a trigger for memory.

and the PSD-95 associated protein SAPAP4. These cytoskeletal/scaffolding protein targets are a potential means by which FMRP might regulate spine structure.

Other well-known and extensively characterized products of local protein synthesis are CaMKII (64) and Arc (65). While the synthesis of these proteins is probably not directly regulated by FMRP, they certainly may play an important role as targets of regulated protein synthesis in dendrites. As we have already discussed in various parts of this book Arc mRNA and protein are selectively localized to active synapses; and Arc as a cytoskeleton-associated protein may serve a morphological/structural role. CaMKII, of course, is a dominant player in post-synaptic function and structure. Thus, while it is quite early to try to synthesize a complete model for the regulation and targets of local dendritic protein synthesis, it is not

unreasonable to think that this process plays a key role in various processes including the regulation of spine structure, morphology, and PSD stabilization, as well as regulating signal transduction locally.

IV. AN OVERVIEW OF THE ROLE OF PROTEIN SYNTHESIS IN MEMORY

In this final section I will summarize a contemporary model proposing how altered protein synthesis is involved in memory formation and its subsequent stabilization. One defining aspect of the model is that altered protein synthesis serves as a trigger for memory consolidation. Thus, specific alterations in the pattern of neuronal protein translation serve as an initial event in long-term memory formation. These specific alterations in protein read-out result in the formation of a protein complex that then serves as a nidus for subsequent perpetuating reinforcement by a positive feedback mechanism. The discussion will emphasize three aspects of the role of altered protein synthesis in memory. First, it is important to note that a relatively short initial time window exists wherein *specific* alterations in the pattern of proteins translated (not overall protein synthesis) is involved in initializing the engram. Second, note that a self-perpetuating positive feedback mechanism maintains the altered pattern of protein expression (synthesis or recruitment) locally. Third, once the formation and subsequent perpetuation of the unique initializing proteins has occurred, ongoing constitutive protein synthesis is all that is necessary for maintenance of the engram.

The model is summarized in Figure 15. In this simplified scheme, a memory-causing event such as a set of appropriately contingent environmental signals leads to NMDA receptor activation and the subsequent formation of a memory engram. You might imagine this as happening at a dendritic spine of a hippocampal pyramidal neuron, for example. The NMDA receptor activation recruits signal transduction mechanisms to precipitate an altered rate of synthesis of a specific subset of synaptic proteins. This altered protein synthesis is in addition to "housekeeping" protein synthesis that contributes to ongoing maintenance of the dendritic spine (the blue pathway in Figure 15). The model specifies that the spine maintains constitutive synthesis of effector proteins that, when in a complex with the appropriate partners, can increase synaptic strength (the green pathway in Figure 15). The "appropriate partners" are the targets of the signal for altered protein synthesis (the red pathway in Figure 15). Thus, the induced proteins interact with a subset of constitutively synthesized proteins in order to increase synaptic strength. In this model, the altered synthesis of a specific subset of proteins in the dendritic spine is the trigger for synaptic potentiation and memory formation, and the "new"proteins interact with other proteins already present to effect the change. The effector protein complex is the read-out of the altered protein synthesis.

How is the elevated level of the effector complex maintained? An absolute requirement is the need for a self-reinforcing positive feedback of some sort. In one alternative (as shown in Figure 15) the elevated synthesis of the red (potentiating) pathway becomes quasi-constitutive by a positive feedback mechanism. In this alternative the triggering mechanism perpetuates itself by promoting its own resynthesis at a new, higher rate locally. This allows the mechanism to perpetuate the altered spectrum (or rate) of synthesis of the new subset of local effector proteins. Alternatively and minimally, the effector complex might perpetuate itself by an increased rate of recruitment to the local subcellular compartment of other copies of itself synthesized elsewhere in the cell. The positive reinforcement mechanism in this second scenario is that a protein, once synthesized in the specific compartment, is able subsequently to capture others of its own species that are synthesized globally in the cell.

Note the mechanistic distinction between the first and second alternatives. The second scenario does not require any long-lasting increase in protein synthesis anywhere in the cell—as long as the relevant protein species are synthesized at an adequate overall basal rate for the entire cell the changes will be persistent. The first scenario involves an increased rate of synthesis of specific proteins and necessitates that the altered rate of synthesis continues perpetually.

In this model one of these two alternative mechanisms is the maintenance mechanism at the molecular level. The self-perpetuating structural/functional change is a component of the engram, and serves as a molecular basis for memory storage.

The altered pattern of proteins translated can be anything from one specific protein species to the entire complement of proteins necessary to form a dendritic spine. The model does not specify the details of this aspect of the mechanism. Indeed, identifying the spectrum of proteins involved in the triggering event is a topic of contemporary research in this field, and the particulars are unclear at this time.

This simple model captures several essential elements to keep in mind when considering how altered protein synthesis might contribute to memory. First, altered protein synthesis serves as a trigger for increased synaptic strength—a persisting increase in overall protein synthesis is not required. Second, a self-perpetuating mechanism of some sort is required to maintain the changes in the face of protein turnover. Finally, some part (or all) of the proteins whose synthesis is changed must impact synaptic function in some fashion in order to participate in memory.

V. SUMMARY

In this chapter we explored several of the fundamentally important issues related to information storage in neurons. How is a persisting biochemical signal generated? How is that signal transmitted to an effector system to alter neuronal function? How is the synthesis of new proteins regulated in memory? Our discussion focused on persistent post-translational modifications and new protein synthesis as *maintenance* mechanisms, and on post-synaptic receptors as target *effectors* of these maintenance signals.

The answers to these various questions provide us with an understanding of the basic underpinnings of molecular information storage in the nervous system. Great progress has been made in defining the basic biochemical mechanisms available to the neuron that allow it to generate a persisting signal and translate that signal into a persisting effect. This work also has begun to define the biochemical processes that can be used by *any* central synapse for augmenting the strength of its synaptic connections.

The following are general take-home points from this chapter:

1. The calcium signal that triggers lasting synaptic plasticity and memory formation first impinges on calcium-binding proteins and their immediate targets. Prominent examples include calmodulin-dependent enzymes and protein kinase C.
2. The MAPK cascade, which is an additional target of calcium-regulated signaling mechanisms, is a prominent regulator of protein synthesis in neurons.
3. CaMKII autophosphorylation and the increased synthesis of PKM-zeta are two prominent mechanisms for generating a persisting biochemical signal in plasticity and memory. These persistently activated species are mechanisms for maintenance of plasticity and memory.
4. Post-synaptic AMPA receptors are targets of the maintenance mechanisms. Effects on AMPA receptors include increased membrane insertion, augmented trafficking, and direct phosphorylation to increase ionic currents through these channels.
5. The existence of localized dendritic protein synthesis and synaptic tags solves the issues of how a cell-wide response such as increased synthesis of proteins can be selectively targeted to the right synapse.
6. As was also discussed in Chapter 3, it is important to remember that all proteins have a half-life due to turnover in the cell, so permanent changes must be mediated by self-reinforcing mechanisms that can perpetuate the molecular signal in the face of protein breakdown.

Further Reading

Adams, J. P., and Sweatt, J. D. (2002). "Molecular psychology: roles for the ERK MAP kinase cascade in memory". *Annu. Rev. Pharmacol. Toxicol.* 42:135–163.

Dineley, K. T., Weeber, E. J., Atkins, C., Adams, J. P., Anderson, A. E., and Sweatt, J. D. (2001). "Leitmotifs in the biochemistry of LTP induction: amplification, integration and coordination". *J. Neurochem.* 77:961–971.

Hayashi, Y., Shi, S. H., Esteban, J. A., Piccini, A., Poncer, J. C., and Malinow, R. (2000). "Driving AMPA receptors into synapses by LTP and CaMKII: requirement for GluR1 and PDZ domain interaction". *Science* 287:2262–2267.

Klann, E., Chen, S. J., and Sweatt, J. D. (1991). "Persistent protein kinase activation in the maintenance phase of long-term potentiation". *J. Bio.l Chem.* 266:24253–24256.

Lee, H. K., Barbarosie, M., Kameyama, K., Bear, M. F., and Huganir, R. L. (2000). "Regulation of distinct AMPA receptor phosphorylation sites during bidirectional synaptic plasticity". *Nature* 405:955–959.

Lisman, J., Schulman, H., and Cline, H. (2002). "The molecular basis of CaMKII function in synaptic and behavioural memory". *Nat. Rev. Neurosci.* 3:175–190.

Lisman, J. E., and Zhabotinsky, A. M. (2001). "A model of synaptic memory: a CaMKII/PP1 switch that potentiates transmission by organizing an AMPA receptor anchoring assembly". *Neuron* 31:191–201.

Malenka, R. C., and Bear, M. F. (2004). "LTP and LTD: an embarrassment of riches". *Neuron* 44:5–21.

Malinow, R., and Malenka, R. C. (2002). "AMPA receptor trafficking and synaptic plasticity". *Annu. Rev. Neurosci.* 25:103–126.

Malinow, R., Madison, D. V., and Tsien, R. W. (1988). "Persistent protein kinase activity underlying long-term potentiation". *Nature* 335:820–824.

Martin, K. C., Casadio, A., Zhu, H., Rose, J. C., Chen, M., Bailey, C. H., and Kandel, E. R. (1997). "Synapse-specific, long-term facilitation of *Aplysia* sensory to motor synapses: a function for local protein synthesis in memory storage". *Cell* 91:927–938.

Scannevin, R. H., and Huganir, R. L. (2000). "Postsynaptic organization and regulation of excitatory synapses". *Nat. Rev. Neurosci.* 1:133–141.

Steward, O., and Schuman, E. M. (2001). "Protein synthesis at synaptic sites on dendrites". *Annu. Rev. Neurosci.* 24:299–325.

Steward, O., and Worley, P. F. (2001). "A cellular mechanism for targeting newly synthesized mRNAs to synaptic sites on dendrites". *Proc. Natl. Acad. Sci. USA*, 98:7062–7068.

Journal Club Articles

Blitzer, R. D., Wong, T., Nouranifar, R., Iyengar, R., and Landau, E. M. (1995). "Postsynaptic cAMP pathway gates early LTP in hippocampal CA1 region". *Neuron* 15:1403–1414.

Frey, U., and Morris, R. G. (1997). "Synaptic tagging and long-term potentiation". *Nature* 385:533–536.

Pastalkova, E., Serrano, P., Pinkhasova, D., Wallace, E., Fenton, A. A., and Sacktor, T. C. (2006). "Storage of spatial information by the maintenance mechanism of LTP". *Science* 313:1141–1144.

Takahashi, T., Svoboda, K., and Malinow, R. (2003). "Experience strengthening transmission by driving AMPA receptors into synapses". *Science* 299:1585–1588.

For more information—relevant topic chapters from: John H. Byrne (Editor-in-Chief) (2008). *Learning and Memory: A Comprehensive Reference*. Oxford: Academic Press (ISBN 978-0-12-370509-9). (4.02 Bailey, C. H., Barco, A., Hawkins, R. D., and Kandel, E. R. *Molecular Studies of Learning and Memory in Aplysia and the Hippocampus: A Comparative Analysis of Implicit and Explicit Memory Storage*. pp. 11–29; 4.11 Schafe, G. E., and LeDoux, J. E. *Neural and Molecular Mechanisms of Fear Memory*. pp. 157–192; 4.13 Rosenblum, K. *Conditioned Taste Aversion and Taste Learning: Molecular Mechanisms*. pp. 217–234; 4.17 Giles, A. C., and Rankin, C. H. *Behavioral Analysis of Learning and Memory in C. elegans*. pp. 629–640; 4.21 Eckel-Mahan, K. L., and Storm, D. R. *Second Messengers: Calcium and cAMP Signaling*. pp. 427–448; 4.22 Sacktor, T. C. *PKM[zeta], LTP Maintenance, and Long-Term Memory*

Storage. pp. 449–467; 4.23 Colbran, R. J. *CaMKII: Mechanisms of a Prototypical Memory Model.* pp. 469–488; 4.25 Kelleher, R. J. III, *Mitogen-Activated Protein Kinases in Synaptic Plasticity and Memory.* pp. 501–523; 4.26 Hegde, A. N. *Proteolysis and Synaptic Plasticity.* pp. 525–545; 4.29 Dynes, J. L., and Steward, O. *Dendritic Transport of mRNA, the IEG Arc, and Synaptic Modifications Involved in Memory Consolidation.* pp. 587–610; 4.30 Alvestad, R. M., Goebel, S. M., Coultrap, S. J., and Browning, M. D. *Glutamate Receptor Trafficking in LTP.* pp. 611–632; 4.31 Lee, H. -K., and Huganir, R. L. *AMPA Receptor Regulation and the Reversal of Synaptic Plasticity—LTP, LTD, Depotentiation, and Dedepression.* pp. 633–648; 4.32 Marcora, E., Carlisle, H. J., and Kennedy, M. B. *The Role of the Postsynaptic Density and the Spine Cytoskeleton in Synaptic Plasticity.* pp. 649–673; 4.33 Costa-Mattioli, M., Sonenberg, N., and Klann, E. *Translational Control Mechanisms in Synaptic Plasticity and Memory.* pp. 675–694; 4.34 Chapleau, C. A., and Pozzo-Miller, L. *Activity-Dependent Structural Plasticity of Dendritic Spines.* pp. 695–719; 4.36 Powell, C. M., and Castillo, P. E. *Presynaptic Mechanisms in Plasticity and Memory.* pp. 741–769; 4.37 Lovinger, D. M. *Regulation of Synaptic Function by Endocannabinoids.* pp. 771–792; 4.38 Hawkins, R. D. *Transsynaptic Signaling by NO during Learning-Related Synaptic Plasticity.* pp. 793–802; 4.40 Mozzachiodi, R., and Byrne, J. H. *Plasticity of Intrinsic Excitability as a Mechanism for Memory Storage.* pp. 829–838.)

References

1. Verdaguer, N., Corbalan-Garcia, S., Ochoa, W. F., Fita, I., and Gomez-Fernandez, J. C. (1999). "Ca^{2+} bridges the C2 membrane-binding domain of protein kinase Calpha directly to phosphatidylserine". *Embo. J.* 18:6329–6338.

2. Kolodziej, S. J., Hudmon, A., Waxham, M. N., and Stoops, J. K. (2000). "Three-dimensional reconstructions of calcium/calmodulin-dependent (CaM) kinase IIalpha and truncated CaM kinase IIalpha reveal a unique organization for its structural core and functional domains". *J. Biol. Chem.* 275:14354–14359.

3. Wong, S. T., Athos, J., Figueroa, X. A., Pineda, V. V., Schaefer, M. L., Chavkin, C. C., Muglia, L. J., and Storm, D. R. (1999). "Calcium-stimulated adenylyl cyclase activity is critical for hippocampus-dependent long-term memory and late phase LTP". *Neuron* 23:787–798.

4. Hernandez, A. L., Blace, N., Cary, J. F. et al. (2003). "Protein kinase Mζ synthesis from a brain mRNA encoding an independent protein kinase Cζ catalytic domain. Implications for the molecular mechanism of memory". *J. Biol. Chem.* 278:40305–40316.

5. Serrano, P., Yao, Y., and Sacktor, T. C. (2005). "Persistent phosphorylation by protein kinase M maintains late-phase long-term potentiation". *J. Neurosci.* 25:1979–1984.

6. Lisman, J., Schulman, H., and Cline, H. (2002). "The molecular basis of CaMKII function in synaptic and behavioural memory". *Nat. Rev. Neurosci.* 3:175–190.

7. Strack, S., and Colbran, R. J. (1998). "Autophosphorylation-dependent targeting of calcium/ calmodulin-dependent protein kinase II by the NR2B subunit of the N-methyl-D-aspartate receptor". *J. Biol. Chem.* 273:20689–20692.

8. Leonard, A. S., Lim, I. A., Hemsworth, D. E., Horne, M. C., and Hell, J. W. (1999). "Calcium/calmodulin-dependent protein kinase II is associated with the N-methyl-D-aspartate receptor". *Proc. Natl. Acad. Sci. USA* 96:3239–3244.

9. Lisman, J. E., and Zhabotinsky, A. M. (2001). "A model of synaptic memory: a CaMKII/PP1 switch that potentiates transmission by organizing an AMPA receptor anchoring assembly". *Neuron* 31:191–201.

10. Hvalby, O., Hemmings, H. C., Jr., Paulsen, O., Czernik, A. J., Nairn, A. C., Godfraind, J. M., Jensen, V., Raastad, M., Storm, J. F., Andersen, P. et al. (1994). "Specificity of protein kinase inhibitor peptides and induction of long-term potentiation". *Proc. Natl. Acad. Sci. USA,* 91:4761–4765.

11. Otmakhov, N., Griffith, L. C., and Lisman, J. E. (1997). "Postsynaptic inhibitors of calcium/calmodulin-dependent protein kinase type II block induction but not maintenance of pairing-induced long-term potentiation". *J. Neurosci.* 17: 5357–5365.

12. Silva, A. J., Stevens, C. F., Tonegawa, S., and Wang, Y. (1992). "Deficient hippocampal long-term potentiation in alpha-calcium-calmodulin kinase II mutant mice". *Science* 257:201–206.

13. Hinds, H. L., Tonegawa, S., and Malinow, R. (1998). "CA1 long-term potentiation is diminished but present in hippocampal slices from alpha-CaMKII mutant mice". *Learn. Mem.* 5:344–354.

14. Mayford, M., Wang, J., Kandel, E. R., and O'Dell, T. J. (1995). "CaMKII regulates the frequency-response function of hippocampal synapses for the production of both LTD and LTP". *Cell* 81:891–904.

15. Chen, H. X., Otmakhov, N., Strack, S., Colbran, R. J., and Lisman, J. E. (2001). "Is persistent activity of calcium/calmodulin-dependent kinase required for the maintenance of LTP?". *J. Neurophysiol.* 85:1368–1376.

16. De Koninck, P., and Schulman, H. (1998). "Sensitivity of CaM kinase II to the frequency of Ca^{2+} oscillations". *Science* 279:227–230.

17. Poser, S., and Storm, D. R. (2001). "Role of Ca^{2+}-stimulated adenylyl cyclases in LTP and memory formation". *Int. J. Dev. Neurosci.* 19:387–394.

18. Roberson, E. D., and Sweatt, J. D. (1996). "Transient activation of cyclic AMP-dependent protein kinase during hippocampal long-term potentiation". *J. Biol. Chem.* 271:30436–30441.

19. Garthwaite, J., and Boulton, C. L. (1995). "Nitric oxide signaling in the central nervous system". *Annu. Rev. Physiol.* 57:683–706.

20. Kleppisch, T., Pfeifer, A., Klatt, P., Ruth, P., Montkowski, A., Fassler, R., and Hofmann, F. (1999). "Long-term potentiation in the hippocampal CA1 region of mice lacking cGMP-dependent kinases is normal and susceptible to inhibition of nitric oxide synthase". *J. Neurosci.* 19:48–55.

21. Bon, C. L., and Garthwaite, J. (2001). "Nitric oxide-induced potentiation of CA1 hippocampal synaptic transmission during baseline stimulation is strictly frequency-dependent". *Neuropharmacology* 40:501–507.

22. Selig, D. K., Segal, M. R., Liao, D., Malenka, R. C., Malinow, R., Nicoll, R. A., and Lisman, J. E. (1996). "Examination of the role of cGMP in long-term potentiation in the CA1 region of the hippocampus". *Learn. Mem.* 3:42–48.

23. Schuman, E. M., and Madison, D. V. (1991). "A requirement for the intercellular messenger nitric oxide in long-term potentiation". *Science* 254:1503–1506.

24. Arancio, O., Antonova, I., Gambaryan, S., Lohmann, S. M., Wood, J. S., Lawrence, D. S., and Hawkins, R. D. (2001). "Presynaptic role of cGMP-dependent protein kinase during long-lasting potentiation". *J. Neurosci.* 21:143–149.

25. Lovinger, D. M., Wong, K. L., Murakami, K., and Routtenberg, A. (1987). "Protein kinase C inhibitors eliminate hippocampal long-term potentiation". *Brain Res.* 436:177–183.

26. Colley, P. A., Sheu, F. S., and Routtenberg, A. (1990). "Inhibition of protein kinase C blocks two components of LTP persistence, leaving initial potentiation intact". *J. Neurosci.* 10:3353–3360.

27. Malinow, R., Madison, D. V., and Tsien, R. W. (1988). "Persistent protein kinase activity underlying long-term potentiation". *Nature* 335:820–824.

28. Wang, J. H., and Feng, D. P. (1992). "Postsynaptic protein kinase C essential to induction and maintenance of long-term potentiation

in the hippocampal CA1 region". *Proc. Natl. Acad. Sci. USA,* 89:2576–2580.

29. Klann, E., Chen, S. J., and Sweatt, J. D. (1991). "Persistent protein kinase activation in the maintenance phase of long-term potentiation". *J. Biol. Chem.* 266:24253–24256.

30. Klann, E., Chen, S. J., and Sweatt, J. D. (1993). "Mechanism of protein kinase C activation during the induction and maintenance of long-term potentiation probed using a selective peptide substrate". *Proc. Natl. Acad. Sci. USA* 90:8337–8341.

31. Leahy, J. C., Luo, Y., Kent, C. S., Meiri, K. F., and Vallano, M. L. (1993). "Demonstration of presynaptic protein kinase C activation following long-term potentiation in rat hippocampal slices". *Neuroscience* 52:563–574.

32. Lovinger, D. M., Akers, R. F., Nelson, R. B., Barnes, C. A., McNaughton, B. L., and Routtenberg, A. (1985). "A selective increase in phosporylation of protein F1, a protein kinase C substrate, directly related to three day growth of long term synaptic enhancement". *Brain Res.* 343:137–143.

33. Gianotti, C., Nunzi, M. G., Gispen, W. H., and Corradetti, R. (1992). "Phosphorylation of the presynaptic protein B-50 (GAP-43) is increased during electrically induced long-term potentiation". *Neuron* 8:843–848.

34. Sacktor, T. C., Osten, P., Valsamis, H., Jiang, X., Naik, M. U., and Sublette, E. (1993). "Persistent activation of the zeta isoform of protein kinase C in the maintenance of long-term potentiation". *Proc. Natl. Acad. Sci. USA,* 90:8342–8346.

35. Schwartz, J. H. (1993). "Cognitive kinases". *Proc. Natl. Acad. Sci. USA,* 90:8310–8313.

36. Powell, C. M., Johnston, D., and Sweatt, J. D. (1994). "Autonomously active protein kinase C in the maintenance phase of N-methyl-D-aspartate receptor-independent long term potentiation". *J. Biol. Chem.* 269:27958–27963.

37. Malenka, R. C., Madison, D. V., and Nicoll, R. A. (1986). "Potentiation of synaptic transmission in the hippocampus by phorbol esters". *Nature* 321:175–177.

38. Malenka, R. C., Ayoub, G. S., and Nicoll, R. A. (1987). "Phorbol esters enhance transmitter release in rat hippocampal slices". *Brain Res.* 403:198–203.

39. Hvalby, O., Reymann, K., and Andersen, P. (1988). "Intracellular analysis of potentiation of CA1 hippocampal synaptic transmission by phorbol ester application". *Exp. Brain Res.* 71:588–596.

40. Hu, G. Y., Hvalby, O., Walaas, S. I., Albert, K. A., Skjeflo, P., Andersen, P., and Greengard, P. (1987). "Protein kinase C injection into hippocampal pyramidal cells elicits features of long term potentiation". *Nature* 328:426–429.

41. Abeliovich, A., Chen, C., Goda, Y., Silva, A. J., Stevens, C. F., and Tonegawa, S. (1993). "Modified hippocampal long-term potentiation in PKC gamma-mutant mice". *Cell* 75:1253–1262.

42. Weeber, E. J., Atkins, C. M., Selcher, J. C., Varga, A. W., Mirnikjoo, B., Paylor, R., Leitges, M., and Sweatt, J. D. (2000). "A role for the beta isoform of protein kinase C in fear conditioning". *J. Neurosci.* 20:5906–5914.

43. Goda, Y., Stevens, C. F., and Tonegawa, S. (1996). "Phorbol ester effects at hippocampal synapses act independently of the gamma isoform of PKC". *Learn. Mem.* 3:182–187.

44. Klann, E., and Thiels, E. (1999). "Modulation of protein kinases and protein phosphatases by reactive oxygen species: implications for hippocampal synaptic plasticity". *Prog. Neuropsychopharmacol. Biol. Psychiatry,* 23:359–376.

45. Knapp, L. T., and Klann, E. (2002). "Potentiation of hippocampal synaptic transmission by superoxide requires the oxidative activation of protein kinase C". *J. Neurosci.* 22:674–683.

46. Osten, P., Valsamis, L., Harris, A., and Sacktor, T. C. (1996). "Protein synthesis-dependent formation of protein kinase Mzeta in long-term potentiation". *J. Neurosci.* 16:2444–2451.

47. Ling, D. S., Benardo, L. S., Serrano, P. A., Blace, N., Kelly, M. T., Crary, J. F., and Sacktor, T. C. (2002). "Protein kinase Mzeta is necessary and sufficient for LTP maintenance". *Nat. Neurosci.* 5:295–296.

48. Hrabetova, S., and Sacktor, T. C. (1996). "Bidirectional regulation of protein kinase M zeta in the maintenance of long-term potentiation and long-term depression". *J. Neurosci.* 16:5324–5333.

49. Williams, J. H., Errington, M. L., Lynch, M. A., and Bliss, T. V. (1989). "Arachidonic acid induces a long-term activity-dependent enhancement of synaptic transmission in the hippocampus". *Nature* 341:739–742.

50. O'Dell, T. J., Hawkins, R. D., Kandel, E. R., and Arancio, O. (1991). "Tests of the roles of two diffusible substances in long-term potentiation: evidence for nitric oxide as a possible early retrograde messenger". *Proc. Natl. Acad. Sci. USA,* 88:11285–11289.

51. Scannevin, R. H., and Huganir, R. L. (2000). "Postsynaptic organization and regulation of excitatory synapses". *Nat. Rev. Neurosci.* 1:133–141.

52. Derkach, V., Barria, A., and Soderling, T. R. (1999). "Ca^{2+}/calmodulin-kinase II enhances channel conductance of alpha-amino-3-hydroxy-5-methyl-4-isoxazolepropionate type glutamate receptors". *Proc. Natl. Acad. Sci. USA,* 96:3269–3274.

53. Benke, T. A., Luthi, A., Isaac, J. T., and Collingridge, G. L. (1998). "Modulation of AMPA receptor unitary conductance by synaptic activity". *Nature* 393:793–797.

54. Barria, A., Muller, D., Derkach, V., Griffith, L. C., and Soderling, T. R. (1997). "Regulatory phosphorylation of AMPA-type glutamate receptors by CaM-KII during long-term potentiation". *Science* 276:2042–2045.

55. Shi, S. H. (2001). "Amersham Biosciences & Science Prize. AMPA receptor dynamics and synaptic plasticity". *Science* 294:1851–1852.

56. Malinow, R., and Malenka, R. C. (2002). "AMPA receptor trafficking and synaptic plasticity". *Annu. Rev. Neurosci.* 25:103–126.

57. Poncer, J. C., Esteban, J. A., and Malinow, R. (2002). "Multiple mechanisms for the potentiation of AMPA receptor-mediated transmission by alpha-Ca^{2+}/calmodulin-dependent protein kinase II". *J. Neurosci.* 22:4406–4411.

58. Lee, H. K., Barbarosie, M., Kameyama, K., Bear, M. F., and Huganir, R. L. (2000). "Regulation of distinct AMPA receptor phosphorylation sites during bidirectional synaptic plasticity". *Nature* 405:955–959.

59. Hayashi, Y., Shi, S. H., Esteban, J. A., Piccini, A., Poncer, J. C., and Malinow, R. (2000). "Driving AMPA receptors into synapses by LTP and CaMKII: requirement for GluR1 and PDZ domain interaction". *Science* 287:2262–2267.

60. Ehlers, M. D. (2000). "Reinsertion or degradation of AMPA receptors determined by activity-dependent endocytic sorting". *Neuron* 28:511–525.

61. Luscher, C., Xia, H., Beattie, E. C., Carroll, R. C., von Zastrow, M., Malenka, R. C., and Nicoll, R. A. (1999). "Role of AMPA receptor cycling in synaptic transmission and plasticity". *Neuron* 24:649–658.

62. Grosshans, D. R., Clayton, D. A., Coultrap, S. J., and Browning, M. D. (2002). "LTP leads to rapid surface expression of NMDA but not AMPA receptors in adult rat CA1". *Nat. Neurosci.* 5:27–33.

63. Martin, K. C., Casadio, A., Zhu, H., Rose, J. C., Chen, M., Bailey, C. H., and Kandel, E. R. (1997). "Synapse-specific, long-term facilitation of aplysia sensory to motor synapses: a function for local protein synthesis in memory storage". *Cell* 91:927–938.

64. Ouyang, Y., Rosenstein, A., Kreiman, G., Schuman, E. M., and Kennedy, M. B. (1999). "Tetanic stimulation leads to increased

accumulation of $Ca^{(2+)}$/calmodulin-dependent protein kinase II via dendritic protein synthesis in hippocampal neurons". *J. Neurosci.* 19:7823–7833.

65. Steward, O., and Worley, P. F. (2001). "A cellular mechanism for targeting newly synthesized mRNAs to synaptic sites on dendrites". *Proc. Natl. Acad. Sci. USA* 98:7062–7068.

66. Steward, O., and Schuman, E. M. (2001). "Protein synthesis at synaptic sites on dendrites". *Annu. Rev. Neurosci.* 24:299–325.

67. Frey, U., Krug, M., Reymann, K. G., and Matthies, H. (1988). "Anisomycin, an inhibitor of protein synthesis, blocks late phases of LTP phenomena in the hippocampal CA1 region *in vitro*". *Brain Res.* 452:57–65.

68. Raught, B., Gingras, A. C., and Sonenberg, N. (2001). "The target of rapamycin (TOR) proteins". *Proc. Natl. Acad. Sci. USA,* 98:7037–7044.

69. Stanton, P. K., and Sarvey, J. M. (1984). "Blockade of long-term potentiation in rat hippocampal CA1 region by inhibitors of protein synthesis". *J. Neurosci.* 4:3080–3088.

70. Angenstein, F., Greenough, W. T., and Weiler, I. J. (1998). "Metabotropic glutamate receptor-initiated translocation of protein kinase p90rsk to polyribosomes: a possible factor regulating synaptic protein synthesis". *Proc. Natl. Acad. Sci. USA* 95:15078–15083.

71. Greenough, W. T., Klintsova, A. Y., Irwin, S. A., Galvez, R., Bates, K. E., and Weiler, I. J. (2001). "Synaptic regulation of protein synthesis and the fragile X protein". *Proc. Natl. Acad. Sci. USA* 98:7101–7106.

72. Gao, F. B. (2002). "Understanding fragile X syndrome: insights from retarded flies". *Neuron* 34:859–862.

73. Huber, K. M., Gallagher, S. M., Warren, S. T., and Bear, M. F. (2002). "Altered synaptic plasticity in a mouse model of fragile X mental retardation". *Proc. Natl. Acad. Sci. USA* 99:7746–7750.

74. Frey, U., and Morris, R. G. (1998). "Synaptic tagging: implications for late maintenance of hippocampal long-term potentiation". *Trends Neurosci.* 21:181–188.

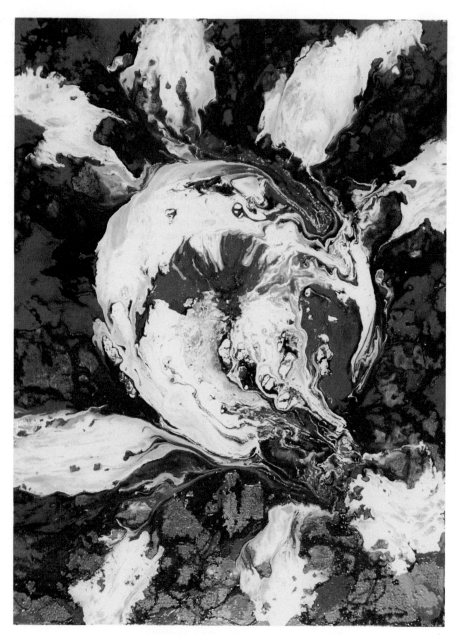

Chromatin Remodeling in Memory Formation
J. David Sweatt, acrylic on canvas, 2008–2009

Molecular Genetic Mechanisms for Long-Term Information Storage at the Cellular Level

I. INTRODUCTION

In this chapter we will discuss the mechanisms unique to inducing and maintaining long-lasting memory and its likely cellular correlate, the late phase of LTP (L-LTP). This is an exciting contemporary area of memory research, and one of those areas where it is clear that additional important discoveries will be made in the near future.

For our purposes in this chapter L-LTP will be defined in terms of an enduring, gene-transcription-dependent form of synaptic potentiation. However, L-LTP is also a correlate of long-term memory in the behaving animal. The particular mechanisms that have been worked out to explain L-LTP are highly relevant to hippocampus-dependent long-term memory

in vivo. Thus, L-LTP is frequently discussed as an analogue of long-term memory, as opposed to being limited to a description of a specific neuronal plasticity phenomenon. Many investigators study L-LTP to understand the general role of altered gene expression, protein synthesis, and structural changes in mediating long-term changes at synapses, and in mediating long-term memory in the animal.

This chapter will be divided into four basic sections. The first major section of the chapter deals with NMDA receptor coupling to the genome, and also deals with receptor-effector coupling mechanisms in the context of transcriptional regulation. We will then proceed in the second section to some identified gene targets in long-term memory, and raise the issue of how the products of these genes get to the right synapses. In the third section we will discuss likely read-outs of altered expression of these target genes, suggesting that these changes mediate structural and morphological changes in the neuron. Thus, the basic model for the third section is that altered expression of gene products gets translated into structural changes at the synaptic spine and altered connectivity of the neuron. Ultimately these changes are manifest as changes in the synaptic circuit in which the neuron resides. In the final major section we will discuss an emerging new topic in long-term memory—the role of *epigenetic* molecular mechanisms in synaptic plasticity and memory formation.

In the context of our systematic nomenclature, in this chapter we will focus largely on the induction mechanisms of L-LTP and long-term memory, exploring how a triggering calcium signal gets converted into a genomic read-out. This is a fascinating area of current investigation and the area for which the most relevant data are available. The maintenance and expression mechanisms of L-LTP and long-term memory are still highly speculative at this point and for this reason will be dealt with in less detail.

II. ALTERED GENE EXPRESSION IN LATE-LONG-TERM POTENTIATION AND LONG-TERM MEMORY

In some of the earliest studies of LTP *in vitro* it was discovered that there is a uniquely definable stage of LTP, L-LTP, which is blocked by inhibition of new gene transcription. Three unique attributes of L-LTP make it distinct from E-LTP.

First, L-LTP is defined as that phase of LTP that is dependent on altered gene expression and protein synthesis for its induction. As we noted in the last chapter when we discussed the role of altered protein synthesis in memory, "altered" is the key word here. In the limit, every cellular process depends on ongoing gene expression, if only to replenish mRNAs as they turn over. What defines L-LTP is a requirement, for its induction, of changes in gene expression, different from a pre-existing baseline.

The maintenance and expression mechanisms for L-LTP are still mysterious, and it is not clear if specifically altered gene expression is necessary for L-LTP maintenance. It is possible that the ongoing maintenance of altered levels of expression of specific genes is necessary for L-LTP maintenance, but this is not clear at this point. At a minimum, however, available data can be interpreted to indicate that alterations in gene and protein expression are necessary for the induction of L-LTP. Thus, we will use this as the first

and defining attribute of L-LTP for the purposes of this chapter.

How then is L-LTP maintained? The working model of L-LTP maintenance that I will use posits a local, self-reinforcing alteration of protein synthesis and synaptic structure (broadly defined) as the maintenance mechanism for L-LTP and memory. I will describe some specific possibilities for molecular players in this scenario later in this chapter.

A second attribute of L-LTP is that it generally is induced, selectively, by multiple trains of tetanic stimuli, or in some cases by more prolonged theta-type stimulation or stimulation paired with dopamine (DA) or other neuromodulators. The fact that L-LTP can be selectively induced with specific protocols suggests that unique molecular events are associated with its induction. Also, the unique L-LTP-inducing stimuli serve a practical purpose, in that one can design experiments to see what molecular events are uniquely associated with these stimuli. I should also note in passing that all of the data I will discuss here will concern NMDA receptor-dependent L-LTP, using data from Schaffer collateral synapses or data from studies of the perforant path inputs to the dentate gyrus.

A third attribute of L-LTP is, of course, its "lateness." Late LTP is generally held to be LTP beginning at about 90 minutes post-tetanus. However, it is worth noting that there is not typically a precipitous drop-off of LTP at any specific time point when L-LTP induction is blocked (see Figure 1). In addition, L-LTP is studied in a wide variety of preparations and at various temperatures, ranging from room temperature in *in vitro* slices to 37°C in intact animal *in vivo* recording. Of course, some *in vivo* experiments go on for days to weeks as well, and what we monolithically call Late LTP is likely subserved by multiple processes. For these various reasons we will define L-LTP mechanistically in terms of altered gene and protein expression, versus temporally in terms of any particular time point. Nevertheless, a working definition of L-LTP is synaptic potentiation in the 90 minutes to 4 hour time range.

With these attributes in mind, we can proceed to consider the experimental evidence supporting a role of altered gene expression in L-LTP and long-term memory. As usual, we will consider this in the context of the block, measure, and mimic criteria (see Table 1). Thus, the hypothesis of a role for altered gene expression in L-LTP and long-term memory predicts that: blocking changes in protein and RNA synthesis should block L-LTP and memory induction; that changes in gene and protein expression should occur with L-LTP and memory-inducing stimulation; and that artificially increasing the synthesis of the appropriate genes should lead to an enhancement of synaptic plasticity and augmented memory formation. We will discuss

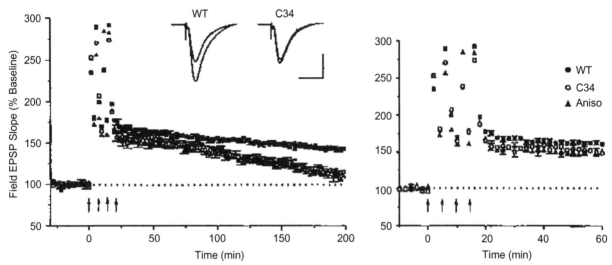

FIGURE 1 Protein synthesis dependence of L-LTP; L-LTP is disrupted in dominant negative CaMKIV transgenic mice. Late-phase LTP (L-LTP) was induced by four trains of tetanic stimulation spaced by five minute intervals. The left panel illustrates the effects of application of the protein synthesis inhibitor anisomycin (filled triangles) and genetic suppression of CaMKIV (C34, open circles) on late-phase LTP. Note that later-developing stages of LTP are selectively lost. The right panel illustrates the same data in greater detail, focusing on the first 60 minutes of LTP. Filled triangles indicate L-LTP obtained with wildtype slices in the presence of anisomycin (Aniso). Superimposed representative EPSPs shown were recorded five minutes before and three hours after L-LTP induction. Calibration bars, 1 mV and 20 ms. As has been routinely observed, only modest effects of protein synthesis inhibitors are observed in E-LTP. Figure and legend adapted from (8).

each of these hypothesis-driven predictions in turn in the next few paragraphs.

Prediction One: blocking changes in gene transcription should block L-LTP induction. In addition to the variety of experiments described in the last chapter demonstrating that protein synthesis inhibitors can block L-LTP and memory, it is also known that inhibition of RNA synthesis blocks these phenomena. Thus, the transcription inhibitor actinomycin D blocks L-LTP induction and long-term memory (1–2). Similarly, knocking out or inhibiting the transcription factor *CREB* and homologous family members can block L-LTP induction and long-term memory, although again there is some disagreement in the reported effects (3–5). (Interpretation of the CREB knockout results is complicated because of compensatory mechanisms that occur with CREB knockouts, and there is an apparent specificity of the effects on L-LTP that are dependent on the L-LTP induction paradigm used.) Finally, knocking out the transcriptional regulators zif268 and c-rel leads to a loss of L-LTP and long-term memory (6,21). Overall, these results indicate that dynamic regulation of gene expression and RNA synthesis is necessary to elicit lasting plastic change and stable memory.

There are also more inferential findings that are consistent with a necessity for transcriptional regulation for L-LTP induction and memory formation. Knockout of CaMKIV, a calmodulin-dependent kinase that regulates the activity of the CREB/CREB binding

protein complex, also leads to a loss of L-LTP and long-term memory (see Figure 1 and references 7–8). Given the prominent role of ERK in regulating gene expression, it is intriguing that ERK activation also is necessary for L-LTP and long-term memory (9–12).

A final piece of more direct block evidence comes from investigating expression of the immediate early gene (IEG) Arc. Arc mRNA is normally present at low levels, and is up-regulated by L-LTP-inducing stimulation. Inhibition of Arc message with antisense to that message leads to an attenuation of L-LTP (13). This finding indicates a necessity for Arc up-regulation in L-LTP. As Arc is one of the genes known to be up-regulated with L-LTP-inducing stimulation and memory formation, this is additional evidence for a requirement for altered gene expression in the induction of these phenomena. Overall, published results using the "block" experimental approach are consistent with a necessity for altered regulation of gene expression in L-LTP induction and long-term memory consolidation.

Prediction Two: changes in gene and protein expression should occur with L-LTP-inducing stimulation and memory formation. There are a wide variety of published experiments that demonstrate that alterations in gene expression occur with L-LTP and memory. The following mRNAs have been documented to increase after L-LTP-inducing stimulation, long-term memory formation, or both: zif268/krox24; krox20; Arc; fos; and related proteins, BDNF; C/EBP; MAP2;

TABLE 1   The Case for Gene Expression in Late-Long-Term Potentiation

Experiment Type	Finding	References
Block	Block of L-LTP with protein synthesis inhibitors	(76)
	Block of L-LTP with RNA synthesis inhibitors	(1–2, 77)
	Loss of L-LTP with CREB KOs	(1–3)
	Block of L-LTP with Arc antisense	(13)
	Loss of L-LTP with CaMKIV KO	(7–8, 78)
	Loss of L-LTP with zif268 KO	(6)
	Loss of L-LTP with c-rel KO	(21)
Measure	Increased zif268/krox24 mRNA	(40)
	Increased krox20	(44)
	Increased expression of fos, jun IEG mRNAs	(40, 42–43)
	Increased CREB phosphorylation	(24, 34–35)
	Increased CRE read-out	(12, 79)
	Increased elk-1 phosphorylation	(35)
	Increased Arc/Arg3.1 mRNA expression	(13, 54, 59)
	Increased AMPA receptor protein	(51)
	Increased BDNF message	(46, 80)
	Increased tissue plasminogen activator message	(47)
	Increased C/EBP beta (in long-term memory)	(45)
	Increased HOMER	(11, 53, 72)
	Increased MAP kinase phosphatase-1	(35, 50)
	Increased SSAT message	(49)
	Increased MAP2 message	(81)
Mimic	Constitutively active CREB augments L-LTP induction	(14)

HOMER; and the GluR1 AMPA receptor (see references in Table 1). In addition, phosphorylation of the transcription factors CREB and elk-1 are known to increase with L-LTP and memory, again indicative of an acute activation of transcriptional regulation. An elegant series of studies from Dan Storm's laboratory demonstrated increased read-out of CREB-regulated genes with L-LTP and memory. These investigators engineered a CRE-driven beta-galactosidase express-ing transgenic mouse that allows monitoring of CREB-mediated gene expression. Use of this mouse allowed a direct demonstration of a CRE-mediated increase in gene expression with LTP-inducing stimulation and long-term memory formation. Thus, overall the data supporting the "measure" approach are quite solid, and indicative of a role for altered gene expression in L-LTP and memory.

Prediction Three: artificially increasing the capacity of the CNS for transcription of the appropriate genes should lead to an enhancement of L-LTP and long-term memory. In a fascinating series of studies two groups have shown that genetically-engineered mice that have augmented CREB function have increased L-LTP and improved memory formation. Hippocampal slices from these mice exhibit a decreased threshold for L-LTP induction. These important observations are in agreement with the idea that altered CREB-mediated gene expression is involved in long-term memory, and are a general test of the "mimic" experi-mental prediction.

III. SIGNALING MECHANISMS

Having reviewed, in a very general sense, the data supporting a role for altered gene expression in long-term memory, we now turn our attention to discussing the mechanisms by which memory-associated changes in gene expression are achieved. How does the plas-ticity-triggering calcium elevation at the synaptic spine get a signal to the nucleus? By way of starting to answer this question it is important to emphasize that this is a complex multi-stage process. The core signal transduction component is calcium activation of kinase cascades that phosphorylate transcription factors and thereby regulate gene expression.

However, many other signals get integrated into this basic process. There are pathways controlling nuclear translocation of transcription factors and kinases. Action potential firing that is a result of the initial synaptic depolarization is important for gener-ating calcium signals in the cell body. "Transcription factors" should really be thought of as multipro-tein complexes that integrate a variety of signals in order to compute whether gene expression should be altered. A single gene can integrate the output of mul-tiple transcriptional regulatory elements. Once the gene is transcribed there are mRNA processing and trafficking mechanisms that are subject to additional layers of regulation. Translation of the mRNA into pro-tein is subject to regulation, as we discussed in the last chapter. In L-LTP and long-lasting forms of memory

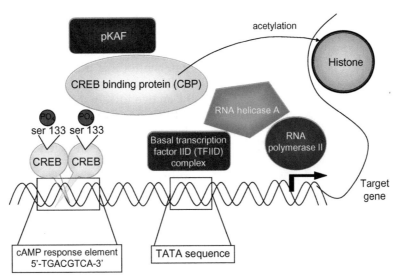

FIGURE 2 The CREB/CRE gene regulation system. Phosphorylated CREB recruits a supramolecular complex to the cyclicAMP response element (CRE) in DNA, triggering increased expression of downstream target genes. CBP, an accessory to CREB, facilitates gene expression by modulation of RNA polymerase activity and histone acetylation. Adapted from Shajwitz and Greenberg, (16).

there are likely multiple waves of altered gene expression, in part because one category of regulated genes codes for transcription factors which when expressed can lead to secondary alterations in gene expression. There are mysterious but clearly extant mechanisms for temporal and spatial integration of signals in the nucleus. There are mechanisms for controlling gene expression that involve relief of inhibitory constraints, such as histone acetylation. Transcriptional repressors also impinge on mechanisms for expression of target genes, and these are themselves subject to regulation.

Instead of discussing all these processes in detail, we will distill the essential processes into a working model of how gene expression is regulated in long-term memory. Thus, it is helpful to break down memory-related mechanisms for regulating gene expression into several basic components to help organize your thinking:

1. A core signal transduction cascade linking calcium to the transcription factor CREB.
2. Modulatory influences that impinge on this cascade.
3. Additional transcription factors besides CREB that may be involved.
4. Genes targeted in memory.
5. mRNA targeting and transport.

Of course, the altered mRNA expression must be converted into a physiologic read-out by some mechanism, giving us a more hypothetical sixth category:

6. Effects of the gene products on synaptic structure.

I will organize the following sections around these six topics.

A. A Core Signal Transduction Cascade Linking Calcium to the Transcription Factor CREB

Introduction to Gene Transcription

Genes are stretches of DNA that have the capacity to code for a functional protein. Transcription of the DNA into a protein-encoding mRNA begins with a transcriptional promoter complex binding to a TATA sequence ("TATA Box") in the DNA sequence, which promotes association of the RNA polymerase II complex with the DNA and transcription at the transcription start site (see Figure 2 and references 15–16). This transcription machinery is regulated by transcription factors that bind to upstream regulatory elements (REs), i.e., DNA sequences that the transcription factors specifically recognize. The transcription factors and their associated co-activators bind to their REs and enable gene transcription of the downstream target gene. Transcription factor activity is regulated by a variety of post-translational processes including phosphorylation, redox state, ubiquitination, and degradation of associated inhibitory proteins. Co-activators, whose activity is typically necessary for the transcription factor *per se* to be active, typically bind to the promoter complex, and/or acetylate histones locally to free up DNA for transcription. We will discuss this mechanism in more detail in Section IV of this chapter.

A diagram of the basic structure of the cyclicAMP response element binding protein (CREB) transcriptional complex is given in Figure 2 for reference purposes. A more realistic picture of CREB bound to the DNA double helix is given in Figure 3. The CRE (5'-TGACGTCA-3') is the DNA sequence identified by

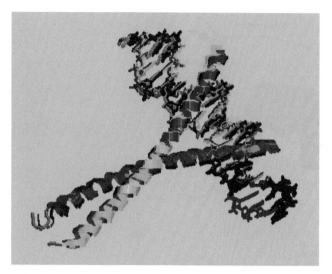

FIGURE 3 Crystal structure of CREB bound to the CRE. Data obtained from the Brookhaven national protein structure data bank and rendered with Rasmol. Figure courtesy of Jennifer Gatchel.

CREB. The activity of CREB is regulated by phosphorylation at Ser133, which can be phosphorylated by PKA, CaMKII and CaMKIV, MSK1, and RSK2 (among many others). This phosphorylation event, however, is not sufficient for transcriptional activation; binding of CREB binding protein (CBP) is also necessary. CBP binding and activation is itself regulated by phosphorylation, in particular phosphorylation and activation by CaMKIV is relevant in the present context. CBP does a number of things—it binds to phosphorylated CREB, it helps bridge CREB to the promoter complex structurally, and it is a histone acetyl transferase (HAT) enzyme that acetylates histone lysine residues to free up bound DNA (see Figure 2).

I use CREB as an example because, as described above, it has been directly implicated in long-term memory formation. In the next section we will focus our discussion on how the calcium trigger for long-term memory signals to CREB and its associated proteins. The relevant pathways are summarized in Figure 4. However, it is very important to note that CREB is just one transcription factor that has been implicated in long-term memory, and we are using it as an example. Other transcription factors that are known to be involved in memory include the serum response element (SRE)-recognizing transcription factor elk-1, nuclear factor kappa B (NFκB), c-rel (an NFκB family member), C/EBP, krox20, and zif268.

In our model, memory-inducing calcium elevation post-synaptically activates adenyl cyclase I/VIII, and via b-raf activates MEK (reviewed in reference 17). In addition, as described in the last chapter, ras-coupled receptors and PKC-coupled receptors can also feed into the MEK pathway. The product of MEK activation,

dually phosphorylated ERK (ppERK) is then translocated into the nucleus. This nuclear translocation of ppERK is a regulated process—both BDNF and PKA can control this translocation by mechanisms that are still being investigated.

Active ERK in the nucleus is most likely coupled to CREB phosphorylation either via activation of a member of the pp90rsk family of S6 kinases, RSK2, or via activation of the mitogen-and-stress activated Kinase MSK1, or both. Ser133 of CREB is not a substrate for ERK; ERK's effect is indirect through activating RSK2 or MSK1. Phosphorylation of Ser133 by these kinases recruits the CREB binding protein, CBP, to the initiator complex, and thereby promotes transcription. CBP activation is itself regulated by CaMKIV phosphorylation, and most likely both CBP activation by CaMKIV, and ERK regulation of RSK2/MSK1/CREB are necessary events for L-LTP induction (see Figure 4 and references 7,18).

This model is consistent with a wide variety of evidence demonstrating that AC knockouts, inhibition of PKA and ERK, and loss of CaMKIV function all lead to loss of L-LTP and long-term memory (see Table 1 and reference 19). Also, the various positive data demonstrating CREB phosphorylation and CRE-mediated gene expression with memory, described in Table 1, motivate this model.

However, one might wonder what happened to CaMKII and PKA phosphorylation of CREB, since these kinases are perfectly capable of phosphorylating ser133 in CREB. The short answer is that available data do *not* indicate that PKA and CaMKII have access to CREB, at least in rat hippocampus and dentate gyrus. A variety of experiments have shown that CaMKII inhibitors do not affect synaptic activity-dependent CREB phosphorylation in these systems, in fact if anything, CaMKII is an inhibitor of CREB through phosphorylation at a site other than Ser133. Also, PKA cannot cause elevated CREB phosphorylation without going through the ERK cascade (20). Surprisingly, the cAMP pathway utilizes the MAPK cascade as an obligatory intermediate in regulating CREB phosphorylation in the hippocampus.

B. Modulatory Influences that Impinge on this Cascade

One of the most important co-regulators of this cascade is CaMKIV. Mice deficient in CaMKIV signaling have deficits in long-term synaptic plasticity, memory, hippocampal CREB phosphorylation, and CREB-mediated gene expression (see Figure 1 and references 7–8,22). As mentioned above, CaMKIV acts by phosphorylating ser 301 in CBP, co-regulating the CREB/CBP complex (7). Regulation of CaMKIV likely

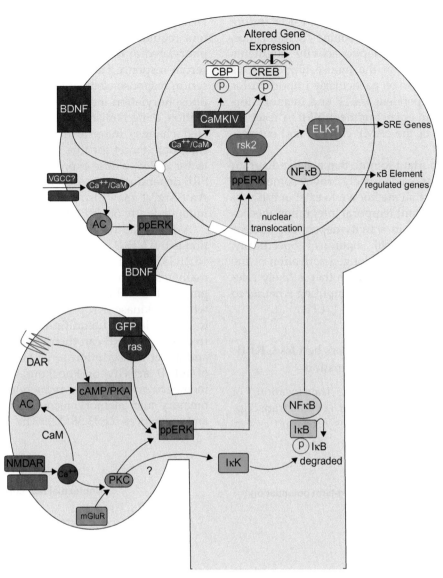

FIGURE 4 Activity-dependent regulation of gene expression in neurons. See text for details and discussion.

depends on calmodulin translocation to the nucleus, an interesting attribute that may confer a capacity for temporal integration onto the nuclear read-out of cellular calcium signals (23). The pathways for nuclear calcium signaling are still being worked out, but they may be initiated by local action-potential-dependent calcium flux at the cell body coupled with ancillary signals from the synapse (24–26). The bottom line of all this is that it is important to remember that increased CREB phosphorylation at Ser133 is not sufficient to give altered gene expression—an additional CaMKIV-mediated signal through the CREB co-activator CBP is also necessary for altered gene expression (7). Thus, the ERK and CaMKIV pathways act in concert to trigger memory-associated altered gene expression.

The growth factor BDNF also triggers modulatory mechanisms that feed into the CREB regulation cascade.

BDNF is released with L-LTP inducing stimulation (27–28) and likely contributes to L-LTP induction and long-term memory by two means (see Figure 4). First, it may act via *ras* to help directly activate the MEK/ERK pathway, a mechanism for augmenting ERK-dependent gene expression (29). In addition, BDNF, by mechanisms still being worked out, controls phospho-ERK translocation into the nucleus, providing a gate-keeping role for triggering lasting changes (30–31).

Additional modulatory signal integration mechanisms also can operate at the synaptic level by augmenting activation of the ERK/CREB pathway. Many possibilities along these lines have already been discussed in earlier chapters, when we talked about the numerous complexities of regulating the level of calcium achieved post-synaptically with LTP-inducing stimulation. One specific example that has received attention experimentally is regulation of L-LTP induction by dopamine (DA; 32). Dopamine co-application during theta-frequency synaptic activity augments the induction of L-LTP. In the mouse hippocampus this pathway appears to be particularly important for generating CREB-dependent L-LTP and memory formation (5). Dopamine may augment NMDA receptor activation by way of the cAMP cascade and enhancing ERK activation.

Finally, it is important to note that a static diagram such as Figure 4 cannot adequately convey some of the kinetic complexities that are known to exist in this system. There are important temporal integration mechanisms that play a role in activity-dependent nuclear signaling in hippocampal neurons. Specifically, repeated stimuli lead to a prolonged activation of the ERK/CREB pathway, a mechanism that is likely relevant for the system in its role of computing whether to trigger altered gene expression and L-LTP.

C. Additional Transcription Factors besides CREB that are Involved in Memory Formation

The activation and nuclear translocation of ERK can lead to the activation of several transcription factors besides CREB, such as *Elk*-1 and *c-Myc*.

Historically prominent among the transcription factors regulated by ERK is Elk-1 which, when phosphorylated at multiple sites by ERK, cooperates with serum response factor (SRF) to drive transcription of serum response element (SRE)-controlled genes. Elk-1 phosphorylation increases with L-LTP-inducing stimulation, a mechanism which likely triggers SRE-mediated changes in gene expression (35). One specific candidate target for this pathway is the transcription factor zif268, whose expression is mediated by Elk-1/SRE dependent processes. In addition, the target gene Arc/Arg3.1 may also be regulated by this pathway independently of CREB (36).

A final pathway contributing to memory formation is the NFκB pathway (see Figure 4 and references 15,21,33,37). NFκB is a transcription factor that normally resides in the cytoplasm, bound to an inhibitory partner IκB (inhibitor of kappaB). NFκB is activated when the kinase IKK phosphorylates IκB, which leads to loss of IκB by ubiquitin-mediated proteolysis. The free, active, NFκB can then translocate to the nucleus and affect transcription of its target genes. Inhibition of NFκB activity or knockout of the NFκB family member *c-rel* leads to a reduction of both long-term memory and memory reconsolidation (see Figure 5 and references 21,33,38–39). The precise mechanism

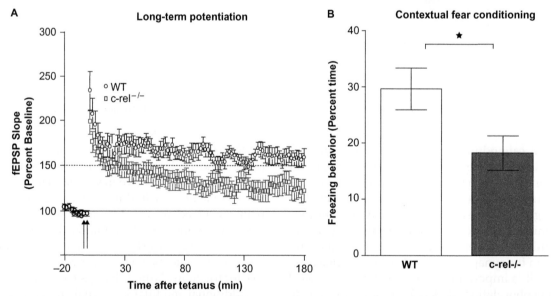

FIGURE 5   Impaired long-term synaptic plasticity in c-rel$^{-/-}$ mice. (A) LTP at Schaffer collateral synapses in hippocampal slices of c-rel$^{-/-}$ mice was compared with wildtype littermate controls, after two trains of 100 Hz stimulation for 1 second separated by 20 seconds at 30 °C. c-rel$^{-/-}$ slices exhibited significantly less potentiation after LTP induction relative to wildtype littermate slices. F[1,1504] = 433.00, P <0.0001; n = 10 wildtype and 9 c-rel$^{-/-}$ (male only). c-rel$^{-/-}$ mice have impaired hippocampus-dependent fear memory. c-rel$^{-/-}$ and wildtype littermate mice were trained in two different fear conditioning paradigms, and then tested for freezing behavior. Hippocampus-dependent long-term memory formation was assessed via a contextual fear conditioning paradigm, and amygdala-dependent long-term memory formation was assessed via a cued fear conditioning paradigm. Mice were trained with modest training protocol (one exposure to cue and shock), and freezing behavior was measured 24 hours after training. (B) In the contextual test, c-rel$^{-/-}$ mice had a significant deficit in freezing behavior assessed 24 hours after training (*P <0.05). n = 9 wildtype (seven male, two female) and 9 c-rel$^{-/-}$ (seven male, two female). Figure and legend from (21). Copyright Cold Springs Harbor Laboratory Press 2008.

of NFκB activation in memory is unclear at this time; however, interesting possible mechanisms include activation by reactive oxygen species like superoxide, direct phosphorylation of IκB by PKC, or indirect activation of IKK by PKC.

D. Gene Targets in Late-Long-Term Potentiation

This is one of the most fascinating aspects of investigation of the role of transcription-regulating processes in memory formation. This is also an area where we have just started to scratch the surface in uncovering the relevant players. Identifying the gene targets of activity-dependent transcriptional regulation in L-LTP specifically, and in long-term memory generally, will be a watershed event in understanding the molecular basis of memory. Clearly, identifying the genes whose expression changes with LTP (and learning) will give us needed clues concerning how very long-lasting changes in synaptic function are achieved in the CNS.

I have already listed some known gene targets in memory as part of the measure-related experiments supporting a role for altered gene expression in L-LTP and long-term memory (see Table 1). In the following section I will reorganize the list along some functional lines. The take-home message from this section is three-fold. First, we are clearly at an early stage with these studies because not many candidates have been identified. Second, where target genes have been identified, the functions of their gene products suggest that there are many complex post-gene-read-out layers of signal transduction involved in memory. Third, even with the paucity of targets that have been identified so far, some interesting themes have begun to emerge.

Transcription Factors

It is notable that a prominent category of L-LTP-associated genes encode transcription factors (see Figure 6). One member of this category is one of the first memory-associated genes identified: zif/268 (aka krox24 and NGFI-A (6,11,40–43)). Zif/268 encodes a transcription factor of the zinc finger family, and recent findings indicate that zif/268 may be a target of the elk-1 transcription factor cascade (35). The zif268 homolog krox20, another zinc-finger transcription factor, is also regulated in L-LTP (44). The target genes regulated by zif/268 and krox20 are still being investigated.

Zif/268 is a member of the immediate early gene (IEG) family of proteins, as are many of the other gene targets we will discuss such as BDNF, t-PA, and others. IEGs are rapidly responding activity- and signal-regulated genes in a wide variety of cell types. Transcription factors of the fos/jun family are prototype IEGs and a variety of early work showed that fos- and jun-family members were also regulated in memory. However, subsequent work has suggested that fos/jun regulation may be more of a general activity-related read-out as opposed to a specific signal associated with memory *per se*. Nevertheless, fos/jun signaling appears to be a likely component of the cascades set

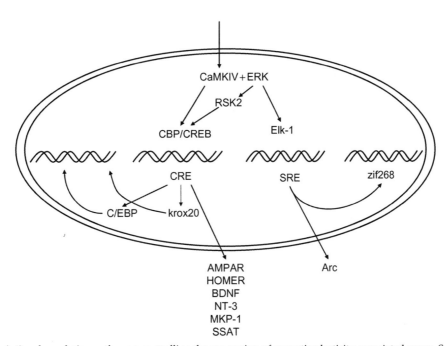

FIGURE 6 Transcriptional regulation pathways controlling the expression of synaptic plasticity-associated genes. See text for discussion.

off by memory-inducing stimulation, adding another example of transcription factor regulation to the list of gene targets in play in memory formation.

An additional transcription factor worth noting in the context of secondary waves of transcription factor regulation is C/EBP. C/EBP is the CCAAT enhancer binding protein, a known secondary target of CREB regulation in *Aplysia* sensory neurons. Cristina Alberini's laboratory has shown that the consolidation of mammalian long-term memory is associated with a relatively late (several hours post-training) elevation of C/EBP that is necessary for memory consolidation (45). These interesting findings support the idea that late waves of altered gene expression contribute to memory consolidation involving hippocampal neurons.

Thus, we see that at least three (C/EBP, zif/268, and krox 20) and probably several more transcription factor-encoding genes are up-regulated in long-term memory. Overall, these findings that transcription factors are targets of the gene expression system of long-term memory suggest that plasticity-associated gene regulation will be quite complex. The findings indicate the likelihood that the initial triggering of altered gene expression with memory-inducing stimulation sets off secondary waves of altered gene expression. The potential for exponential expansion of altered gene expression in memory, along with combinatorics for secondary signals impinging on these mechanisms, appears somewhat daunting. However, parsing out these complex pathways will be necessary to answer a fundamental question in biology—how neuronal cell surface activity impinges on the genome in order to trigger lasting functional changes.

Signaling Molecules

A second category of memory-associated genes encode signaling molecules. As with the transcription factors regulated in memory, increased production of signaling molecules and regulators of signal transduction cascades suggests the triggering of a variety of post-genome secondary effects by memory-inducing stimulation.

One of the most interesting molecules in this category is brain-derived neurotrophic factor (BDNF). BDNF gene expression increases with L-LTP-inducing stimulation, along with that of a related growth factor, neurotrophin-3 (46). This likely occurs via CRE-regulated expression as the BDNF gene has the necessary sequence in its upstream region. BDNF is particularly intriguing because, as we have already discussed, it is a modulator of LTP induction and is furthermore capable of triggering lasting increases in synaptic strength in its own right. Thus, increased BDNF expression could play a role in modulating subsequent

memory-associated plasticity in a temporal integration fashion, or could itself trigger lasting plastic change. In the limit, BDNF, which couples to the ERK/CREB cascade, could trigger a self-perpetuating feedback mechanism for perpetually maintaining increased synaptic strength. While this idea is quite speculative, it provides an appealing example of a potential self-reinforcing mechanism that could survive protein turnover and last the lifetime of the animal.

Another signaling molecule gene regulated by L-LTP-inducing stimulation codes is for tissue plasminogen activator (t-PA). t-PA is a secreted protease that has the capacity to modulate the extracellular matrix structure. t-PA knockout mice have defects in L-LTP and memory (47). Potentially, t-PA could serve in a long-term regulatory role through increasing active products in the extracellular space via its known role of converting pro-hormones into hormones. Another molecule that has been proposed to play a similar role is matrix metalloprotease-9, whose gene is regulated in an activity-dependent fashion and which cleaves extracellular matrix molecules (48). Both t-PA and MMP-9 might also play a role in regulating the structure of the synaptic region.

Overall, no clear and simple model for the role of memory-associated genes affecting signal transduction emerges at this time. However, some interesting possibilities exist, and the available data are consistent with diverse secondary effects downstream of altered gene regulation. Similarly with the transcription factor category of targets, the regulation of signaling molecules with long-term memory suggests that complicated cascades of biochemical sequelae will be triggered by memory-inducing stimulation.

Structural Proteins

In contrast to the signaling molecules described above, the few structural proteins that have been identified as potential gene targets in memory bring us back to tried-and-true functional players in synaptic transmission. Most straightforward in this context is the AMPA receptor itself (51). L-LTP is associated with increased AMPA receptor synthesis at the protein level (although the genetic basis for this has not been worked out). This translates in a conceptually straightforward way into a mechanism for increasing synaptic strength.

The metabotropic receptor scaffolding protein HOMER has also been identified as a gene regulated in L-LTP (11,52–53). This is interesting, because this protein is a part of the synaptic spine structural complex interacting with metabotropic glutamate receptors, as we discussed in an earlier chapter. In addition, mGluRs have been implicated as controlling dendritic spine protein synthesis, and increased HOMER expression might play a role in facilitating or regulating local protein synthesis as one component of a mechanism for maintaining increased synaptic strength.

This last idea is reasonable, considering that there is another target of memory-associated gene expression that is involved in the same types of processes—Arc. We have already discussed Arc in the context of local dendritic protein synthesis (see Chapter 9 and reference 54 for a review). Arc mRNA is rapidly induced by LTP-inducing stimulation and memory formation. Moreover, as we will discuss in the next section, this mRNA is selectively localized to recently-active synaptic regions, and is subject to selective expression by local protein synthesis mechanisms. Arc is a cytoskeleton-associated protein that may be involved in stabilizing structural changes at potentiated synapses, as inhibition of Arc synthesis disrupts maintenance of LTP and memory (13).

Thus, it is palatable to think that increased expression of AMPA receptors, HOMER and Arc, might contribute to a stable increase in synaptic strength as a mechanism for expressing long-term memory. As more pieces of the puzzle become available the applicability of this model will become clear.

Overall, while we are at a very early stage with these types of studies, some tantalizing themes have begun to emerge from the identified gene targets in memory. First, transcription factors are up-regulated, suggesting that secondary waves of gene expression will be involved in memory induction and consolidation. Second, structural proteins at the synapse appear to be targets that are up-regulated, suggesting the hypothesis that altered gene expression is a component of triggering and maintaining long-term structural changes at the synapse in memory (55–56). We will return to this idea in more general terms in a subsequent section of this chapter. Finally, signaling molecules and modulators of plasticity-related signal transduction mechanisms are targets of altered gene expression in memory. Particularly intriguing molecules in this context are molecules like BDNF, which are themselves capable of triggering long-term change and promoting activity-dependent long-term change. This suggests the interesting idea that positive feedback mechanisms might be triggered that provide a self-reinforcing component necessary for perpetually maintaining synaptic potentiation. Indeed, the general necessity for this type of mechanism in memory stabilization was discussed in Chapter 3 of this book.

E. mRNA Targeting and Transport

L-LTP, a protein-synthesis-dependent phenomenon, can be selectively induced at particular synapses, or at least particular dendritic regions. Considering these data leads us to the hypothetical necessity for localization of newly-synthesized mRNAs (or proteins) at recently activated synapses, so that the altered mRNA expression necessary for memory is manifest appropriately at these potentiated synapses. This brings us to the final question that we will think about in the context of the cell biology of memory: how is it that the new gene products get expressed at the right place among the multitude of synapses in a neuronal dendritic tree? It is known that L-LTP is synapse-specific—how is it that the gene products get targeted to the right synapses in order to increase synaptic strength appropriately? This process is still mysterious, but it is actively under investigation. However, several useful insights are already available, in large part from studies of regulation of induction and expression of the mRNA for Arc/Arg3.1.

It is useful to think of the Arc messenger RNA as a prototype for studying the regulation of the distribution of new gene products in the neuron (reviewed in references 57–58). As we have already discussed, Arc/Arg3.1 was discovered as a gene product induced by activity in general and LTP in particular (13,54,59). Arc, like many of the other L-LTP-associated gene products we have been discussing, is an immediate early gene. Like the other IEGs, its increased expression is transient, which facilitates experimental study because there is a low pre-stimulus level of its mRNA. Finally and most importantly, once Arc mRNA is expressed, the mRNA is selectively localized to active synapses, or synapses that have been potentiated (see Figure 7). Thus, Arc regulation likely represents a microcosm of activity-dependent, selectively targeted gene products in the neuron.

Returning to our original question: how is it that mRNAs end up at the right synapses? Two broad possibilities present themselves. One possibility is that mRNAs leave the nucleus with "addresses" that send them to the right spot. The second possibility is that mRNAs are sent throughout the neuron and are selectively captured at the appropriate synapses. Studies of Arc indicate that the second scenario is the correct one. Newly-synthesized Arc mRNA is distributed throughout the dendrites, presumably by diffusion but also potentially by mRNA carrier proteins associated with the cytoskeleton. The Arc mRNA is then "captured," or concentrated, at active synapses.

Thus, the targeting process appears to be locally initiated and controlled, and dependent on biochemical processes restricted to a particular synaptic region. The mRNA is not targeted specifically to a predefined dendritic region as it leaves the nucleus. There is no address on the mRNA when it leaves the nucleus—the mRNA is sent out globally and sequestered locally.

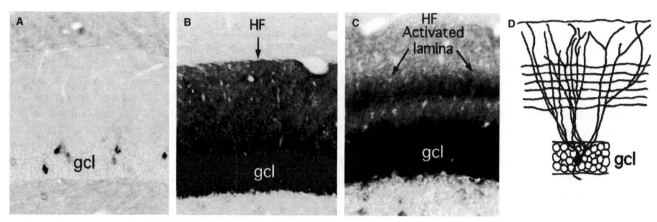

FIGURE 7   Activity-dependent ARC expression and dendritic localization. Newly-synthesized Arc mRNA is selectively targeted to dendritic domains that have been synaptically activated. The photomicrographs illustrate the distribution of Arc mRNA as revealed by *in situ* hybridization in: (A) nonactivated dentate gyrus; (B) two hours after a single electroconvulsive seizure; and (C) and after delivering high-frequency trains to the medial perforant path over a two hour period. Note the uniform distribution of Arc mRNA across the dendritic laminae after an ECS, and the prominent band of labeling in the middle molecular layer after high-frequency stimulation of the perforant path. (D) Schematic illustration of the dendrites of a typical dentate granule cell and the pattern of termination of medial perforant path projections. HF, hippocampal fissure; GCL, granule cell layer. Figure from Steward and Worley, (57). (A) and (B) reproduced with permission. Copyright Elsevier Science 2001. (D) reproduced with permission. Copyright Elsevier Science 1998.

If this is the general mechanism for neuronal mRNA targeting (and there is no reason to think it isn't), this type of mechanism eliminates an enormously complex trafficking problem. mRNAs do not have to have to be pre-addressed—local demands can dictate their disposition.

An additional implication of this finding is that induction signals from the dendrites to the nucleus, such as those processes we discussed in Section I of this chapter, can also be "unaddressed." The synapse-to-nucleus signal does not need a return address on it, a signal arriving at the genome can originate from any synapse or dendritic region and its point of origin is immaterial. The genome simply has to respond appropriately to the signal with an increased read-out, and local activity-dependent mechanisms in the dendrites will ensure that the right synapses capture the product.

The mechanism for the appropriate capture of mRNAs at potentiated synapses is unknown, but the basic phenomenon is, of course, highly reminiscent of the synaptic tagging observation described in the last chapter. As we discussed earlier, a parsimonious model for synaptic capture is simply to invoke persisting signals already localized at potentiated synapses, such as autonomously active CaMKII or PKC, as the root of the capture signal. A similar mechanism has already been proposed to operate in site-specific facilitation of *Aplysia* sensory neuron synapses by Wayne Sossin and his colleagues (60).

One aspect of the targeting and capture mechanism that seems clear is that an mRNA-binding protein of some sort must be involved. After all, *a priori* it is clear that an mRNA must bind to something in order

to have its diffusion restricted to a particular domain. There are several interesting candidate molecules that are known mRNA-binding proteins, and thus might participate in mRNA capture at dendrites (reviewed in references 58 and 61). One appealing possibility is the fragile X mRNA binding protein (FMRP) that we discussed in the last chapter. Activity-dependent synthesis of FMRP might provide a mechanism for mRNA capture. Another candidate that, at a minimum, is involved in dendritic mRNA trafficking (if not synapse-specific localization) is the staufen protein (62). Staufen is an mRNA-binding protein localized to dendrites that is involved in mRNA targeting in a variety of systems. A final possibility is the cytoplasmic polyadenylation element binding protein (CPEB, *not* to be confused with the transcription factor C/EBP (33). The CPEBs are mRNA-binding proteins that also regulate translation of mRNAs. Again, I emphasize that the mechanisms for targeting are unknown, and that these are just possibilities that have been identified as potential players.

Although the mechanisms are unknown, it is clear that the specifically localized Arc mRNA is converted into a localized increase in Arc protein. There is no need to invoke a specific mechanism for this—it can simply be accomplished by local protein synthesis. Arc might be handled by the same mechanisms that are used for the synthesis of proteins from mRNAs that are expressed constitutively, such as CaMKII and MAP2.

What is it that the Arc protein does once it is made at the right synapses? Although the function of Arc is unknown, there are tantalizing clues. It is known from various studies that Arc is part of the NMDAR supramolecular complex. Also, Arc is known to be a cytoskeleton-associated protein, which is part of how it got its name (*Activity-regulated cytoskeleton-associated protein*). Thus, Arc may be part of a local receptor-complex stabilizing structure or even a component of the specific NMDAR/AMPAR stabilizing mechanism that was described in the last chapter. This is, of course, speculative, but it at least allows the possibility of directly translating an increase in Arc protein into an increase in synaptic strength.

In summary, Arc is an interesting proof-of-principle molecule. Studies of Arc have demonstrated that activity-dependent mechanisms of mRNA localization exist in neurons. They have given important initial insights into some of the strategies the neuron uses to solve the problem of targeting altered gene products to the right synapses, and highlight an important role for localized protein synthesis at activated synapses. What remains is to figure out the detailed biochemical mechanisms for these processes, and to increase our understanding of how local protein synthesis gets converted into potentiated synaptic transmission locally. Also, it is clear that identifying the molecular identity of the "synaptic tag" is a high priority, in order to understand the bridging mechanisms for the transition of short-term plasticity into long-term functional changes.

F. Effects of the Gene Products on Synaptic Structure

Consideration of Arc as a molecule contributing to L-LTP also introduces a number of very important considerations about constraints on maintenance mechanisms for very long-lasting synaptic potentiation. The half-life of the Arc protein is a few hours: think about the implications of this fact. The Arc message increases transiently (about half an hour) and returns to a low basal level. The mRNA is concentrated at the right synapses and translated into protein, which is broken down with a half-life of a few hours. In the absence of Arc mRNA, which has already decayed to basal levels, this protein cannot be replenished. Thus, if Arc (or any other protein with similar regulation and kinetics) participates in synaptic potentiation, this mechanism can only allow potentiation to be maintained for less than a day. Induction of Arc or any similar protein is clearly not a maintenance mechanism for very long-lasting events.

While we have discussed this concept specifically in the context of Arc, because it is well-studied and known to be necessary for L-LTP (13), the generalization applies to any protein involved in very long-lasting effects in neurons. This consideration highlights the fact that triggering altered gene expression and protein synthesis is likely an induction mechanism for long-lasting changes, but not necessarily a maintenance mechanism. All proteins have a finite half-life; thus, maintaining long-lasting change requires an ongoing process. As we discussed in Chapter 3 of this book, in biochemical systems the route for achieving persisting effects in the face of breakdown and resynthesis of the component molecules involved is via a self-reinforcing chemical reaction. This is a controlled positive feedback loop wherein the activated molecule promotes its own resynthesis.

Given the constraint of protein turnover, how is it that really long-lasting changes in synaptic strength are achieved in long-term memory? In this section I will present a very general model for how this might happen. The model has two components: a change in synaptic structure due to altered expression of structural proteins; and a positive feedback mechanism to maintain these changes in the face of protein turnover.

The Structural Change

The structural change will be left undefined. It could be an increased number of AMPA receptors at a pre-existing spine, with its multitudinous receptor binding partners and cytoskeletal/PSD associations. It could be a new spine that splits off by spine fission, as has been proposed by a number of investigators (reviewed in reference 56). It could be the growth of entirely new spines from the dendritic shaft (55–56,63–66). These are variations of the same issue from a biochemical perspective—doubling the surface area of a spine is basically placing the same demand on the protein synthesis machinery as splitting off a second spine or growing a new spine from the dendrite. It's not that the question of which of these actually happens is uninteresting, or that they are even functionally identical, it's just that for the purposes of the present discussion they are equivalent in their impact. However, for ease of presenting the model I will take the case of increasing the post-synaptic size (equivalent to an increased number of receptors) in a pre-existing spine.

The mechanisms we have talked about so far in Sections III.C and III.E of this chapter have gotten us to the point of having a spine with increased AMPA receptor protein, hypothetically through Arc-dependent signaling mechanisms. What happens when the Arc signal decays and all of the newly synthesized AMPA receptors, etc., are undergoing continual breakdown and resynthesis? The new, larger PSD complex must have some way to perpetuate itself in its new, larger state. This requires some ongoing feedback signal that says "stay big." This could happen by any of a number of specific mechanisms, but this basic point is the important concept for this section of the chapter. Maintaining an increased synaptic connection over many protein half-lives in the face of complete breakdown and resynthesis of all the protein components that make up that synapse requires a self-reinforcing maintenance signal.

The specific mechanisms for this self-perpetuating signal are unknown at this point, but the possibilities fall into two broad categories. One possibility is that there is an ongoing activity integration mechanism that keeps the size of the synapse scaled to its pre-existing level. Variations of this idea are such things as a mechanism integrating the average spine calcium level (which would vary dependent on net synaptic activity, larger in a potentiated synapse), or a mechanism reading out the existing amount of receptor subunits present and maintaining it at a constant level. These are just specific examples for illustrative purposes; there are of course many other possibilities.

The second general possibility is that there is a unique molecule that is introduced into a potentiated synapse that makes a unique signal that is self-perpetuating. This molecule would, of course, need to have the capacity to increase synaptic size in parallel through impinging on the protein synthesis and receptor insertion machinery, etc.

We will focus our discussion on this second model, because there are some appealing specific candidate molecules that can perform the necessary functions that have been implicated experimentally as playing a role in memory. These are the cell adhesion molecules, specifically the integrins and cadherins (see Figures 8 and 9), and there are a number of appealing findings in this context. First, blocking the function of either cadherins or integrins blocks L-LTP (67–71). Second, this category of molecules functions in transducing signals from one cell directly to another, allowing for direct pre-synaptic-to-post-synaptic communication. Third, integrins couple to MAPK cascades in many cells to trigger local changes at the submembranous compartment, similar to what would be required to allow them to communicate locally with the protein synthesis machinery at synapses. This local control of protein synthesis could allow for both pleiotropic effects on synaptic function, and for self-reinforcing stimulation of their own synthesis. ERK coupling could also be used to communicate with the genome if necessary, for example allowing the nucleus to integrate total metabolic needs for ongoing gene expression across a large number of synapses. Fourth, these molecules classically function in regulating cell morphology through controlling the cytoskeleton (see Figure 8, also reviewed in reference 72), and in fact in

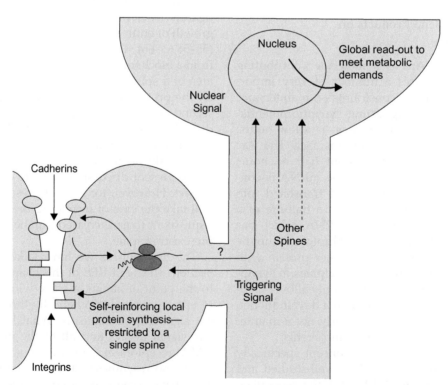

FIGURE 8 Hypothetical mechanisms contributing to activity-dependent changes in synaptic structure. Both local effects and nuclear signaling are likely involved in triggering and maintaining very long-term structural changes in synaptic spines. See text for additional discussion.

most cells these molecules are involved in maintaining long-lasting morphological differentiation. Thus, while the case for integrins and cadherins in maintaining long-lasting synaptic change is somewhat circumstantial at this point, these molecules appear to have all the attributes necessary to serve as self-perpetuating maintenance signals at dendritic spines.

Thus, the basic model for maintaining perpetual synaptic strengthening is as follows. Specific integrin and cadherin molecules have their mRNA expression increased and targeted to the right synapse in a fashion similar to Arc. The synthesis and insertion of these molecules into a synapse (hypothetically where they did not previously exist) leads to the following consequences: morphological changes and increased contact with the pre-synaptic terminal; enhanced ongoing AMPA receptor insertion; and localized self-stimulation of their ongoing synthesis and membrane insertion via stimulation of ERK or other signal transduction pathways. This last point fulfills the requirement for the generation of a self-perpetuating signal that can outlast the triggering events and maintain the potentiated state indefinitely.

While I have presented this brief model using specific molecules as examples, please keep in mind that the model is more in the vein of a thought experiment than a specific hypothesis. It serves to illustrate some of the important functions that must be subserved in

maintaining a life-long change in synaptic strength, especially the necessity of a self-perpetuating signal that can impinge on synaptic transmission. The specific candidate molecules I outlined are appealing possibilities, but they are still candidates at this point in time.

IV. EXPERIENCE-DEPENDENT EPIGENETIC MODIFICATIONS IN THE CENTRAL NERVOUS SYSTEM

In this section we will discuss recent discoveries demonstrating that experience can drive the production of *epigenetic* marks in the adult nervous system, and that the experience-dependent regulation of epigenetic molecular mechanisms in the mature CNS participates in the control of gene transcription underlying the formation of long-term memories. In the mammalian experimental systems investigated thus far, epigenetic mechanisms have been linked to associative fear conditioning, extinction of learned fear, and hippocampus-dependent spatial memory formation. Intriguingly, in one experimental system epigenetic marks at the level of chromatin structure (histone acetylation) have been linked to the recovery of memories that had appeared to be "lost," i.e., not available

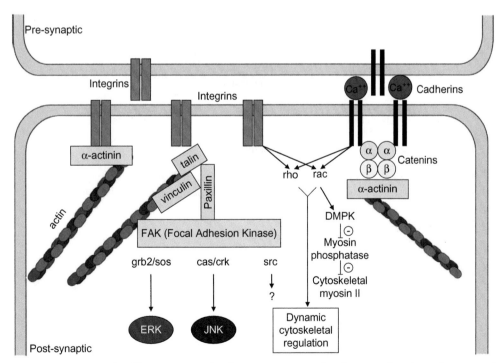

FIGURE 9   Signaling mechanisms utilized by integrins and cadherins. Integrins and cadherins, cell surface adhesions molecules, are prominent regulators of the cytoskeleton. Both families of molecules serve as cytoskeletal anchors and also regulate various signal transduction mechanisms. One role of activating these signal transduction processes is to dynamically regulate cytoskeletal structure and function. Via other pathways such as ERK, they might regulate local protein synthesis.

for recollection. In addition, environmental enrichment has long been known to have positive effects on memory capacity, and recent studies have suggested that these effects are at least partly due to the recruitment of epigenetic mechanisms by environmental enrichment. Taken together, these eclectic findings suggest a new perspective on experience-dependent dynamic regulation of epigenetic mechanisms, and their relevance to memory formation.

A. What is Epigenetics?

The term "epigenetics" is derived from Waddington (75). Waddington coined the term to describe a conceptual solution to a conundrum, a puzzle that arises as a fundamental consideration in developmental biology. All the different cells in your body have exactly the same genome, i.e., exactly the same DNA nucleotide sequence, with only a few exceptions in your reproductive and immune systems. Thus, your liver cells have exactly the same DNA as your neurons. However, those two types of cells are clearly vastly different in terms of the gene products that they produce. How can two cells have exactly the same DNA, but be so different? Especially when what *makes* them

different is that they produce different gene transcripts that are read directly from the identical DNA? Waddington coined the term epigenesis to describe the conceptual solution to this problem. Some level of mechanism must exist, he reasoned, that was above the level of the genes encoded by the DNA sequence, which controlled the DNA read-out. These are what we now refer to as epigenetic mechanisms. These epigenetic mechanisms specify in a neuron that genes A, C, D, L, … are turned into functional products, and in a liver cell that genes A, B, C, E, … are turned into functional products. Epigenetic marks are put in place during cell fate determination, and serve as a cellular information storage system perpetuating cellular phenotype over the lifespan (see Figure 10 and Box 1).

However, an additional aspect of epigenetic control of gene expression is now emerging from recent studies of epigenetic molecular mechanisms in the nervous system. Thus, evidence is accumulating that epigenetic mechanisms do not just contribute to phenotypic hard-wiring at the cellular level. Rather, in the nervous system, with its abundance of terminally-differentiated, non-dividing cells, epigenetic mechanisms also play a role in acute regulation of gene expression in response to memory-inducing experience. In addition, epigenetic

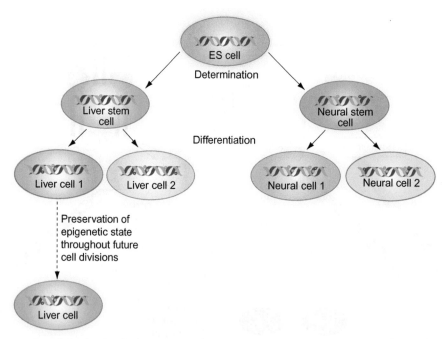

FIGURE 10   Memory at the cellular level. All embryonic cells begin with identical genotypes and phenotypes. External signals trigger developmental events that lead to the differentiation of cells. Mature cells become phenotypically distinct, but remain genotypically identical. The differences in gene expression persist in the face of numerous cell divisions, which indicate that they are self-sustaining. These developmentally-induced changes in gene expression in mature cells are mediated by epigenetic regulation of gene expression. Reproduced with permission from Levenson and Sweatt, *Nature Reviews Neuroscience*. Copyright Macmillan Publishers Ltd 2005.

BOX 1

NEURAL DEVELOPMENT AND DIFFERENTIATION

Neurons express a complement of proteins that are important for their function, but would be detrimental to other cell types. These include proteins that are involved in excitability, transmitter release, and the maintenance of transmembrane potential. Genes that are to be expressed in neurons, but not in other cell types, have a neuron-restrictive silencer element (NRSE) in their promoter (124–126). This regulatory element, which is approximately 21–24 base pairs long, can completely silence a gene in non-neuronal cells (126).

The first step toward understanding how NRSEs confer tissue-specific regulation of gene expression was identification of the transcription factors that bind to this regulatory element (see Figure). The RE1-silencing transcription factor (REST or NRSF) was the first transcription factor that was shown to bind to NRSEs and repress gene expression (127). The REST protein is ubiquitously expressed in cells outside the nervous system, where it acts to repress the expression of neuronal genes (127). Deletion of the REST gene or functional inhibition of the protein in non-neuronal tissues leads to erroneous expression of neuronal genes and embryonic lethality, whereas ectopic expression of REST in the nervous system inhibits expression of neuronal genes, and results in developmental dysfunction (127–129). Therefore, REST is important in determining whether a cell has a neuronal phenotype.

REST-dependent gene silencing requires the action of transcriptional co-repressors, two of which have been identified as the REST-binding proteins Sin3A and CoREST (130–132). The cellular expression pattern of Sin3A is nearly identical to that of REST, which indicates that most REST-dependent gene repression might be co-mediated by Sin3A (133). The expression of CoREST is more restricted, which indicates that it might be important in mediating specific gene expression patterns in subtypes of cells.

REST-mediated gene silencing requires modulation of chromatin structure. REST/Sin3A repressor complexes are associated with HDAC1, whereas REST/CoREST

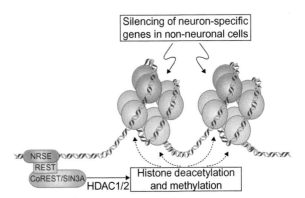

BOX 1 Epigenetics in nervous system development. The RE1-silencing transcription factor (REST)/REST Co-Repressor (CoREST) system. The NRSE upstream of genes to be silenced in non-neuronal cells recruits REST as a mediator of transcriptional repression. Sin3A, CoREST, and REST, acting in concert with additional factors such as HDAC1 and 2, leads to chromatin condensation and gene silencing. Reproduced with permission from Levenson and Sweatt, *Nature Reviews Neuroscience*. Copyright Macmillan Publishers Ltd 2005.

complexes with HDAC2 (131–132,134–135). Thus, REST-dependent gene silencing with either co-repressor seems to involve decreases in histone acetylation. CoREST has also been shown to associate with members of the hSWI-SNF complex, which is an ATP-dependent chromatin remodeling complex (136). Interestingly, REST/CoREST-dependent chromatin remodeling, including decreases in histone acetylation and increases in DNA methylation, does not seem to be restricted to the immediate region around an NRSE silencer sequence; rather, the formation of heterochromatin extends across several genes that flank an NRSE (137). These observations indicate that REST-dependent gene silencing, and thus cellular differentiation, involves the action of several proteins, which, through decreases in histone acetylation and/or increases in DNA methylation, ultimately mark DNA epigenetically for repression.

mechanisms appear to contribute to both psychiatric and neurological disorders. In retrospect, these roles for epigenetic molecular mechanisms are perhaps not surprising. Epigenetic mechanisms, even in their role in development, sit at the interface of the environment and the genome.

B. What are Epigenetic Marks and What do they do?

There are two basic molecular epigenetic mechanisms that are widely studied at present—regulation of chromatin structure through histone post-translational modifications and DNA methylation. Other epigenetic molecular mechanisms, such as regulation of gene expression through non-coding RNAs and prion protein-based mechanisms, are also known to exist, but we will not discuss them here.

The first major mechanism whereby the genome can be epigenetically marked is DNA methylation. Methylation of DNA is a direct chemical modification of a cytosine side-chain that adds a –CH$_3$ group through a covalent bond (see Figure 11). Methylation of DNA is catalyzed by a class of enzymes known as DNA methyltransferases (DNMTs) (76). DNMTs transfer methyl groups to cytosine residues within a continuous stretch of DNA, specifically at the 5′-position of the pyrimidine ring (82–83). Not all cytosines can be methylated; usually cytosines must be immediately followed by a guanine in order to be methylated (84–85). These "CpG" dinucleotide sequences are highly underrepresented in the genome relative to what would be predicted by random chance; however, about 70% of the CpG dinucleotides that are present are methylated (86). The rest of the normally unmethylated CpG dinucleotides occur in small clusters, known as "CpG islands" (see Figure 12 and references 87–88).

There are two variants of DNMTs: maintenance DNMTs and *de novo* DNMTs. The DNMT1 enzymatic isoform is the maintenance DNMT, DNMTs 3a and 3b are the *de novo* DNMT isoforms. Both maintenance and *de novo* DNMTs are expressed in most cells in the body. The two variants of DNMTs differ in one important respect, related to the conditions under which they will methylate DNA. *De novo* DNMTs methylate previously unmethylated CpG sites in DNA—sites which have no methyl-cytosine on either DNA strand. The maintenance DNMT isoform methylates hemi-methylated DNA—DNA which has a methylated CpG already present on one strand, but no methyl-cytosine on the complementary strand. These two different isoforms thereby serve two distinct roles in the cell. *De novo* DNMTs place new methylation marks on DNA, for example when specific genes are first silenced as part of cell fate determination. Maintenance DNMTs perpetuate methylation marks after cell division. They regenerate the methyl-cytosine marks on the newly-synthesized complementary DNA strand that arises from DNA replication. Thus, in summary: DNMT1, the maintenance DNMT, propagates epigenetic marks through cell generations in dividing cells, while DNMTs 3a and 3b, the *de novo* DNMTs, are responsible for laying down the initial patterns of DNA methylation when cell fate is determined.

What are the functional consequences of DNA methylation? In most cases that have been studied so far, methylation of DNA is associated with suppression of gene transcription, and in many cases extensive DNA methylation triggers complete silencing of the associated gene. In other words, methylation is a process whereby a gene can be functionally shut off. The precise molecular processes through which this occurs are complex, and an area of intense investigation at present. However, one simplified model is shown in Figure 13. In essence, methylation

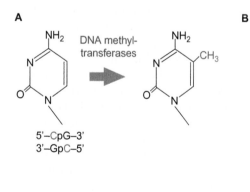

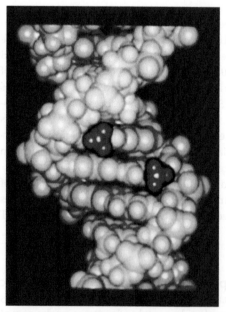

FIGURE 11   Methylation of cytosine side-chains in DNA. (A) The biochemical reaction catalyzed by DNA methyltransferases. (B) Methyl-cytosines in sites in a DNA double helix. The methyl groups are marked in red. Figure courtesy of the Environmental Mutagenesis Society, used with permission.

AGGGGAATTAGGGATACCCCAAGGGCTTCCGAGGGCTGAATCC**CG**GCAAGGGAAAAGG**CGCG**T**CG**TCCCC**T**T

TAAGCAGC**CG**CCCCGAATGGGTAT**CG**GTGG**CGCG**GCTGAGCAGGGAGGGGATAGGGG**CG**GCGCTGTCTG**A**C

CAAT**CG**AAGCTCAAC**CG**AAGAGCTAAATAATGTCTGACCCCAGTGCCTGG**CG**CTGGCTGAGCTCTGGGTGC

C**CG**CCGCTGC**CG**C**CG**GC**GCCG**GGG**CG**CACC**CG**CTGGCTGGCTGT**CG**CAC**GG**TCCCCATT**GCG**CC**CG**GGACTC

CC**CG**GCTTGGAGAAGGAAAC**CG**CCTGGGG**CGGCGCG**CCACCTC**CG**CCTGGCAGGCTTTGATGAGAC**CG**GGT

TCCCTCAGCT**CG**CCAC**CG**CTGCTTTGGGGCAGA**CG**AGAAAG**CG**CAC**GG**GGCCCAGGGCAGGG**CG**CAGGGAC

CAGGAGCGTGACAACAATGTGACTCCACTGC**CG**GGGATC**CG**AGAGCTTTGTGTGGACCCTGAGGTAGG**CG**A

CTGC**CG**GGG**CG**TGGGGCTAAG**CGCG**AGAGCTGGAGG**CGCG**TG**CG**CC**CG**GGAAAGTTGGCTAGGGGACTGAGA

AGTTGTGGGAC**CG**CATAACTT**CG**GCTTCACCTT**CG**TCC**CG**GGACAGC**GG**AGGG**CG**GGGTTGCTCCTGAGGA

G**CG**TTCTCC**CG**GGAGCCCACGACCC**CG**AGAGACAGC**GCG**ACCC**CG**GGAATCCCTTCAGTG**CG**AGAGAAAAA

GCCAAGGGAAGAGGACGACTTG**CG**CCATGGGAGCAAAGCCTG**CG**TCC**CG**GGGATCCC**CG**AAGTCCTCC**CG**C

AGA**CG**AGGAAGGGTGGTGAGAGAGATGTAGGGCAACAGCTG

FIGURE 12 A "CpG island" in the BDNF gene. CpG's are marked in red, and transcription start site is indicated by the arrow. Figure courtesy of Tania Roth and Farah Lubin.

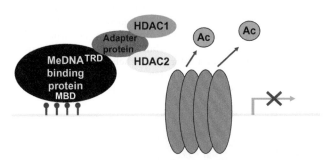

FIGURE 13 A simplified scheme for DNA methylation-dependent gene silencing. Methylation of cytosines at CpG dinucleotides (red lollipops) recruits methyl-DNA binding proteins locally to specific sites in the genome. All proteins that bind to methylated DNA have both a methyl-DNA binding domain (MBD) and a transcription-regulatory domain (TRD). The TRD recruits adapter proteins which in turn recruit histone deacetylases (HDACs). The HDACs alter chromatin structure locally through removing acetyl groups (Ac) from histone core proteins (gray spheres), leading to compaction of chromatin and transcriptional suppression. It is important to note that while this is the traditional and well-established role of methyl-DNA binding proteins in transcriptional regulation recent findings support the idea that DNA methylation can also be associated with transcriptional activation. Adapted from "Experience-dependent epigenetic modifications in the central nervous system." *Biological Psychiatry* 65:7. Copyright Elsevier 2009.

of cytosines at CpG dinucleotides recruits methyl-DNA binding proteins, at specific sites in the genome. Proteins that bind to methylated DNA have both a methyl-DNA binding domain (MBD, see Figure 14) and a transcription-regulatory domain (TRD). The TRD recruits adapter/scaffolding proteins, which in turn recruit histone deacetylases (HDACs) to the site.

The HDACs alter chromatin structure locally— "chromatin" is the term describing nuclear DNA/protein complexes (see Figure 15). HDACs alter chromatin structure through removing acetyl groups from histone core proteins, leading to compaction of chromatin and transcriptional suppression. Thus, through this complex and highly-regulated biochemical machinery, methylation of DNA triggers localized regulation of the three-dimensional structure of DNA and its associated histone proteins, resulting in a higher-affinity interaction between DNA and the histone core, and transcriptional repression by allosteric means. It is important to note that while DNA methylation is usually (and historically) associated with transcriptional suppression, recent studies have indicated that DNA methylation can also be associated with transcriptional activation, by mechanisms that have not yet been determined (89–90).

Consideration of the mechanism of transcriptional silencing by DNA methylation thus leads us to the second major category of epigenetic marks, histone post-translational modifications.

C. Epigenetic Tagging of Histones

Histones are highly basic proteins whose function is to organize DNA within the nucleus. As mentioned above, in the nucleus DNA is tightly packaged into chromatin, a DNA-protein complex that consists of DNA in a double helix, histone proteins, and various associated regulatory proteins. The interaction between

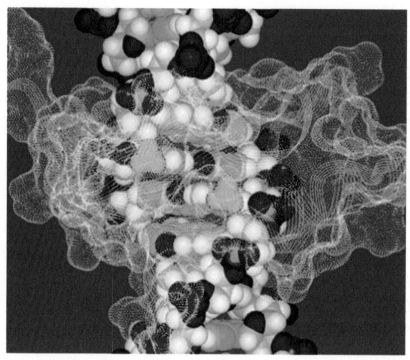

FIGURE 14 A homology model of the methyl-binding domain (MBD) of MECP2 interacting with a symmetrically methylated CpG within a DNA duplex. To construct this model, the NMR solution structure of the MBD of MeCP2 (Wakefield et al. (1999). *J. Mol. Biol.* 291:1055–1065) was superimposed on the solution structure of the MBD of MBD1 bound to a symmetrically methylated DNA sequence (Ohki et al. (2001). *Cell* 105:487–497) using the Insight computer package. The methyl groups of the 5-methylcytosine residues are in yellow. The white ribbon represents the secondary structure of the backbone of the protein, and the remainder of the protein is the white mesh. This model illustrates the proximity of the methyl groups on the complementary strands within the major groove of a B-form DNA helix, as well as points of hydrophobic interactions between the methyl groups and the MBD. Oxidative damage to major contact points within the methyl-CpG dinucleotide significantly inhibits MBD binding. Figure and legend from Valinluck et al. (2004). *Nucleic Acids Res.* 32:4100–4108. Copyright Oxford University Press 2004.

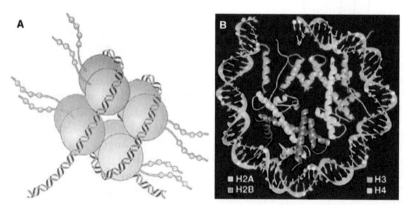

FIGURE 15 The nucleosome. (A) Each nucleosome is comprised of an octamer of histone molecules, which consists of an $H3_2$-$H4_2$ tetramer and two H2A-H2B dimers. The N-termini of histones project out of the nucleosome core and interact with DNA. These histone tails can be epigenetically modified, and act as signal integration platforms. (B) Crystal structure of the nucleosome depicting the interaction of DNA with histones. Reproduced with permission from Levenson and Sweatt, *Nature Reviews Neuroscience*. Copyright Macmillan Publishers Ltd 2005.

histones which form the core of the chromatin particle and DNA is mediated in part by the N-terminal tail of histone proteins. One can imagine chromatin as a core of eight histone proteins (histones 2A, 2B, 3, and 4, with two copies of each molecule, see Figure 15) with DNA wrapped around it like rope on a windlass.

Structural studies indicate that the N-terminal tails of histones protrude beyond the DNA, and are available for post-translational modifications (91).

Several specific sites of post-translational modification exist within the N-terminal tails of histone proteins, and modification of these sites modulates

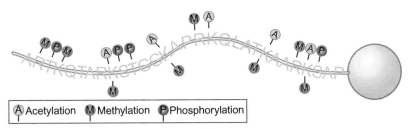

FIGURE 16 The histone code. The first 30 amino acids in the N-terminus of the human histone H3 are illustrated. Many sites in the N-terminus can be targets for epigenetic tagging such as acetylation (A), phosphorylation (P) and methylation (M). Regulation of each site is independent, and the integration of epigenetic tags elicits a finely-tuned transcriptional response. The integration of signalling at the level of epigenetics is commonly referred to as the histone code. Figure from Levenson and Sweatt, *Nature Reviews Neuroscience*. Copyright Macmillan Publishers Ltd 2005.

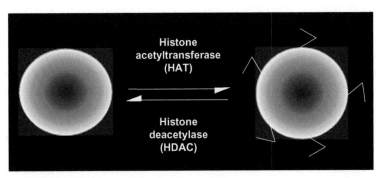

FIGURE 17 Bidirectional regulation of histone acetylation by HAT's and HDAC's. Reproduced with permission from Levenson and Sweatt, *Nature Reviews Neuroscience*. Copyright Macmillan Publishers Ltd 2005.

the overall structure of chromatin (see Figure 16). Currently, four distinct post-translational modifications of histone tails have been well-characterized: acetylation; methylation; ubiquitination; and phosphorylation. All of these modifications serve as epigenetic tags (92). However, for our purposes I will only discuss histone acetylation, because it has been most extensively studied in the CNS.

Acetylation of histones occurs at lysine residues, specifically on their side-chain amino group, which effectively neutralizes their positive charge. Histone acetyltransferases (HATs) catalyze the direct transfer of an acetyl group from acetyl-CoA to the ε-NH$^+$ group of the lysine residues within a histone (93–96). Histone acetylation is a reversible process, and the enzymes that catalyze the reversal of histone acetylation are known as histone deacetylases (HDACs, see Figure 17). By way of background, there are a total of eleven different classical HDAC isoforms, broadly divided into two classes. HDACs 1, 2, 3, and 8 are Class I HDACs, while Class II encompasses HDAC isoforms 4, 5, 6, 7, 9, 10, and 11. The newly-characterized SIR2 family of HDACs (the "sirtuins") are another major category of HDAC, but I will not discuss them here (97).

HDAC inhibitors are the principal method of manipulating the epigenome pharmacologically at present. In terms of some commonly available HDAC inhibitors, trichostatin A (TsA) inhibits HDACs broadly across both Class I and Class II, while the inhibitors sodium butyrate and suberoylanylide hydroxamic acid (SAHA, also known as Vorinostat or Zolinza) select for Class I HDACs.

It is important to remember when considering HDAC inhibitors that "histone deacetylase" is actually a misnomer. Histone deacetylase enzymes should be more accurately described as "lysine deacetylases." Lysine amino acid side-chains are acetylated in a wide variety of different cellular proteins as well as histones. The list of known lysine-acetylated proteins is quite long, including transcription factors, cytoskeletal proteins, and a wide variety of metabolic enzymes. HDACs operate on all these proteins, not just their prototype substrate, histones.

D. Signaling Systems that Control Histone Modifications

The signal transduction processes controlling histone acetylation in the mature CNS are just beginning to be investigated. However, two signaling cascades have been implicated in controlling histone acetylation and chromatin structure in the mature CNS so far. One pathway is in the mitogen-activated protein kinase

(MAPK) superfamily—exemplified by the ERK/ MSK/CREB pathway. In this pathway the extracellular-signal regulated kinase (ERK) activates its downstream target mitogen- and stress-activated kinase (MSK), which in turn phosphorylates CREB (98–101). This phosphorylation and activation of CREB recruits CREB binding protein (CBP), which is a histone acetyltransferase that regulates local chromatin structure as part of CREB-dependent activation of nuclear gene transcription, as we discussed earlier in this chapter.

The second known category of signaling pathway regulating chromatin structure in the mature CNS is the nuclear factor kappa B (NFκB) signaling pathway. Exactly how NFκB controls histone acetylation and chromatin structure in the CNS is still being investigated (33,102). It is known that NFκB is controlled by its upstream regulator inhibitor of kappa B kinase (IKK), which itself is a target of multiple upstream regulatory signaling cascades, as we discussed earlier in this chapter. Thus, overall it is known at this point that both the ERK/MSK/CREB pathway and the IKK/NFκB pathway actively regulate chromatin structure in the mature CNS. One suspects that many important additional mechanisms await discovery (103–105).

E. Epigenetic Mechanisms in Learning and Memory

Formation of long-term memory is associated with epigenetic marking of the genome. For example, in contextual fear conditioning acetylation of hippocampal histone H3 is significantly increased. This epigenetic marking requires NMDA-receptor-dependent synaptic transmission and the ERK MAPK signaling cascade in the hippocampus (106–109), as does the memory itself; thus, epigenetic tagging of the genome occurs during consolidation of hippocampus-dependent long-term memory (110–111).

If acetylation of histones is functionally significant for consolidation of long-term memory, then disruption of HAT activity would be predicted to interfere with long-term memory formation. Several studies have investigated long-term memory formation in genetically-manipulated mice with impaired CBP function, and these have demonstrated that CBP/ HAT-deficient mice have both L-LTP and long-term memory deficits (112–115).

Thus, histone acetylation is regulated in long-term memory, and disruption of HAT activity impairs long-term memory formation. Together, these observations suggest that perturbations in the processes that regulate chromatin structure can influence long-term memory formation in the behaving animal *in vivo*. However, can augmentation of histone acetylation *enhance* memory formation? Several studies have investigated the effect of HDAC inhibitors on long-term memory formation, and found that, indeed, HDAC inhibition improves memory formation in paradigms such as fear conditioning, Morris water maze, and extinction of conditioned fear (106,115–118).

A recent series of studies has investigated the capacity of DNA methylation, the other major epigenetic molecular mechanism besides histone modification, to regulate synaptic plasticity and memory in adult animals (119–120). Inhibitors of DNMTs that likely block the net effects of both maintenance and *de novo* DNMTs alter DNA methylation in adult CNS tissue and block hippocampal LTP *in vitro*, and block fear conditioning *in vivo* (119). In addition, fear conditioning is associated with rapid methylation and transcriptional silencing of the memory suppressor gene protein phosphatase 1 (PP1), and demethylation and transcriptional activation of the synaptic plasticity gene reelin. These findings have the surprising implication that both DNA methylation and demethylation might be involved in long-term memory consolidation. Overall, these results suggest that DNA methylation is dynamically-regulated in the adult nervous system and that this cellular mechanism is a crucial step in memory formation. Taken together, all these studies of histone acetylation and DNA methylation indicate that long-term behavioral memory processes regulate, and are regulated by, the epigenome (see Figure 18).

Finally, the preceding section discussed results from animal models implicating epigenetic mechanisms in learning and memory. However, there is a considerable body of evidence, albeit indirect, implicating disruption of epigenetic mechanisms as a causal basis for human cognitive dysfunction as well. Some examples where derangements in molecular components of the epigenetic apparatus have been implicated in human cognitive disorders are listed in Table 2. We will return to several of these in the next chapter.

In interpreting these findings in the present context, an important caveat applies. When considering these cases it is important to distinguish between a *developmental* need for epigenetic mechanisms, to allow formation of a normal nervous system, versus an *ongoing* need for these mechanisms as part of cognitive processing *per se* in the adult. The majority of the attention to date has justifiably focused on developmental roles for epigenetics in establishing the capacity for cognitive function in the adult. However, the experimental results outlined above also suggest the possibility of an ongoing and active role for epigenetic mechanisms in adult cognition.

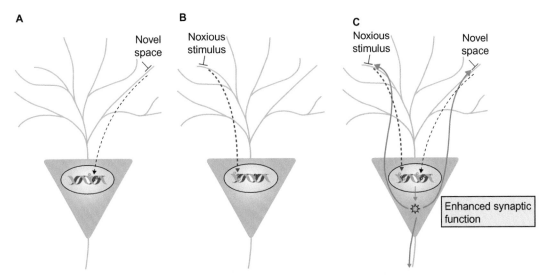

FIGURE 18 Model for epigenetics in contextual fear memory—a histone code for memory formation? Exposure of a test subject to various environmental conditions leads to changes in the epigenetic profile of the genome in neurons residing in relevant brain regions. In this example, we focus on pyramidal neurons in area CA1 of the hippocampus. In this speculative model: (A) Exposure of a subject to a novel environment leads to epigenetic changes and formation of novel spatial memories; (B) Exposure to a noxious stimulus leads to epigenetic changes and formation of novel fear memory; (C) Coupling the presentation of the novel environment with the noxious stimulus results in integration of the epigenetic responses, contributing to the formation of a specific contextual fear memory. Figure from Levenson and Sweatt, *Nature Reviews Neuroscience*. Copyright Macmillan Publishers Ltd 2005.

TABLE 2   Epigenetics in Human Cognitive Disorders

Disease	Gene	Function	Epigenetic Effect
Rubinstein-Taybi Syndrome	CBP	Histone acetyltransferase	↑ histone acetylation
Rett Syndrome	MECP2	Binds to CpG dinucleotides and recruits HDACs	↓ histone acetylation
Fragile X mental retardation	FMR1 and FMR2*	Expansion of CGG or CCG repeats results in aberrant DNA methylation around *FMR1* and *FMR2* genes	↑ DNA methylation ↑ histone acetylation
Alzheimer's disease	APP	*APP* intracellular domain acts as a notch-like transcription factor; associated with the HAT TIP60	↓ histone acetylation
Schizophrenia	reelin	An extracellular matrix protein, involved in synapse development	↑ DNA methylation around the reelin gene

*Trinucleotide expansions in *FMR1* and *FMR2*. *APP*, amyloid precursor protein; *CBP*, cyclic-AMP response-element-binding protein; *FMR*, fragile X mental retardation; *HAT*, histone acetyltransferases; *HDAC*, histone deacetylase; *MECP2*, methyl CpG-binding protein 2; *TIP60*, HIV-1 Tat interactive protein, 60kDa.

F. Environmental Enrichment and Recovery of Lost Memories

As described above, HDAC inhibitors have been identified as being capable of improving memory formation in studies of normal rats and mice. In addition, a wide variety of prior laboratory animal studies pioneered by Bill Greenough's laboratory (121) have demonstrated that environmental enrichment, i.e., making available a wide variety of toys, exercise apparatus, and socially complex housing, also boosts memory capacity.

Thus, two very different types of treatments, environmental enrichment and inhibition of histone deacetylases (HDACs), boost memory function in rodents. Might these two observations be mechanistically related? Indeed, recent studies provide evidence that environmental enrichment achieves its effects through elevating histone acetylation in the hippocampus. In this vein, Tsai and colleagues found that environmental enrichment is associated with increased histone acetylation in the hippocampus (122). Tsai and co-workers confirmed in these studies that environmental enrichment improves spatial memory capacity

BOX 2

MOTHER'S DAY—EVERY DAY OF YOUR LIFE

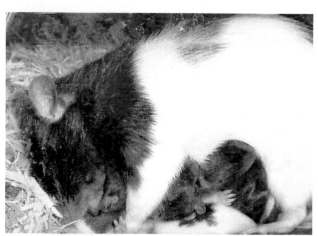

BOX 2   Figure courtesy of Tania Roth, UAB.

Historically, mothers have not been prone to underestimate their lasting impact on their children's behaviors. A recent finding should strengthen their conviction even further (138).

Mother rats that exhibit strong nurturing behaviors toward their pups, for example by frequently licking and grooming their offspring, produce lasting alterations in the patterns of DNA methylation in the CNS of their pups which apparently persist throughout adulthood (138). There is evidence that these changes in DNA structure result in decreased anxiety and a strong maternal nurturing instinct in the adult offspring.

There are several interesting implications of these studies. First, the study indicates that alterations in DNA methylation affect behaviors in the adult. Second, the persistence of neonatally-acquired patterns of DNA methylation in the mature CNS is consistent with the hypothesis that epigenetic mechanisms contribute to lasting cellular effects, i.e., cellular memory in the CNS. Finally, and perhaps most importantly, the study suggests a specific epigenetic mechanism in the CNS for perpetuating an acquired behavioral characteristic across generations—a particularly robust example of behavioral memory that is potentially subserved by epigenetics.

in mice, and that this improvement in spatial memory was mimicked by HDAC inhibitors. These findings strongly suggest that environmental enrichment acts via increasing histone acetylation in the CNS.

In their studies, Tsai and colleagues also found that HDAC inhibitors not only improve the capacity to form new memories, they also restore the capacity to form memories in a mouse model of neurodegenerative disorders (122). They generated these findings by using a genetically-engineered mouse model that they produced, that exhibits inducible neurodegeneration in its CNS. These engineered mice have neuronal loss in their hippocampus, and indeed Tsai and her colleagues have previously demonstrated that these mice have pronounced deficits in long-term spatial memory, as assessed using a variety of behavioral assays. In their studies, they demonstrated that both HDAC inhibitors

and environmental enrichment restored spatial memory capacity in these mice with neurodegeneration. These studies therefore implicate HDAC inhibitors as a potential new therapeutic approach to human cognitive disorders arising from neurodegeneration. Indeed, their work and others' suggests that HDAC inhibitors might be a useful general therapy for aging-related memory dysfunction as a broadly defined category (123).

In their studies, Tsai and colleagues also asked an intriguing question: are HDAC inhibitors capable of allowing an animal undergoing memory loss through neurodegeneration to recover memories that had apparently already been lost? This would seem almost beyond the realm of possibility, but that is exactly what they observed to be an effect of HDAC inhibition in their mouse model of neurodegeneration. In a particularly fascinating set of experiments they trained a group of animals, let their memory for that training event decay over time (due directly or indirectly to neurodegeneration in their mouse model), and confirmed that the animals had lost the capacity to recall that memory. Amazingly, administration of an HDAC inhibitor then restored the capability of the animals to recall that memory, restoring access to a memory that had apparently already been lost. This is an extremely surprising finding, and its cellular and neuronal circuit basis is quite mysterious. Apparently the drug is restoring sufficient robustness of function to the remaining cells in the memory circuit such that they are able to unmask a latent memory trace. Future studies into the basis of this effect may well lead to fundamental new insights into the molecular and cellular basis of memory recall.

G. Section Summary

In this brief overview I have presented an emerging new view of the epigenome and its role in the adult CNS. New studies are rapidly being published demonstrating that epigenetic mechanisms are involved in mediating diverse experience-driven changes in the CNS. These experience-driven changes in the adult CNS are manifest at the molecular, cellular, circuit, and behavioral levels. Overall, these diverse observations support the view that the epigenome resides at the interface of the environment and the genome (see Box 2). Furthermore, it is now becoming clear that epigenetic mechanisms can influence behavior. Future studies geared toward understanding the role of the epigenome in experience-dependent behavioral modification will clearly be important for, and relevant to, the memory field.

V. NEUROGENESIS IN THE ADULT CENTRAL NERVOUS SYSTEM

Finally, as if the processes for establishing and maintaining long-term memory weren't already complicated enough, recent findings indicate that other novel mechanisms may also play a role. Specifically, *neurogenesis* has entered the picture. Not too long ago the widely held dogma was that there is no new generation of neurons in the adult CNS. However, fascinating recent results have shown that neurogenesis does indeed continue into adulthood, particularly in the dentate gyrus. One key publication by Fred Gage and his colloborators showed specifically that new neurons are generated in the adult human brain (73). How might this fact be ascertained? Cancer patients sometimes receive treatment with the drug bromo-deoxy uridine (BrdU). It selectively affects dividing

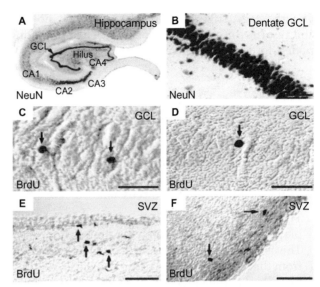

FIGURE 19 Neurogenesis in the adult human hippocampus. Newly-generated cells can be detected in the adult human brain in patients previously treated with BrdU. (A) The hippocampal region of the adult human brain immunoperoxidase-stained for the neuronal marker NeuN. (B) The hippocampal dentate gyrus granule cell layer (GCL) visualized with immunoperoxidase staining for NeuN. (C) Differential interference contrast photomicrograph showing BrdU-labeled nuclei (arrows) in the dentate granule cell layer (GCL). (D) Differential interference contrast photomicrograph showing a BrdU-labeled nucleus (arrow) in the human dentate GCL. BrdU-positive nuclei have a rounded appearance and resemble the chromatin structure of mature granule cells and are found within the granule cell layer. (E) Differential interference contrast photomicrograph showing BrdU-positive cells (arrows) adjacent to the ependymal lining in the subventricular zone of the human caudate nucleus. Cells with elongated nuclei resembling migrating cells are in the rat subventricular zone (SVZ). (F) Differential interference contrast photomicrograph showing BrdU-positive cells (arrows) with round to elongated nuclei in the subventricular zone of the human caudate nucleus. All scale bars represent 50 μm. Figure and legend from (73). Reprinted by permission from Macmillan Publishers Ltd: *Nature Medicine*. Copyright Macmillan Publishers Ltd 1998.

cells by being incorporated into their DNA on *de novo* DNA synthesis. An ancillary aspect of this is, therefore, that BrdU selectively labels freshly-divided cells. Post-mortem analysis of the brains of cancer patients that had received BrdU as a chemotherapeutic treatment revealed that, indeed, new dentate granule cells are produced in an ongoing fashion in the adult human brain (see Figure 19).

Are these newly-generated cells important for memory? Work by Tracy Shors, Elizabeth Gould, and their collaborators, has suggested that these new cells are necessary for memory formation, in rodents at a minimum (73–74). Thus, both Morris water maze training and trace eye-blink conditioning lead to enhanced neurogenesis in rats. Moreover, inhibiting neurogenesis attenuates memory formation in these same paradigms. These fascinating studies, while at an early stage, suggest we need to consider the possibility of a role for neurogenesis when formulating models for long-term memory.

VI. SUMMARY

In this chapter we considered those molecular mechanisms that are uniquely involved in triggering very long-lasting changes in synaptic transmission in memory. There are a number of central concepts that we can take away from this discussion.

1. The PKA/ERK/MSK/CREB pathway is a principal player in memory-associated gene regulation. This is a core signaling cascade for getting a signal from the synapse to the genome. However, it is important to remember that a multitude of various transcription factors and gene products are also clearly involved in memory formation.

2. An intriguing problem in the cell biology of memory is how altered gene expression becomes manifest selectively at the appropriate synapse. Studies of Arc mRNA trafficking in the mammalian nervous system serve as a prototype system in beginning to address these issues. Importantly, studies of Arc trafficking indicate that local synaptic signals likely direct activity-dependent trafficking of mRNAs in memory formation.

3. Epigenetic molecular mechanisms are emerging as an important component of gene regulation in memory. This role in memory reprises their role as cellular information storage devices in development, and suggests an important conservation of function as molecular information storage devices.

4. Neurogenesis, the generation of new neurons in the adult CNS, is also emerging as a potential site important for memory formation or storage.

5. It is important to keep in mind that the available data support the model that altered gene expression is an induction mechanism for L-LTP and memory. The question of whether altered gene expression contributes to the maintenance of L-LTP and memory is still, by and large, an open one at present.

6. We also talked about how changes in gene expression become manifest as changes at the synapse. We discussed two different models for how this happens. The first was based on increased AMPA receptors and associated proteins at the synapse, dependent on a triggering event such as Arc arrival at the synapse. These changes then manifested themselves as an increase in synaptic strength. This proposed mechanism is a fairly straightforward read-out of increased production of synaptic components, with Arc-like molecules serving as a nucleating event.

7. However, considering the limitations of proteins like Arc with a half-life of a few hours led us to conclude that later stages of long-term memory must involve additional processes. In response to this consideration we formulated a speculative model for how self-perpetuating changes in local protein synthesis might underlie weeks-long or life-long synaptic changes.

8. Finally, it is very important to remember that the types of synaptic changes we have discussed in this chapter are functionally manifest as an alteration in the properties of a neuronal circuit in the CNS. Clearly, self-perpetuating molecular changes are necessary for very long-lasting effects, but the lasting effects are not the entirety of the memory. The maintenance of the synaptic change in the context of the circuit is what constitutes the memory. The self-perpetuating synaptic change is the mechanism for the maintenance of the memory.

Further Reading

Alberini, C. M. (2009). "Transcription factors in long-term memory and synaptic plasticity." *Physiol. Rev.* 89:121–145.

Barco, A., Alarcon, J. M., and Kandel, E. R. (2002). "Expression of constitutively active CREB protein facilitates the late phase of long-term potentiation by enhancing synaptic capture." *Cell* 108:689–703.

Bourtchuladze, R., Frenguelli, B., Blendy, J., Cioffi, D., Schutz, G., and Silva, A. J. (1994). "Deficient long-term memory in mice with a targeted mutation of the cAMP-responsive element-binding protein." *Cell* 79:59–68.

Brivanlou, A. H., and Darnell, J. E., Jr. (2002). "Signal transduction and the control of gene expression." *Science* 295:813–818.

Cole, A. J., Saffen, D. W., Baraban, J. M., and Worley, P. F. (1989). "Rapid increase of an immediate early gene messenger RNA in hippocampal neurons by synaptic NMDA receptor activation." *Nature* 340:474–476.

Eisch, A. J., Cameron, H. A., Encinas, J. M., Meltzer, L. A., Ming, G. L., and Overstreet-Wadiche, L. S. (2008). "Adult neurogenesis, mental health, and mental illness: hope or hype?." *J. Neurosci.* 28:11785–11791.

Flavell, S. W., and Greenberg, M. E. (2008). "Signaling mechanisms linking neuronal activity to gene expression and plasticity of the nervous system." *Annu. Rev. Neurosci.* 31:563–590.

Gass, P., Wolfer, D. P., Balschun, D., Rudolph, D., Frey, U., Lipp, H. P., and Schutz, G. (1998). "Deficits in memory tasks of mice with CREB mutations depend on gene dosage." *Learn. Mem.* 5:274–288.

Gräff, J., and Mansuy, I. M. (2008). "Epigenetic codes in cognition and behaviour." *Behav. Brain Res.* 192:70–87.

Greer, P. L., and Greenberg, M. E. (2008). "From synapse to nucleus: calcium-dependent gene transcription in the control of synapse development and function." *Neuron* 59:846–860.

Guzowski, J. F., Lyford, G. L., Stevenson, G. D., Houston, F. P., McGaugh, J. L., Worley, P. F., and Barnes, C. A. (2000). "Inhibition of activity-dependent arc protein expression in the rat hippocampus impairs the maintenance of long-term potentiation and the consolidation of long-term memory." *J. Neurosci.* 20:3993–4001.

Huang, F., Chotiner, J. K., and Steward, O. (2007). "Actin polymerization and ERK phosphorylation are required for Arc/Arg3.1 mRNA targeting to activated synaptic sites on dendrites." *J. Neurosci.* 27:9054–9067.

Levenson, J. M., and Sweatt, J. D. (2005). "Epigenetic mechanisms in memory formation." *Nat. Rev. Neurosci.* 6:108–118.

Lubin, F. D., and Sweatt, J. D. (2008). "The IkappaB kinase regulates chromatin structure during reconsolidation of conditioned fear memories." *Neuron* 55:942–957.

Nguyen, P. V., Abel, T., and Kandel, E. R. (1994). "Requirement of a critical period of transcription for induction of a late phase of LTP." *Science* 265:1104–1107.

Roberson, E. D., English, J. D., Adams, J. P., Selcher, J. C., Kondratick, C., and Sweatt, J. D. (1999). "The mitogen-activated protein kinase cascade couples PKA and PKC to cAMP response element binding protein phosphorylation in area CA1 of hippocampus." *J. Neurosci.* 19:4337–4348.

Schuman, E. M., Dynes, J. L., and Steward, O. (2006). "Synaptic regulation of translation of dendritic mRNAs." *J. Neurosci.* 26:7143–7146.

Weaver, I. C. et al. (2004). "Epigenetic programming by maternal behavior." *Nat. Neurosci.* 7:847–854.

Wood, M. A., Hawk, J. D., and Abel, T. (2006). "Combinatorial chromatin modifications and memory storage: a code for memory." *Learn. Mem.* 13:241–244.

Zhao, C., Deng, W., and Gage, F. H. (2008). "Mechanisms and functional implications of adult neurogenesis." *Cell* 132:645–660.

Journal Club Articles

Atkins, C. M., Selcher, J. C., Petraitis, J. J., Trzaskos, J. M., and Sweatt, J. D. (1998). "The MAPK cascade is required for mammalian associative learning." *Nat. Neurosci.* 1:602–609.

Borrelli, E., Nestler, E. J., Allis, C. D., and Sassone-Corsi, P. (2008). "Decoding the epigenetic language of neuronal plasticity." *Neuron* 60(6):961–974.

Fischer, A., Sananbenesi, F., Wang, X., Dobbin, M., and Tsai, L. H. (2007). "Recovery of learning and memory is associated with chromatin remodeling." *Nature* 447:178–182.

Reijmers, L. G., Perkins, B. L., Matsuo, N., and Mayford, M. (2007). "Localization of a stable neural correlate of associative memory." *Science* 317:1230–1233.

Shema, R., Sacktor, T. C., and Dudai, Y. (2007). "Rapid erasure of long-term memory associations in the cortex by an inhibitor of PKM zeta." *Science* 317:951–953.

For more information—relevant topic chapters from: John H. Byrne (Editor-in-Chief) (2008). *Learning and Memory: A Comprehensive Reference.* Oxford: Academic Press (ISBN 978-0-12-370509-9). (4.02 Bailey, C. H., Barco, A., Hawkins, R. D., and Kandel, E. R. *Molecular Studies of Learning and Memory in Aplysia and the Hippocampus: A Comparative Analysis of Implicit and Explicit Memory Storage.* pp. 11–29; 4.11 Schafe, G. E., and LeDoux, J. E. *Neural and Molecular Mechanisms of Fear Memory.* pp. 157–192; 4.12 Winstanley, C. A., and Nestler, E. J. *The Molecular Mechanisms of Reward.* pp. 193–215; 4.13 Rosenblum, K. *Conditioned Taste Aversion and Taste Learning: Molecular Mechanisms.* pp. 217–234; 4.14 Alberini, C. M., and Taubenfeld, S. M. *Memory Reconsolidation.* pp. 235–244; 4.21 Eckel-Mahan, K. L., and Storm, D. R. *Second Messengers: Calcium and cAMP Signaling.* pp. 427–448; 4.22 Sacktor, T. C. *PKM[zeta], LTP Maintenance, and Long-Term Memory Storage.* pp. 449–467; 4.25 Kelleher, R. J. III, *Mitogen-Activated Protein Kinases in Synaptic Plasticity and Memory.* pp. 501–523; 4.26 Hegde, A. N. *Proteolysis and Synaptic Plasticity.* pp. 525–545; 4.27 Cole, C. J., and Josselyn, S. A. *Transcription Regulation of Memory: CREB, CaMKIV, Fos/Jun, CBP, and SRF.* pp. 547–566; 4.28 Shrum, C. K., and Meffert, M. K. *The NF-[kappa]B Family in Learning and Memory.* pp. 567–585; 4.29 Dynes, J. L., and Steward, O. *Dendritic Transport of mRNA, the IEG Arc, and Synaptic Modifications Involved in Memory Consolidation.* pp. 587–610; 4.32 Marcora, E., Carlisle, H. J., and Kennedy, M. B. *The Role of the Postsynaptic Density and the Spine Cytoskeleton in Synaptic Plasticity.* pp. 649–673; 4.33 Costa-Mattioli, M., Sonenberg, N., and Klann, E. *Translational Control Mechanisms in Synaptic Plasticity and Memory.* pp. 675–694; 4.34 Chapleau, C. A., and Pozzo-Miller, L. *Activity-Dependent Structural Plasticity of Dendritic Spines.* pp. 695–719; 4.35 Chan, C. -S., and Davis, R. L. *Integrins and Cadherins—Extracellular Matrix in Memory Formation.* pp. 721–740; 4.40 Mozzachiodi, R., and Byrne, J. H. *Plasticity of Intrinsic Excitability as a Mechanism for Memory Storage.* pp. 829–838; 4.41 Jessberger, S., Aimone, J. B., and Gage, F. H. *Neurogenesis.* pp. 839–858; 4.42 Levenson, J. M., and Wood, M. A. *Epigenetics—Chromatin Structure and Rett Syndrome.* pp. 859–878.)

References

1. Nguyen, P. V., Abel, T., and Kandel, E. R. (1994). "Requirement of a critical period of transcription for induction of a late phase of LTP." *Science* 265:1104–1107.

2. Frey, U., Frey, S., Schollmeier, F., and Krug, M. (1996). "Influence of actinomycin D, a RNA synthesis inhibitor, on long-term potentiation in rat hippocampal neurons *in vivo* and *in vitro*." *J. Physiol.* 490(Pt 3):703–711.

3. Bourtchuladze, R., Frenguelli, B., Blendy, J., Cioffi, D., Schutz, G., and Silva, A. J. (1994). "Deficient long-term memory in mice with a targeted mutation of the cAMP-responsive element-binding protein." *Cell* 79:59–68.

4. Gass, P., Wolfer, D. P., Balschun, D., Rudolph, D., Frey, U., Lipp, H. P., and Schutz, G. (1998). "Deficits in memory tasks of mice with CREB mutations depend on gene dosage." *Learn. Mem.* 5:274–288.

5. Pittenger, C., Huang, Y. Y., Paletzki, R. F., Bourtchouladze, R., Scanlin, H., Vronskaya, S., and Kandel, E. R. (2002). "Reversible inhibition of CREB/ATF transcription factors in region CA1 of the dorsal hippocampus disrupts hippocampus-dependent spatial memory." *Neuron* 34:447–462.

6. Jones, M. W., Errington, M. L., French, P. J., Fine, A., Bliss, T. V., Garel, S., Charnay, P., Bozon, B., Laroche, S., and Davis, S. (2001). "A requirement for the immediate early gene Zif268 in the expression of late LTP and long-term memories." *Nat. Neurosci.* 4:289–296.

7. Impey, S., Fong, A. L., Wang, Y., Cardinaux, J. R., Fass, D. M., Obrietan, K., Wayman, G. A., Storm, D. R., Soderling, T. R., and Goodman, R. H. (2002). "Phosphorylation of CBP mediates transcriptional activation by neural activity and CaM kinase IV." *Neuron* 34:235–244.

8. Kang, H., Sun, L. D., Atkins, C. M., Soderling, T. R., Wilson, M. A., and Tonegawa, S. (2001). "An important role of neural activity-dependent CaMKIV signaling in the consolidation of long-term memory." *Cell* 106:771–783.

9. English, J. D., and Sweatt, J. D. (1996). "Activation of p42 mitogen-activated protein kinase in hippocampal long term potentiation." *J. Biol. Chem.* 271:24329–24332.

10. English, J. D., and Sweatt, J. D. (1997). "A requirement for the mitogen-activated protein kinase cascade in hippocampal long term potentiation." *J. Biol. Chem.* 272:19103–19106.

11. Rosenblum, K., Futter, M., Voss, K., Erent, M., Skehel, P. A., French, P., Obosi, L., Jones, M. W., and Bliss, T. V. (2002). "The role of extracellular regulated kinases I/II in late-phase long-term potentiation." *J. Neurosci.* 22:5432–5441.

12. Impey, S., Obrietan, K., Wong, S. T., Poser, S., Yano, S., Wayman, G., Deloulme, J. C., Chan, G., and Storm, D. R. (1998). "Cross talk between ERK and PKA is required for Ca^{2+} stimulation of CREB-dependent transcription and ERK nuclear translocation." *Neuron* 21:869–883.

13. Guzowski, J. F., Lyford, G. L., Stevenson, G. D., Houston, F. P., McGaugh, J. L., Worley, P. F., and Barnes, C. A. (2000). "Inhibition of activity-dependent arc protein expression in the rat hippocampus impairs the maintenance of long-term potentiation and the consolidation of long-term memory." *J. Neurosci.* 20:3993–4001.

14. Barco, A., Alarcon, J. M., and Kandel, E. R. (2002). "Expression of constitutively active CREB protein facilitates the late phase of long-term potentiation by enhancing synaptic capture." *Cell* 108:689–703.

15. Brivanlou, A. H., and Darnell, J. E., Jr. (2009). "Signal transduction and the control of gene expression." *Science* 295:813–818.

16. Shaywitz, A. J., and Greenberg, M. E. (1999). "CREB: a stimulus-induced transcription factor activated by a diverse array of extracellular signals." *Annu. Rev. Biochem.* 68:821–861.

17. Poser, S., and Storm, D. R. (2001). "Role of Ca^{2+}-stimulated adenylyl cyclases in LTP and memory formation." *Int. J. Dev. Neurosci.* 19:387–394.

18. Kornhauser, J. M., Cowan, C. W., Shaywitz, A. J., Dolmetsch, R. E., Griffith, E. C., Hu, L. S., Haddad, C., Xia, Z., and Greenberg, M. E. (2002). "CREB transcriptional activity in neurons is regulated by multiple, calcium-specific phosphorylation events." *Neuron* 34:221–233.

19. Ohno, M., Frankland, P. W., Chen, A. P., Costa, R. M., and Silva, A. J. (2001). "Inducible, pharmacogenetic approaches to the study of learning and memory." *Nat. Neurosci.* 4:1238–1243.

20. Roberson, E. D., English, J. D., Adams, J. P., Selcher, J. C., Kondratick, C., and Sweatt, J. D. (1999). "The mitogen-activated protein kinase cascade couples PKA and PKC to cAMP response element binding protein phosphorylation in area CA1 of hippocampus." *J. Neurosci.* 19:4337–4348.

21. Levenson, J. M., Choi, S., Lee, S. Y., Cao, Y. A., Ahn, H. J., Worley, K. C., Pizzi, M., Liou, H. C., and Sweatt, J. D. (2004). "A bioinformatics analysis of memory consolidation reveals involvement of the transcription factor c-rel." *J. Neurosci.* 24(16):3933–3943.

22. Ho, N., Liauw, J. A., Blaeser, F., Wei, F., Hanissian, S., Muglia, L. M., Wozniak, D. F., Nardi, A., Arvin, K. L., Holtzman, D. M., Linden, D. J., Zhuo, M., Muglia, L. J., and Chatila, T. A. (2000). "Impaired synaptic plasticity and cAMP response element-binding protein activation in Ca^{2+}/calmodulin-dependent protein kinase type IV/Gr-deficient mice." *J. Neurosci.* 20:6459–6472.

23. Mermelstein, P. G., Deisseroth, K., Dasgupta, N., Isaksen, A. L., and Tsien, R. W. (2001). "Calmodulin priming: nuclear translocation of a calmodulin complex and the memory of prior neuronal activity." *Proc. Natl. Acad. Sci. USA*, 98:15342–15347.

24. Deisseroth, K., Bito, H., and Tsien, R. W. (1996). "Signaling from synapse to nucleus: postsynaptic CREB phosphorylation during multiple forms of hippocampal synaptic plasticity." *Neuron* 16:89–101.

25. Deisseroth, K., and Tsien, R. W. (2002). "Dynamic multiphosphorylation passwords for activity-dependent gene expression." *Neuron* 34:179–182.

26. Dudek, S. M., and Fields, R. D. (2002). "Somatic action potentials are sufficient for late-phase LTP-related cell signaling." *Proc. Natl. Acad. Sci. USA*, 99:3962–3967.

27. Gooney, M., and Lynch, M. A. (2001). "Long-term potentiation in the dentate gyrus of the rat hippocampus is accompanied by brain-derived neurotrophic factor-induced activation of TrkB." *J. Neurochem.* 77:1198–1207.

28. Hall, J., Thomas, K. L., and Everitt, B. J. (2000). "Rapid and selective induction of BDNF expression in the hippocampus during contextual learning." *Nat. Neurosci.* 3:533–535.

29. Yin, Y., Edelman, G. M., and Vanderklish, P. W. (2002). "The brain-derived neurotrophic factor enhances synthesis of Arc in synaptoneurosomes." *Proc. Natl. Acad. Sci. USA*, 99:2368–2373.

30. Patterson, S. L., Pittenger, C., Morozov, A., Martin, K. C., Scanlin, H., Drake, C., and Kandel, E. R. (2001). "Some forms of cAMP-mediated long-lasting potentiation are associated with release of BDNF and nuclear translocation of phospho-MAP kinase." *Neuron* 32:123–140.

31. Ying, S. W., Futter, M., Rosenblum, K., Webber, M. J., Hunt, S. P., Bliss, T. V., and Bramham, C. R. (2002). "Brain-derived neurotrophic factor induces long-term potentiation in intact adult hippocampus: requirement for ERK activation coupled to CREB and upregulation of Arc synthesis." *J. Neurosci.* 22:1532–1540.

32. Matthies, H., Becker, A., Schroeder, H., Kraus, J., Hollt, V., and Krug, M. (1997). "Dopamine D1-deficient mutant mice do not express the late phase of hippocampal long-term potentiation." *Neuroreport* 8:3533–3535.

33. Lubin, F. D., and Sweatt, J. D. (2007). "The IkappaB kinase regulates chromatin structure during reconsolidation of conditioned fear memories." *Neuron* 55(6):942–957.

34. Schulz, S., Siemer, H., Krug, M., and Hollt, V. (1999). "Direct evidence for biphasic cAMP responsive element-binding protein phosphorylation during long-term potentiation in the rat dentate gyrus *in vivo*." *J. Neurosci.* 19:5683–5692.

35. Davis, S., Vanhoutte, P., Pages, C., Caboche, J., and Laroche, S. (2000). "The MAPK/ERK cascade targets both Elk-1 and cAMP response element-binding protein to control long-term potentiation-dependent gene expression in the dentate gyrus *in vivo*." *J. Neurosci.* 20:4563–4572.

36. Waltereit, R., Dammermann, B., Wulff, P., Scafidi, J., Staubli, U., Kauselmann, G., Bundman, M., and Kuhl, D. (2001). "Arg3.1/Arc mRNA induction by Ca^{2+} and cAMP requires protein kinase A and mitogen-activated protein kinase/extracellular regulated kinase activation." *J. Neurosci.* 21:5484–5493.

37. Mattson, M. P., Culmsee, C., Yu, Z., and Camandola, S. (2000). "Roles of nuclear factor kappaB in neuronal survival and plasticity." *J. Neurochem.* 74:443–456.

38. Albensi, B. C., and Mattson, M. P. (2000). "Evidence for the involvement of TNF and NF-kappaB in hippocampal synaptic plasticity." *Synapse* 35:151–159.

39. Meberg, P. J., Kinney, W. R., Valcourt, E. G., and Routtenberg, A. (1996). "Gene expression of the transcription factor NF-kappa B in hippocampus: regulation by synaptic activity." *Brain Res. Mol. Brain Res.* 38:179–190.

40. Cole, A. J., Saffen, D. W., Baraban, J. M., and Worley, P. F. (1989). "Rapid increase of an immediate early gene messenger RNA in hippocampal neurons by synaptic NMDA receptor activation." *Nature* 340:474–476.

41. Wisden, W., Errington, M. L., Williams, S., Dunnett, S. B., Waters, C., Hitchcock, D., Evan, G., Bliss, T. V., and Hunt, S. P. (1990). "Differential expression of immediate early genes in the hippocampus and spinal cord." *Neuron* 4:603–614.

42. Abraham, W. C., Dragunow, M., and Tate, W. P. (1991). "The role of immediate early genes in the stabilization of long-term potentiation." *Mol. Neurobiol.* 5:297–314.

43. Abraham, W. C., Mason, S. E., Demmer, J., Williams, J. M., Richardson, C. L., Tate, W. P., Lawlor, P. A., and Dragunow, M. (1993). "Correlations between immediate early gene induction and the persistence of long-term potentiation." *Neuroscience* 56:717–727.

44. Williams, J., Dragunow, M., Lawlor, P., Mason, S., Abraham, W. C., Leah, J., Bravo, R., Demmer, J., and Tate, W. (1995). "Krox20

may play a key role in the stabilization of long-term potentiation." *Brain Res. Mol. Brain Res.* 28:87–93.

45. Taubenfeld, S. M., Wiig, K. A., Monti, B., Dolan, B., Pollonini, G., and Alberini, C. M. (2001). "Fornix-dependent induction of hippocampal CCAAT enhancer-binding protein [beta] and [delta] co-localizes with phosphorylated cAMP response element-binding protein and accompanies long-term memory consolidation." *J. Neurosci.* 21:84–91.

46. Patterson, S. L., Grover, L. M., Schwartzkroin, P. A., and Bothwell, M. (1992). "Neurotrophin expression in rat hippocampal slices: a stimulus paradigm inducing LTP in CA1 evokes increases in BDNF and NT-3 mRNAs." *Neuron* 9:1081–1088.

47. Huang, Y. Y., Bach, M. E., Lipp, H. P., Zhuo, M., Wolfer, D. P., Hawkins, R. D., Schoonjans, L., Kandel, E. R., Godfraind, J. M., Mulligan, R., Collen, D., and Carmeliet, P. (1996). "Mice lacking the gene encoding tissue-type plasminogen activator show a selective interference with late-phase long-term potentiation in both Schaffer collateral and mossy fiber pathways." *Proc. Natl. Acad. Sci. USA*, 93:8699–8704.

48. Szklarczyk, A., Lapinska, J., Rylski, M., McKay, R. D., and Kaczmarek, L. (2002). "Matrix metalloproteinase-9 undergoes expression and activation during dendritic remodeling in adult hippocampus." *J. Neurosci.* 22:920–930.

49. Ingi, T., Worley, P. F., and Lanahan, A. A. (2001). "Regulation of SSAT expression by synaptic activity." *Eur. J. Neurosci.* 13:1459–1463.

50. Qian, Z., Gilbert, M., and Kandel, E. R. (1994). "Temporal and spatial regulation of the expression of BAD2, a MAP kinase phosphatase, during seizure, kindling, and long-term potentiation." *Learn. Mem.* 1:180–188.

51. Nayak, A., Zastrow, D. J., Lickteig, R., Zahniser, N. R., and Browning, M. D. (1998). "Maintenance of late-phase LTP is accompanied by PKA-dependent increase in AMPA receptor synthesis." *Nature* 394:680–683.

52. Kato, A., Ozawa, F., Saitoh, Y., Hirai, K., and Inokuchi, K. (1997). "vesl, a gene encoding VASP/Ena family related protein, is upregulated during seizure, long-term potentiation and synaptogenesis." *FEBS Lett.* 412:183–189.

53. Matsuo, R., Murayama, A., Saitoh, Y., Sakaki, Y., and Inokuchi, K. (2000). "Identification and cataloging of genes induced by long-lasting long-term potentiation in awake rats." *J. Neurochem.* 74:2239–2249.

54. Steward, O., and Worley, P. F. (2001). "Selective targeting of newly synthesized Arc mRNA to active synapses requires NMDA receptor activation." *Neuron* 30:227–240.

55. Bolshakov, V. Y., Golan, H., Kandel, E. R., and Siegelbaum, S. A. (1997). "Recruitment of new sites of synaptic transmission during the cAMP-dependent late phase of LTP at CA3-CA1 synapses in the hippocampus." *Neuron* 19:635–651.

56. Luscher, C., Nicoll, R. A., Malenka, R. C., and Muller, D. (2000). "Synaptic plasticity and dynamic modulation of the postsynaptic membrane." *Nat. Neurosci.* 3:545–550.

57. Steward, O., and Worley, P. F. (2001). "A cellular mechanism for targeting newly synthesized mRNAs to synaptic sites on dendrites." *Proc. Natl. Acad. Sci. USA*, 98:7062–7068.

58. Steward, O., and Schuman, E. M. (2001). "Protein synthesis at synaptic sites on dendrites." *Annu. Rev. Neurosci.* 24:299–325.

59. Link, W., Konietzko, U., Kauselmann, G., Krug, M., Schwanke, B., Frey, U., and Kuhl, D. (1995). "Somatodendritic expression of an immediate early gene is regulated by synaptic activity." *Proc. Natl. Acad. Sci. USA*, 92:5734–5738.

60. Khan, A., Pepio, A. M., and Sossin, W. S. (2001). "Serotonin activates S6 kinase in a rapamycin-sensitive manner in *Aplysia* synaptosomes." *J. Neurosci.* 21:382–391.

61. Raught, B., Gingras, A. C., and Sonenberg, N. (2001). "The target of rapamycin (TOR) proteins." *Proc. Natl. Acad. Sci. USA*, 98:7037–7044.

62. Tang, S. J., Meulemans, D., Vazquez, L., Colaco, N., and Schuman, E. (2001). "A role for a rat homolog of staufen in the transport of RNA to neuronal dendrites." *Neuron* 32:463–475.

63. Engert, F., and Bonhoeffer, T. (1999). "Dendritic spine changes associated with hippocampal long-term synaptic plasticity." *Nature* 399:66–70.

64. Maletic-Savatic, M., Malinow, R., and Svoboda, K. (1999). "Rapid dendritic morphogenesis in CA1 hippocampal dendrites induced by synaptic activity." *Science* 283:1923–1927.

65. Toni, N., Buchs, P. A., Nikonenko, I., Bron, C. R., and Muller, D. (1999). "LTP promotes formation of multiple spine synapses between a single axon terminal and a dendrite." *Nature* 402:421–425.

66. Yuste, R., and Bonhoeffer, T. (2001). "Morphological changes in dendritic spines associated with long-term synaptic plasticity." *Annu. Rev. Neurosci.* 24:1071–1089.

67. Bozdagi, O., Shan, W., Tanaka, H., Benson, D. L., and Huntley, G. W. (2000). "Increasing numbers of synaptic puncta during late-phase LTP: N-cadherin is synthesized, recruited to synaptic sites, and required for potentiation." *Neuron* 28:245–259.

68. Tang, L., Hung, C. P., and Schuman, E. M. (1998). "A role for the cadherin family of cell adhesion molecules in hippocampal long-term potentiation." *Neuron* 20:1165–1175.

69. Chun, D., Gall, C. M., Bi, X., and Lynch, G. (2001). "Evidence that integrins contribute to multiple stages in the consolidation of long term potentiation in rat hippocampus." *Neuroscience* 105:815–829.

70. Kramar, E. A., Bernard, J. A., Gall, C. M., and Lynch, G. (2002). "Alpha3 integrin receptors contribute to the consolidation of long-term potentiation." *Neuroscience* 110:29–39.

71. Bliss, T., Errington, M., Fransen, E., Godfraind, J. M., Kauer, J. A., Kooy, R. F., Maness, P. F., and Furley, A. J. (2000). "Long-term potentiation in mice lacking the neural cell adhesion molecule L1." *Curr. Biol.* 10:1607–1610.

72. Juliano, R. L. (2002). "Signal transduction by cell adhesion receptors and the cytoskeleton: functions of integrins, cadherins, selectins, and immunoglobulin-superfamily members." *Annu. Rev. Pharmacol. Toxicol.* 42:283–323.

73. Eriksson, P. S., Perfilieva, E., Bjork-Eriksson, T., Alborn, A. M., Nordborg, C., Peterson, D. A., and Gage, F. H. (1998). "Neurogenesis in the adult human hippocampus." *Nat. Med.* 4:1313–1317.

74. Gould, E., Beylin, A., Tanapat, P., Reeves, A., and Shors, T. J. (1999). "Learning enhances adult neurogenesis in the hippocampal formation." *Nat. Neurosci.* 2:260–265.

75. Waddington, C. H. (1957). *The Strategy of the Genes.* New York: MacMillan.

76. Okano, M., Xie, S., and Li, E. (1998). "Cloning and characterization of a family of novel mammalian DNA (cytosine-5) methyltransferases." *Nat. Genet.* 19:219–220.

77. Nguyen, P. V., and Kandel, E. R. (1997). "Brief theta-burst stimulation induces a transcription-dependent late phase of LTP requiring cAMP in area CA1 of the mouse hippocampus." *Learn. Mem.* 4:230–243.

78. Wei, F., Qiu, C. S., Liauw, J., Robinson, D. A., Ho, N., Chatila, T., and Zhuo, M. (2002). "Calcium calmodulin-dependent protein kinase IV is required for fear memory." *Nat. Neurosci.* 5:573–579.

79. Impey, S., Mark, M., Villacres, E. C., Poser, S., Chavkin, C., and Storm, D. R. (1996). "Induction of CRE-mediated gene expression by stimuli that generate long-lasting LTP in area CA1 of the hippocampus." *Neuron* 16:973–982.

80. Gartner, A., and Staiger, V. (2002). "Neurotrophin secretion from hippocampal neurons evoked by long-term-potentiation-inducing electrical stimulation patterns." *Proc. Natl. Acad. Sci. USA*, 99:6386–6391.

81. Roberts, L. A., Large, C. H., Higgins, M. J., Stone, T. W., O'Shaughnessy, C. T., and Morris, B. J. (1998). "Increased expression of dendritic mRNA following the induction of long-term potentiation." *Brain Res. Mol. Brain Res.* 56:38–44.

82. Chen, L., MacMillan, A. M., Chang, W., Ezaz-Nikpay, K., Lane, W. S., and Verdine, G. L. (1991). "Direct identification of the active-site nucleophile in a DNA (cytosine-5)-methyltransferase." *Biochemistry* 30:11018–11025.

83. Santi, D. V., Garrett, C. E., and Barr, P. J. (1983). "On the mechanism of inhibition of DNA-cytosine methyltransferases by cytosine analogs." *Cell* 33:9–10.

84. Bird, A. P. (1978). "Use of restriction enzymes to study eukaryotic DNA methylation: II. The symmetry of methylated sites supports semi-conservative copying of the methylation pattern." *J. Mol. Biol.* 118:49–60.

85. Cedar, H., Solage, A., Glaser, G., and Razin, A. (1979). "Direct detection of methylated cytosine in DNA by use of the restriction enzyme MspI." *Nucleic Acids Res.* 6:2125–2132.

86. Cooper, D. N., and Krawczak, M. (1989). "Cytosine methylation and the fate of CpG dinucleotides in vertebrate genomes." *Hum. Genet.* 83:181–188.

87. Gardiner-Garden, M., and Frommer, M. (1987). "CpG islands in vertebrate genomes." *J. Mol. Biol.* 196:261–282.

88. Bird, A. P. (1986). "CpG-rich islands and the function of DNA methylation." *Nature* 321:209–213.

89. Chahrour, M., Jung, S. Y., Shaw, C., Zhou, X., Wong, S. T., Qin, J., and Zoghbi, H. Y. (2008). "MeCP2, a key contributor to neurological disease, activates and represses transcription." *Science* 320:1224–1229.

90. Cohen, S., Zhou, Z., and Greenberg, M. E. (2008). "Activating a repressor." *Science* 320:1172–1173.

91. Luger, K., Mader, A. W., Richmond, R. K., Sargent, D. F., and Richmond, T. J. (1997). "Crystal structure of the nucleosome core particle at 2, 8, A resolution." *Nature* 389:251–260.

92. Strahl, B. D., and Allis, C. D. (2000). "The language of covalent histone modifications." *Nature* 403:41–45.

93. Tanner, K. G., Langer, M. R., and Denu, J. M. (1999). "Catalytic mechanism and function of invariant glutamic acid 173 from the histone acetyltransferase GCN5 transcriptional coactivator." *J. Biol. Chem.* 274:18157–18160.

94. Tanner, K. G., Langer, M. R., Kim, Y., and Denu, J. M. (2000). "Kinetic mechanism of the histone acetyltransferase GCN5 from yeast." *J. Biol. Chem.* 275:22048–22055.

95. Lau, O. D., Courtney, A. D., Vassilev, A., Marzilli, L. A., Cotter, R. J., Nakatani, Y., and Cole, P. A. (2000). "p300/CBP-associated factor histone acetyltransferase processing of a peptide substrate. Kinetic analysis of the catalytic mechanism." *J. Biol. Chem.* 275:21953–21959.

96. Tanner, K. G., Langer, M. R., and Denu, J. M. (2000). "Kinetic mechanism of human histone acetyltransferase P/CAF." *Biochemistry* 39:11961–11969.

97. Buck, S. W., Gallo, C. M., and Smith, J. S. (2004). "Diversity in the Sir2 family of protein deacetylases." *J. Leukoc. Biol.* 75:939–950.

98. Swank, M. W., and Sweatt, J. D. (2001). "Increased histone acetyltransferase and lysine acetyltransferase activity and biphasic activation of the ERK/RSK cascade in insular cortex during novel taste learning." *J. Neurosci.* 21:3383–3391.

99. Chwang, W. B., O'Riordan, K. J., Levenson, J. M., and Sweatt, J. D. (2006). "ERK/MAPK regulates hippocampal histone phosphorylation following contextual fear conditioning." *Learn. Mem.* 13:322–328.

100. Brami-Cherrier, K., Valjent, E., Hervé, D., Darragh, J., Corvol, J. C., Pages, C., Arthur, S. J., Girault, J. A., and Caboche, J. (2005). "Parsing molecular and behavioral effects of cocaine in mitogen- and stress-activated protein kinase-1-deficient mice." *J. Neurosci.* 25:11444–11454.

101. Chwang, W. B., Arthur, J. S., Schumacher, A., and Sweatt, J. D. (2007). "The nuclear kinase mitogen- and stress-activated protein kinase 1 regulates hippocampal chromatin remodeling in memory formation." *J. Neurosci.* 27:12732–12742.

102. Yeh, S. H., Lin, C. H., and Gean, P. W. (2004). "Acetylation of nuclear factor-kappaB in rat amygdala improves long-term but not short-term retention of fear memory." *Mol. Pharmacol.* 65:1286–1292.

103. Oliveira, A. M., Wood, M. A., McDonough, C. B., and Abel, T. (2007). "Transgenic mice expressing an inhibitory truncated form of p300 exhibit long-term memory deficits." *Learn. Mem.* 14:564–572.

104. Kim, S. Y., Levenson, J. M., Korsmeyer, S., Sweatt, J. D., and Schumacher, A. (2007). "Developmental regulation of Eed complex composition governs a switch in global histone modification in brain." *J. Biol. Chem.* 282:9962–9972.

105. Chandramohan, Y., Droste, S. K., and Reul, J. M. (2007). "Novelty stress induces phospho-acetylation of histone H3 in rat dentate gyrus granule neurons through coincident signalling via the N-methyl-D-aspartate receptor and the glucocorticoid receptor: relevance for c-fos induction." *J. Neurochem.* 101:815–828.

106. Levenson, J. M., O'Riordan, K. J., Brown, K. D., Trinh, M. A., Molfese, D. L., and Sweatt, J. D. (2004). "Regulation of histone acetylation during memory formation in the hippocampus." *J. Biol. Chem.* 279:40545–40559.

107. Fanselow, M. S., Kim, J. J., Yipp, J., and De Oca, B. (1994). "Differential effects of the N-methyl-D-aspartate antagonist DL-2-amino-5-phosphonovalerate on acquisition of fear of auditory and contextual cues." *Behav. Neurosci.* 108:235–240.

108. Atkins, C. M., Selcher, J. C., Petraitis, J. J., Trzaskos, J. M., and Sweatt, J. D. (1998). "The MAPK cascade is required for mammalian associative learning." *Nat. Neurosci.* 1:602–609.

109. Selcher, J. C., Atkins, C. M., Trzaskos, J. M., Paylor, R., and Sweatt, J. D. (1999). "A necessity for MAP kinase activation in mammalian spatial learning." *Learn. Mem.* 6:478–490.

110. Gräff, J., and Mansuy, I. M. (2008). "Epigenetic codes in cognition and behaviour." *Behav. Brain Res.* 192(1):70–87.

111. Wood, M. A., Hawk, J. D., and Abel, T. (2006). "Combinatorial chromatin modifications and memory storage: a code for memory." *Learn. Mem.* 13:241–244.

112. Korzus, E., Rosenfeld, M. G., and Mayford, M. (2004). "CBP histone acetyltransferase activity is a critical component of memory consolidation." *Neuron* 42:961–972.

113. Alarcon, J. M., Malleret, M., Vronskava, S., Ishii, S., Kandel, E. R., and Barco, A. (2004). "Chromatin acetylation, memory, and LTP are impaired in CBP +/− mice: a model for the cognitive deficit in Rubinstein-Taybi syndrome and its amelioration." *Neuron* 42:947–959.

114. Wood, M. A., Attner, M. A., Oliveira, A. M., Brindle, P. K., and Abel, T. (2006). "A transcription factor-binding domain of the coactivator CBP is essential for long-term memory and the expression of specific target genes." *Learn. Mem.* 13:609–617.

115. Vecsey, C. G., Hawk, J. D., Lattal, K. M., Stein, J. M., Fabian, S. A., Attner, M. A., Cabrera, S. M., McDonough, C. B., Brindle, P. K., Abel, T., and Wood, M. A. (2007). "Histone deacetylase inhibitors enhance memory and synaptic plasticity via CREB:CBP-dependent transcriptional activation." *J. Neurosci.* 27:6128–6140.

116. Bredy, T. W., Wu, H., Crego, C., Zellhoefer, J., Sun, Y. E., and Barad, M. (2007). "Histone modifications around individual

BDNF gene promoters in prefrontal cortex are associated with extinction of conditioned fear." *Learn. Mem.* 14:268–276.

117. Bredy, T. W., and Barad, M. (2008). "The histone deacetylase inhibitor valproic acid enhances acquisition, extinction, and reconsolidation of conditioned fear." *Learn. Mem.* 15:39–45.

118. Lattal, K. M., Barrett, R. M., and Wood, M. A. (2007). "Systemic or intrahippocampal delivery of histone deacetylase inhibitors facilitates fear extinction." *Behav. Neurosci.* 121:1125–1131.

119. Levenson, J. M., Roth, T. L., Lubin, F. D., Miller, C. A., Huang, I. C., Desai, P., Malone, L. M., and Sweatt, J. D. (2006). "Evidence that DNA (cytosine-5) methyltransferase regulates synaptic plasticity in the hippocampus." *J. Biol. Chem.* 281:15763–15773.

120. Miller, C. A., Campbell, S. L., and Sweatt, J. D. (2008). "DNA methylation and histone acetylation work in concert to regulate memory formation and synaptic plasticity." *Neurobiol. Learn. Mem.* 89:599–603.

121. Greenough, W. T., Wood, W. E., and Madden, T. C. (1972). "Possible memory storage differences among mice reared in environments varying in complexity." *Behav. Biol.* 7: 717–722.

122. Fischer, A., Sananbenesi, F., Wang, X., Dobbin, M., and Tsai, L. H. (2007). "Recovery of learning and memory is associated with chromatin remodeling." *Nature* 447:178–182.

123. Abel, T., and Zukin, R. S. (2008). "Epigenetic targets of HDAC inhibition in neurodegenerative and psychiatric disorders." *Curr. Opin. Pharmacol.* 8:57–64.

124. Maue, R. A., Kraner, S. D., Goodman, R. H., and Mandel, G. (1990). "Neuron-specific expression of the rat brain type II sodium channel gene is directed by upstream regulatory elements." *Neuron* 4:223–231.

125. Li, L., Suzuki, T., Mori, N., and Greengard, P. (1993). "Identification of a functional silencer element involved in neuron-specific expression of the synapsin I gene." *Proc. Natl. Acad. Sci. USA*, 90:1460–1464.

126. Mori, N., Schoenherr, C., Vandenbergh, D. J., and Anderson, D. J. (1992). "A common silencer element in the SCG10 and type II Na^+ channel genes bind a factor present in nonneuronal cells but not in neuronal cells." *Neuron* 9:45–54.

127. Chong, J. A., Tapia-Ramirez, J., Kim, S., Toledo-Aral, J. J., Zheng, Y., Boutros, M. C., Altshuller, Y. M., Frohman, M. A., Kraner, S. D., and Mandel, G. (1995). "REST: a mammalian silencer protein that restricts sodium channel gene expression to neurons." *Cell* 80:949–957.

128. Chen, Z. F., Paquette, A. J., and Anderson, D. J. (1998). "NRSF/ REST is required *in vivo* for repression of multiple neuronal target genes during embryogenesis." *Nat. Genet.* 20:136–142.

129. Paquette, A. J., Perez, S. E., and Anderson, D. J. (2000). "Constitutive expression of the neuron-restrictive silencer factor (NRSF)/REST in differentiating neurons disrupts neuronal gene expression and causes axon pathfinding errors *in vivo*." *Proc. Natl. Acad. Sci. USA*, 97:12318–12323.

130. Andres, M. E., Burger, C., Peral-Rubio, M. J., Battaglioli, E., Anderson, M. E., Grimes, J., Dallman, J., Ballas, N., and Mandel, G. (1999). "CoREST: a functional corepressor required for regulation of neural-specific gene expression." *Proc. Natl. Acad. Sci. USA*, 96:9873–9878.

131. Huang, Y., Myers, S. J., and Dingledine, R. (1999). "Transcriptional repression by REST: recruitment of Sin3A and histone deacetylase to neuronal genes." *Nat. Neurosci.* 2:867–872.

132. Naruse, Y., Aoki, T., Kojima, T., and Mori, N. (1999). "Neural restrictive silencer factor recruits mSin3 and histone deacetylase complex to repress neuron-specific target genes." *Proc. Natl. Acad. Sci. USA*, 96:13691–13696.

133. Grimes, J. A., Nielsen, S. J., Battaglioli, E., Miska, E. A., Speh, J. C., Berry, D. L., Atouf, F., Holdener, B. C., Mandel, G., and Kouzarides, T. (2000). "The co-repressor mSin3A is a functional component of the REST-CoREST repressor complex." *J. Biol. Chem.* 275:9461–9467.

134. Roopra, A., Sharling, L., Wood, I. C., Briggs, T., Bachfischer, U., Paquette, A. J., and Buckley, N. J. (2000). "Transcriptional repression by neuron-restrictive silencer factor is mediated via the Sin3-histone deacetylase complex." *Mol. Cell Biol.* 20:2147–2157.

135. Ballas, N., Battaglioli, E., Atouf, F., Andres, M. E., Chenoweth, J., Anderson, M. E., Burger, C., Moniwa, M., Davie, J. R., Bowers, W. J., Federoff, H. J., Rose, D. W., Rosenfeld, M. G., Brehm, P., and Mandel, G. (2001). "Regulation of neuronal traits by a novel transcriptional complex." *Neuron* 31:353–365.

136. Battaglioli, E., Andrés, M. E., Rose, D. W., Chenoweth, J. G., Rosenfeld, M. G., Anderson, M. E., and Mandel, G. (2002). "REST repression of neuronal genes requires components of the hSWI. SNF complex." *J. Biol. Chem.* 277:41038–41045.

137. Lunyak, V. V., Burgess, R., Prefontaine, G. G., Nelson, C., Sze, S. H., Chenoweth, J., Schwartz, P., Pevzner, P. A., Glass, C., Mandel, G., and Rosenfeld, M. G. (2002). "Corepressor-dependent silencing of chromosomal regions encoding neuronal genes." *Science* 298:1747–1752.

138. Weaver, I. C., Cervoni, N., Champagne, F. A., D'Alessio, A. C., Sharma, S., Seckl, J. R., Dymov, S., Szyf, M., and Meaney, M. J. (2004). "Epigenetic programming by maternal behavior." *Nat. Neurosci.* 7:847–854.

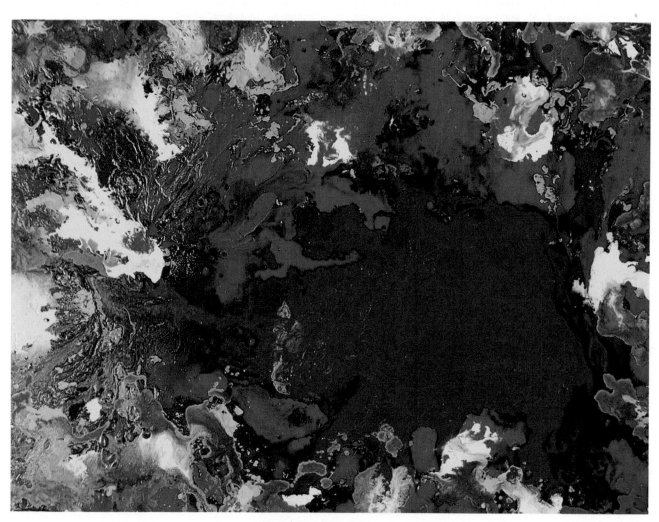

Mental Retardation Syndromes
J. David Sweatt, acrylic on canvas, 2008–2009

11

Inherited Disorders of Human Memory—Mental Retardation Syndromes

As human beings, our great capacity for learning and remembering plays an enormous role in forming our personal potential. Moreover, our personal experiences, where we have learned and remembered specific items and events, define us as individuals. These truths are nowhere more evident than when we consider individuals with pronounced learning and memory deficits present from birth. In this chapter we consider human mental retardation syndromes and their underlying molecular basis. In some instances we will actually be able to tie mechanisms for these disorders back into fundamental mechanisms for synaptic plasticity and learning that we have already discussed.

There is another point that is important to make in the context of this chapter. Of all the various areas of cognitive neurobiology, the field of learning and memory has advanced the farthest into studies at the molecular level, based on a reductionist approach of using model systems simpler than the human one. But how can one bridge the enormous distance from specific molecules to *human* cognition? Over the past few years a number of research groups have undertaken bridging this gap by studying naturally-occurring human mental retardation syndromes. The philosophy of the approach is to use identified human genetic mutations that result in mental retardation and learning disorders, and use these identified genes as an entry to start understanding the molecular basis of human cognition. As a practical matter, this translates into taking an identified human gene linked to a mental retardation syndrome or learning disability and making knockout and transgenic mouse models of that disorder to study in the laboratory. These models are then used to generate insights into the underlying molecular and cellular basis of the defect. The rationale is that this gives one insights into the analogous "knockout humans," and hence gives insights into the molecular neurobiology of human cognitive processing related to learning and memory formation. Some specific examples of mental retardation syndromes where this approach has been applied are given in Table 1.

TABLE 1   Mouse Models of Human Mental Retardation Syndromes

Human Mental Retardation Syndromes	Gene Product	Potential Targets	Mouse Model		References
			Learning defects?	LTP change?	
Neurofibromatosis	Neurofibromin 1 (NF1)	ras/ERK, adenylyl cyclase, cytoskeleton	+	+	Costa et al. (4, 39) Tong et al. (9)
Coffin-Lowry Syndrome	Ribosomal S6 Kinase2 (rsk2)	CREB, ribosomal S6 protein	+	?	Dufresne et al. (12) Harum et al. (13)
Angelman Syndrome	Ubiquitin ligase (E6AP)	p53 tumor suppressor protein, others?	+	+	Jiang et al. (40)
Fragile X mental retardation 1	FMR1 protein (RNA binding protein)	protein synthesis machinery, mRNA targeting, spine structure, LTD	+ (strain dependent)	?	Bardoni et al. (17)
Fragile X mental retardation 2	FMR2 protein (putative transcription factor)	Unknown—gene expression	+	+	Gu et al. (41)
Rett Syndrome	Methyl-CpG binding protein 2 (MeCP$_2$)	Transcriptional repressors— regulation of unknown genes	?	?	Shahbazian et al. (23)
Myotonic dystrophy	Dystrophin protein kinase (DMPK)	Na$^+$ channels, Tau, many others	?	?	Mistry et al. (42)
Down Syndrome (Trisomy 21)	DS critical locus	Multiple genes including DYRK1A and SOD	+	+	Siarey et al. (36)
	DYRK1A (minibrain kinase homolog)	unknown	+	?	Altafaj et al. (35)
	Superoxide dismutase (SOD)	Superoxide-dependent processes—redox regulation of PKC, ras, transcription factors	+	+	Gahtan et al. (43)
Williams Syndrome	WS critical locus: LIMK-1 Elastin Syntaxin 1A FKBP6 EIFH4	cytoskeleton extracellular matrix spine morphology	+	+	Morris et al. (44)

Even though this approach is at a very early stage, it is interesting that different studies of this sort have already begun to converge on two common signal transduction cascades as being involved in human learning and memory: the ras/ERK cascade and its associated upstream regulators and downstream targets (see Figures 1 and 2); and the CaMKII system. In the first section of this chapter I will describe exciting recent findings implicating dysfunction of the ras/ERK cascade in human learning disabilities. I should emphasize that several of the ideas I will present in this section, where I present potential mechanistic links between various different human mental retardation syndromes, are at best educated guesses. However, considering these studies allows us to begin to synthesize a unified picture of critical molecular events in human learning, which extend perfectly the sorts of studies we have been discussing where learning was studied in rodent models.

In the second section of this chapter I will discuss recent findings implicating CaMKII in a form of human learning and memory disorder, Angelman Syndrome.[1]

[1]Before getting down to the serious business of this chapter I want to relate a personal anecdote that illustrates the funny way that things sometime evolve in science. Alcino Silva and I are of the same scientific generation, and as such have been competitors in a certain sense—we both set out as naïve, optimistic young scientists to "solve memory," of course ideally before anyone else did. While I'm oversimplifying, Alcino basically staked his claim with CaMKII and I grabbed MAP kinases, each of us working on basic mechanisms of synaptic plasticity and memory that were described earlier in this book. Essentially as side projects, Alcino started working on neurofibromatosis mental retardation and my laboratory started working on Angelman mental retardation syndrome. In the first section of this chapter I'm going to describe work from Alcino's laboratory highlighting the likely importance of MAP kinase in human memory, based on his studies of neurofibromatosis. In the second section, I am going to describe studies from my laboratory suggesting the importance of CaMKII in human memory, based on our studies of Angelman Syndrome. In my mind these are very satisfying examples of how following the clues that Nature gives us will always lead us to common ground.

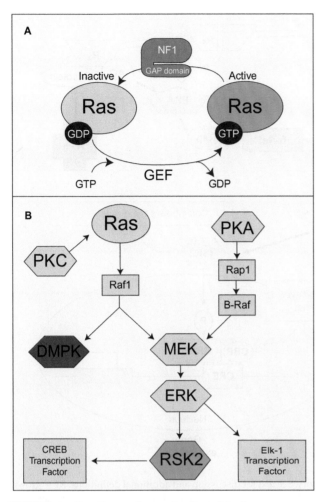

FIGURE 1 Signaling pathways implicated in human memory formation. (A) Ras is a small GTPase whose activity is regulated by the presence of GTP or GDP. When bound to GDP, Ras is inactive. Guanine nucleotide exchange factors (GEF) catalyze the exchange of a molecule of GDP for a molecule of GTP. Once bound to GTP, Ras is activated. GTPase activating proteins (GAP) promote the hydrolysis of GTP to GDP, inactivating Ras. NF1 contains a GAP, and is involved in inactivation of Ras. (B) Signaling through PKA and PKC leads to activation of ERK/MAPK. In parallel, Raf-1 also activates the DM1-associated protein kinase (DMPK) involved in myotonic dystrophy. RSK2 is activated by ERK, and regulates gene transcription. CLS is due to disruption of RSK2. Figure and legend adapted from Weeber et al. (2002). *Molecular Interventions* 2(6):376–391. Copyright American Society for Pharmacology and Experimental Therapeutics 2002.

In the final section I will discuss fragile X retardation syndromes, and we will see yet another instance of where basic studies of synaptic plasticity have run head-on into studies of a human learning disorder. In this last section I will highlight work that has begun to tie mechanisms of local dendritic protein synthesis in with molecular mechanisms of fragile X mental retardation type 1.

I. NEUROFIBROMATOSIS, COFFIN-LOWRY SYNDROME, AND THE RAS/ERK CASCADE

Neurofibromatosis is an autosomal dominant disease that exhibits a variety of clinical features, principally neurofibromas, or benign tumors of neural origin. Other characteristics can include skin discoloration (café au lait spots) and skeletal malformation. The gene that causes neurofibromatosis when mutated in humans is the neurofibromatosis type 1 oncogene, NF1. NF1 is distinct from the gene coding for a second type of neurofibroma-related gene, NF2, which causes a different type of neurofibromatosis.

Heterozygous NF1 mutations result in human mental retardation in about 50% of cases. The heterogeneity of mutations in the NF1 gene is likely to contribute to its lack of complete penetrance for various phenotypes, including the mental retardation phenotype. Thus, while *neurofibromatosis* was initially identified and named for the neurofibroma tumor phenotype, the genetic mutation also causes *mental retardation* in humans (2–3).

The product of the NF1 gene is neurofibromin, a multidomain molecule that has the capacity to regulate several intracellular processes, including the ERK MAP kinase cascade, adenylyl cyclase, and cytoskeletal assembly. *In vivo* human neurofibromin is expressed as the product of four different mRNA splice variants, and the type I and type II variants are abundantly expressed in brain. Alternative splicing of exon 23a in the gene results in the type I and type II variants; type II neurofibromin includes the 23a exon product, while type I does not. In a sophisticated study using knockout mouse technology, Alcino Silva and his colleagues identified the 23a exon product as being critical for learning (4). Mice lacking the 23a product exhibited learning problems, but no apparent developmental abnormalities or tumor predisposition, thus implicating the 23a-encoded protein domain as being involved in learning. The 23a-encoded domain of neurofibromin type I protein contributes to regulating the GAP (GTPase activating protein) domain of NF1, a domain that regulates interaction with the NF1 target ras (5–6). As was described in an earlier chapter, ras is a low-molecular-weight G protein coupled to downstream activation of the ERK cascade (see Figure 1).

In considering that the learning-associated exon of NF1 controlled its GAP activity, Silva and his group proposed that loss of NF1 regulation of ras, specifically hyperactivation of ras, caused the learning disorder phenotype in Nf1 exon 23a−/− animals. However, due to the complexities of NF1 protein function, and indeed even the complexities of how the 23a exon

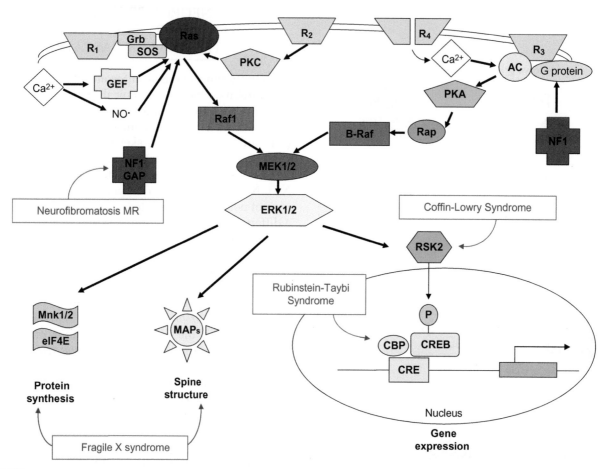

FIGURE 2 Signal transduction pathways involved in learning and memory. See text for discussion and additional definitions. R1 = growth factor receptor tyrosine kinases; R2 = phospholipase C coupled receptors; R3 = adenylyl cyclase coupled receptors; R4 = ligand-gated calcium channels. MAPs = microtubulin associated proteins. CBP = CREB binding protein. CRE = cAMP response element. Figure reproduced from Weeber et al. (1).

product might itself regulate GAP activity in NF1, the conclusion was inferential. Thus, it was necessary to come up with an independent line of evidence that the NF-1 mutation-associated learning deficits were indeed due to mis-regulation of ras. In impressive follow-up studies Silva's laboratory directly tested their hypothesis that ras hyperactivation caused learning deficiencies in NF1-deficient animals. In this series of studies they used the classical genetic approach of diminishing ras function through heterozygous ras gene deletion, as well as using a pharmacologic inhibitor of ras activity *in vivo*, to probe for interactions of the NF1 gene product with the ras pathway (7).

The mouse model that they used was an NF1 knockout mouse with a heterozygous deficiency. Silva et al. assessed learning using the Morris water maze paradigm which, as we have already discussed, measures hippocampus-dependent spatial learning. They observed that heterozygous NF1-deficient animals

exhibited deficits in the Morris maze task, as assessed using a probe trial and by quantitating quadrant search time. Thus, as expected, heterozygous NF1-deficient mice mimicked aspects of the human learning defects associated with NF1 deficiency. Prior studies by another group (8) had shown directly that loss of NF1 led to aberrant activation of the ras/ERK cascade, specifically that NF1 heterozygous deficient animals exhibited increased ras/ERK activity in non-neuronal cells. This observation directly suggested that alterations is ras activity occurred in these mice, and thus could be causative of the learning phenotype, as they had hypothesized based on their earlier studies with exon 23a-deficient mice.

To test this idea, Silva et al. crossed NF1 heterozygous knockout animals with animals deficient in ras, reasoning appropriately that if hyperactive ras caused the NF1+/− learning phenotype, then genetically-diminishing ras activity should rescue the

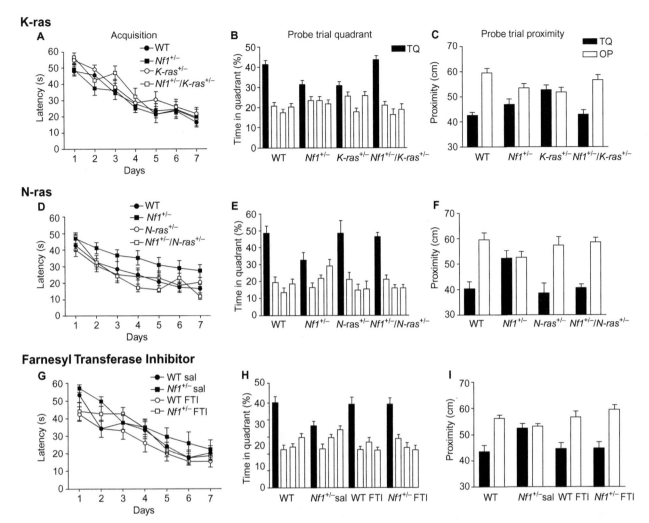

FIGURE 3 RAS-dependent spacial learning in *Nf1^{+/-}* animals. These data illustrate learning deficits of Nf1+/− mice are Ras dependent. Results shown are from the hidden version of the water maze for the Nf1+/−/K-ras+/− population, n=11 (wildtype (WT), n=24; Nf1+/−, n=15; K-ras+/−, n=15). (A) Latency to get to the platform over days. (B) Percent time spent in each quadrant during a probe trial. (C) Average proximity to the exact position where the platform was during training, compared with proximity to the opposite position in the pool. (D)–(F) Illustrate acquisition, percent time in quadrant, and proximity data for the Nf1+/−/N-ras+/− population (WT, n=10; Nf1+/−, n=10; N¡ras, n=7; Nf1+/−/N-ras+/−, n=9). (G)–(I) Illustrate data obtained with acute pharmacologic inhibition of ras by use of a farnesyl transferase inhibitor (abbreviated FTI). Acquisition, percent time in quadrant, and proximity data for the different genotypes and treatments during the FTI rescue experiment (WT+FTI, n=19; WTsaline, n=18; Nf1+/− FTI , n=18; Nf1+/− saline, n=18). Quadrants are training quadrant (TQ), adjacent right, adjacent left and opposite quadrant (OP). Figure reproduced from Costa et al. (39).

animals to normal learning behavior. Costa et al. identified both N-ras and K-ras heterozygous deficiencies as rescuing the learning defect in NF1+/− mice (see Figure 3). These data strongly implicate ras, specifically N-ras and K-ras, as downstream effectors of NF1 *in vivo*. Moreover, these findings implicate hyperactivation of this pathway as causative of learning deficiencies in NF1-deficient mammals, including, of course, the human.

In all studies using animal models constitutively deficient in a gene product it is important to distinguish between the acute, ongoing need for the activity

of the gene product, versus a developmental necessity for the same protein. Silva and his collaborators addressed this issue by acutely administering a farnesyl transferase inhibitor (which inhibits ras activity by disrupting its membrane association), and demonstrating that transient inhibition of ras in adult animals rescued the learning phenotype in NF1 heterozygous animals. Of course, farnesyl transferases act on other proteins besides ras, so a caveat to this experiment is the possibility of the inhibitor affecting other targets than ras. However, their interpretation of a need for acute ras-dependent processes for adult learning and memory is also consistent with the wide variety of additional evidence we have already discussed implicating the ras/ERK cascade in learning and memory.

Silva et al. next used their NF1+/− animal models to assess hippocampal long-term potentiation (LTP), using theta-burst stimulation. They found deficits in theta-burst LTP in NF1-deficient animals which, like the learning defects, were rescued by heterozygous deletion of ras (see Figure 4). One twist to the story is that Silva found that alterations in GABA-ergic function are likely involved in the LTP phenotype, specifically GABA-ergic feedforward inhibitory neurons in area CA1 that regulate cellular excitability and the likelihood of LTP induction under some conditions such as theta-burst stimulation. They observed that blocking this system rescued the effects of NF1 deficiency on LTP, suggesting that NF1 functioned to control this GABA-ergic system, and through this mechanism controlled the likelihood of LTP induction. They also directly observed enhanced GABA-ergic function in the NF1+/− animals in whole-cell recording of GABA inputs onto CA1 pyramidal neurons. Thus, the critical locus of NF1 function may be GABA-ergic interneurons. However, in additional, more recent studies, Silva's group has observed derangement of LTP in the pyramidal neurons of area CA1 as well, using other types of LTP induction protocols that don't involve GABA-ergic interneurons. Thus, there is also an effect of NF1/ras in pyramidal neuron dendrites.

Having found that diminishing ras function led to a rescue of the phenotype, we are compelled to ask: what is the target of ras that leads to these derangements? As described earlier, ras regulates the MEK/ERK MAPK cascade in hippocampal neurons, and Ingram et al. (8) had previously reported elevated ERK activity in NF1-deficient animals. Thus, the most likely target is the raf/MEK/ERK signal transduction cascade. Moreover, other work by Silva has also nicely demonstrated an interaction of ras with the ERK cascade using an approach they termed "pharmacogenetics." They found that mice heterozygous for a null mutation of the K-ras gene (K-ras+/−) showed normal hippocampal ERK activation, LTP, and contextual conditioning in a conditioned place preference task. However, treatment with a low dose of MEK inhibitor, ineffective in wildtype controls, blocked MAPK activation, LTP, and contextual learning in K-ras+/− mutants. These data strongly indicated that K-Ras is upstream of MEK/ERK signaling in the hippocampus, and that acute activation of this pathway is involved in synaptic plasticity and memory.

Aside from direct ras/ERK cascade regulation, another potential function of NF1 is regulating adenylyl cyclase; Tong et al. demonstrated that NF1 also regulates adenylyl cyclase in mammalian neurons (see Figure 1 and reference 9). They showed that neuropeptide and G-protein-stimulated adenylyl cyclase activity were reduced in mice completely deficient in NF1 activity. While the effects on adenylyl cyclase seen by Tong et al. were selective for animals with homozygous deletions of NF1, it is certainly worthwhile considering that attenuation of subtle forms of regulation of adenylyl cyclase might also play a role in learning deficits in heterozygous NF1-deficient animals. Of course, adenylyl cyclase is also upstream of the ERK MAP kinase cascade in hippocampal neurons (see Figure 1). Thus, NF1 may couple to ERK via two pathways in the hippocampus, and both these effects may contribute to dysregulation of ERK in NF1-deficient mice and humans.

One of the targets of ERK in the hippocampus is CREB, and as we discussed in the last chapter this molecule has been widely implicated in learning and memory in many species. ERK can couple to CREB through the intervening kinase ribosomal S6 kinase (RSK2), which phosphorylates CREB at ser133 just like PKA. As I described in the last chapter, in the mammalian hippocampus it has been found that PKA cannot elicit CREB phosphorylation without going through ERK, thus ERK/RSK2 may be an obligatory step in PKA regulation of CREB-mediated gene expression in mammalian hippocampal neurons (10–11). The important implication of this in the present context is that rsk2 is the gene disrupted in human Coffin-Lowry Mental Retardation Syndrome (12–13). Thus, the same pathway implicated in studies of neurofibromatosis mental retardation, ERK/RSK2/CREB, has also been implicated as being involved in human learning and memory in an independent line of studies (see also Box 1).

Overall, while our current thinking is likely oversimplified, it is interesting that two different human mental retardation or learning deficiency-associated syndromes impinge on the same signal transduction cascade, the ras/ERK/CREB cascade, which is coupled to regulation of gene expression in neurons. As we have discussed earlier, it is noteworthy that this same cascade has been implicated in learning and memory in a wide variety of different species—it is now safe in my opinion to add the human to the list.

It is also interesting to speculate about another potential downstream target of the ERK cascade, the protein synthesis machinery (see Figure 2). This target is appealing, given the widespread documentation of a role for protein synthesis in learning that we have discussed. As was described in Chapter 9, ERK is known to regulate protein synthesis through regulating the activity of eIF4E, via the intervening kinase

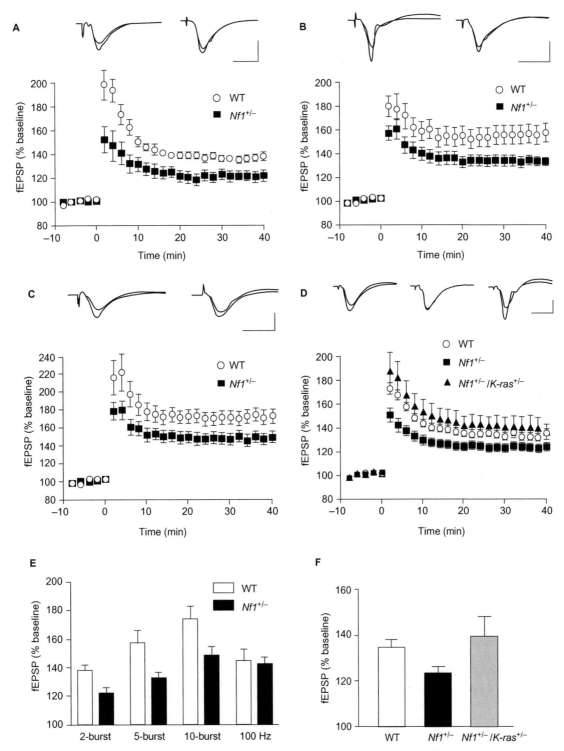

FIGURE 4 RAS-dependent LTP deficits in *NF1*[+/−] animals. (A)–(D) Neurofibromin 1 heterozygous deficiency animals exhibit LTP deficits for a variety of LTP induction protocols. (D) Illustrates that K-ras heterozygous deficiency rescues the Nf1-associated LTP deficit, indicating that it results from an overactivation of ras. For each panel percentage of baseline field EPSE is plotted over time. (A) Two burst induction protocol (wild type (WT), n = 5; *Nf1*[+/−], n = 8). (B) Five-burst induction protocol (WT, n = 7; *NF1*[+/−], n = 8). (C) Ten-burst induction protocol (WT, n = 7; *Nf1*[+/−], n = 11). (D) Two burst induction protocol ras rescue experiment, where heterozygous deficiency of K-ras rescues the LTP in *Nf1*-deficient animals. Thus, LTP deficits in *Nf1*[+/−] mice are Ras dependent (WT, n = 13; *Nf1*[+/−], n = 13; *Nf1*[+/−]/K-ras[+/−], n = 8). Representative traces are shown from left to right for WT, *Nf1*[+/−] and *Nf1*[+/−]/K-ras [+/−]. Horizontal bar, 10 ms; vertical bar 1 mV. (E) Summarizes the amount of LTP measured 40 minutes after induction under the different stimulation protocols. (F) Illustrates that LTP measured 40 minutes after induction in the *Nf1*[+/−]/K-ras[+/−] rescue experiment is comparable to wildtype. Data, figure and legend reproduced from Costa et al. (39).

BOX 1

RUBINSTEIN-TAYBI SYNDROME

As we discussed in the last chapter, one human mental retardation syndrome associated with the PKA/ERK/CREB pathway is Rubinstein-Taybi Syndrome (RTS). RTS patients have some facial abnormalities, broad big toes and thumbs, and mental retardation. The RTS gene has been mapped to chromosome 16 and identified as CREB binding protein (CBP). As described earlier, CBP is a transcriptional co-activator with CREB that obligatorily participates with phospho-CREB to regulate gene expression downstream of the CRE (20). As described in much more detail in the last chapter, CBP is a histone acetyl transferase (HAT), and one mechanism by which CBP promotes gene expression is through histone acetylation, which promotes exposure of DNA for transcription. Loss of this HAT function of CBP likely is one important contributing factor in RTS, through derangements of the normal mechanisms controlling CREB-mediated gene expression.

MNK. Also, a known role for RSK2, the Coffin-Lowry Syndrome gene product, is regulation of protein synthesis. It is intriguing to consider protein synthesis as a potential target downstream of the gene products for neurofibromatosis and Coffin-Lowry Syndrome, because the fragile X mental retardation type 1 (FMR1) gene product (FMRP) likely also contributes to regulating protein synthesis (14); we will discuss this in Section III of this chapter. This potentially would tie yet a third human mental retardation gene product, the fragile X protein, to a common signaling/regulatory cascade.

II. Angelman Syndrome

The use of traditional (i.e., non-inducible) knockout mouse models to try to study the signal transduction events involved in synaptic plasticity and memory has been widely and legitimately criticized, because of the great confound of secondary effects of loss of the gene. In particular, developmental derangements can contribute to any observed phenotype, and there is a real concern that the effect of loss of the gene product is not an indication of the protein having any necessary role in an acute, learning-related signal transduction event. Need for caution in interpreting these types of experiments is highlighted by the numerous demonstrations that these types of developmental and secondary effects do occur in knockout animals.

However, this weakness in the context of one type of experiment is a strength of knockout models in another context. In making a model of a human inherited (i.e., genetic) disorder such as a mental retardation syndrome, one wishes to have the defect present from the point of conception, as is typically the case for the analogous human. The generation of secondary molecular and developmental effects is desirable, in that they model the same secondary effects that are likely to occur in the human. Thus, a strength of the knockout approach in mouse models of human mental retardation is that by characterizing the knockout mice one can gain insights into the entire range of molecular and anatomical effects that contribute to the human learning disorder.

In this section we will be discussing a mouse model for human Angelman Mental Retardation Syndrome. Current thinking in the area is that the Angelman gene product is not itself directly involved in signaling events necessary for learning and memory (although it is too early to really rule this out!), but that secondary changes in targets of the gene product lead to disruption of signaling events necessary for memory. Tracking down these secondary changes has been an interesting detective story: while we are only part of the way to the solution, recent results suggest that one culprit in Angelman Syndrome is dysregulation of CaMKII.

Angelman Syndrome is a fairly rare (about 1 per 15,000 people) but severe human learning and behavioral disorder characterized by four principal features:

1. Developmental delay and pronounced mental retardation;
2. Near or total absence of the capacity for language and speech;
3. Motor dysfunction; and
4. An abnormally cheerful disposition, propensity for laughter, and cheerful affect.

In addition, a history of seizures often presents. The principal features of Angelman Syndrome led

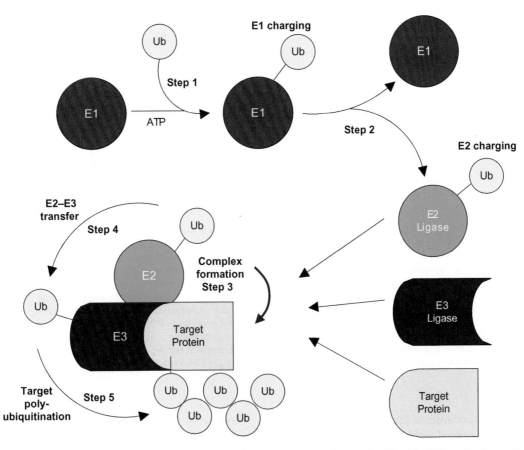

FIGURE 5   The ubiquitination pathway. Covalent association of an E1 subunit with a single ubiquitin (Ub) molecule results in the ATP-dependent activation of Ub (step 1). Ub is then transferred to an E2 subunit (step 2). Association of the E2 and/or E3 plus the target protein results in the formation of a complex (step 3). Complex formation results in the transfer of Ub by E2 either directly to the target protein or through the transfer of the Ub to an E3 (step 4). E3 transfers successive UB molecules to the target protein forming poly-UB chains (step 5). Reproduced from Weeber and Sweatt, (45).

to the unfortunate use of the term "Happy Puppet Syndrome" to describe these patients at one point in time. As with most mental retardation syndromes, the underlying genetic etiology is mixed, in large part due to heterogeneity of deletion mutations that can lead to the disorder. Despite this complexity, recent efforts have identified the gene for Angelman Syndrome as UBE3A, which codes for the E6-AP ubiquitin ligase. E6-AP is an E3 ubiquitin ligase, which covalently attaches the low molecular weight protein ubiquitin to substrate proteins (see Figure 5), a complex process involving other proteins that serve as intermediates and modulators of the final ubiquitination step. Ubiquitination, of course, by and large serves to control trafficking of proteins to the proteasome for degradation. However, it is important to keep in mind that new functions for ubiquitination are being discovered that play a signal transduction role conceptually similar to other post-translational processes, such as phosphorylation.

The Angelman Syndrome E6-AP E3 ligase is one member of a large family of around 60 different E3 ligases, each of which has different substrate selectivities. The E6-AP protein has very restricted substrate specificity—known substrates include the p53 tumor suppressor protein, E6-AP itself, and one additional protein of unknown function.

Expression of the UBE3A gene, in both human and mouse, exhibits a phenomenon called *imprinting*. Imprinting is a general term to describe epigenetic phenomena that can result in silencing the expression of a particular gene. In the case of the UBE3A gene, imprinting, through complex epigenetic molecular mechanisms that are not entirely clear at this point, results in selective silencing of the paternal copy of the gene in the hippocampus and cerebellum. The upshot of this is that the maternal copy of the gene is selectively expressed in these brain subregions. Thus, offspring who inherit a defective copy of UBE3A from their mother have a selective loss of the E6-AP ubiquitin

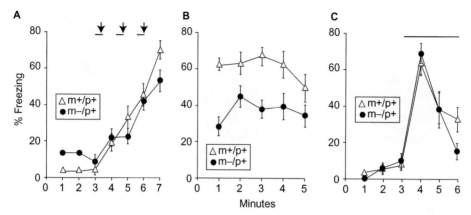

FIGURE 6 Selective deficit in context-dependent fear conditioning in ubiquitin ligase maternal deficiency mice. The E6AP ubiquitin ligase gene (the Angelman Syndrome gene) exhibits imprinting, such that the maternal copy of the gene is selectively expressed in the hippocampus. Offspring of a female mouse deficient in the E6AP ubiquitin ligase thus have a selective hippocampal loss of the E6AP subtype of E3 ubiquitin ligase. In these experiments wildtype mice or maternal deficiency mice were assessed for both contextual (B) or cued (C) fear conditioning 24 hours after training (A). The same group of maternal deficiency mice (n = 12) and wildtype mice (n = 12) were assessed for both context- and tone-dependent freezing. (A) Wildtype and maternal deficiency mice showed comparable freezing during and after the tone and foot shock were administered. (B) Context-dependent fear conditioning: maternal deficiency mice displayed significantly less freezing than wildtype when returned to the test chamber 24 hours later. Significant p values (<0.001) were seen at each sampling period and for the total data by X^2 test. (C) Tone-dependent fear conditioning: maternal deficiency mice and wildtype mice showed comparable freezing when presented with the tone in a novel context immediately after context-dependent testing. Tone is shown by horizontal bar and shock is indicated by arrows. Data and figures reproduced from Jiang et al. (40). Copyright Cell Press.

ligase in their hippocampus and cerebellum. Put in genetics jargon, maternal deficiency (m−/p+) results in a brain subregion-specific knockout of E6AP in both the mouse and human. Angelman Syndrome patients have a rare defect—a brain subregion-selective loss of a specific protein. This imprinting pattern and subregion-selective defect is, of course, consistent with the deficits observed in these patients, which selectively involve learning and motor control.

It seems clear on the face of it that understanding the underlying pathology of Angelman Syndrome patients will give insights into the effects of hippocampal lesions in humans, much like studies of other patients such as H.M. have done. In the case of Angelman Syndrome patients, however, the lesion is genetic and not anatomical—in fact there appear to be no discernible anatomical malformations in the CNS of AS patients. In Angelman Syndrome patients the defect is, of course, also present from birth, in contrast to lesions such as those experienced by H. M.

After Kishino et al. discovered that the UBE3A gene was the Angelman Syndrome gene, ube3a knockout mice were developed in order to make a murine model for Angelman Syndrome. These studies utilized the maternal deficiency mice, as opposed to other types of heterozygous or homozygous knockout animals, in order to model the human syndrome as accurately as possible.

Yong-hui Jiang discovered that mice with a maternal deficiency in ube3a ubiquitin ligase exhibited a selective deficit in contextual fear conditioning, consistent with the selective loss of *hippocampal* ubiquitin ligase due to the maternal imprinting (see Figure 6 and reference 15). The same mice did not exhibit any deficit in cued conditioning, this data serving as a nice positive control for the animals having normal capacity in the amygdala-dependent, hippocampus-independent component of the task.

In addition, hippocampal slices prepared from maternal deficiency mice exhibited a loss of long-term potentiation of Schaffer collateral inputs in area CA1, but normal stimulus-response relationships and paired-pulse facilitation (see Figure 7). Thus, the hippocampus-dependent learning deficit apparently can be accounted for by a selective loss of LTP in the hippocampus—a striking finding considering that hippocampal baseline synaptic transmission, short-term plasticity, and hippocampal anatomy all appear normal in these mice.

In a broad sense these findings implicate the ubiquitin/proteosome pathway in mammalian associative learning and hippocampal long-term potentiation. This represents an interesting parallel to a variety of evidence demonstrating a role for the ubiquitin pathway in long-term facilitation and long-term memory in *Aplysia*. In this system, long-term behavioral sensitization is in part subserved by ubiquitin-mediated proteolysis of PKA regulatory subunits, which elicits long-term increases in PKA activity and long-term facilitation of neurotransmitter release (21–22) (see Chapter 3). In the future it will be interesting to determine to what

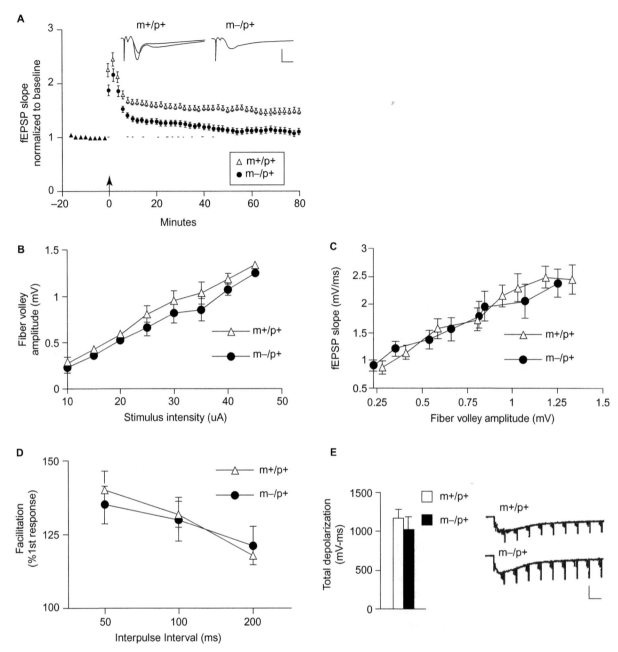

FIGURE 7 Impairment of hippocampal LTP in ubiquitin ligase maternal deficiency mice. (A) Summary of field potential recordings from the CA1 region (mean±SEM) from wildtype (n=17 slices, 11 animals) and E6AP maternal deficiency mice (14 slices, 6 animals). Baseline measurements were taken for at least 20 minutes to confirm stability. Stimulation intensity was adjusted for responses that were ~50% of the maximal fEPSP. Two 100 Hz, 1 second stimuli were given at time 0. Each point is a 2 minute average of six individual fEPSP measurements. The inset presents extracellular field recordings from a representative experiment during a baseline interval and 60 minutes after induction of LTP for a wildtype (m+/p+) and a maternal deficiency (m−/p+) slice. Scale bars for inset, 2 mV and 4 ms. (B) and (C) Baseline synaptic responses were similar for maternal deficiency and wildtype mice. Plots of fiber volley amplitude versus stimulus strength and fEPSP slope versus fiber volley amplitude revealed no difference between wildtype and maternal deficiency mice. Results shown are from nine slices for wildtype and eight slices for maternal deficiency mice. (D) Paired-pulse facilitation is not impaired in maternal deficiency mice. The magnitude of the second response is presented as a percentage of the first response. Results shown are from five slices for wildtype and seven slices for maternal deficiency animals. (E) Responses to tetanic stimulation are no different between maternal deficiency and wildtype mice. Total depolarization (the integral of the tetanic depolarization response) is presented for wildtype (n=6, upper trace) and maternal deficiency (n=6, lower trace) animals. Scale bars for inset, 2 mV and 90 ms. Reproduced from Jiang et al. (40).

extent the roles of the ubiquitin system in mammals parallel those in *Aplysia*.

To the extent that deficiencies in the mouse model for Angelman Syndrome reflect those in human Angelman Syndrome patients, available data suggest that defects in hippocampal long-term potentiation may underlie the learning defects exhibited in Angelman Syndrome. Angelman mice have normal synaptic transmission, short-term plasticity, and hippocampal morphology. Anatomical studies of humans indicate that their hippocampal morphology is similarly normal. Thus, Angelman Syndrome humans appear to have a selective deficit in synaptic plasticity with normal baseline function, based on their anatomical characterization and extrapolating from the mouse model findings. Due to the imprinting of the UBE3A gene Angelman patients likely have this loss of synaptic plasticity restricted to their hippocampus (and cerebellum). Thus, these patients appear to have a very precise and selective lesion, in contrast to patients such as H. M., where there is extensive and imprecise anatomical derangement and, of course, loss of all anatomical connections to and from the hippocampus. To the best of our ability to determine what is happening in the human based on studies of the mouse model, selective deficits in hippocampal long-term synaptic plasticity are what lead to the profound learning and memory deficits of Angelman Syndrome. In my mind this is one of the most important findings to come out of this work.

What are the targets of the E6-AP ubiquitin ligase pathway that lead to this striking memory dysfunction? One possibility, as mentioned above, is that this E3 ligase is serving as a signal transduction pathway that modulates downstream targets acutely. Although this is a possibility, there is no direct evidence to suggest this at present, and a much more parsimonious hypothesis is that the E6-AP is playing the more traditional role of controlling the level of target proteins through sending them to the proteasome. In this scenario, loss of E6-AP will secondarily lead to elevations in the levels of downstream targets due to loss of this mechanism for their degradation.

In considering this hypothesis, I note that it does not immediately lead to a lot of specific possibilities. The E6AP E3 ligase apparently has a quite restricted set of substrates, as mentioned above, so not many candidates come to mind as downstream targets. One known substrate is the p53 tumor suppressor. In fact, maternal deficiency mice exhibit altered levels of p53 in hippocampal pyramidal neurons, so this is one potential mechanism. Disappointingly, however, p53 function is difficult to tie in to synaptic plasticity based on our present state of knowledge. In short, nothing specific about the function of p53

suggests how it could lead to a derangement of LTP and memory.

To try to address the problem in a different way, Ed Weeber in my laboratory decided to test for derangements in the signal transduction mechanisms that we already knew were involved in normal memory formation (see Futher Reading). For these studies we used hippocampal tissue from the Angelman mouse model in western blotting screens, in order to see if any candidate molecules known to function in LTP could be identified. To make a long story very short, after looking at a wide variety of specific proteins and protein kinases, we found an alteration in hippocampal CaMKII.

The alteration was in Thr286 autophosphorylation, not total protein level, which was quite surprising to us because we had expected the loss of proteolysis of a target protein to lead to an increase in the level of that protein. Nevertheless, we observed that hippocampal extracts from Angelman mice exhibited a selective increase in Thr286 autophosphorylation with no change in total protein.

Based on the known property of Thr286 autophosphorylation to render the kinase autonomously active, we next tested these hippocampal extracts for increases in CaMKII activity. In fact, to our further surprise in these studies we found that Angelman mice had *decreased* CaMKII activity. Further studies in collaboration with Ype Elgersma and Alcino Silva indicated the answer to this mystery. These studies showed that there was aberrant hyperphosphorylation of CaMKII at the inhibitory site, thr305/306. This increased inhibitory autophosphorylation is the likely mechanism through which there is a diminution of CaMKII activity in Angelman hippocampus.

Is this single molecular change, increased autophosphorylation at thr305, sufficient to cause Angelman Syndrome? In a complementary series of studies Silva's laboratory converged on this same hypothesis using a transgenic point mutant animal that mimicked hyperphosphorylation at the 305 site, a transgenic animal expressing a thr-to-asp CaMKII point mutant. Their motivation for generation of this animal arose from their years of work investigating the details of CaMKII function and phosphorylation in synaptic plasticity and memory. Strikingly, the data from Silva's laboratory indicated that the 305 hyperphosphorylation is indeed sufficient to give an LTP and learning phenotype reminiscent of Angelman Syndrome.

Finally, in an interesting series of studies, Ed Weeber and Ype Elgersma performed a "rescue" experiment using a double-transgenic approach. In these studies they genetically introduced a mutated form of CaMKII into the Angelman Syndrome mouse line (see Journal Club Articles). The mutated CaMKII they introduced lacked the Thr305 inhibitory auto-phosphorylation site. In an impressive series of studies they found that eliminating the aberrant Thr305 autophosphorylation rescued the plasticity and memory deficits in the Angelman Syndrome mice. Thus, Angelman Syndrome/Thr305 double-mutant animals exhibited normal LTP and normal contextual fear conditioning. These results greatly solidified the hypothesis that aberrant hyperphosphorylation of CaMKII underlies the plasticity and memory deficits in Angelman Syndrome.

We do not know the basis of the hyperphosphorylation. One current working hypothesis, which is very speculative, is that E6AP regulates the level of some protein(s) that control phosphatase activity, perhaps a phosphatase inhibitor. This would link proteolysis, which presumably controls the steady-state level of some protein in the cell, with the phosphorylation increase that has been observed in the Angelman Syndrome mouse model. As mentioned above, certainly at this point one cannot rule out the involvement of a more acute, signal-transduction type process wherein ubiquitination acutely controls a target's catalytic activity.

Overall, in the broadest context, these data strongly indicate that normal function of the CaMKII cascade is necessary for human synaptic plasticity and memory. Specifically, these findings implicate subtle derangement of regulatory mechanisms for CaMKII as being involved in the pronounced memory dysfunction of Angelman Syndrome. As was the case with studies of neurofibromatosis and the ras/ERK cascade, once again decades of study of the basic signal transduction mechanisms for synaptic plasticity and memory converged with studies of human mental retardation.

III. FRAGILE X SYNDROMES

A. Fragile X Mental Retardation Syndrome Type 1

In the late 1980s, an interesting new mechanism for gene disruption was discovered as an outgrowth of studies investigating the genetic basis of human degenerative CNS disorders—the *triplet repeat* mechanism. The essential discovery was that in humans there are repetitive DNA sequences, specifically CGG or similar trinucleotide sequences, that can expand in length (i.e., number of CGG repeats) from generation to generation. In general, once a triplet repeat sequence in or around a gene reaches a critical length normal expression of the gene product is disrupted. Thus, from one generation to the next a family can go from normal expression of a gene product to loss of that same gene due to triplet repeat expansion.

In another variation of triplet repeat-based disorders, the loss of gene function is not precipitous. For example, in a number of neurodegenerative disorders the family exhibits *anticipation*, which refers to a progressive decrease in age-of-onset for the disorder from generation to generation. The decrease in age-of-onset is highly correlated with the length of the triplet repeat expansion.

The exact mechanisms by which triplet repeats disrupt gene expression and gene product function are complex and subject to vigorous investigation at present. If the CGG triplet repeat lies within a coding region of a gene it can result in the expression of a protein product containing polyglutamine. The presence of the polyglutamine stretch can, of course, disrupt the normal function of the protein in which it resides. Alternatively, the expression in cell of polyglutamine itself can be toxic, essentially (or theoretically even directly) resulting in a toxic "gain of function" gene product. Once again, the exact mechanisms by which cellular expression of polyglutamine-containing proteins in neurons lead to neurodegeneration is unclear at present and an active area of investigation.

There also are a number of ways the presence of triplet repeats has been found to affect gene expression. In myotonic dystrophy, the disorder in which triplet repeats were first identified, the mechanism appears to be due to disruption of the function of upstream regulatory DNA sequences that control expression of a protein kinase referred to as dystrophin protein kinase (DMPK; see Table 1 and Figure 1), although other genes may also be affected (Box 2).

For other triplet repeat-based disorders the mechanism is also due to loss of gene/protein expression, but through more complex mechanisms (see Box 3). One example in this category is fragile X mental retardation type 1 (14, 16–17). Fragile X mental retardation syndrome, often abbreviated FRAXA, is one of the most common and debilitating forms of human mental retardation, with a frequency of occurrence in the 1 per 2000 range. The FMR1 gene promoter region in normal humans has 5–50 CGG repeats, which do not adversely affect gene expression. Expansion of the repeats into the 200-repeat range leads to loss of gene expression, and the mechanism for this gene loss is complex (see Figure 8). With expanded repeat numbers, the FMR1 gene promoter region undergoes DNA methylation at C residues of CpG dinucleotides, resulting in gene silencing. Of course, loss of gene transcription leads to loss of mRNA and protein synthesis.

The product of the FMR1 gene is referred to as FMRP, the fragile X mental retardation protein.

BOX 2

RETT SYNDROME

Rett Syndrome was introduced when we discussed DNA methylation and methyl-DNA binding proteins. Rett Syndrome is an unusual disorder in girls that manifests itself as an age-dependent progressive decline in cognitive function, starting after the first year of life. Among its attributes are diminished brain size, mental retardation, the development of stereotyped hand-wringing movements, and ultimately autism-like features. The gene for Rett Syndrome is on the X-chromosome, and embryonic lethality in males (which of course have only one copy of the X-chromosome) likely leads to the syndrome being selectively observed in girls. However, recent findings of Rett gene mutations in boys may lead to identification of a new homologous syndrome in males.

The Rett gene encodes methyl-CpG binding protein 2 (MECP2; 23). As discussed in the last chapter, DNA methylation plays a role in transcriptional silencing of genes and MECP2 is a protein that binds to methylated DNA sequencing and contributes to suppressing the expression of genes in the vicinity. Thus, loss of MECP2 leads to aberrant expression of genes that are normally silent. There is, of course, the potential that a large number of genes are affected secondarily to loss of MECP2, and experiments are underway to determine target genes of this pathway. Studies in this area are also giving important new insights into the mechanisms involved in DNA methylation-associated transcriptional silencing.

BOX 3

WILLIAMS SYNDROME

Another mental retardation-associated syndrome is Williams Syndrome. Williams Syndrome (WS) patients exhibit an interesting idiosyncratic social behavioral syndrome—they are overly friendly. They have been described as "never meeting a stranger," that is, they treat even people that they have just met with great familiarity. Behavioral studies of WS patients show that they manifest an abnormal positive bias toward unknown individuals (24). They also exhibit spatio-visual processing deficits and mild to severe mental retardation. Williams Syndrome arises from deletions in chromosome 7 that typically include multiple genes. Given the complex behavioral manifestations in WS patients, Williams Syndrome provides an interesting example of genetic contributions to complex social behaviors.

One identified gene in the WS locus on chromosome 7 is LIM Kinase 1 (LIMK-1; 25–26), thus WS is associated with a heterozygous deficiency in LIMK-1. LIMK-1 is a target of the rac, rho, and PKC cascades that controls cytoskeletal organization (see Figure). LIMK-1 exerts its effects through phosphorylating and inhibiting actin depolymerization factor (ADF)/cofilin. ADF/cofilin binds directly to actin and promotes actin depolymerization. Thus, the LIMK-1 pathway is one of the specific mechanisms whereby the rho system regulates cytoskeletal structure.

LIMK-1 homozygous knockout mice, as might be expected, have alterations in actin microfilaments due to derangements of actin turnover (27). They also manifest altered dendritic spine morphology at Schaffer collateral synapses in the hippocampus. Specifically, they have fewer actin microfilaments than the normally actin-dense spines, and the dendritic spines in LIMK-1 knockout mice lack the normal bulbous ending that dendritic spines exhibit. However, there are no apparent alterations in synaptic number or baseline synaptic function. Like FMR2 knockout mice, LIMK-1 knockouts exhibit LTP that saturates at a higher level than controls—a higher maximal level of potentiation is achieved with repetitive LTP-inducing stimulation.

BOX 3—cont'd

WILLIAMS SYNDROME

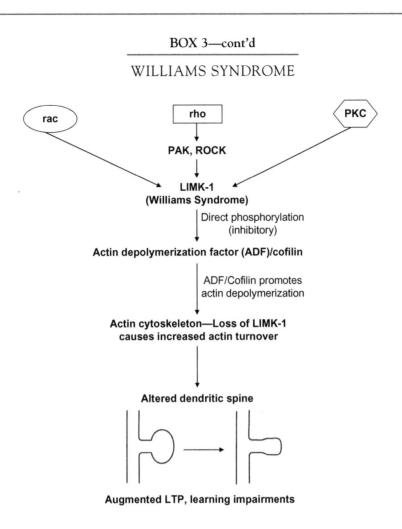

This alteration in synaptic plasticity is also associated with impaired learning. Specifically, LIMK-1 knockouts show a decrease in their capacity to "unlearn" the location of a hidden platform in a Morris water maze task, once they have learned that a platform is associated with a particular location. This is assessed using a platform reversal variation of the water maze, where the hidden platform is moved to a new location after the animal has been repeatedly trained with the platform in one place. The effects on LTP and dendritic spine morphology in the LIMK-1 knockout mouse suggest a possible basis for the cognitive effects in Williams Syndrome. They also point to the growing understanding of the importance of morphological regulation in learning and synaptic plasticity, including apparently those processes occurring in the human CNS.

Although the function of this protein is still being investigated, several studies have indicated that FMRP is an RNA binding protein. As we have already discussed, a current model proposes that, through binding a variety of mRNA species, FMRP regulates protein synthesis (see Chapters 9 and 10). Moreover, several groups have found that FMRP function is necessary for metabotropic glutamate receptor regulation of protein synthesis in synapses (see Further Reading and reference 14). Other studies have also indicated derangements of dendritic spine numbers and morphology in fragile X tissue samples, and in a fragile X mouse model (see Box 4 and reference 18). Thus, while studies in this area are still at a relatively early stage, the intriguing hypothesis is emerging that FMRP plays a key role in local protein synthesis in dendrites, and helps

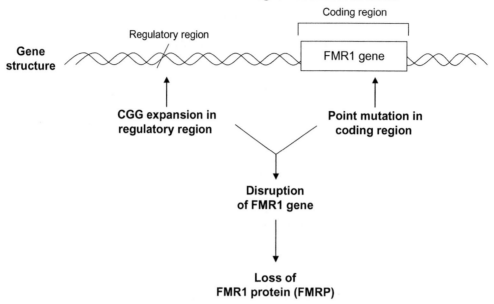

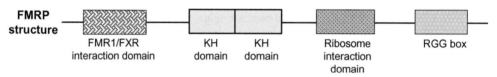

FIGURE 8 A model for fragile X mental retardation syndrome. Triplet repeats in the regulatory region, or mutations in the coding region, of the FMR1 gene lead to (among other things) a loss of the FMR1 gene product, FMRP. FMRP is an RNA binding protein proposed to be involved in dendritic mRNA localization and local protein synthesis (see text for additional discussion).

BOX 4

NON-SYNDROMIC X-LINKED MENTAL RETARDATION

There are a variety of different forms of mental retardation that are not "syndromic," or linked to a specific and consistent spectrum of clinical features other than cognitive impairment, and there have been a number of different genes identified as contributing to these non-syndromic forms of mental retardation. Some of the interesting genes on the X chromosome that have been associated with mental retardation include the L1 neural cell adhesion molecule and three different

genes involved in the rho signal transduction cascade (28–31). Rho stands for ras homolog, which like ras is a low molecular weight G protein linked to a variety of downstream targets (see Figure and reference 32). While the details of the molecular components of this cascade in neurons are still being investigated, three different members of this general cascade have been identified as loci for mental retardation. These include the rho target PAK3 (p21-Activated Kinase; 31, 33), the rho guanine

BOX 4—cont'd

NON-SYNDROMIC X-LINKED MENTAL RETARDATION

nucleotide exchange factors ARHGEF6 (30) and oligophrenin 1 (OPHN1; 34). In general, the rho cascades control cytoskeleton arrangement, cell migration, and gene expression. Current working models for the rho

cascade-associated mental retardation, as well as the retardation associated with L1 protein deficiency, hypothesize the involvement of derangements of cell migration and neuronal process extension.

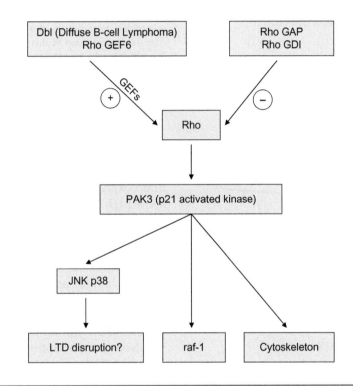

mediate the function of metabotropic glutamate receptors (mGluRs) at the synapse. The mGluR theory of fragile X mental retardation proposes that disruption of this process leads to an excess of mGluR-dependent LTD in the hippocampus, and thus to the learning derangements of fragile X (see Figures 9 and 10). Therefore, once again, we see an example of how detailed studies of the molecular mechanisms of synaptic plasticity have converged with studies of a human learning disorder.

B. Fragile X Mental Retardation Type 2

Fragile X mental retardation type 2, similar to the case with FMR1, results from expansion and methylation of a CCG trinucleotide repeat located in exon 1 of the X-linked FMR2 gene, which results in transcriptional silencing. While the FMR1 syndrome and FMR2

mental retardation share a similar name and mechanism of mutation, FMR2 (also known as FRAXE) is "non-syndromic" (see Box 4). Also, in contrast to the profound mental retardation of FMR1, loss of the FMR2 gene product is associated with a milder mental impairment. Among those with the FMR2 phenotype delays in language development are particularly prominent, and some FMR2 patients also have behavioral deficits, such as attention deficit, hyperactivity, and autistic-like behavior. Also, in contrast to fragile X type 1, which is likely the most common form of mental retardation, expansion of the FMR2-associated CCG repeat is quite rare, with an incidence estimated at less than 1 per 50,000.

Expansion and methylation of a CCG repeat in the 5′ untranslated region (UTR) of exon 1 of FMR2 is the most common lesion, and results in the reduction of FMR2 gene expression. The product of FMR2 is a

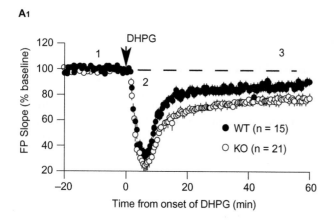

A1

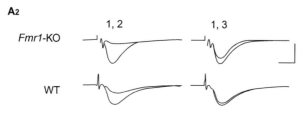

A2

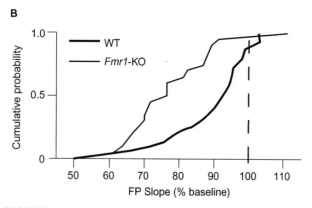

B

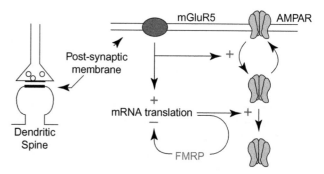

FIGURE 10 A model for the role of mGluR5 in fragile X mental retardation. Previous research has shown that activation of mGluR5 stimulates the internalization of AMPA receptors and NMDARs. The stable expression of this modification requires protein synthesis, which we propose is negatively regulated by FMRP synthesized in response to mGluR activation. Therefore, in the absence of FMRP, LTD magnitude is increased. Figure and legend adapted from Huber et al. (2002). *PNAS* 99:7746–7750. Copyright 2002 National Academy of Sciences, USA.

FIGURE 9 Brief application of the mGluR agonist DHPG (5 minutes; 100 μM) induces greater LTD of synaptic responses in hippocampus of Fmr1-KO mice as compared with WT littermate controls. (A1) Plotted are average (± SEM) FP slope values over the time-course of the experiment. In Fmr1-KO animals, the response 60 minutes after treatment was depressed to 77 ± 3% of preDHPG baseline (n = 21 slices from 9 mice; open circles); in interleaved WT controls, the response was depressed to 88 ± 4% of baseline (n = 15 slices from 8 mice; filled circles; different at P = 0.02; t test). (A2) Representative FPs (2 minutes average) taken at the times indicated by the numbers on the graph. (Bar = 1 mV; 5 msec.) (B) Cumulative probability distributions of FP slope values (% of baseline), measured 1 hour after DHPG in individual slices from both KO and WT groups. The distribution in KO mice is significantly different from that in WT mice, as determined by Kolmolgarov–Smirnov test (P <0.05). Figure and legend adapted from Huber et al. (2002). *PNAS* 99:7746–7750. Copyright 2002 National Academy of Sciences, USA.

novel member of a family of proteins, and the gene encodes a 1311 amino acid protein with a predicted molecular mass of 141 kDa. As described in the next paragraph, the current hypothesis for the function of the FMR2 protein is that the protein functions as a transcription factor or transcriptional regulator. Adult brain expression studies using northern blots in mice show high expression of fmr2 (the mouse homolog) in the hippocampus and amygdale (Box 5).

As mentioned, while the function of FMR2 has yet to be directly determined, FMR2 is hypothesized to be a transcriptional activator. It shares significant homology (20–35% amino acid identity) with three autosomal genes: AF4; LAF4; and AF5Q31. All four proteins of the FMR2 family share several highly similar regions that are homologous to functional motifs involved in transcriptional regulation.

David Nelson's laboratory developed a murine Fmr2 gene knockout model for FRAXE (19). Mice lacking Fmr2 showed impairment of both contextual and cued fear conditioning, suggesting a similarity of learning deficiencies in the mouse and human. The contextual fear impairment was found to be time-dependent. Fmr2 knockout mice displayed significantly less conditioned fear in the 24-hour delay context test; however, levels of contextual fear conditioning were similar between Fmr2-deficient and wildtype control mice when the test occurred 30 minutes after training. These findings indicate that the Fmr2-deficient mice learn to associate the shock with the training context, and can remember the context over a short delay interval, but that these same mice have impaired conditioned fear that is delay-dependent. Overall, these data indicate that the Fmr2 protein may play a role in the memory consolidation process for contextual memory.

Ironically, long-term potentiation (LTP) in area CA1 was found to be *enhanced* in hippocampal slices of Fmr2 KO compared to their wildtype littermates (see Figure 11), although the mechanism of enhanced

BOX 5

DOWN'S SYNDROME

Mental retardation can arise not only from loss or derangement of the function of a gene product, but also from aberrant overproduction of a gene product. One example of mental retardation in this category is Down's Syndrome. Down's Syndrome results not from a genetic mutation, but from aberrant chromosome duplication, specifically duplication of one copy of chromosome 21. For this reason, Down's Syndrome is also referred to as Trisomy 21. Because of this unique mechanism, Down's Syndrome is not a heritable disorder in the usual sense— it arises as an epigenetic phenomenon as part of the initial stages of chromosome replication during oocyte generation or oocyte fertilization.

Thus, Down's Syndrome arises due to the overproduction of proteins encoded by the genes on chromosome 21. Obviously, the molecular basis of the syndrome is quite complex due to the plethora of gene products potentially involved. However, portions of chromosome 21 (region q22.2 specifically) have been identified that are critical for the development of Down's Syndrome, a region referred to as the Down's Syndrome "critical locus" or "critical region." In part, this region was identified by characterizing Down's Syndrome patients who had not undergone complete duplication of chromosome 21. It is not clear at present precisely which genes in the critical region (or combination of genes) result in Down's Syndrome, and this is an area of active research at present.

There are two genes on chromosome 21 that are receiving particular attention at this point that are interesting in

the context of known signal transduction mechanisms that we have been discussing as related to learning and memory. These are DYRK1 and superoxide dismutase (35–37). DYRK1 is the human homolog to *Drosophila* minibrain kinase, which was identified in that species as a nervous system development-related gene. DYRK1 is homologous to members of the MAP kinase superfamily. The targets and mechanisms for regulation of DYRK1/minibrain kinase are unclear at present, but are under active investigation. Superoxide dismutase (SOD) is another interesting candidate. As we discussed in Chapters 8 and 9, superoxide has been implicated as a signaling molecule in hippocampal LTP, hypothesized to act through its capability to lead to autonomous PKC activation. Thus, the interesting model arises that part of the defects in Down's Syndrome are due to overexpression of SOD and attenuation of superoxide signaling in the nervous system. In fact, transgenic animal models have indicated that this is a viable hypothesis, as SOD-overproducing mice have deficits in LTP and hippocampus-dependent memory formation.

A final chromosome 21 gene worth noting is the gene for amyloid precursor protein (APP). As we will discuss in more detail in the next chapter of this book, overproduction of the APP-derived product amyloid beta peptide likely leads to Alzheimer's Disease. Gene duplication of the APP gene in Down's Syndrome patients leads to overproduction of amyloid beta peptide, and unfortunately almost all Down's Syndrome patients who live past the age of 35 also develop Alzheimer's Disease-like pathology.

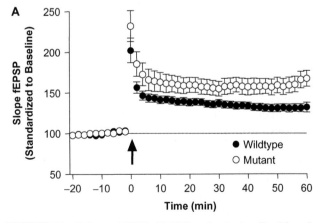

FIGURE 11 Enhanced LTP in FMR2 knockout mice. Fmr2 knockout hippocampal slices showed enhanced LTP compared with wildtypes after a modest LTP-inducing protocol consisting of a single set of tetani while maintaining slices at 25°C (60 minutes after tetanus: n (KO, male) = 9, 167 ± 9%; n (WT, male) = 14, 132 ± 6%; p = 0.003). Reproduced from Gu et al. (41).

LTP in Fmr2 knockout mice is not clear at this time. Interestingly, this knockout is an example of an animal model of human mental retardation with impaired learning and memory performance and *increased* LTP. These findings highlight the importance of keeping in mind that increases in LTP may be a fundamental mechanism that leads to impaired cognitive processing, just like loss of LTP (Box 6).

IV. SUMMARY

In this chapter we have covered a topic of pronounced importance—disorders of human cognition, specifically related to memory formation. In this chapter we saw three examples of convergence of basic memory research with clinical investigation, highlighting neurofibromatosis mental retardation, Angelman

---

BOX 6

NURTURE VERSUS NATURE: ENRICHED ENVIRONMENTS CAN HELP OVERCOME INHERITED LEARNING DISORDERS

Coffin-Lowry Syndrome, neurofibromatosis mental retardation, and fragile X syndrome—these devastating forms of mental retardation arise from defects in genes whose normal functioning is critical for learning and memory. From the moment of conception children with these disorders face an uphill battle to overcome their inherited disadvantage. Can their environment help compensate for their being short-changed by Nature? Studies by Joe Tsien and his colleagues suggest that there is indeed cause for hope.

Tsien and colleagues capitalized on genetic engineering to construct a general mouse model for inherited learning defects—they created a mouse strain missing the NMDA receptor. In an additional refinement, Tsien and colleagues engineered their mouse so that the NMDA receptor was selectively lost in the hippocampus.

As expected, in behavioral tests these mice demonstrated a decrease in learning capacity in several tasks linked to hippocampal function, such as identifying new foodstuffs appropriately, recognizing objects, and recognizing their environment (38).

The investigators then set out to determine if enriching the animals' environment could help compensate for their inborn loss of learning capacity. In their studies, they made the important discovery that raising these animals in an environment rich in sensory stimuli, toys, and opportunities for exploration resulted in a significant improvement in their learning capacity. These results are one of the most convincing demonstrations to date that an enriched environment can help overcome learning deficiencies, even those deficiencies arising from defects in the genetic hard-wiring of an individual.

Syndrome, and fragile X mental retardation. It is quite striking how the detailed analysis of the basic signal transduction mechanisms underlying rodent learning and memory have converged on many of the same molecular systems recently identified using human genetic characterization approaches in the study of mental retardation syndromes. I am cautiously optimistic that this convergence will ultimately lead to an improvement in the human condition, through identifying new therapeutic approaches to treating mental retardation.

On the abstract, intellectual side, the findings we have covered in this chapter have interesting cognitive neurobiological implications. It appears that the last decades of parsing the esoteric details of synaptic plasticity and rodent memory mechanisms may well have lived up to its promise. In my opinion, it is not too early to begin to think of the types of mechanisms we have been covering in this book in the context of giving insights into human cognitive processing as well. The convergence of human and basic studies onto the same molecular cascades suggests that, indeed, we may be in the process of generating insights into the molecular basis of human cognition.

This line of thinking also raises an interesting issue; the distinction between a developmental necessity for the gene products versus an acute, ongoing necessity as part of the signal transduction mechanisms subserving cognition. Many of the mutations we have discussed do not lead to gross morphological changes

in the human CNS. Moreover, mouse studies, where available, indicate that baseline synaptic transmission is normal after loss of these gene products. These observations are consistent with a necessity for *ongoing* need for the gene products in human learning and memory. In addition, in the case of the ERK/CREB/CBP system and the CaMKII system, there is direct evidence from animal studies that acute inhibition of these systems in adults is sufficient to cause learning deficiencies. These types of considerations suggest a rethinking of our outlook on human learning disorders, changing from the traditional view of them as purely developmental problems, to a new view of them as cognitive deficiencies. This sea-change in outlook may be one of the most important outcomes of new and ongoing discoveries concerning the basic signal transduction processes subserving learning and memory.

In overview, there are several specific take-home messages from this chapter:

1. Studies of NF1-associated learning deficits, Coffin-Lowry Syndrome, and Rubinstein-Taybi Syndrome have implicated the ras/ERK pathway and its targets in human memory formation.
2. Studies of Angelman Mental Retardation Syndrome have implicated hippocampal LTP and CaMKII regulation as necessary for human learning and memory formation.

3. Disruptions of the regulation of metabotropic glutamate receptor-mediated LTD in the hippocampus, along with related alterations in the control of protein synthesis, have led to the mGluR theory of fragile X mental retardation.

4. All of these studies illustrate a striking convergence of animal studies of the roles of specific molecular and cellular processes underlying memory with recent studies of the molecular and cellular basis of human learning and memory disorders.

Further Reading

Abel, T., and Zukin, R. S. (2008). "Epigenetic targets of HDAC inhibition in neurodegenerative and psychiatric disorders." *Curr. Opin. Pharmacol.* 8:57–64.

Alarcon, J. M., Malleret, G., Touzani, K., Vronskaya, S., Ishii, S., Kandel, E. R., and Barco, A. (2004). "Chromatin acetylation, memory, and LTP are impaired in CBP + / − mice: a model for the cognitive deficit in Rubinstein-Taybi syndrome and its amelioration." *Neuron* 42:947–959.

Bear, M. F., Huber, K. M., and Warren, S. T. (2004). "The mGluR theory of fragile X mental retardation." *Trends Neurosci.* 27(7):370–377.

Chahrour, M., Jung, S. Y., Shaw, C., Zhou, X., Wong, S. T., Qin, J., and Zoghbi, H. Y. (2008). "MeCP2, a key contributor to neurological disease, activates and represses transcription." *Science* 320:1224–1229.

Costa-Mattioli, M., Sossin, W. S., Klann, E., and Sonenberg, N. (2009). "Translational control of long-lasting synaptic plasticity and memory." *Neuron* 61:10–26.

Dölen, G., Osterweil, E., Rao, B. S., Smith, G. B., Auerbach, B. D., Chattarji, S., and Bear, M. F. (2007). "Correction of fragile X syndrome in mice." *Neuron* 56:955–962.

Greer, P. L., Zieg, J., and Greenberg, M. E. (2009). "Activity-dependent transcription and disorders of human cognition." *Am. J. Psychiatry* 166(1):14–15.

Guy, J., Gan, J., Selfridge, J., Cobb, S., and Bird, A. (2007). "Reversal of neurological defects in a mouse model of Rett syndrome." *Science* 315:1143–1147.

Korzus, E., Rosenfeld, M. G., and Mayford, M. (2004). "CBP histone acetyltransferase activity is a critical component of memory consolidation". *Neuron* 42:961–972.

Levenson, J. M., O'Riordan, K. J., Brown, K. D., Trinh, M. A., Molfese, D. L., and Sweatt, J. D. (2004). "Regulation of histone acetylation during memory formation in the hippocampus." *J. Biol. Chem.* 279:40545–40559.

Silva, A. J., Frankland, P. W., Marowitz, Z., Friedman, E., Lazlo, G., Cioffi, D., Jacks, T., and Bourtchuladze, R. (1997). "A mouse model for the learning and memory deficits associated with neurofibromatosis type I." *Nat. Genet.* 15:281–284.

Sweatt, J. D. (2001). "Protooncogenes subserve memory formation in the adult CNS." *Neuron* 31:671–674.

Vaillend, C., Poirier, R., and Laroche, S. (2008). "Genes, plasticity and mental retardation." *Behav. Brain Res.* 192:88–105.

Weeber, E. J., and Sweatt, J. D. (2002). "Molecular neurobiology of human cognition." *Neuron* 33:845–848.

Journal Club Articles

Amir, R. E., Van den Veyver, I. B., Wan, M., Tran, C. Q., Francke, U., and Zoghbi, H. Y. (1999). "Rett syndrome is caused by mutations in X-linked MECP2, encoding methyl-CpG-binding protein 2." *Nat. Genet.* 23:185–188.

Jiang, Y. H., Armstrong, D., Albrecht, U., Atkins, C. M., Noebels, J. L., Eichele, G., Sweatt, J. D., and Beaudet, A. L. (1998). "Mutation of the Angelman ubiquitin ligase in mice causes increased cytoplasmic p53 and deficits of contextual learning and long-term potentiation." *Neuron* 21:799–811.

Petrij, F. et al. (1995). "Rubinstein-Taybi syndrome caused by mutations in the transcriptional co-activator CBP." *Nature* 376:348–351.

Van Woerden, G. M., Harris, K. D., Hojjati, M. R., Gustin, R. M., Qiu, S., de Avila Freire, R., Jiang, Y. H., Elgersma, Y., and Weeber, E. J. (2007). "Rescue of neurological deficits in a mouse model for Angelman syndrome by reduction of alphaCaMKII inhibitory phosphorylation." *Nat. Neurosci.* 10:280–282.

For more information—relevant topic chapters from: John H. Byrne (Editor-in-Chief) (2008). *Learning and Memory: A Comprehensive Reference*. Oxford: Academic Press (ISBN 978-0-12-370509-9). (2.37 Ornstein P. A., Haden, C. A., and San Souci, P. *The Development of Skilled Remembering in Children*. pp. 715–744; 2.38 Grigorenko, E. L. *Developmental Disorders of Learning*. pp. 745–758; 2.39 Dawson, M., Mottron, L., and Gernsbacher, M. A. *Learning in Autism*. pp. 759–772; 2.40 Kane, M. J., and Miyake, T. M. *Individual Differences in Episodic Memory*. pp. 773–785; 2.43 McDaniel, M. A., and Callender, A. A. *Cognition, Memory, and Education*. pp. 235–244; 3.04 Squire, L. R., and Shrager, Y. *Declarative Memory System: Amnesia*. pp. 67–78; 3.05 Voss, J. L., and Paller, K. A. *Neural Substrates of Remembering—Electroencephalographic Studies*. pp. 79–97; 3.27 Gold, P. E. *Memory-Enhancing Drugs*. pp. 555–575; 4.19 Shilyansky, C., Wiltgen, B. J., and Silva, A. J. *Neurofibromatosis Type I Learning Disabilities*. pp. 387–407; 4.24 Banko, J. L., and Weeber, E. J. *Angelman Syndrome*. pp. 489–500; 4.25 Kelleher, R. J. III, *Mitogen-Activated Protein Kinases in Synaptic Plasticity and Memory*. pp. 501–523; 4.26 Hegde, A. N. *Proteolysis and Synaptic Plasticity*. pp. 525–545; 4.42 Levenson, J. M., and Wood, M. A. *Epigenetics—Chromatin Structure and Rett Syndrome*. pp. 859–878.

References

1. Weeber, E. J., and Sweatt, J. D. (2002). "Molecular neurobiology of human cognition." *Neuron* 33:845–848.

2. Ozonoff, S. (1999). "Cognitive impairment in neurofibromatosis type 1." *Am. J. Med. Genet.* 89:45–52.

3. Silva, A. J., Frankland, P. W., Marowitz, Z., Friedman, E., Lazlo, G., Cioffi, D., Jacks, T., and Bourtchuladze, R. (1997). "A mouse model for the learning and memory deficits associated with neurofibromatosis I." *Nat. Genet.* 15:281–284.

4. Costa, R. M., Yang, T., Huynh, D. P., Pulst, S. M., Viskochil, D. H., Silva, A. J., and Brannan, C. I. (2001). "Learning deficits, but normal development and tumor predisposition, in mice lacking exon 23a of Nf1." *Nat. Genet.* 27:399–405.

5. Andersen, L. B., Ballester, R., Marchuk, D. A., Chang, E., Gutmann, D. H., Saulino, A. M., Camonis, J., Wigler, M., and Collins, F. S. (1993). "A conserved alternative splice in the von Recklinghausen neurofibromatosis (NF1) gene produces two neurofibromin isoforms, both of which have GTPase-activating protein activity." *Mol. Cell Biol.* 13:487–495.

6. Zhu, Y., and Parada, L. F. (2001). "A particular GAP in mind." *Nat. Genet.* 27:354–355.

7. Ohno, M., Frankland, P. W., Chen, A. P., Costa, R. M., and Silva, A. J. (2001). "Inducible, pharmacogenetic approaches to the study of learning and memory." *Nat. Neurosci.* 4:1238–1243.

8. Ingram, D. A., Hiatt, K., King, A. J., Fisher, L., Shivakumar, R., Derstine, C., Wenning, M. J., Diaz, B., Travers, J. B., Hood, A., Marshall, M., Williams, D. A., and Clapp, D. W. (2001). "Hyperactivation of p21(ras) and the hematopoietic-specific Rho

GTPase, Rac2, cooperate to alter the proliferation of neurofibromin-deficient mast cells *in vivo* and *in vitro*." *J. Exp. Med.* 194:57–69.

9. Tong, J., Hannan, F., Zhu, Y., Bernards, A., and Zhong, Y. (2002). "Neurofibromin regulates G protein-stimulated adenylyl cyclase activity." *Nat. Neurosci.* 5:95–96.

10. Impey, S., Obrietan, K., Wong, S. T., Poser, S., Yano, S., Wayman, G., Deloulme, J. C., Chan, G., and Storm, D. R. (1998). "Cross talk between ERK and PKA is required for Ca^{2+} stimulation of CREB-dependent transcription and ERK nuclear translocation." *Neuron* 21:869–883.

11. Roberson, E. D., English, J. D., Adams, J. P., Selcher, J. C., Kondratick, C., and Sweatt, J. D. (1999). "The mitogen-activated protein kinase cascade couples PKA and PKC to cAMP response element binding protein phosphorylation in area CA1 of hippocampus." *J. Neurosci.* 19:4337–4348.

12. Dufresne, S. D., Bjorbaek, C., El-Haschimi, K., Zhao, Y., Aschenbach, W. G., Moller, D. E., and Goodyear, L. J. (2001). "Altered extracellular signal-regulated kinase signaling and glycogen metabolism in skeletal muscle from p90 ribosomal S6 kinase 2 knockout mice." *Mol. Cell Biol.* 21:81–87.

13. Harum, K. H., Alemi, L., and Johnston, M. V. (2001). "Cognitive impairment in Coffin-Lowry syndrome correlates with reduced RSK2 activation." *Neurology* 56:207–214.

14. Greenough, W. T., Klintsova, A. Y., Irwin, S. A., Galvez, R., Bates, K. E., and Weiler, I. J. (2001). "Synaptic regulation of protein synthesis and the fragile X protein." *Proc. Natl. Acad. Sci. USA* 98:7101–7106.

15. Jiang, Y. H., Armstrong, D., Albrecht, U., Atkins, C. M., Noebels, J. L., Eichele, G., Sweatt, J. D., and Beaudet, A. L. (1998). "Mutation of the Angelman ubiquitin ligase in mice causes increased cytoplasmic p53 and deficits of contextual learning and long-term potentiation." *Neuron* 21:799–811.

16. Hagerman, R. J., and Hagerman, P. J. (2001). "Fragile X syndrome: a model of gene-brain-behavior relationships." *Mol. Genet. Metab.* 74:89–97.

17. Bardoni, B., Schenck, A., and Mandel, J. L. (2001). "The Fragile X mental retardation protein." *Brain Res. Bull.* 56:375–382.

18. Zhang, Y. Q., Bailey, A. M., Matthies, H. J., Renden, R. B., Smith, M. A., Speese, S. D., Rubin, G. M., and Broadie, K. (2001). "*Drosophila* fragile X-related gene regulates the MAP1 B homolog Futsch to control synaptic structure and function". *Cell* 107:591–603.

19. Gu, Y., McIlwain, K., Weeber, E. J., Yamagata, T., Xu, B., Antalffy, B., Reye, C., Yuva-Paylor, L., Armstrong, D., Zoghbi, H., Sweatt, J. D., Paylor, R., and Nelson, D. (2002). "Impaired conditioned fear and enhanced long-term potentiation in Fmr2 knockout mice." *Journal of Neuroscience* 22(7):2753–2763.

20. Oike, Y., Hata, A., Mamiya, T., Kaname, T., Noda, Y., Suzuki, M., Yasue, H., Nabeshima, T., Araki, K., and Yamamura, K. (1999). "Truncated CBP protein leads to classical Rubinstein-Taybi syndrome phenotypes in mice: implications for a dominant-negative mechanism." *Hum. Mol. Genet.* 8:387–396.

21. Hegde, A. N., Inokuchi, K., Pei, W., Casadio, A., Ghirardi, M., Chain, D. G., Martin, K. C., Kandel, E. R., and Schwartz, J. H. (1997). "Ubiquitin C-terminal hydrolase is an immediate-early gene essential for long-term facilitation in *Aplysia*." *Cell* 89:115–126.

22. Chain, D. G., Hegde, A. N., Yamamoto, N., Liu-Marsh, B., and Schwartz, J. H. (1965). "Persistent activation of cAMP-dependent protein kinase by regulated proteolysis suggests a neuron-specific function of the ubiquitin system in *Aplysia*." *J. Neurosci.* 15:7592–7603.

23. Shahbazian, M. D., Antalffy, B., Armstrong, D. L., and Zoghbi, H. Y. (2002). "Insight into Rett syndrome: MeCP2 levels display tissue- and cell-specific differences and correlate with neuronal maturation." *Hum. Mol. Genet.* 11:115–124.

24. Bellugi, U., Adolphs, R., Cassady, C., and Chiles, M. (1999). "Towards the neural basis for hypersociability in a genetic syndrome." *Neuroreport* 10:1653–1657.

25. Donnai, D., and Karmiloff-Smith, A. (2000). "Williams syndrome: from genotype through to the cognitive phenotype." *Am. J. Med. Genet.* 97:164–171.

26. Korenberg, J. R., Chen, X. N., Hirota, H., Lai, Z., Bellugi, U., Burian, D., Roe, B., and Matsuoka, R. (2000). "VI. Genome structure and cognitive map of Williams syndrome." *J. Cogn. Neurosci.* 12(Suppl 1):89–107.

27. Meng, Y., Zhang, Y., Tregoubov, V., Janus, C., Cruz, L., Jackson, M., Lu, W. Y., MacDonald, J. F., Wang, J. Y., Falls, D. L., and Jia, Z. (2002). "Abnormal spine morphology and enhanced LTP in LIMK-1 knockout mice." *Neuron* 35:121–133.

28. Bienvenu, T., des Portes, V., McDonell, N., Carrie, A., Zemni, R., Couvert, P., Ropers, H. H., Moraine, C., van Bokhoven, H., Fryns, J. P., Allen, K., Walsh, C. A., Boue, J., Kahn, A., Chelly, J., and Beldjord, C. (2000). "Missense mutation in PAK3, R67, C, causes X-linked nonspecific mental retardation." *Am. J. Med. Genet.* 93:294–298.

29. Schmid, R. S., Pruitt, W. M., and Maness, P. F. (2000). "A MAP kinase-signaling pathway mediates neurite outgrowth on L1 and requires Src-dependent endocytosis." *J. Neurosci.* 20:4177–4188.

30. Kutsche, K., Yntema, H., Brandt, A., Jantke, I., Nothwang, H. G., Orth, U., Boavida, M. G., David, D., Chelly, J., Fryns, J. P., Moraine, C., Ropers, H. H., Hamel, B. C., van Bokhoven, H., and Gal, A. (2000). "Mutations in ARHGEF6, encoding a guanine nucleotide exchange factor for Rho GTPases, in patients with X-linked mental retardation." *Nat. Genet.* 26:247–250.

31. Allen, K. M., Gleeson, J. G., Bagrodia, S., Partington, M. W., MacMillan, J. C., Cerione, R. A., Mulley, J. C., and Walsh, C. A. (1998). "PAK3 mutation in nonsyndromic X-linked mental retardation." *Nat. Genet.* 20:25–30.

32. Ridley, A. J. (2001). "Rho family proteins: coordinating cell responses." *Trends Cell Biol.* 11:471–477.

33. King, A. J., Sun, H., Diaz, B., Barnard, D., Miao, W., Bagrodia, S., and Marshall, M. S. (1998). "The protein kinase Pak3 positively regulates Raf-1 activity through phosphorylation of serine 338." *Nature* 396:180–183.

34. Billuart, P., Bienvenu, T., Ronce, N., des Portes, V., Vinet, M. C., Zemni, R., Roest Crollius, H., Carrie, A., Fauchereau, F., Cherry, M., Briault, S., Hamel, B., Fryns, J. P., Beldjord, C., Kahn, A., Moraine, C., and Chelly, J. (1998). "Oligophrenin-1 encodes a rhoGAP protein involved in X-linked mental retardation." *Nature* 392:923–926.

35. Altafaj, X., Dierssen, M., Baamonde, C., Marti, E., Visa, J., Guimera, J., Oset, M., Gonzalez, J. R., Florez, J., Fillat, C., and Estivill, X. (2001). "Neurodevelopmental delay, motor abnormalities and cognitive deficits in transgenic mice overexpressing Dyrk1 A (minibrain), a murine model of Down's syndrome." *Hum. Mol. Genet.* 10:1915–1923.

36. Siarey, R. J., Carlson, E. J., Epstein, C. J., Balbo, A., Rapoport, S. I., and Galdzicki, Z. (1999). "Increased synaptic depression in the Ts65Dn mouse, a model for mental retardation in Down syndrome." *Neuropharmacology* 38:1917–1920.

37. Thiels, E., Urban, N. N., Gonzalez-Burgos, G. R., Kanterewicz, B. I., Barrionuevo, G., Chu, C. T., Oury, T. D., and Klann, E. (2000). "Impairment of long-term potentiation and associative memory in mice that overexpress extracellular superoxide dismutase." *J. Neurosci.* 20:7631–7639.

38. Rampon, C., Tang, Y. P., Goodhouse, J., Shimizu, E., Kyin, M., and Tsien, J. Z. (2000). "Enrichment induces structural changes and recovery from nonspatial memory deficits in CA1 NMDAR1-knockout mice." *Nat. Neurosci.* 3:238–244.

39. Costa, R. M., Federov, N. B., Kogan, J. H., Murphy, G. G., Stern, J., Ohno, M., Kucherlapati, R., Jacks, T., and Silva, A. J. (2002).

"Mechanism for the learning deficits in a mouse model of neurofibromatosis type 1." *Nature* 415:526–530.

40. Jiang, Y. H., Armstrong, D., Albrecht, U., Atkins, C. M., Noebels, J. L., Eichele, G., Sweatt, J. D., and Beaudet, A. L. (1998). "Mutation of the Angelman ubiquitin ligase in mice causes increased cytoplasmic p53 and deficits of contextual learning and long-term potentiation." *Neuron* 21:799–811.

41. Gu, Y., McIlwain, K. L., Weeber, E., Yamagata, T., Xu, B., Antalffy, B. A., Reyes, C., Yuva-Paylor, L., Armstrong, D., Zoghbi, H., Sweatt, J. D., Paylor, R., and Nelson, D. L. (2002). "Impaired conditioned fear and enhanced long-term potentiation in Fmr2 knock-out mice." *J. Neurosci.* 22:2753–2763.

42. Mistry, D. J., Moorman, J. R., Reddy, S., and Mounsey, J. P. (2001). "Skeletal muscle Na currents in mice heterozygous for Six5 deficiency." *Physiol. Genomics* 6:153–158.

43. Gahtan, E., Auerbach, J. M., Groner, Y., and Segal, M. (1998). "Reversible impairment of long-term potentiation in transgenic Cu/Zn-SOD mice." *Eur. J. Neurosci.* 10:538–544.

44. Morris, C. A., and Mervis, C. B. (2000). "Williams syndrome and related disorders." *Annu. Rev. Genomics Hum. Genet.* 1:461–484.

45. Weeber, E. J., and Sweatt, J. D. (2000). "Disruptions of signal transduction pathways in mental retardation: Angelman and Coffin-Lowry syndrome." *Recent Research Developments in Neurochemistry* 3:289–299.

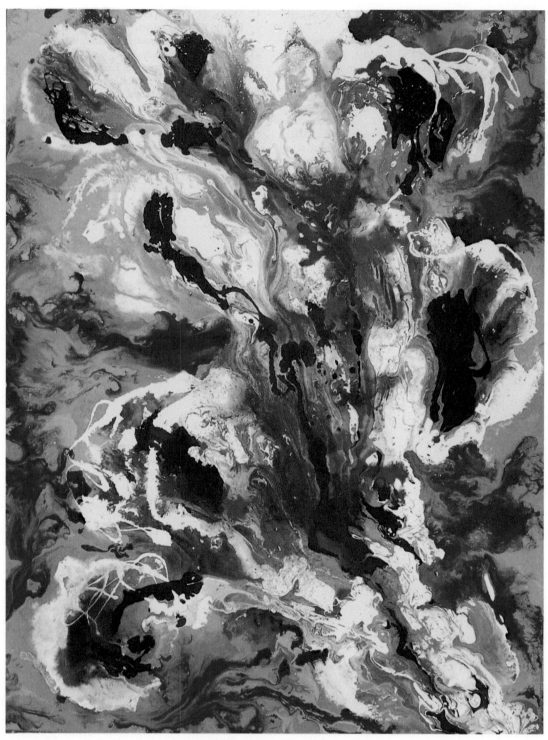

Amyloid Plagues and Neurofibrillary Tangles
J. David Sweatt, acrylic on canvas, 2008–2009

Aging-Related Memory
Disorders—Alzheimer's Disease

In the last chapter we talked about human mental retardation syndromes—inherited deficiencies in learning and memory that manifest from birth. In this chapter we move to the other end of the developmental spectrum and discuss aging-related memory dysfunction. In particular we will focus on Alzheimer's disease (AD) as an example of an inherited memory disorder that does not manifest itself until adulthood is reached. We will focus on inherited forms of AD not because they are the most prevalent, but rather because they are the forms most tractable for experimental investigation at present. This is because inherited forms of AD, being gene-based, lend themselves to investigation using genetically-engineered mice. As we have seen throughout the book, the recent advent of the capacity for genetic engineering in animal models holds the promise of a watershed of new insights into all aspects of memory, including investigating aging-related memory dysfunction such as AD.

In this chapter I will present an overview of the clinical and pathological manifestations of AD, and discuss in particular the emerging hypothesis that amyloid beta (Aβ) is the proximal causative agent. I will also discuss other important molecular events involved in AD pathogenesis, always with an eye toward how these events might impinge on the molecular mechanisms for learning and memory that we have been discussing in detail throughout the book. I will spend some time going over new mouse models that are relevant to AD, in keeping with our motif of considering rodent models and behavioral paradigms of relevance to human memory disorders.

I. AGING-RELATED MEMORY DECLINE

As most people over the age of 60 will attest, a decline in learning and memory is a part of the "normal" aging process (see reference 1 for a review). Most noticeable in humans is the decline in hippocampus-dependent forms of memory, the learning and remembering of new names, recent events, and even spatial information. For the most part in normal individuals these memory deficits are not debilitating, but they are quite noticeable because they are involved so directly in human conscious behavior.

These types of hippocampus-dependent memory dysfunction are recapitulated in aging rodents, as assessed using various learning paradigms that we have discussed throughout this book. Carol Barnes has been a leader in this area, and in fact developed her maze learning task specifically to probe for memory deficits in aged animals, as was described in Chapter 4. *In vivo* recordings have also demonstrated deficiencies in hippocampal place field stabilization in aged rats (2). Thus, an aging-related decline in behavioral and cellular manifestations of hippocampus-dependent learning is well-established in humans and other mammals.

Trying to understand the molecular and cellular basis of aging-related memory decline is an active area of research at present. No one unifying hypothesis for aging-related memory decline has yet to emerge, but several intriguing observations have been made in this regard. For example, hippocampal LTP is diminished in aged animals (3). The basis for these declines remains mysterious, although decreased synaptic inputs or diminished NMDA receptor function are possibilities, depending on the hippocampal region under consideration (3–4). In addition, Marina Lynch's group has executed a series of studies implicating excessive production of reactive oxygen species as a contributing factor in aging-related memory and synaptic plasticity dysfunction (5). Given the ambiguous nature of the molecular process we call "aging," the biochemical mechanisms underlying aging-related memory decline are likely to remain enigmatic for some period of time. This does not diminish the importance of understanding them, but rather highlights their complexity.

A. Mild Cognitive Impairment

More pronounced aging-related memory dysfunction, beyond that observed with normal aging, can lead to a clinically diagnosable disorder referred to as mild cognitive impairment (MCI). MCI, despite what the name might suggest, is a diminution of memory and executive function that *significantly* disrupts a person's capacity for normal daily function. MCI is a loss of overall cognitive function that can be distinguished and diagnosed using behavioral psychological testing. Individuals diagnosed with MCI are at a higher-than-average risk of subsequently developing more pronounced and serious forms of aging-related memory impairments.

B. Age-Related Dementias

In terms of cognitive decline, beyond MCI there exist much more dramatic insults to the human capacity for hippocampus- and prefrontal cortex-dependent learning and memory. These can arise for a number of reasons—stroke, vascular problems, psychiatric disorders, Parkinson's disease, and Alzheimer's disease (AD) principal among them. These all can lead to dementia much more pronounced than ever occurs with normal aging or MCI. The focus of the remainder of this chapter will be the Alzheimer's type of dementia, as this is the form of aging-related memory dysfunction that we have the most mechanistic information about.

Please keep in mind that "dementia" does not mean the same thing in the clinical realm that it does in general parlance. "Demented" is generally used by the lay public synonymously with "mad" or "insane." In clinical terms, dementia refers to a specific and pronounced decline of cognitive function in humans—a decline in mentation. Among the symptoms of dementia are: loss of learning and memory capacity; decline in reasoning ability; attention problems; language difficulties; and problems with perception.

AD is the most common of the tragically debilitating senile (i.e., age-related) dementias, and in the United States alone AD is projected to affect approximately 5 million people in total in the next few years. In the United States, about 1 in 10 people over the age of 65 have AD. If you live to age 85 you have about a 1 in 2 chance of developing AD. As human longevity increases worldwide, the ironic and at-present unavoidable consequence of that fact is that the prevalence of AD will similarly increase on a global scale. AD is projected to affect nearly 20 million people worldwide by 2025. These are sobering statistics, given that at present there is no effective treatment for the disease.

II. WHAT IS ALZHEIMER'S DISEASE?

Of the various dementing illnesses, our understanding of AD has progressed the farthest at the molecular level. That is not to say that our molecular understanding of AD is good, but rather that we have at least a few clues as to what is happening. As we will discuss below, a number of specific genes have been identified which, when mutated, essentially invariably lead to an individual developing AD. We will discuss these genes and gene products in more detail later, but for now I raise the issue to make two points. First, even considering the already-identified genes for AD, we can still only account mechanistically for factors contributing to about 30% of AD cases.

TABLE 1   Stages of Alzheimer's Disease

AD Stage	Areas First Affected	Symptoms
I, II	Trans-entorhinal region entorhinal cortex area CA1	Can be clinically silent; subtle loss of episodic memory and difficulty executing complex progressive tasks; anecdotal repetition; some spatial disorientation
III, IV	Entirety of hippocampus	Early-stage AD; loss of episodic memory, difficulty with spatial reasoning and recognition, difficulty with coherent speech and planning
V, VI	Neocortex	Fully developed AD; pronounced decline in cognition, frank dementia, can include psychosis or depression, ultimately a complete inability to communicate or care for themselves

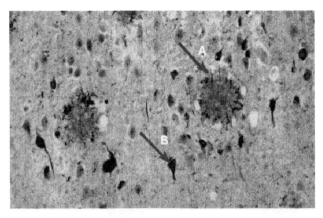

FIGURE 1   Amyloid plaques and neurofibrillary tangles, the two principal neuropathologic markers for AD. (A) indicates an amyloid plaque and (B) indicates a neurofibrillary tangle. See text for additional discussion. Figure courtesy of Poul Jørgensen,[1] Claus Bus,[1] Niels Pallisgaard,[1] Marianne Bryder,[3] and Arne Lund Jørgensen[2,3] ([1]Department of Molecular Biology, C.F. Møllers Allé 130, DK 8000 Aarhus C, Denmark; [2]Institute of Human Genetics, The Bartholin Building, University of Aarhus, DK 8000 Aarhus C, Denmark; and [3] Cytogenetic Laboratory, Psychiatric Hospital in Aarhus, Skovagervej 2, DK 8240 Risskov, Denmark. (Electronic mail address: POUL@BIOBASE.DK.) Copyright Elsevier 2003.

Second, among the known genes, there are heterogeneous mechanisms by which they lead one to arrive in the AD state. Thus, it appears certain that AD is in fact more than one disease. As our understanding of the molecular bases of AD increases, it is likely that AD subtypes will be diagnosable, and perhaps differentially treatable. For our purposes in this chapter, because of the present limited state of understanding, I will refer to AD monolithically.

Despite the clear molecular heterogeneity of AD, there are commonalities to AD that are defined clinically. AD is a pathological state with defined associated molecular and cellular changes in the human CNS. A number of different schema have emerged for describing the progression of AD (see Table 1). The one that I will follow here is based on the system promulgated by Heiko and Eva Braak (6–9) that is based on histopathological criteria, specifically the development of neurofibrillary tangles in various brain regions, and associated clinical symptomology (see Figures 1 and 2).

A. Stages of Alzheimer's Disease

In the final stages (stages V and VI), typically about 8–10 years after the initial diagnosis of AD, patients are completely bedridden and unable to care for themselves. There is complete dementia and an inability to communicate effectively. Perpetual confusion, incontinence, and an inability to execute the most basic cognitive functions are the hallmarks of this final stage of AD.

This final stage is preceded by a period of progressive loss of reasoning and cognitive ability (stages III and IV). There is profound anterograde episodic memory loss. In many cases, additional symptoms such as psychosis, delusional behavior, and depression are present. Reading and writing are essentially

impossible, as is watching a movie or television program, because episodic and declarative memory are so impaired. Verbal communication becomes progressively incoherent. Recognition of known individuals progressively declines.

The earlier stages of AD (stages I and II) typically read like a textbook case of hippocampal dysfunction.[1] Episodic memory formation is lost—a patient typically has no recollection of their ongoing experiences on a daily basis. Spatial disorientation is pronounced, both in the sense of navigation and also in place recognition. For example, AD patients in this stage may

[1]Consider the following description taken verbatim from "Diagnosis of Alzheimer's Disease" by John C. Morris (in *Alzheimer's Disease*, Khachaturian and Radebaugh, 1996. New York: CRC Press, p. 78), and compare it to the roles of hippocampal synaptic plasticity that we have been discussing throughout the book. "Probable AD begins insidiously, and it is often impossible to precisely date its onset. Several years may pass before the family recognizes that everyday functioning has been sufficiently compromised to the point that medical attention is sought. Forgetfulness is the typical presenting symptom. Common examples of memory deficits in this stage are the repetition of questions or statements and the misplacement of items without independent retrieval. Impaired acquisition of new information is manifest by inability to recall recent conversations or events, whereas highly learned material from years gone by may be remembered with seeming clarity. Minor geographic and temporal disorientation also may be early symptoms; the patient may need directions to find even familiar locations, or may ask for frequent reminders of the date. Poor judgment and impaired problem solving occur as part of the dysexecutive syndrome wherein patients lack insight (often being unaware of their deficits), have poor attention, and experience uncharacteristic difficulty in completing tasks that involve sequencing of information, such as operating an automatic coffee maker or balancing the checkbook."

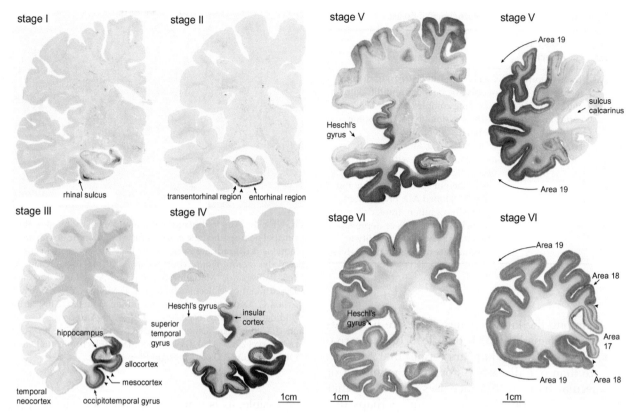

FIGURE 2 Stages of neurofibrillary pathology in Alzheimer's disease. Whole-brain sections were immunostained with antibody to phosphorylated tau. In stage I, involvement is limited to the transentorhinal region. Neurofibrillary pathology spreads to the entorhinal cortex in stage II. Stage III involves the hippocampus. Stage IV involves spread to the insula and inferior temporal neocortex. Finally, in stages V–VI even more neocortical areas are affected. From Braak, H., Rüb, U., Schultz, C., et al. (2006). "Vulnerability of cortical neurons to Alzheimer's and Parkinson's diseases." *J. Alzheimers Dis.* 9:35–44, with permission from IOS Press. However, other glial activities protect neurons against dysfunction and degeneration. ApoE4 and tau promote Aβ-induced neuronal injury and also have independent adverse effects. From Roberson, E. D., and Mucke, L. (2006). "100 years and counting: Prospects for defeating Alzheimer's disease." *Science* 314:781–784. Figure courtesy of Erik Roberson. Copyright Elsevier 2008.

regularly ask when they are "going home," when in fact they are at home already. The capacity to remember new individuals and other specific named items becomes increasingly difficult. The execution of complex serial tasks is affected, as would be expected if ordering of episodic events is impaired. Cooking, for example, or other serial tasks, become difficult, then impossible, to execute.

The increasing frequency over time of these types of hippocampal memory deficits are what lead the patient and their family members to suspect that AD might be present, and to go to a physician to have themselves clinically evaluated. These types of memory deficits are also the basis for the initial diagnosis of early AD by the clinician (see Box 1). I emphasize this because, while later stages of AD are a manifestation of a horrible dementing illness, the early stages of AD are a much more subtle derangement of normal hippocampus-dependent memory formation and hippocampal function.

While later stages of AD clearly involve extensive cell death across broad areas of the CNS, investigating the basis of hippocampus-dependent synaptic plasticity and learning has much to offer toward our understanding mechanisms of early AD. It is important to consider the concept of thinking of AD, at least in its early stages, as a memory disorder. This is in contrast to thinking of AD in its later stages as a dementing illness with wide-ranging cognitive and perceptual effects. These broad changes and extensive cell loss clearly are the case in later stages of the disease, and this is an important area of investigation. However, as an adjunct to these lines of investigation one should also consider how we can capitalize on ongoing discoveries of the cellular and molecular basis of hippocampal function, in order to improve our understanding of the earliest stages of AD.

For the rest of the chapter I will proceed with this perspective in mind—biasing the discussion toward early molecular events of relevance to the hippocampus and hippocampal synaptic plasticity. This is

BOX 1

DIAGNOSING ALZHEIMER'S DISEASE

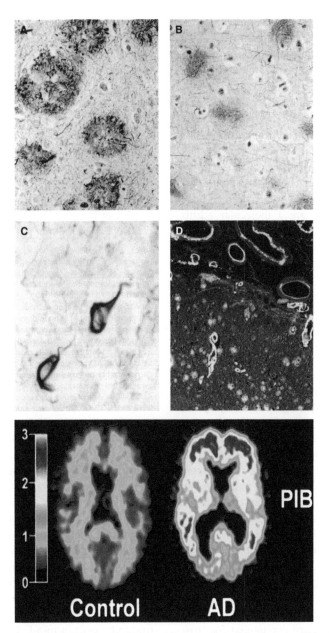

BOX 1 Diagnosis. Microscopic features of Alzheimer's disease. (A) Several neuritic plaques within the cerebral cortex are seen on this silver stain. (B) Diffuse plaques predominate in this field of cerebral cortex. Silver stain. (C) Two neurofibrillary tangles are seen on silver stain. (D) A fluorescent stain (thioflavin S) reveals the ring-like profiles of amyloid within blood vessel walls in the meninges or coverings of the brain. The underlying cortical blood vessels also evidence amyloid angiopathy. Senile plaques in the cortex are also seen in this preparation. Reproduced from Khachaturian and Radebaugh, *Alzheimer's Disease Cause(s), Diagnosis, Treatment, and Care* (113). Top panel: Figure courtesy of Erik Roberson. Adapted from *Learning and Memory: A Comprehensive Reference*, Volume 4: Molecular Mechanisms of Memory. Copyright Elsevier 2008.
Lower panel: *In vivo* imaging of amyloid plaques with Pittsburgh compound B (PIB). PIB–positron emission tomography scan of a 79-year-old patient with AD shows a robust signal attributable to amyloid plaque binding, compared with a 67-year-old control subject. From Klunk, W. E., Engler, H., Nordberg, A., et al. (2004) "Imaging brain amyloid in Alzheimer's disease with Pittsburgh Compound-B." *Ann. Neurol.* 55:306–319. Reprinted with permission of John Wiley & Sons, Inc.

Continued

BOX 1—cont'd

DIAGNOSING ALZHEIMER'S DISEASE

At present there is no definitive method for pre-mortem diagnosis of AD. Accepted practice is for AD to be diagnosed post-mortem by pathological examination of autopsy tissue. Histopathological analysis of post-mortem tissue uses criteria not appreciably different from those described by Alois Alzheimer himself in 1907 (10). The gross hallmarks are cortical atrophy, enlargement of the ventricles, and shrinkage of the hippocampus and surrounding areas of the medial temporal lobe.

Microscopic examination reveals diffuse neuronal death, and the presence of "senile plaques" and "neurofibrillary tangles" (see Figure A and Figure 1 from the text). The plaques are a molecular admixture of amyloid peptides and other constituents, and they can be subdivided into two categories. *Neuritic plaques* contain a dense core of amyloid peptide aggregate and are surrounded by distressed neuronal processes. *Diffuse plaques* lack associated neuronal processes and exhibit a more diffuse deposition of amyloid. Plaques can be seen readily using silver stains or thioflavin stains—the advent of silver staining chemistry is in fact what allowed Alzheimer to make his landmark discovery.

Microscopy of post-mortem AD tissue also reveals the presence of neurofibrillary tangles in the cytoplasm of neurons in affected brain areas. Neurofibrillary tangles are insoluble deposits of hyperphosphorylated tau protein (see text). An additional feature of AD is the presence of angiopathy, that is, pathology of the cerebral vasculature. Blood vessels in the AD patient exhibit amyloid deposition to varying degrees, an attribute that has been termed "hardening of the arteries."

Pre-mortem diagnosis of AD is a more difficult proposition. Established criteria have been published under the aegis of the NIH (78) that, when adhered to, can give about 90% accuracy versus post-mortem assessment of the same individual.

Clinical diagnosis of AD requires the availability of a spouse or other frequent companion for cross-reference. Inaccurate recollection on the part of the patient themselves is a great confound, so that an informed acquaintance needs to be available to give an objective description of the patient's symptoms. Preliminary diagnosis of AD revolves around assessment of hippocampus-dependent memory function, for the most part. For example, a typical test battery

involves giving a list of three words and then asking the patient to recall them at some later point in the interview (79). The general degree of orientation and attention on the part of the patient are also evaluated. A commonly utilized test battery is the "Mini Mental State" battery, which evaluates orientation, memory, concentration, and language usage (80). A slightly more detailed exam is the "Blessed" battery, also known as the Information-Memory-Concentration Test (81), performance on which has been correlated with post-mortem assessments in the same individual.

A thorough neurological examination is also requisite as part of the diagnostic process. This is because diagnosis of AD is, in large part, an elimination of other possible explanations—a diagnosis by serial elimination. Other possibilities that need to be excluded are stroke, trauma, diffuse vascular insult, transient delirium due to metabolic imbalance, Parkinson's disease, psychosis, and "pseudodementia" associated with depression. Brain imaging is a necessary adjunct to assess specific anatomical pathologies such as tumors and strokes. Although brain imaging techniques do not allow independent diagnosis of AD, there are specific metabolic changes in the temporal lobes associated with AD that can be detected with PET scans (82), and through the use of a plaque-binding agent termed Pittsburgh compound B (PIB, see Figure B).

The state-of-the-art in diagnosing AD is steadily improving. The rapid expansion of our understanding of the genetic components contributing to AD will no doubt allow further refinements in pre-mortem diagnosis of AD. The irony of the present situation is that, because no effective treatments for AD pathogenesis are available at present (see Box 2), a definitive diagnosis of AD is of little direct benefit to the patient. This might lead one to ask the question "What's the point?" If nothing else, it helps the patient and their families prepare for what lies ahead. However, there is also a larger picture to be kept in mind. There are many ongoing clinical trials related to various aspects of AD, including trials related to the development of new AD treatments. Patients diagnosed with AD will potentially benefit themselves by participating in these trials, and through their participation will definitely benefit the greater society in which we all live. Diagnosis opens the door for this opportunity.

because understanding these processes is critical to understanding and potentially developing treatments for AD. Ideally, one would like to develop treatments that intervene before any extensive cell death begins to occur. Focusing on processes involved in early-stage AD provides the promise of early intervention. Understanding the basis for the more subtle disruptions in hippocampal function that are the hallmarks of early AD is a key to finding the first line of attack in developing new therapies.

B. Pathological Hallmarks of Alzheimer's Disease

It has been known for over a century now (10) that AD clinical signs and symptoms are correlated with

selective dysfunction (and ultimately death) of neurons in brain regions and neural circuits critical for memory and cognition (see Table 1). These include the hippocampus, amygdala, neocortex, anterior thalamus, the basal forebrain cholinergic system (see Box 2 and Figure 2) and the mono-aminergic brainstem system (6, 11–15). Areas initially affected are the entorhinal and transentorhinal cortex, and parts of the hippocampus. This progresses to increasing hippocampal involvement. This is followed by spread to the amygdala and limbic nuclei of the thalamus, and is accompanied by a worsening of initially affected areas. Final stages involve various areas of the cerebral cortex with subsequent cellular pathology in the association areas.

BOX 2

THE CHOLINERGIC HYPOTHESIS OF ALZHEIMER'S DISEASE AND CURRENT PHARMACOTHERAPIES

In the mid- to late-1970s and early 1980s, there were a series of landmark papers published describing a loss of cholinergic neurons in the brains of AD patients (11,83–84). This led to the formulation of the "cholinergic hypothesis" of AD (85–87) which, briefly stated, posited that loss of cholinergic function in the CNS was the basis for the dementia in AD. There was palpable optimism in the papers published during that period, which is poignant in retrospect. The feeling was that this might be the breakthrough in AD that would be analogous to the dopaminergic hypothesis of Parkinson's disease—perhaps treatment with cholinomimetics or acetylcholinesterase inhibitors might do for AD patients what L-DOPA had done for Parkinson's patients.

It is now clear that this is not going to be the case. AD has a complex pathophysiology and the cholinergic treatment route is not nearly as efficacious as it was hoped it would be. Nevertheless, augmenting cholinergic function does provide symptomatic ameliorative effects in a subpopulation of patients. In other words, augmenting acetylcholine function helps improve some of the cognitive effects in earlier stages of AD, for some of the patients. The efficacy of the treatment declines as the disease progresses. Acetylcholine-targeted treatments do not affect or slow the underlying pathogenesis of AD (88).

The currently-available drugs commonly prescribed for AD act to augment acetylcholine function in the CNS by inhibiting acetylcholinesterase, which is the enzyme

that breaks down acetylcholine, converting it to acetate and choline. The specific drugs available at present are donepezil (Aricept), rivastigmine (Exelon), galantamine (Reminyl), and tacrine (Cognex).

Aside from providing a rationale for drug development, the selective loss of cholinergic neurons in AD raises an additional interesting point. How is it that cholinergic neurons get selectively targeted? Some AD-related process is clearly picking cholinergic neurons out of the diverse array of central neurons in a highly selective manner. Recent work from a number of groups has suggested a partial answer to this question. It turns out that amyloid beta peptide binds with extremely high affinity to CNS nicotinic acetylcholine receptors (see Figure, from reference 89). This provides an insight into how cholinergic neurons might be targeted—amyloid beta peptide selectively binds to cholinergic autoreceptors on their cell surface. The precise mechanisms for how this might lead to neuron loss or derangement is actively under investigation. Possibilities include direct effects of Aβ on the receptors themselves, which are ligand-gated ion channels (77), or elevated intracellular levels of Aβ in cholinergic neurons due to nicotinic receptor-mediated endocytosis (90–91).

Additional detailed discussions of current molecular models for AD are given in Chin, Roberson and Mucke, Chapter 15 of *Learning and Memory: A Comprehensive Review*, Elsevier 2008.

Continued

THE CHOLINERGIC HYPOTHESIS OF ALZHEIMER'S DISEASE AND CURRENT PHARMACOTHERAPIES

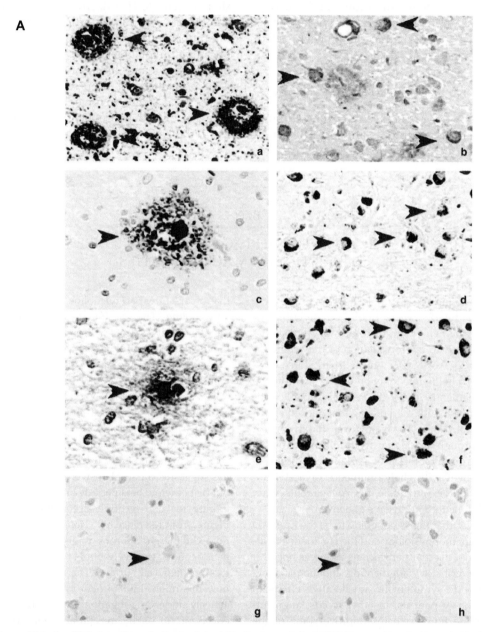

BOX 2 Immunohistochemical detection of α7 nicotinic ACh Receptor (α7nAChR) in neuritic plaques of AD hippocampus. Upper photographs. (A) Tissues were stained with a modified Bielschowsky silver stain technique. Arrowheads indicate areas of neuritic plaques. Tissues were then stained with the appropriate antibodies to either amyloid beta peptide or α7nAChR. (B) Arrowheads indicate neurofibrillary tangles. (C) Presence of Aβ_{1-42} (arrowheads) in a dense core plaque and (D) in neurons. (E) Presence of α7nAChR (arrowheads) in a neuritic plaque and (F) in neurons. (G) Lack of α4nAChR immunoreactivity in a plaque (arrowhead) in a section stained with an alpha4 nicotinic receptor-selective antibody. (H) Lack of N-methyl-D-aspartate R1 glutamate receptor immunoreactivity in a plaque (arrowhead) stained with an NMDAR antibody. Magnification: (A) × 20; (B)–(H) × 40. All 12 AD brain samples showed identical results, and representative data from two cases of sporadic AD are shown.

BOX 2—cont'd

THE CHOLINERGIC HYPOTHESIS OF ALZHEIMER'S DISEASE AND CURRENT PHARMACOTHERAPIES

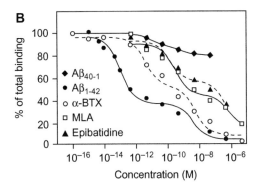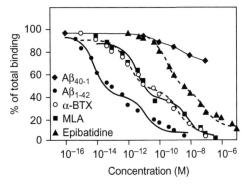

BOX 2   In other studies (lower graphs), the interaction of Aβ peptides with the α7nicotinic ACh receptor was assessed by ligand receptor binding assay using the α7nAChR-selective ligand alpha-bungarotoxin (89). Left panel: ^{125}I-α-bungarotoxin (BTX) binding to α7 receptor-containing cell membranes was assessed. Amyloid beta peptide competes for bungarotoxin binding to the alpha-7 receptor with high affinity. In the right-hand panel ^{125}I-Aβ$_{1-40}$ binding to α7 receptor-containing membrane was also assessed. Alpha-7 selective antagonists (BTX, MLA, and epibatidine) compete for ^{125}I-Aβ$_{1-40}$ binding with high affinity. Overall, these data indicate a high-affinity interaction of amyloid beta peptide with the alpha7 nicotinic acetylcholine receptor. Mean data from at least three experiments are presented. Nonlinear regression data curve fit was performed by Prism. Reproduced from Wang et al. (2000) *The Journal of Biological Chemistry* 275:5626–5632. Copyright Elsevier 2003.

At the cellular level, a predictable sequence of damage to these brain regions occurs. A principal pathologic feature of AD brain is the presence of "senile plaques" (Figures 1 and 2). Senile plaques exhibit several features. Plaque formation is associated with the accumulation of dystrophic neurites in the areas surrounding senile plaques. At the core of the senile plaque is a structure known as the amyloid plaque (10). An additional neuropathological feature of AD is neurofibrillary tangles (NFTs). Progression of the disease is marked by an increase in the number of amyloid plaques and neurofibrillary tangles in affected neurons and brain areas, accompanied ultimately by neuronal loss (see Figure 3). In the next two sections we will cover the molecular composition of NFTs and amyloid plaques. A number of the most important findings in the history of AD research were related to discovering the chemical nature of these materials.

Neurofibrillary Tangles

One of the principal cytopathological diagnostic features of AD are NFTs. NFTs are located in the soma, dendrites, and dystrophic neurites (abnormal neuronal processes and axon terminals) of affected neurons. NFTs comprise aggregates of poorly soluble filaments, the principal component being hyperphosphorylated isoforms of the microtubule-associated protein tau (see Figures 1 and 4, and reference 16).

Hyperphosphorylated tau from human AD tissue can be phosphorylated at more than 20 different sites. Tau is a substrate for a variety of protein kinases, including ERK and JNK MAP kinases, cyclin-dependent kinase 5 (cdk5) and glycogen synthase kinase 3 (GSK3). The relevant kinases that phosphorylate tau in AD and other pathologic states are currently under investigation, but all these kinases are viable candidates for mediating increased tau phosphorylation in AD. Similarly, the basis for aberrant kinase activation (or aberrant phosphatase inhibition) in AD is an area of ongoing investigation.

Current hypotheses invoke the idea that hyperphosphorylation of tau has two effects. First, it causes dissociation of tau from the microtubule cytoskeleton, and hence leads to cytoskeletal disarrangement. Second, hyperphosphorylated tau aggregates into a cytopathologic feature known as paired helical filaments (PHFs). These intracellular protein aggregates may themselves be cytotoxic, by mechanisms yet to be discerned (see reference 17 for a review). Thus, the combination of architectural derangement and neuronal inclusions is hypothesized to lead to neuronal dysfunction, and ultimately neuron death. It should not escape our attention that many of the identified tau kinases are ones that we discussed in previous chapters in terms of their involvement in synaptic plasticity and memory formation.

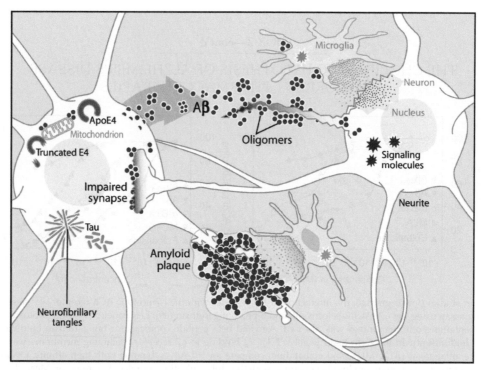

FIGURE 3 Key molecules involved in Alzheimer's disease pathogenesis. Aβ peptides produced by neurons and other brain cells aggregate into a variety of assemblies, including amyloid plaques containing Aβ fibrils, and soluble nonfibrillar oligomers. Some of these Aβ assemblies impair synapses and neuronal dendrites, either directly or through the engagement of pathogenic glial loops. However, other glial activities protect neurons against dysfunction and degeneration. ApoE4 and tau promote Aβ-induced neuronal injury and also have independent adverse effects. From Roberson, E. D., and Mucke, L. (2006). "100 years and counting: Prospects for defeating Alzheimer's disease." *Science* 314:781–784. Figure courtesy of Erik Roberson. Copyright Elsevier 2008.

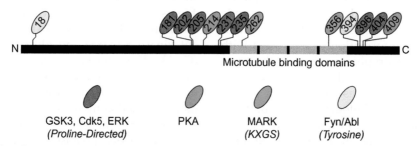

FIGURE 4 Tau phosphorylation sites. The four microtubule-binding domains are indicated by shading in a schematic line drawing of tau protein. Most tau phosphorylation sites surround the microtubule-binding regions. Figure and legend from Chin, Roberson, and Mucke, "Learning and Memory: A Comprehensive Review." *Science* 314:781–784. Figure courtesy of Erik Roberson. Copyright Elsevier 2008.

The neurofibrillary tangle is a cytopathological feature associated with several neuropathological disorders besides AD, such as amyotrophic lateral sclerosis/Parkinsonism dementia complex, Pick's disease, corticobasal degeneration, and progressive supranuclear palsy. This spectrum of disorders is now known as the "Tauopathies" (17). It is likely that NFTs are a hallmark of neurodegeneration, however as mentioned above, the causative role that hyperphosphorylated tau and NFTs play in neurodegeneration is not well understood.

Amyloid Plaques

Senile plaques are composed of dystrophic neurites displayed around extracellular deposits of amyloid. A key breakthrough, and perhaps the key breakthrough, in understanding the molecular pathology of AD came with the identification of the chemical structure of amyloid by George Glenner in 1984 (18). This work, along with subsequent studies (19, 20), made clear that AD-associated amyloid in both the vascular system and in amyloid plaques is comprised of aggregates of a peptide termed amyloid beta (Aβ) peptide.

"Amyloid beta peptide" is actually a mixture of peptides *in vivo*. Aβ comprises peptides with a length of 40 to 43 amino acids, all of which are identical except for the carboxy-terminal 3 amino acids. The sequence of the longest (43 amino acid) peptide is:

DAEFR(G)HDSGY(F) EVH(R)HQKLVFF
AEDVGSNKGA I IGLMVGGVV IAT.

This is the human amino acid sequence. In keeping with our focus on rodent models, I have also included in parentheses the rat (and mouse) sequence, which differs only at the three indicated amino acids. Current work focuses on the 42-amino acid variant (Aβ42) as a principal culprit in AD, as we will return to later.

Aβ42, being a fairly small peptide, can assume a number of different conformations in solution and even in protein crystals. One three-dimensional structure of an Aβ peptide that has been determined is shown in Figure 5 for your reference. However, Aβ42 is highly "fibrillogenic," that is, it is subject to not remaining as a monomer in solution, but rather forms oligomers, multimers, and aggregates. It is these polymerized forms of Aβ42, in complex with Aβ40, that make up the amyloid plaques that are characteristic of AD. Exactly which state of Aβ (monomer versus multimer versus aggregate) is involved in AD pathogenesis is an area of much debate at present.

Work subsequent to the discovery of the sequence of Aβ revealed that Aβ is derived from β-amyloid precursor proteins (APPs; 20), yet another finding that has catalyzed progress in understanding the cellular and molecular underpinnings of AD. APPs are type I integral membrane proteins that are expressed at the cell surface (see Figures 6 and 7). The APP gene is located on chromosome 21 and contains 19 exons—over ~400 kb of DNA (21). Several alternatively spliced mRNAs encode APP in neurons and, to a lesser extent, glia. The 695 amino acid splice variant (APP695) is expressed exclusively in neurons—the APP751 and APP770 variants are more widely expressed.

In axons of the peripheral and central nervous system, APP is transported by the fast anterograde system to nerve terminals, where Aβ peptides are generated and released into the extracellular space by mechanisms that are not clear at present (22–23). Aβ peptide is a normal constituent of the extracellular milieu, and is present in your brain and CSF as you are reading this sentence. It is only when it is aberrantly overproduced (or under-degraded) that amyloid plaques form. The normal physiologic role of Aβ peptide and its precursor APP are completely unknown at present. Not surprisingly, almost all the work in this area has focused on the role of these proteins in AD pathogenesis.

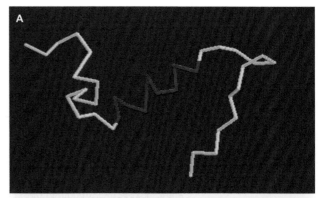

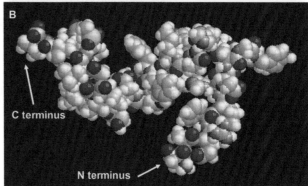

FIGURE 5 A crystal structure of a fragment of amyloid beta peptide. These two panels show a peptide backbone (A) and spacefill (B) rendering of amino acids 1–39 of amyloid beta peptide. Figures rendered using Rasmol and file 1BA6 from the Brookhaven National Protein Database. Note that amyloid beta peptide can assume many different conformations, and this particular structure is only representative of one known conformation of the peptide. In (A) the shaded region indicates a central alpha-helical domain. Both panels are the same perspective of the molecule. The amino terminus of the molecule is at the lower right. Data for image is published in Watson et al. (111). Copyright Elsevier 2003.

Given that the overproduction of Aβ appears to be such a critical factor in the development of AD, much important effort has been invested in understanding the production of this peptide. APPs are subject to alternative proteolytic processing by a family of "secretase" activities which are still in the process of being defined at the molecular level (24–26). The three relevant secretases for processing APP and other similar proteins (the developmental regulator Notch is another example) are termed alpha, beta, and gamma secretase (see Figure 6). The α-secretase cleaves APP within the Aβ sequence to release the N-terminal ectodomain of APP (APPˢa); thus, α-secretase cleavage within the Aβ domain *precludes* production of Aβ peptides (see Figure 7). The alpha-secretase activity therefore dictates a route of APP processing distinct from the amyloidogenic, AD-related process.

However, the actions of the beta and gamma secretases lead to production of Aβ peptides (reviewed

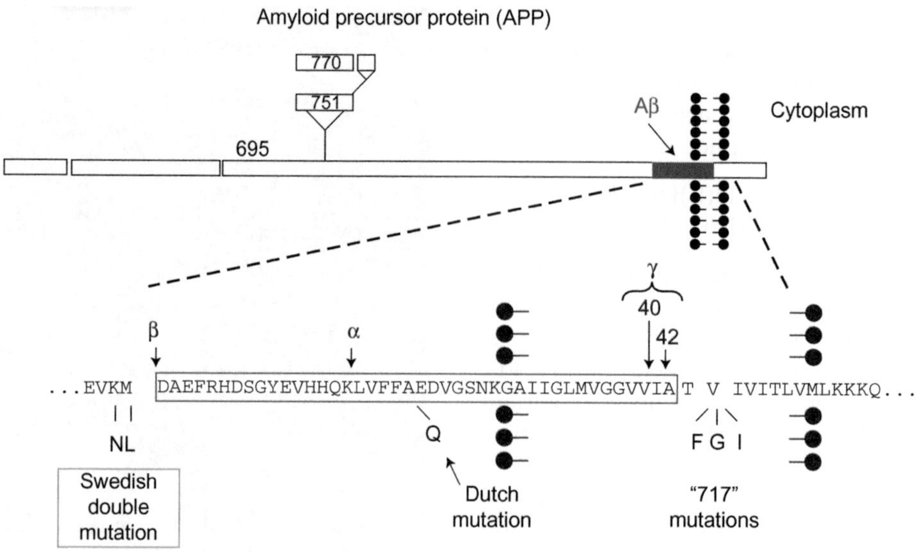

Amyloid precursor protein (APP)

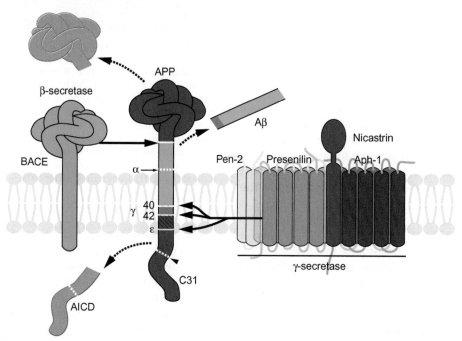

FIGURE 6 Amyloid precursor protein. The basic structure of APP is shown (upper section), along with several known mutations and the sites of alpha, beta, and gamma secretase cleavage (marked α, β, and γ, lower section). See text for additional discussion. Adapted from Price et al. (112). Copyright Elsevier 2003.

FIGURE 7 APP, Aβ, and the secretases. Aβ production depends on sequential proteolytic cleavage of APP by β-secretase, also known as β-site APP-cleaving enzyme 1 (BACE1), and the γ-secretase complex, composed of presenilin and other proteins. γ-secretase can cleave APP at different locations to generate Aβ40, Aβ42, or the APP intracellular domain (AICD). Caspase cleavage at the carboxy-terminus yields the C31 fragment. Modified from Roberson, E. D., and Mucke, L. (2006). "100 years and counting: Prospects for defeating Alzheimer's disease." *Science* 314:781–784. Figure courtesy of Erik Roberson. Copyright Elsevier 2008.

in reference 27). The γ-secretase is unusual, because it cleaves proteins, including APP, within the lipid bilayer. That is, this protease actually acts to cut the APP at its alpha-helical transmembrane domain while it is still in the membrane. The β-secretase is more pedestrian, cleaving the APP in a soluble

domain. However, even the β-secretase has the unusual attribute that it is an ecto-protease, that is, it acts on the extracellular domain of the APP molecule.

The β-secretase has been identified and termed BACE (for Beta-site APP Cleaving Enzyme) (reviewed in reference 29, see also reference 28). BACE is a single-transmembrane domain aspartyl protease that can cleave APP at several sites, including the one responsible for generating Aβ peptide. BACE also cleaves other proteins. Knockout mice deficient in BACE produce essentially no amyloid beta peptide (30). These knockout mice also have no discernible behavioral or developmental phenotype, a good sign in terms of the possibility of utilizing BACE inhibitors as a potential AD therapy.

What about the γ-secretase? There is a clear and compelling candidate for the γ-secretase; a family of proteins termed the presenilins (PS). There are two homologous human PS genes, PS1 and PS2. As might be expected for an enzyme capable of proteolyzing a transmembrane alpha helix, PSs have multiple transmembrane domains (31). These proteins also undergo proteolysis themselves as part of their conversion to the active state. Presenilins are hypothesized to be *the* gamma secretase, although there is some discussion in the literature that PSs might instead act indirectly to promote gamma secretase activity. Certainly other proteins such as nicastrin are necessary in addition to presenilins in order to achieve full gamma-secretase activity.

Presenilins act not only on APP, but also on other proteins such as Notch, a general role referred to as regulated intramembrane proteolysis (RIP, reviewed in reference 32). PS-mediated RIP is involved in a variety of cellular signaling processes that are important in neurodevelopment and homeostasis. For our purposes, we will focus on the role of presenilins in regulating the production of Aβ peptides in AD.

The APP fragments produced by the combined activities of the beta- and gamma-secretases are generally 40 or 42–43 amino acids in length. This is because there is some variability in the site of cleavage of the gamma secretase—it can cleave APP at any of three sites. A240 comprises ~90% of the Aβ population, while the rest is usually made up of Aβ42(43) (33). The minor Aβ species (42/43) is highly fibrillogenic, readily aggregates, and is neurotoxic (34–39).

C. Aβ42 as the Cause of Alzheimer's Disease

Briefly stated, decades of work indicate that Aβ42 is the likely causative agent of AD. This idea is commonly referred to as the amyloid hypothesis of AD (see reference 31 for a review). The essential findings supporting this hypothesis are as follows:

1. As we have already discussed, amyloid senile plaque number (i.e., Aβ deposition) in the neocortex is the primary criterion for the post-mortem diagnosis of Alzheimer's disease (AD) (40–43). The initial deposits in senile plaques are the Aβ42 and Aβ43 peptides (39).

Moreover, Aβ burden is an early indicator of cognitive decline in AD. Post-mortem studies of total Aβ (non-aggregate and aggregates in diffuse or mature senile plaques combined) in the brains of recently deceased patients correlate with recent pre-morbid Clinical Dementia Rating scale values for those individuals. Quantitative histopathological studies have shown that the number of senile plaques correlates with dementia scores in AD patients (44). This is true even for patients not yet in advanced stages of the disease. These findings support the idea that extracellular Aβ levels are elevated in at-risk individuals, even prior to gross plaque deposition and severe cognitive impairment.

2. Recent studies from animal and *in vitro* models have made clear the capacity of aberrant Aβ production to elicit pathological features of AD. For example, animals genetically-engineered to overproduce Aβ exhibit some of the pathological features of AD, such as amyloid plaque production (see Figure 8 and references 45–46). *In vitro* studies have shown that Aβ can elicit cytotoxic effects as well.

3. The genetics of AD also support the hypothesis. Familial AD (FAD) is associated with the inheritance of specific genes, be they mutated genes or the presence of specific allele types. All known FAD gene products directly or indirectly impinge on Aβ peptide production, resulting in increased Aβ levels in the CNS—we will return to this in more detail in the next section (see also Box 3).

If Aβ causes AD, how does this happen? The basic mechanisms underlying Aβ-mediated neuronal dysfunction and neuronal loss are unknown and, of course, a topic of much vigorous investigation. There are a number of scenarios in play at present. A variety of evidence suggests the involvement of senile plaque components in triggering inflammatory responses that culminate in neuronal death. Plaque structures appear to act as irritants and initiate inflammatory responses. For example, hypertrophic astrocytes and activated microglia often surround plaques (47), and these responses likely lead to localized cell death. The overproduction of reactive oxygen species by inflammatory process or even direct chemical catalysis by the Aβ peptide, with resulting oxidative toxicity, is another hypothesis. A large number of research groups are working in the general area of testing for effects of Aβ as causing altered activation of cellular signaling processes such as protein kinases and phosphatases. The idea is that derangement of these signaling cascades can lead to both derangements of synaptic physiology and altered phosphorylation of

Tg 2576   Tg 2576 +
                           PS1 A246E

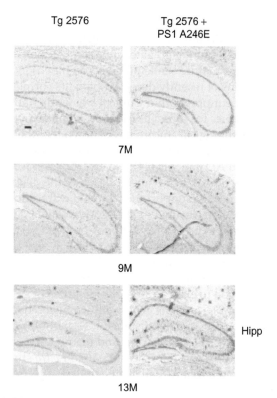

7M

9M

Hipp

13M

FIGURE 8 PS1 A246 E FAD mutant transgene greatly accelerates amyloid plaque pathology of Tg2576 transgenic mice. Brain sections of the hippocampus of transgenic mice coexpressing APP K670N/M671 L (the Tg 2576 line) and PS1 A246 E FAD mutant transgenes were immunostained with Aβ specific mAb 6E10, and compared to that of age-matched Tg2576 transgenic animals. Panels are hippocampus of mice 7, 9, and 13 months of age. At all ages examined, both the density and the size of plaques in heterozygous doubly transgenic mice far exceeded that of heterozygous APP mice at comparable ages. Consistent plaque deposits were detected in 7 month old heterozygous doubly transgenic mice when the APP transgenic mice were free of plaques. At 9 months of age, while APP transgenic mice exhibit occasional diffuse Aβ plaques, doubly transgenic mice showed numerous Aβ deposits in various regions of the brain, including cerebral cortex (data not shown) and hippocampus. Aβ load was further enhanced in 13-month-old doubly transgenic mice and multiple brain areas were covered with plaques. Wildtype human PS1 transgene does not accelerate plaque deposition when coexpressed with the mutant APP transgene (data not shown). Littermates that express PS1 A246 E alone do not develop detectable amyloid plaques up to 14 months of age (data not shown). Data courtesy of Kelly Dineley et al. (74). Copyright Elsevier 2003.

proteins such as tau, that are known to be associated with cell death. Another idea is that Aβ peptide binds to cell-surface receptors in order to trigger its deleterious effects. A number of laboratories are currently working on the idea that neuronal nicotinic acetylcholine receptors are targets of Aβ peptide (see Box 3). Misregulation of these surface ion channels could lead to both synaptic and cellular derangement; this mechanism could also provide an explanation for the selective loss of cholinergic fibers and their targets in AD.

Although the processes that Aβ peptide triggers still remain mysterious, a parsimonious explanation consistent with most of the available data is the idea that amyloid beta peptide causes AD. In the next section we will review some of the strongest evidence available supporting this idea—findings that gene mutations known to invariably cause AD in humans occur in genes directly linked to the production of amyloid beta peptide.

III. GENES—FAMILIAL AND LATE-ONSET ALZHEIMER'S DISEASE

AD is broadly divided into two types. The first and relatively better understood category is early-onset familial AD, which I will abbreviate as FAD. FAD is relatively rare, accounting in aggregate for a few percent of total AD cases (see reference 48 for a review). FAD is inherited in an autosomal dominant fashion, and is highly penetrant, meaning that if you inherit a single copy of the gene you are highly likely to develop AD before age 60. So far FAD-causing mutations have been identified in the human genes for APP, presenilin 1, and presenilin 2 (PS1 and PS2).

The second category of AD is late-onset AD, commonly abbreviated LOAD. LOAD is associated with several risk factors, the most common of which are age and the inheritance of specific genes. The LOAD-related genetic factor that has been unambiguously demonstrated to date is the inheritance of the epsilon4 (ε4) allele type of apolipoprotein E (ApoE4; 49–51). ApoE alleles vary normally among individuals. If you inherit the ε4 allele you have an increased *likelihood* of developing LOAD (see Figure 9). Interestingly, if you inherit the less-common ε2 allele there is a small protective effect against AD.

The existence of inherited factors in AD, of course, indicates that subtypes of the disease do in fact have a genetic component. This is not as obvious as it might at first sound, given that even familial AD patients do not develop AD until age 40 or so at the earliest. Thus, even the inherited forms of AD are time-dependent and multi-factorial.

One mystery for FAD is how an inherited disorder, present from conception, can take so long to develop clinical manifestations. FAD may require a second (albeit common) environmental insult, perhaps even one that can accumulate over time. An alternative model is that the kinetics of the underlying biochemistry are extremely slow. Finally, it may be that the underlying process is one for which appreciable compensatory capacity exists relative to the rate of insult accumulation (see Box 4). At present, these temporal aspects of AD development remain inexplicable.

BOX 3

Aβ PEPTIDE IMMUNIZATION AS A POTENTIAL THERAPY FOR ALZHEIMER'S DISEASE

In 1999 Shenk et al. discovered that immunization with amyloid β peptide protects against amyloid βplaque deposition in a mutant mouse model for Alzheimer's disease (92). In these studies, they used the "PDAPP" transgenic mouse expressing human APP mutated at amino acid 717. The approach was a fairly straightforward application of traditional immunization—they injected the Aβ peptide into the animals, using an adjuvant carrier to boost the immune response. In this first study, the investigators documented significant prevention of plaque formation in the immunized mice. This was a very exciting finding concerning a new potential therapy for AD—immunization with Aβ, allowing the body's normal immune response to do the rest.

How does the immunization effect a decrease in amyloid plaque formation? These immunization procedures produce active anti-Aβ antibodies in the bloodstream, a fraction of which can apparently penetrate into the CNS. The idea is that microglia in the CNS clear the antibody-Aβ complexes, reducing Aβ burden. Alternatively, decreased Aβ in the bloodstream due to immune clearance outside the brain may result in lowered CNS Aβ levels, by passive diffusion of the Aβ peptide out of the CNS.

A year later, two groups continued these efforts and published further exciting and encouraging results. Janus et al. and Morgan et al. (93–94) both reported ameliorative effects of the immunization protocol on the development of aging-related deficits in learning and memory in AD mouse models. This took the observations to the next level, demonstrating important symptomatic relief, as least as assessed using the currently available tools. Also encouraging was that similar results were obtained using a variation of the immunization approach. "Passive" immunization involves the

perfusion of previously isolated and purified antibodies into the test subject. Like the active immunization studies described above, passive immunization with anti-Aβ antibodies similarly improves memory performance in AD model mice (95–96).

Overall, these findings precipitated great hope that an immunization approach might prove of practical utility in humans. Unfortunately, work in this area is at somewhat of a standstill at present. Pilot immunization studies in normal humans indicated no deleterious effects of Aβ immunization. However, in the initial study of immunization therapy using human AD patients, a small number of study subjects developed brain inflammation. This side-effect, while perhaps not entirely unexpected, necessitated a halt to the study, and at present there is a moratorium on this specific line of human studies.

The potential of immunotherapy as an effective treatment for Alzheimer's disease is one of the most exciting developments in the recent history of Alzheimer's research, offering real hope for effective therapy in the aging human. However, at present it is clear that significant work lies ahead in evaluating whether the approach will be clinically adaptable to the human.

There is an additional reason to highlight these studies, independent of their significance as a potential new therapeutic approach. As we discussed in the main text, much work is currently underway aimed at testing various predictions of the amyloid beta hypothesis of AD. The behavioral studies with Aβ immunization test one key prediction of this hypothesis—the block prediction. The observation that decreasing Aβ burden in the CNS ameliorates behavioral deficiencies is strong support for the hypothesis that Aβ is a causative agent in the memory defects associated with early AD.

One commonality across all forms of AD is the involvement of the metabolism of APP and its products. All the FAD autosomal dominant mutations, and the inheritance of the ApoE-ε4 allele, result in altered metabolism of the amyloid precursor protein (APP). These inherited factors, moreover, have in common that their major consequence is elevated production of Aβ42 in the CNS. In the following sections, I will briefly review how this is thought to happen.

A. APP Mutations

There are two categories of mutations in APP that lead to early-onset familial AD (see Figure 3). One is the so-called "Swedish double mutation," named for the Swedish kindred in which it was first identified. The Swedish mutation is a K670M, N671L double mutation in the APP gene (52–53). This double mutation results in higher levels of secreted Aβ peptides

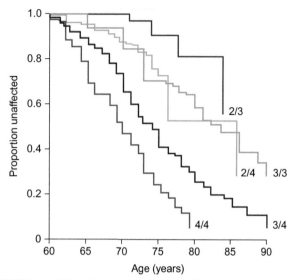

FIGURE 9 Effect of apoE genotype on AD risk. ApoE4 increases AD risk in a gene dose-dependent manner, while apoE2 lowers risk. Numbers at the ends of the graphs refer to the two ApoE allele forms present in the individual, for example, 4/4 indicates that those individuals express two copies of the ApoE4 gene, 2/3 indicates one copy of 2 and one copy of 3, etc. From Strittmatter, W. J., and Roses, A. D. (1996). "Apolipoprotein E and Alzheimer's disease." *Annu. Rev. Neurosci.* 19:53–77. Figure courtesy of Erik Roberson. Copyright Elsevier 2008.

in the CNS. The second type of AD-associated APP mutation results in a higher fraction of the longer Aβ peptides being produced. These are the missense mutations at residue 717 in the APP gene (38, 53–54). Both these categories of mutations affect the endoproteolytic cleavage pattern during APP processing, promoting the β- and γ-secretase cleavage activities over the α-secretase (55–56). A final type of APP mutation, commonly referred to as the "Dutch" type of mutation, does not cause AD *per se*. These are mutations in and around amino acid 693 in the APP sequence. These mutations also elicit overproduction of amyloid, but result in variations of a syndrome known as Dutch-type hereditary cerebral hemorrhage with amyloidosis, a vascular disorder.

B. Presenilin Mutations

As you might have guessed from the name, the presenilin gene that likely codes for the APP-processing endoprotease was first identified as an AD candidate gene and termed presenilin on that basis (reviewed in reference 48). Only later was it identified as a strong candidate for being the actual gamma secretase that helps process APP into Aβ. Mutations in both the PS-1 and PS-2 genes (PSEN-1 and -2 in the human) result in early onset FAD, but PS-1 mutations result in a slightly earlier onset of FAD than PS-2 mutations.

Most of the known FAD-causing mutations that have been identified to date, several dozen distinct mutations, are mutations in PS-1 (31). These mutations in PS-1 and PS-2 all have in common the fact that they lead to alterations in APP processing. Transgenic mouse studies indicate that PS1 FAD mutations do not inactivate normal PS1 activity (57), but rather alter APP processing in such a way as to enhance Aβ42 synthesis (57–59). The net result is that the ratio of secreted Aβ42 (43) to Aβ40 in individuals with PS-1 or PS-2 mutations are elevated relative to unaffected family members (52). Furthermore, in transfected mammalian cells and the brains of transgenic (Tg) mice that co-express APP and mutant PS1 variants, levels of secreted Aβ42 are also elevated (see Figure 4 and reference 59). These observations are consistent with the interpretation that changes in APP metabolism, due to altered secretase cleavage patterns, result in an increased burden of extracellular Aβ peptide. In essence, PS-1 and PS-2 mutations that lead to AD are "gain of function" mutations, leading to elevated Aβ peptide production.

Mutations in the APP and PSEN1/2 genes account for only about 5% of AD cases. Moreover, they account for only about 40% or so of autosomal dominant AD cases—that is those that are clearly and proximally caused by inherited mutations. Clearly, much is left to be learned from pursuing the identification of new AD genes. One promising category of genes left to be identified are those encoding for the enzymes that break down Aβ. Specifically, it appears to be the case that Insulin Degrading Enzyme or a gene near it on chromosome 10 may be involved in regulating Aβ levels and thus linked to LOAD (60–62).

C. ApoE4 Alleles in Alzheimer's Disease

Current estimates are that the ApoE ε4 allele is a contributing factor to about 20% of AD cases. The basis for ApoE alleles contributing to AD is much less clear than the APP and PSEN mutations (51). For one thing, the ApoE-E4 allele is neither necessary nor sufficient to cause AD. It is a contributing risk factor, when present, which decreases the average age of onset of AD, and presumably by this mechanism increases the incidence of AD in that population (see Figure 9).

One unifying attribute, which at least allows for a consistent model in the context of the APP and PSEN mutations, is that the presence of the ApoE ε4 allele clearly leads to elevated Aβ burden in the CNS. This is true in both the human brain (63) and in emerging mouse models for AD (64). This gives a unifying model across the known genetic factors contributing to AD: elevation of Aβ in the CNS.

BOX 4

THE NUN STUDY

One of the most interesting studies ever published on the epidemiology of AD is the "Nun Study." In pursuing this work, David Snowdon undertook an amazingly sophisticated scientific and personal mission in order to help understand the epidemiologic factors involved in AD (97). He did this with the help and commitment of 678 Catholic Sisters of the "School Sisters of Notre Dame" Order, an order devoted to education, teaching, and service. They took as one of their missions to help us all learn about AD, by opening their personal lives and histories to prying scientific eyes, and by donating their brains for scientific study post-mortem.

David Snowdon and his colleagues had the insight to assess a large group of Catholic nuns as an epidemiologic cohort. This is about as scientifically well-controlled a group of humans as is imaginable, practically speaking. Most of them have lived their entire adult lives alongside their Sisters, eating the same foods and living in the same environment. Detailed personal histories are available, including very early records from when they joined the order in their late teens. Confounding vices, such as illicit drug use, are understandably of minimal concern with a group of this sort. A constant and comparable level of healthcare applies across the group as well. Comparison within this group to assess who develops AD and who doesn't allows new insights into individual attributes that correlate with a risk of AD.

An additional important component of the nun study is that each nun wrote a brief autobiography before taking her final vows to join the order. These writing samples were obtained, on average, from study participants when they were in their late teens or early twenties. This served as a critical point of reference concerning language usage by each of the study participants. One astounding finding from the Nun Study came from comparing language usage in their youth with the development of AD later in life. In brief, this type of analysis convincingly demonstrated that complex cognitive skills and abilities at a relatively young age correlate with a *decreased* likelihood of developing AD in late adulthood. These findings are in general agreement with a number of prior studies correlating college-level education or higher with a decreased incidence of AD.

It is not clear how a high level of cognitive ability in youth might relate mechanistically to developing late-onset AD. Three general possibilities have been suggested. First, AD may in fact start developing at a young age, manifesting subtle effects even in individuals in their late teens. Second, the two findings may be correlative but not causally-related—for example the same genes that predispose one to AD may also impinge negatively on cognitive function, for reasons unrelated to AD pathology. Finally, higher baseline abilities in cognitive function may allow a "reserve" of brain capacity, helping delay the detectable onset of AD. Which of these possibilities is relevant will hopefully become clear as the molecular underpinnings of AD are determined.

How ApoE might do this is the unclear part (reviewed in reference 51). The initial discovery of a role for ApoE in AD grew out of studies of a direct interaction of ApoE with Aβ, so direct effects on amyloid deposition are a clear possibility (49,65–66, reviewed in reference 67). ApoE has also been classically studied in terms of cholesterol handling, and this role might somehow play a part. However, more recent work has demonstrated that ApoE also binds directly to a number of neuronal cell surface receptors, and effects via this mechanism might also contribute to AD pathogenesis (see reference 68 for a review). In Section IV I will provide a brief overview of the ApoE system in order to give some context for how ApoE isoforms and their receptors might contribute to AD pathogenesis.

IV. APOLIPOPROTEIN E IN THE NERVOUS SYSTEM

Lipoproteins are complexes of carrier proteins and lipids, including cholesterol, that in the cardiovascular and digestive systems are involved in the trafficking of dietary lipids. Apolipoprotein E (ApoE) is a component of lipoproteins, and mediates the uptake of these lipoprotein particles into target tissues. In the liver, ApoE is incorporated into very low density lipoproteins (VLDLs), which carry triglycerides and cholesterol to peripheral tissues, mainly muscle and adipose tissue. In the gut, ApoE becomes a component of chylomicrons and mediates the transport of dietary fat to the liver. In macrophages, the scavenger cells of the immune system, ApoE is involved in the resecretion of absorbed cholesterol. However, ApoE is also expressed in cells of the nervous system, predominantly in astrocytes. The role of ApoE secretion and its binding to the ApoE receptors (ApoERs) that are present on the surface of neurons is unclear at this point.

ApoE occurs in three major isoforms in the general human population, ApoE2, ApoE3, and ApoE4. As described earlier, the ApoE4 isoform, also known as ApoE ε4, is associated with AD.

There are a variety of ApoE receptors that are expressed on the surface of neurons that may be involved in the pathological process by which ApoE contributes to AD. Two members of this neuronal family of ApoE receptors warrant particular attention: the very-low-density lipoprotein receptor (VLDLR); and the apolipoprotein E receptor 2 (ApoER2). Both these receptors participate in neuronal signaling pathways related to memory formation. These receptors bind not only ApoE, but also the signaling molecule Reelin, a large protein of approximately 400 kDa that is secreted by interneurons dispersed throughout the neocortex and the hippocampus.

The ApoE/Reelin receptors ApoER2 and VLDLR couple to the adaptor protein Dab1, that is essential to ApoE/Reelin signaling. As I mentioned in a prior chapter, these receptors couple via Dab1 to the src pathway and potentially via this mechanism contribute to NMDA receptor regulation (see Figure 10).

A recent series of experiments found that mice lacking the ApoE/Reelin receptors VLDLR and ApoER2 have pronounced defects in memory formation and hippocampal long-term potentiation (69). Furthermore, Reelin greatly enhances LTP in hippocampal slices. These results thus reveal a role for ApoE receptors in synaptic function and in the formation of long-term memory. These data are also consistent with a hypothetical model in which the promotion of memory dysfunction by ApoE4 might involve an impairment of this ApoE receptor-dependent signaling pathway—how this might be involved in AD is a current line of investigation in several laboratories.

V. MOUSE MODELS FOR ALZHEIMER'S DISEASE

Further progress in understanding and developing new therapies for AD hinges on the availability of suitable model systems for investigating the disease in the laboratory. In this vein, the application of transgenic animal technology to the pursuit of investigating AD appears to be a critically important endeavor. There are several considerations that factor into the critical role of genetic engineering in developing suitable laboratory models for AD. First, AD is an exclusively human disorder—no naturally occurring animal homologs that we can study in the laboratory appear to exist. AD is not transmissible, at least as far as we know, so one cannot attempt to mutate already occurring pathogens in order to generate new models. No environmental factor has yet been identified that is capable of producing AD or even aspects of the disease. Chemical or anatomical lesions to the CNS are unable to mimic the condition adequately. The only clearly identified basis for AD so far is genetic. Therefore, genetic engineering is the only practical route available for modeling AD *in vivo*.

Mouse models for AD fortunately are becoming increasingly available (see Table 2). These mouse models capitalize on the important studies described above that have identified human AD-causing gene mutations. Current mouse models are transgenic mouse models expressing mutated forms of human genes (reviewed in references 27, 70–71). The engineered animals generally use neuron-selective promoters to drive expression of the transgenes in the CNS. Currently available lines that model AD are all derived from transgenic animals expressing mutated human APP, either alone or in combination with mutated human PS1 and/or mutated human tau. Transgenic lines expressing ApoE alleles are still at a relatively early stage of development.

One prominent transgenic mouse model for AD expresses a human splice-variant of APP containing the "Swedish" double mutation. This specific mutation and splice variant was identified in a large family with FAD (45, 53). This model is variously referred to as the "Swedish" mouse (after the mutation), or the "Tg2576" mouse (after the mouse line number). I will refer to it as the Tg2576 mouse.

Another major mouse line that has been extensively characterized so far is the "PDAPP" line. The name derives from the fact that it is a line expressing the human APP transgene (mutated at position 717) driven by a PDGF promoter. Other lines under development and characterization include other 717 APP mutant lines, a mixture variation combining the Swedish and 717 mutations, APP mutants combined with PS-1 mutants, and APP mutants combined with tau mutants.

In addition, an important new transgenic mouse line that has become available in the last few years is the "3xTg-AD" mouse line (114). This mouse is a triple-transgenic mouse expressing three mutated human AD-related genes in its nervous system: the Swedish double-mutation APP gene; the M146V PS1 mutant gene; and the P301L tau gene. This mouse has the unique attribute that it exhibits both amyloid

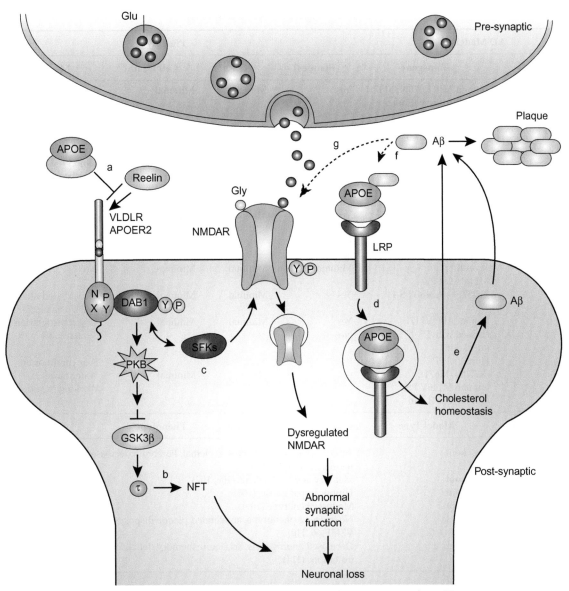

FIGURE 10 Reelin and ApoE signaling—implications for AD. Binding of Reelin to VLDLR and ApoER2 receptors initiates a cascade of events that leads to modulation of NMDA receptor function and enhanced long-term potentiation. ApoE can impede Reelin signaling by competing for receptor binding. Impaired Reelin signaling results in impaired synaptic plasticity, as well as in elevated tau phosphorylation, which could contribute to neurofibrillary tangles associated with AD. Additionally, binding of ApoE to the LRP lipoprotein receptor results in internalization of the ligand-bound receptor. Cholesterol homeostasis modulates the production and trafficking of Aβ. Secreted Aβ can bind apoE and be cleared through receptor-mediated endocytosis, promote the internalization of NMDA receptors, and deposit into plaques. From Herz, J., and Chen, Y. (2006). "Reelin, lipoprotein receptors and synaptic plasticity." *Nat. Rev. Neurosci.* 7:850–859. Figure courtesy of Erik Roberson. Copyright Elsevier 2008.

plaques (from the APP and PS1 mutations) and neurofibrillary tangles (from the mutant tau). These mutant lines, along with a few other related knockout mouse lines and selected references, are summarized in Table 2.

For illustrative purposes, I will discuss some of the attributes of the Tg2576 line in more detail. I choose to focus on the Tg2576 line for two reasons. First, it is one of the lines that have been studied most extensively. Second, its properties seem to be fairly representative of the various mouse lines under investigation at present. In particular, the Tg2576 line and the other major line, the PDAPP line, appear to have similar molecular and behavioral characteristics. Also, the Tg2576 mutation is present in the 3x-Tg mouse line.

A. The Tg2576 Mouse

The Tg2576 strain is a mouse model for AD in which the transgene is the human 695 splice-variant of APP which contains the double mutation K670M,

TABLE 2   Selected Mouse Models for AD

AD Models		Phenotypes			
Mouse model	Transgene	Plaques?	NFT's?	Cell Death?	Memory Deficits?
Tg2576 (APPswe)	human APP K670N/M671L 695 AA splice variant prion promoter	Yes	Minimal	Minimal	Fear conditioning (74) Water maze (73) Forced Alternation (75)
PDAPP	human APP V717F PDGF promotor	Yes	Partial (98)	Minimal	Water maze Spatial series (99) Object recognition (95) Holeboard (95)
Tg2576 + JNPL3	APPswe P301L Tau	Yes	Yes (100)	Minimal	?
TgLRND8	Human APP 670N/671L + V717F (+M146L L286V PS-1 mutant)	Yes / Plaques accelerated	Minimal	Minimal	Water maze (93, 101)
PS-1	several M146L, L286V	Minimal	Minimal	Minimal	No (74)
APP + PS-1	Tg2576 + A246E PS-1	Yes	Minimal	Minimal	Exacerbated relative to Tg2576 alone (74, 102)
V717I V717I	human APP V717I crossed with PS-1 knockout	Yes No	Minimal	Minimal	Object recognition Similar (103)
3xTg-AD	Human APP (K670N/M671L) Human M146V PS1 Human P301L tau	yes	yes	Minimal	Fear conditioning Water maze Working memory (114)

Relevant Molecules	Model Type	Phenotype
PS-1	Knockout	+/- developmental defects, -/- lethal; Forebrain:decreased hippocampal neurogenesis (104, 105)
ApoE	Knockout	Memory and LTP deficits (106, 107)
APP	Knockout	Hippocampal gliosis (108)
PS-2	Knockout	Modest phenotype (109)
ApoE4	Transgenic	No learning phenotype, accelerated plaque disposition when combined with APP V717F(66, 110)
Tau	Transgenic	Decreased neurogeneis, accelerate memory deficits when combined with APP/PS mutations (114)

N671L driven by a hamster prion protein gene promoter (expression is predominantly in neurons). The brains of these animals contain about five times more transgenic mutant human APP than endogenous mouse APP. Transgenic APP expression appears to remain unchanged between 2 and 14 months of age. They exhibit about a five-fold increase in Aβ40 and a 10- to 15-fold increase in Aβ42/43 over levels measured in nontransgenic littermates. Similar to observations in AD brain, and consistent with the notion that elevated Aβ is potentially toxic to brain cells, senile plaques in the brains of these mice are associated with signs of cellular inflammatory responses.

Tg2576 mice exhibit many behavioral and pathological features of AD, including elevated production of Aβ peptides, age-dependent accumulation of amyloid fibrils, and plaque formation with subsequent age-dependent hippocampal learning and memory

deficits (45–46, 70, 72–75). This mouse model demonstrates a correlation between hippocampal dysfunction at both the cellular and behavioral levels versus its increased burden of extracellular Aβ42 (43), as I will describe briefly below.

At six months of age and older, mice exhibit a deficit in spatial memory (Morris water maze). In addition to impairment in spatial memory at 14–16 months of age, mice also exhibit a working memory deficit as measured using a forced-alternation paradigm (75–76). Tg2576 mice also exhibit deficits in contextual fear conditioning (see Figure 11 and references 74, 76). Several AD-like pathologies are not present in these mice. For example, there is no neuronal loss in CA1 or other brain areas (37). Thus, these mice do not model AD-associated neuronal loss. Nonetheless, the age-dependent amyloidogenesis and working memory deficits are powerful correlates of AD, and make this

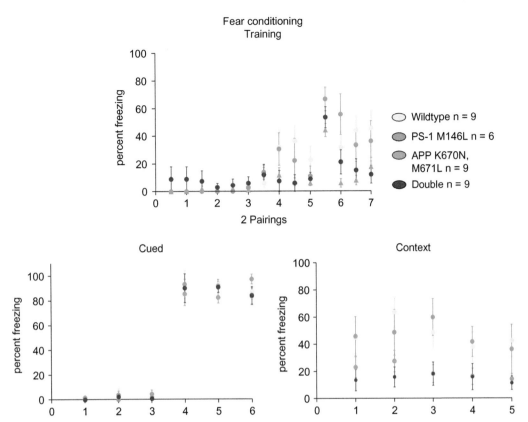

FIGURE 11 Fear conditioning in mouse models of AD. PS-1, APP, doubly-transgenic and control mice were subjected to a standard fear conditioning paradigm in which the animals learn to associate a neutral stimulus with an aversive one. The mice were placed in a novel context (fear conditioning box) and exposed to two pairings of a white-noise cue and mild foot shock. Fear learning was assessed 24 hours later by measuring freezing behavior in response to representation of the context or of the auditory cue within a completely different context.

At five months of age, there were no apparent differences in the freezing behavior of the different mouse genotypes during the two-pairing training phase of fear conditioning (upper panel). In the contextual test for fear learning, the APP and doubly-transgenic animals exhibited decreased freezing behavior compared to both the control littermates and PS-1 transgenic group (lower right). One-way ANOVA and Tukey *post hoc* analysis detected a significant difference in freezing behavior at the 1–4 minute time epochs, compared to control littermates and at the 1, 2, 3, and 5 minute epochs compared to the PS-1 transgenic group (Fig. 7(b; min 1: $F(3, 60) = 5.60$; min 2: $F = 7.68$; min 3: $F = 8.51$; min 4: $F = 4.26$; min 5: $F = 4.35$; $p < 0.05$ all groups). Analysis of overall freezing behavior indicates that APP and doubly-transgenic animals freeze significantly less than control and PS-1 transgenic animals (Fig. 11a; Tukey's multiple comparison test: $F(5, 16) = 27.97$; control versus APP, control versus doubly, APP versus PS-1, doubly versus PS-1 all $p < 0.001$). These data indicate that APP and doubly-transgenic animals have a deficit in contextual fear learning. These same animals did not exhibit a deficit in cued fear conditioning (lower left panel). One-way ANOVA and Tukey *post hoc* analysis determined that all animals displayed similar and significant freezing in the cued test for associative learning, indicating that the impairment in contextual fear learning exhibited by the APP and doubly-transgenic animal groups is not due to an inability to freeze or to an inability to detect the aversive foot shock stimulus (Figure 7c; $p < 0.001$, all groups). Therefore, five-month-old APP and doubly-transgenic mice appear to have a selective hippocampus-dependent impairment in associative learning following two pairings of conditioned and unconditioned stimuli for fear conditioning. Adapted from Dineley et al. (74, 76).

animal model an attractive launching point for investigations into the cellular signaling processes underlying neuronal dysfunction induced by an increased burden of extracellular A-beta.

It has also been reported that accompanying the behavioral deficits in working memory, Tg2576 and similar transgenic mice exhibit disruptions of LTP in both the Schaffer collateral and perforant pathways of the hippocampus. Synaptic transmission and paired-pulse facilitation appear normal (indicating that Ca^{++}-dependent synaptic vesicle release is normal), and there is no decrease in the number of CA1 neurons

or synaptic density in the dentate gyrus (75). Thus, in Tg2576 mice, selective impairments in synaptic plasticity correlate with deficits in cognitive abilities.

Our take-home message from all of this is that the Tg2576 mouse strain exhibits learning deficits and alterations in synaptic plasticity with no neuronal cell loss. In that respect, along with all other available mouse strains modeling AD, it does not recapitulate one of the major hallmarks of late-stage AD—cell death. However, these mouse lines accurately model amyloidosis and likely model early-stage AD. The lack of cell death in all these lines also has an important implication. Because there is no appreciable cell loss or pronounced alterations in neuronal morphology, the impairment that leads to the memory phenotype is likely in the normal cellular signaling cascades involved in learning and synaptic plasticity.

Crossing PS1 transgenic mice carrying the A246E FAD mutation with Tg2576 mice causes acceleration of CNS amyloid accumulation and plaque formation (see Figure 8 and Table 2). The doubly-transgenic animals also have exacerbated associative learning deficits relative to the Tg2576 transgenic mice. These data indicate that, as might be expected, there is an interaction of the APP and PS-1 gene products *in vivo*. The point in raising this observation is two-fold. First, over time there will likely be improvement in modeling AD in mice through these kinds of mix-and-match genetic experiments, as exemplified by the 3x-Tg triple-transgenic mouse line. Second, this result illustrates a use of genetically-engineered mouse models of AD that is independent of their utility as a model for human disease *per se*. That is, the emergence of these various transgenic mouse lines will allow the testing of various specific predictions of current working models for how the various gene products identified as relevant to amyloid beta peptide production interact in the living animal.

Overall, the studies published so far indicate cause for optimism that transgenic mouse models for AD will be of great utility both in studying the biochemistry and physiology of the disease, and in assessing potential new treatment avenues for AD (see Boxes 2 and 3). Important work in the near future will allow further evaluation and optimization of mouse models for investigating AD. In addition, as we obtain further basic information concerning human AD, for example identification of additional genetic factors predisposing us to AD, further enhancement of progress in mouse models is likely.

However, these practical considerations should not completely overshadow the additional important implications of transgenic mouse experiments. The transgenic mouse studies to date can be looked at as experiments testing predictions of the amyloid beta hypothesis of AD. The measure experiments using human AD tissues identified an association of Aβ with AD. Transgenic mouse experiments are the mimic experiments. Thus far, studies of transgenic mice overexpressing Aβ peptide certainly indicate that Aβ is sufficient to cause many of the pathological hallmarks and cognitive features of early AD. These are important experimental results in their own right.

VI. SUMMARY

In this chapter I have promoted viewing the earliest stages of Alzheimer's disease (AD) as a memory disorder, as opposed to thinking of AD as a generalized neuropathologic dementia. The basic hypothesis is that for early stages of AD, which are characterized not by generalized dementia, but rather by much more subtle deficits in memory consolidation, there will be derangements of the normal signal transduction machinery that underlies memory. I am optimistic that this will be a fruitful avenue of pursuit, because the idea is based on the tremendous advances that have been made in the last decade in our understanding of the basic biochemistry of memory. If this is the case, it also means that AD is likely the area where recent progress in understanding the basic science of memory will translate into an improvement in the capacity to attack a clinical disorder of great significance.

There are several additional take-home messages from this chapter.

1. Several studies have indicated that Aβ peptide overproduction in the CNS can elicit cognitive deficits in rodents in the absence of neuronal loss or even Aβ deposition into plaques. These findings are consistent with the idea that memory deficits in early stages of AD may be due to disruption of the neuronal signal transduction machinery that normally subserves memory formation.

2. Great strides have been made in identifying the genetic factors contributing to AD. Specifically, we talked about APP, presenilin, and ApoE4, and how mutations or isoforms of these gene products can cause or predispose one to developing AD.

3. These discoveries of human genes linked to AD have allowed the generation of new mouse models for AD that capitalize on the human findings, in order to allow the production of model systems of utility in the basic science research laboratory.

4. A principal unifying theme of this chapter is the amyloid beta hypothesis of AD. There is a reassuring convergence of many different sorts of data that support the Aβ hypothesis of AD. While I did not organize the chapter around evaluating this hypothesis directly, evaluating the contents of the chapter with this question in mind is a useful exercise. Students in particular might find it useful to recast the section on mouse models of AD in terms of evaluating the block, mimic, and measure predictions of the Aβ hypothesis.

5. More than most other areas of contemporary neuroscience research, the AD field is at the intersection of basic and clinical research—a critically important clinical problem in search of answers that only basic science can provide. AD is a disease of human memory. The complexity of AD pathogenesis is rooted in the complexity of memory itself. Hopefully, advances in

understanding the basic science of memory will soon translate into tangible improvements in treating AD.

Further Reading

Billings, L. M., Oddo, S., Green, K. N., McGaugh, J. L., and LaFerla, F. M. (2005). "Intraneuronal Abeta causes the onset of early Alzheimer's disease-related cognitive deficits in transgenic mice". *Neuron* 45:675–688.

Braak, H., Braak, E., and Bohl, J. (1993). "Staging of Alzheimer-related cortical destruction". *Eur. Neurol.* 33:403–408.

Burke, S. N., and Barnes, C. A. (2006). "Neural plasticity in the ageing brain". *Nat. Rev. Neurosci.* 7:30–40.

Chapman, P. F., White, G. L., Jones, M. W., Cooper-Blacketer, D., Marshall, V. J., Irizarry, M., Younkin, L., Good, M. A., Bliss, T. V., Hyman, B. T., Younkin, S. G., and Hsiao, K. K. (1999). "Impaired synaptic plasticity and learning in aged amyloid precursor protein transgenic mice". *Nat. Neurosci.* 2:271–276.

Herz, J., and Chen, Y. (2006). "Reelin, lipoprotein receptors and synaptic plasticity". *Nat. Rev. Neurosci.* 7:850–859.

Oddo, S., Caccamo, A., Shepherd, J. D., Murphy, M. P., Golde, T. E., Kayed, R., Metherate, R., Mattson, M. P., Akbari, Y., and LaFerla, F. M. (2003). "Triple-transgenic model of Alzheimer's disease with plaques and tangles: intracellular Abeta and synaptic dysfunction". *Neuron* 39:409–421.

Roberson, E. D., and Mucke, L. (2006). "100 years and counting: Prospects for defeating Alzheimer's disease". *Science* 314:781–784.

Roberson, E. D., Scearce-Levie, K., Palop, J. J., Yan, F., Cheng, I. H., Wu, T., Gerstein, H., Yu, G. Q., and Mucke, L. (2007). "Reducing endogenous tau ameliorates amyloid beta-induced deficits in an Alzheimer's disease mouse model". *Science* 316:750–754.

Selkoe, D. J. (2002). "Alzheimer's disease is a synaptic failure". *Science* 298:789–791.

Selkoe, D. J., and Wolfe, M. S. (2007). "Presenilin: running with scissors in the membrane". *Cell* 131:215–221.

Walsh, D. M., and Selkoe, D. J. (2004). "Deciphering the molecular basis of memory failure in Alzheimer's disease". *Neuron* 44:181–193.

Whitehouse, P. J., Price, D. L., Struble, R. G., Clark, A. W., Coyle, J. T., and Delon, M. R. (1982). "Alzheimer's disease and senile dementia: loss of neurons in the basal forebrain". *Science* 215:1237–1239.

Wong, P. C., Cai, H., Borchelt, D. R., and Price, D. L. (2001). "Genetically engineered models relevant to neurodegenerative disorders: their value for understanding disease mechanisms and designing/testing experimental therapeutics". *J. Mol. Neurosci.* 17:233–257.

Wu, W., Brickman, A. M., Luchsinger, J., Ferrazzano, P., Pichiule, P., Yoshita, M., Brown, T., DeCarli, C., Barnes, C. A., Mayeux, R., Vannucci, S. J., and Small, S. A. (2008). "The brain in the age of old: the hippocampal formation is targeted differentially by diseases of late life". *Ann. Neurol.* 64:698–706.

Journal Club Articles

Barnes, C. A., Suster, M. S., Shen, J., and McNaughton, B. L. (1997). "Multistability of cognitive maps in the hippocampus of old rats". *Nature* 388:272–275.

Hsiao, K., Chapman, P., Nilsen, S., Eckman, C., Harigaya, Y., Younkin, S., Yang, F., and Cole, G. (1996). "Correlative memory deficits, Abeta elevation, and amyloid plaques in transgenic mice". *Science* 274:99–102.

Klunk, W. E., Engler, H., Nordberg, A., Wang, Y., Blomqvist, G., Holt, D. P., Bergström, M., Savitcheva, I., Huang, G. F., Estrada, S., Ausén, B., Debnath, M. L., Barletta, J., Price, J. C., Sandell, J., Lopresti, B. J., Wall, A., Koivisto, P., Antoni, G., Mathis, C. A., and Långström, B. (2004). "Imaging brain amyloid in Alzheimer's disease with Pittsburgh Compound-B". *Ann. Neurol.* 55:306–319.

Snowdon, D. A., Kemper, S. J., Mortimer, J. A., Greiner, L. H., Wekstein, D. R., and Markesbery, W. R. (1996). "Linguistic ability in early life and cognitive function and Alzheimer's disease in late life. Findings from the Nun Study". *Jama* 275:528–532.

For more information—relevant topic chapters from: John H. Byrne (Editor-in-Chief) (2008). *Learning and Memory: A Comprehensive Reference*. Oxford: Academic Press (ISBN 978-0-12-370509-9). (2.41 Naveh-Benjamin, S.R. *Old, Aging and Memory*. pp. 787–808; 3.25 Juraska, J. M., and Rubinow, M. J. *Hormones and Memory*. pp. 503–520; 3.26 McGaugh, J. L., and Roozendaal, B. *Memory Modulation*. pp. 521–553; 3.27 Gold, P. E. *Memory-Enhancing Drugs*. pp. 555–575; 3.28 Daselaar, S., and Cabeza, R. *Episodic Memory Decline and Healthy Aging*. pp. 577–599; 3.29 Brickman, A. M., and Buchsbaum, M. S. *Alzheimer's Disease: Neurostructures*. pp. 601–620; 4.15 Chin, J., Roberson, E. D., and Mucke, L. *Molecular Aspects of Memory Dysfunction in Alzheimer's Disease*. pp. 245–293.)

References

1. Barnes, C. A. (1988). "Aging and the physiology of spatial memory". *Neurobiol. Aging* 9:563–568.

2. Barnes, C. A., Suster, M. S., Shen, J., and McNaughton, B. L. (1997). "Multistability of cognitive maps in the hippocampus of old rats". *Nature* 388:272–275.

3. Barnes, C. A., Rao, G., and Houston, F. P. (2000). "LTP induction threshold change in old rats at the perforant path—granule cell synapse". *Neurobiol. Aging* 21:613–620.

4. Barnes, C. A., Rao, G., and Shen, J. (1997). "Age-related decrease in the N-methyl-D-aspartateR-mediated excitatory postsynaptic potential in hippocampal region CA1". *Neurobiol. Aging* 18:445–452.

5. Lynch, M. A. (1998). "Analysis of the mechanisms underlying the age-related impairment in long-term potentiation in the rat". *Rev. Neurosci.* 9:169–201.

6. Braak, H., Braak, E., and Bohl, J. (1993). "Staging of Alzheimer-related cortical destruction". *Eur. Neurol.* 33:403–408.

7. Nagy, Z., Hindley, N. J., Braak, H., Braak, E., Yilmazer-Hanke, D. M., Schultz, C., Barnetson, L., Jobst, K. A., and Smith, A. D. (1999). "Relationship between clinical and radiological diagnostic criteria for Alzheimer's disease and the extent of neuropathology as reflected by 'stages': a prospective study". *Dement. Geriatr. Cogn. Disord.* 10:109–114.

8. Braak, E., and Braak, H. (1997). "Alzheimer's disease: transiently developing dendritic changes in pyramidal cells of sector CA1 of the Ammon's horn." *Acta. Neuropathol.* (Berl) 93:323–325.

9. Braak, H., and Braak, E. (1998). "Evolution of neuronal changes in the course of Alzheimer's disease". *J. Neural. Transm. Suppl.* 53:127–140.

10. Alzheimer, A. (1907). "Uber eine eigenartige Erkrankung der Hirnrinde". *Allgemeine Zeitschrift fur Psychiatrie und Psychisch-gerichtliche Medizin* 64:146–148.

11. Whitehouse, P. J., Price, D. L., Struble, R. G., Clark, A. W., Coyle, J. T., and Delon, M. R. (1982). "Alzheimer's disease and senile dementia: loss of neurons in the basal forebrain". *Science* 215:1237–1239.

12. Braak, H. Braak, E. In: Caine, D. B. (Ed.) (1994). *Neurodegenerative Diseases*: W.B. Saunders Co. Philadelphia, pp. 585–613.

13. Zweig, R. M., Ross, C. A., Hedreen, J. C., Steele, C., Cardillo, J. E., Whitehouse, P. J., Folstein, M. F., and Price, D. L. (1988). "The

neuropathology of aminergic nuclei in Alzheimer's disease". *Ann. Neurol.* 24:233–242.

14. Hyman, B. T., Van Horsen, G. W., Damasio, A. R., and Barnes, C. L. (1984). "Alzheimer's disease: cell-specific pathology isolates the hippocampal formation". *Science* 225:1168–1170.

15. Hyman, B. T., Van Hoesen, G. W., Kromer, L. J., and Damasio, A. R. (1986). "Perforant pathway changes and the memory impairment of Alzheimer's disease". *Ann. Neurol.* 20:472–481.

16. Spillantini, M. G., and Goedert, M. (1998). "Tau protein pathology in neurodegenerative diseases". *Trends Neurosci.* 21:428–433.

17. Taylor, J. P., Hardy, J., and Fischbeck, K. H. (2002). "Toxic proteins in neurodegenerative disease". *Science* 296:1991–1995.

18. Glenner, G. G., and Wong, C. W. (1984). "Alzheimer's disease: initial report of the purification and characterization of a novel cerebrovascular amyloid protein". *Biochem. Biophys. Res. Commun.* 120:885–890.

19. Masters, C. L., Simms, G., Weinman, N. A., Multhaup, G., McDonald, B. L., and Beyreuther, K. (1985). "Amyloid plaque core protein in Alzheimer disease and Down syndrome". *Proc. Natl. Acad. Sci. USA* 82:4245–4249.

20. Kang, J., Lemaire, H. G., Unterbeck, A., Salbaum, J. M., Masters, C. L., Grzeschik, K. H., Multhaup, G., Beyreuther, K., and Muller-Hill, B. (1987). "The precursor of Alzheimer's disease amyloid A4 protein resembles a cell-surface receptor". *Nature* 325:733–736.

21. Lamb, B. T., Sisodia, S. S., Lawler, A. M., Slunt, H. H., Kitt, C. A., Kearns, W. G., Pearson, P. L., Price, D. L., and Gearhart, J. D. (1993). "Introduction and expression of the 400 kilobase amyloid precursor protein gene in transgenic mice [corrected]". *Nat. Genet.* 5:22–30.

22. Koo, E. H., Sisodia, S. S., Archer, D. R., Martin, L. J., Weidemann, A., Beyreuther, K., Fischer, P., Masters, C. L., and Price, D. L. (1990). "Precursor of amyloid protein in Alzheimer disease undergoes fast anterograde axonal transport". *Proc. Natl. Acad. Sci. USA* 87:1561–1565.

23. Buxbaum, J. D., Thinakaran, G., Koliatsos, V., O'Callahan, J., Slunt, H. H., Price, D. L., and Sisodia, S. S. (1998). "Alzheimer amyloid protein precursor in the rat hippocampus: transport and processing through the perforant path". *J. Neurosci.* 18:9629–9637.

24. Haass, C., and Selkoe, D. J. (1993). "Cellular processing of beta-amyloid precursor protein and the genesis of amyloid beta-peptide". *Cell* 75:1039–1042.

25. Sahasrabudhe, S. R., Spruyt, M. A., Muenkel, H. A., Blume, A. J., Vitek, M. P., and Jacobsen, J. S. (1992). "Release of aminoterminal fragments from amyloid precursor protein reporter and mutated derivatives in cultured cells". *J. Biol. Chem.* 267:25602–25608.

26. Sisodia, S. S. (1992). "Beta-amyloid precursor protein cleavage by a membrane-bound protease". *Proc. Natl. Acad. Sci. USA* 89:6075–6079.

27. Wong, P. C., Cai, H., Borchelt, D. R., and Price, D. L. (2002). "Genetically engineered mouse models of neurodegenerative diseases". *Nat. Neurosci.* 5:633–639.

28. Vassar, R., Bennett, B. D., Babu-Khan, S., Kahn, S., Mendiaz, E. A., Denis, P., Teplow, D. B., Ross, S., Amarante, P., Loeloff, R., Luo, Y., Fisher, S., Fuller, J., Edenson, S., Lile, J., Jarosinski, M. A., Biere, A. L., Curran, E., Burgess, T., Louis, J. C., Collins, F., Treanor, J., Rogers, G., and Citron, M. (1999). "Beta-secretase cleavage of Alzheimer's amyloid precursor protein by the transmembrane aspartic protease BACE". *Science* 286:735–741.

29. Vassar, R., and Citron, M. (2000). "Abeta-generating enzymes: recent advances in beta- and gamma-secretase research". *Neuron* 27:419–422.

30. Luo, Y., Bolon, B., Kahn, S., Bennett, B. D., Babu-Khan, S., Denis, P., Fan, W., Kha, H., Zhang, J., Gong, Y., Martin, L., Louis, J. C.,

Yan, Q., Richards, W. G., Citron, M., and Vassar, R. (2001). "Mice deficient in BACE1, the Alzheimer's beta-secretase, have normal phenotype and abolished beta-amyloid generation". *Nat. Neurosci.* 4:231–232.

31. Hardy, J., and Selkoe, D. J. (2002). "The amyloid hypothesis of Alzheimer's disease: progress and problems on the road to therapeutics". *Science* 297:353–356.

32. Ebinu, J. O., and Yankner, B. A. (2002). "A RIP tide in neuronal signal transduction". *Neuron* 34:499–502.

33. Mann, D. M., Iwatsubo, T., Ihara, Y., Cairns, N. J., Lantos, P. L., Bogdanovic, N., Lannfelt, L., Winblad, B., Maat-Schieman, M. L., and Rossor, M. N. (1996). "Predominant deposition of amyloid-beta 42(43) in plaques in cases of Alzheimer's disease and hereditary cerebral hemorrhage associated with mutations in the amyloid precursor protein gene". *Am. J. Pathol.* 148:1257–1266.

34. Pike, C. J., Walencewicz, A. J., Glabe, C. G., and Cotman, C. W. (1991). "Aggregation-related toxicity of synthetic beta-amyloid protein in hippocampal cultures". *Eur. J. Pharmacol.* 207:367–368.

35. Roher, A. E., Lowenson, J. D., Clarke, S., Wolkow, C., Wang, R., Cotter, R. J., Reardon, I. M., Zurcher-Neely, H. A., Heinrikson, R. L., Ball, M. J. et al. (1993). "Structural alterations in the peptide backbone of beta-amyloid core protein may account for its deposition and stability in Alzheimer's disease". *J. Biol. Chem.* 268:3072–3083.

36. Yankner, B. A., Dawes, L. R., Fisher, S., Villa-Komaroff, L., Oster-Granite, M. L., and Neve, R. L. (1989). "Neurotoxicity of a fragment of the amyloid precursor associated with Alzheimer's disease". *Science* 245:417–420.

37. Yankner, B. A. (1996). "Mechanisms of neuronal degeneration in Alzheimer's disease". *Neuron* 16:921–932.

38. Suzuki, N., Cheung, T. T., Cai, X. D., Odaka, A., Otvos, L., Jr., Eckman, C., Golde, T. E., and Younkin, S. G. (1994). "An increased percentage of long amyloid beta protein secreted by familial amyloid beta protein precursor (beta APP717) mutants". *Science* 264:1336–1340.

39. Saido, T. C., Iwatsubo, T., Mann, D. M., Shimada, H., Ihara, Y., and Kawashima, S. (1995). "Dominant and differential deposition of distinct beta-amyloid peptide species, A beta N3(pE), in senile plaques". *Neuron* 14:457–466.

40. Khachaturian, Z. S. (1985). "Diagnosis of Alzheimer's disease". *Arch. Neurol.* 42:1097–1105.

41. Mirra, S. S., Heyman, A., McKeel, D., Sumi, S. M., Crain, B. J., Brownlee, L. M., Vogel, F. S., Hughes, J. P., van Belle, G., and Berg, L. (1991). "The consortium to establish a registry for Alzheimer's disease (CERAD). Part II. Standardization of the neuropathologic assessment of Alzheimer's disease". *Neurology* 41:479–486.

42. Mirra, S. S., Hart, M. N., and Terry, R. D. (1993). "Making the diagnosis of Alzheimer's disease. A primer for practicing pathologists". *Arch. Pathol. Lab. Med.* 117:132–144.

43. Mirra, S. S., Gearing, M., and Nash, F. (1997). "Neuropathologic assessment of Alzheimer's disease". *Neurology* 49:S14–S16.

44. Roth, M., Tomlinson, B. E., and Blessed, G. (1966). "Correlation between scores for dementia and counts of 'senile plaques' in cerebral grey matter of elderly subjects". *Nature* 209:109–110.

45. Hsiao, K., Chapman, P., Nilsen, S., Eckman, C., Harigaya, Y., Younkin, S., Yang, F., and Cole, G. (1996). "Correlative memory deficits, Abeta elevation, and amyloid plaques in transgenic mice". *Science* 274:99–102.

46. Hsiao, K. (1998). "Transgenic mice expressing Alzheimer amyloid precursor proteins". *Exp. Gerontol.* 33:883–889.

47. McGeer, P. L., and McGeer, E. G. (1998). "Mechanisms of cell death in Alzheimer's disease—immunopathology". *J. Neural. Transm. Suppl.* 54:159–166.

48. Tanzi, R. E., and Bertram, L. (2001). "New frontiers in Alzheimer's disease genetics". *Neuron* 32:181–184.

49. Strittmatter, W. J., Saunders, A. M., Schmechel, D., Pericak-Vance, M., Enghild, J., Salvesen, G. S., and Roses, A. D. (1993). "Apolipoprotein E: high-avidity binding to beta-amyloid and increased frequency of type 4 allele in late-onset familial Alzheimer disease". *Proc. Natl. Acad. Sci. USA* 90:1977–1981.

50. Strittmatter, W. J., and Roses, A. D. (1996). "Apolipoprotein E and Alzheimer's disease". *Annu. Rev. Neurosci.* 19:53–77.

51. Strittmatter, W. J. (2001). "Apolipoprotein E and Alzheimer's disease: signal transduction mechanisms". *Biochem. Soc. Symp.* 2001:101–109.

52. Scheuner, D., Eckman, C., Jensen, M., Song, X., Citron, M., Suzuki, N., Bird, T. D., Hardy, J., Hutton, M., Kukull, W., Larson, E., Levy-Lahad, E., Viitanen, M., Peskind, E., Poorkaj, P., Schellenberg, G., Tanzi, R., Wasco, W., Lannfelt, L., Selkoe, D., and Younkin, S. (1996). "Secreted amyloid beta-protein similar to that in the senile plaques of Alzheimer's disease is increased *in vivo* by the presenilin 1 and 2 and APP mutations linked to familial Alzheimer's disease". *Nat. Med.* 2:864–870.

53. Mullan, M., Crawford, F., Axelman, K., Houlden, H., Lilius, L., Winblad, B., and Lannfelt, L. (1992). "A pathogenic mutation for probable Alzheimer's disease in the APP gene at the N-terminus of beta-amyloid". *Nat. Genet.* 1:345–347.

54. Goate, A., Chartier-Harlin, M. C., Mullan, M., Brown, J., Crawford, F., Fidani, L., Giuffra, L., Haynes, A., Irving, N., James, L. et al. (1991). "Segregation of a missense mutation in the amyloid precursor protein gene with familial Alzheimer's disease". *Nature* 349:704–706.

55. Thinakaran, G., Borchelt, D. R., Lee, M. K., Slunt, H. H., Spitzer, L., Kim, G., Ratovitsky, T., Davenport, F., Nordstedt, C., Seeger, M., Hardy, J., Levey, A. I., Gandy, S. E., Jenkins, N. A., Copeland, N. G., Price, D. L., and Sisodia, S. S. (1996). "Endoproteolysis of presenilin 1 and accumulation of processed derivatives *in vivo*". *Neuron* 17:181–190.

56. Perez, R. G., Squazzo, S. L., and Koo, E. H. (1996). "Enhanced release of amyloid beta-protein from codon 670/671 'Swedish' mutant beta-amyloid precursor protein occurs in both secretory and endocytic pathways". *J. Biol. Chem.* 271:9100–9107.

57. Qian, S., Jiang, P., Guan, X. M., Singh, G., Trumbauer, M. E., Yu, H., Chen, H. Y., Van de Ploeg, L. H., and Zheng, H. (1998). "Mutant human presenilin 1 protects presenilin 1 null mouse against embryonic lethality and elevates Abeta1-42/43 expression". *Neuron* 20:611–617.

58. Citron, M., Oltersdorf, T., Haass, C., McConlogue, L., Hung, A. Y., Seubert, P., Vigo-Pelfrey, C., Lieberburg, I., and Selkoe, D. J. (1992). "Mutation of the beta-amyloid precursor protein in familial Alzheimer's disease increases beta-protein production". *Nature* 360:672–674.

59. Borchelt, D. R., Wong, P. C., Sisodia, S. S., and Price, D. L. (1998). "Transgenic mouse models of Alzheimer's disease and amyotrophic lateral sclerosis". *Brain Pathol.* 8:735–757.

60. Bertram, L., Blacker, D., Mullin, K., Keeney, D., Jones, J., Basu, S., Yhu, S., McInnis, M. G., Go, R. C., Vekrellis, K., Selkoe, D. J., Saunders, A. J., and Tanzi, R. E. (2000). "Evidence for genetic linkage of Alzheimer's disease to chromosome 10q". *Science* 290:2302–2303.

61. Ertekin-Taner, N., Graff-Radford, N., Younkin, L. H., Eckman, C., Baker, M., Adamson, J., Ronald, J., Blangero, J., Hutton, M., and Younkin, S. G. (2000). "Linkage of plasma Abeta42 to a quantitative locus on chromosome 10 in late-onset Alzheimer's disease pedigrees". *Science* 290:2303–2304.

62. Myers, A., Holmans, P., Marshall, H., Kwon, J., Meyer, D., Ramic, D., Shears, S., Booth, J., DeVrieze, F. W., Crook, R., Hamshere, M., Abraham, R., Tunstall, N., Rice, F., Carty, S., Lillystone, S., Kehoe, P., Rudrasingham, V., Jones, L., Lovestone, S., Perez-Tur, J., Williams, J., Owen, M. J., Hardy, J., and Goate, A. M. (2000). "Susceptibility locus for Alzheimer's disease on chromosome 10". *Science* 290:2304–2305.

63. Schmechel, D. E., Saunders, A. M., Strittmatter, W. J., Crain, B. J., Hulette, C. M., Joo, S. H., Pericak-Vance, M. A., Goldgaber, D., and Roses, A. D. (1993). "Increased amyloid beta-peptide deposition in cerebral cortex as a consequence of apolipoprotein E genotype in late-onset Alzheimer disease". *Proc. Natl. Acad. Sci. USA* 90:9649–9653.

64. Brendza, R. P., Bales, K. R., Paul, S. M., and Holtzman, D. M. (2002). "Role of apoE/Abeta interactions in Alzheimer's disease: insights from transgenic mouse models". *Mol. Psychiatry* 7:132–135.

65. Corder, E. H., Saunders, A. M., Strittmatter, W. J., Schmechel, D. E., Gaskell, P. C., Small, G. W., Roses, A. D., Haines, J. L., and Pericak-Vance, M. A. (1993). "Gene dose of apolipoprotein E type 4 allele and the risk of Alzheimer's disease in late onset families". *Science* 261:921–923.

66. Holtzman, D. M., Bales, K. R., Tenkova, T., Fagan, A. M., Parsadanian, M., Sartorius, L. J., Mackey, B., Olney, J., McKeel, D., Wozniak, D., and Paul, S. M. (2000). "Apolipoprotein E isoform-dependent amyloid deposition and neuritic degeneration in a mouse model of Alzheimer's disease". *Proc. Natl. Acad. Sci. USA* 97:2892–2897.

67. Holtzman, D. M. (2001). "Role of apoe/Abeta interactions in the pathogenesis of Alzheimer's disease and cerebral amyloid angiopathy". *J. Mol. Neurosci.* 17:147–155.

68. Herz, J., and Beffert, U. (2000). "Apolipoprotein E receptors: linking brain development and Alzheimer's disease". *Nat. Rev. Neurosci.* 1:51–58.

69. Weeber, E. J., Beffert, U., Jones, C., Christian, J. M., Forster, E., Sweatt, J. D., and Herz, J. (2002). "Reelin and ApoE receptors cooperate to enhance hippocampal synaptic plasticity and learning". *J. Biol. Chem.* 277(42):39944–39952.

70. Chapman, P. F., Falinska, A. M., Knevett, S. G., and Ramsay, M. F. (2001). "Genes, models and Alzheimer's disease". *Trends Genet.* 17:254–261.

71. Janus, C., and Westaway, D. (2001). "Transgenic mouse models of Alzheimer's disease". *Physiol. Behav.* 73:873–886.

72. Irizarry, M. C., McNamara, M., Fedorchak, K., Hsiao, K., and Hyman, B. T. (1997). "APPSw transgenic mice develop age-related A beta deposits and neuropil abnormalities, but no neuronal loss in CA1". *J. Neuropathol. Exp. Neurol.* 56:965–973.

73. Westerman, M. A., Cooper-Blacketer, D., Mariash, A., Kotilinek, L., Kawarabayashi, T., Younkin, L. H., Carlson, G. A., Younkin, S. G., and Ashe, K. H. (2002). "The relationship between Abeta and memory in the Tg2576 mouse model of Alzheimer's disease". *J. Neurosci.* 22:1858–1867.

74. Dineley, K. T., Xia, X., Bui, D., Sweatt, J. D., and Zheng, H. (2002). "Accelerated plaque accumulation, associative learning deficits, and up-regulation of alpha 7 nicotinic receptor protein in transgenic mice co-expressing mutant human presenilin 1 and amyloid precursor proteins". *J. Biol. Chem.* 277:22768–22780.

75. Chapman, P. F., White, G. L., Jones, M. W., Cooper-Blacketer, D., Marshall, V. J., Irizarry, M., Younkin, L., Good, M. A., Bliss, T. V., Hyman, B. T., Younkin, S. G., and Hsiao, K. K. (1999). "Impaired synaptic plasticity and learning in aged amyloid precursor protein transgenic mice". *Nat. Neurosci.* 2:271–276.

76. Corcoran, K. A., Lu, Y., Turner, R. S., and Maren, S. (2002). "Overexpression of hAPPswe impairs rewarded alternation and contextual fear conditioning in a transgenic mouse model of Alzheimer's disease". *Learn. Mem.* 9:243–252.

77. Dineley, K. T., Westerman, M., Bui, D., Bell, K., Ashe, K. H., and Sweatt, J. D. (2001). "Beta-amyloid activates the mitogen-activated protein kinase cascade via hippocampal alpha7 nicotinic acetylcholine receptors: *In vitro* and *in vivo* mechanisms related to Alzheimer's disease". *J. Neurosci.* 21:4125–4133.

78. McKhann, G., Drachman, D., Folstein, M., Katzman, R., Price, D., and Stadlan, E. M. (1984). "Clinical diagnosis of Alzheimer's disease: report of the NINCDS-ADRDA Work Group under the auspices of Department of Health and Human Services Task Force on Alzheimer's Disease". *Neurology* 34:939–944.

79. Kuslansky, G., Buschke, H., Katz, M., Sliwinski, M., and Lipton, R. B. (2002). "Screening for Alzheimer's disease: the memory impairment screen versus the conventional three-word memory test". *J. Am. Geriatr. Soc.* 50:1086–1091.

80. Folstein, M. F., Folstein, S. E., and McHugh, P. R. (1975). "'Mini-mental state.' A practical method for grading the cognitive state of patients for the clinician". *J. Psychiatr. Res.* 12:189–198.

81. Blessed, G., Tomlinson, B. E., and Roth, M. (1968). "The association between quantitative measures of dementia and of senile change in the cerebral grey matter of elderly subjects". *Br. J. Psychiatry* 114:797–811.

82. Kumari, V., Mitterschiffthaler, M. T., and Sharma, T. (2002). "Neuroimaging to predict preclinical Alzheimer's disease". *Hosp. Med.* 63:341–345.

83. Whitehouse, P. J., Price, D. L., Clark, A. W., Coyle, J. T., and DeLong, M. R. (1981). "Alzheimer disease: evidence for selective loss of cholinergic neurons in the nucleus basalis". *Ann. Neurol.* 10:122–126.

84. Davies, P., and Maloney, A. J. (1976). "Selective loss of central cholinergic neurons in Alzheimer's disease". *Lancet* 2:1403.

85. Davies, P. (1983). "The neurochemistry of Alzheimer's disease and senile dementia". *Med. Res. Rev.* 3:221–236.

86. Coyle, J. T., Price, D. L., and DeLong, M. R. (1983). "Alzheimer's disease: a disorder of cortical cholinergic innervation". *Science* 219:1184–1190.

87. Bartus, R. T., Dean 3rd, R. L., Beer, B., and Lippa, A. S. (1982). "The cholinergic hypothesis of geriatric memory dysfunction". *Science* 217:408–414.

88. Frolich, L. (2002). "The cholinergic pathology in Alzheimer's disease—discrepancies between clinical experience and pathophysiological findings". *J. Neural. Transm.* 109:1003–1013.

89. Wang, H. Y., Lee, D. H., D'Andrea, M. R., Peterson, P. A., Shank, R. P., and Reitz, A. B. (2000). "beta-Amyloid(1-42) binds to alpha7 nicotinic acetylcholine receptor with high affinity. Implications for Alzheimer's disease pathology". *J. Biol. Chem.* 275:5626–5632.

90. Nagele, R. G., D'Andrea, M. R., Anderson, W. J., and Wang, H. Y. (2002). "Intracellular accumulation of beta-amyloid (1-42) in neurons is facilitated by the alpha 7 nicotinic acetylcholine receptor in Alzheimer's disease". *Neuroscience* 110:199–211.

91. Nordberg, A., Hellstrom-Lindahl, E., Lee, M., Johnson, M., Mousavi, M., Hall, R., Perry, E., Bednar, I., and Court, J. (2002). "Chronic nicotine treatment reduces beta-amyloidosis in the brain of a mouse model of Alzheimer's disease (APPsw)". *J. Neurochem.* 81:655–658.

92. Schenk, D., Barbour, R., Dunn, W., Gordon, G., Grajeda, H., Guido, T., Hu, K., Huang, J., Johnson-Wood, K., Khan, K., Kholodenko, D., Lee, M., Liao, Z., Lieberburg, I., Motter, R., Mutter, L., Soriano, F., Shopp, G., Vasquez, N., Vandevert, C., Walker, S., Wogulis, M., Yednock, T., Games, D., and Seubert, P. (1999). "Immunization with amyloid-beta attenuates Alzheimer-disease-like pathology in the PDAPP mouse". *Nature* 400:173–177.

93. Janus, C., Pearson, J., McLaurin, J., Mathews, P. M., Jiang, Y., Schmidt, S. D., Chishti, M. A., Horne, P., Heslin, D., French, J., Mount, H. T., Nixon, R. A., Mercken, M., Bergeron, C., Fraser, P. E., St George-Hyslop, P., and Westaway, D. (2000). "A beta peptide immunization reduces behavioural impairment and plaques in a model of Alzheimer's disease". *Nature* 408:979–982.

94. Morgan, D., Diamond, D. M., Gottschall, P. E., Ugen, K. E., Dickey, C., Hardy, J., Duff, K., Jantzen, P., DiCarlo, G., Wilcock, D.,

Connor, K., Hatcher, J., Hope, C., Gordon, M., and Arendash, G. W. (2000). "A beta peptide vaccination prevents memory loss in an animal model of Alzheimer's disease". *Nature* 408:982–985.

95. Dodart, J. C., Bales, K. R., Gannon, K. S., Greene, S. J., DeMattos, R. B., Mathis, C., DeLong, C. A., Wu, S., Wu, X., Holtzman, D. M., and Paul, S. M. (2002). "Immunization reverses memory deficits without reducing brain Abeta burden in Alzheimer's disease model". *Nat. Neurosci.* 5:452–457.

96. Bard, F., Cannon, C., Barbour, R., Burke, R. L., Games, D., Grajeda, H., Guido, T., Hu, K., Huang, J., Johnson-Wood, K., Khan, K., Kholodenko, D., Lee, M., Lieberburg, I., Motter, R., Nguyen, M., Soriano, F., Vasquez, N., Weiss, K., Welch, B., Seubert, P., Schenk, D., and Yednock, T. (2000). "Peripherally administered antibodies against amyloid beta-peptide enter the central nervous system and reduce pathology in a mouse model of Alzheimer disease". *Nat. Med.* 6:916–919.

97. Snowdon, D. A., Kemper, S. J., Mortimer, J. A., Greiner, L. H., Wekstein, D. R., and Markesbery, W. R. (1996). "Linguistic ability in early life and cognitive function and Alzheimer's disease in late life. Findings from the Nun Study". *Jama* 275:528–532.

98. Masliah, E., Sisk, A., Mallory, M., and Games, D. (2001). "Neurofibrillary pathology in transgenic mice overexpressing V717F beta-amyloid precursor protein". *J. Neuropathol. Exp. Neurol.* 60:357–368.

99. Chen, G., Chen, K. S., Knox, J., Inglis, J., Bernard, A., Martin, S. J., Justice, A., McConlogue, L., Games, D., Freedman, S. B., and Morris, R. G. (2000). "A learning deficit related to age and beta-amyloid plaques in a mouse model of Alzheimer's disease". *Nature* 408:975–979.

100. Lewis, J., Dickson, D. W., Lin, W. L., Chisholm, L., Corral, A., Jones, G., Yen, S. H., Sahara, N., Skipper, L., Yager, D., Eckman, C., Hardy, J., Hutton, M., and McGowan, E. (2001). "Enhanced neurofibrillary degeneration in transgenic mice expressing mutant tau and APP". *Science* 293:1487–1491.

101. Chishti, M. A., Yang, D. S., Janus, C., Phinney, A. L., Horne, P., Pearson, J., Strome, R., Zuker, N., Loukides, J., French, J., Turner, S., Lozza, G., Grilli, M., Kunicki, S., Morissette, C., Paquette, J., Gervais, F., Bergeron, C., Fraser, P. E., Carlson, G. A., George-Hyslop, P. S., and Westaway, D. (2001). "Early-onset amyloid deposition and cognitive deficits in transgenic mice expressing a double mutant form of amyloid precursor protein 695". *J. Biol. Chem.* 276:21562–21570.

102. Arendash, G. W., King, D. L., Gordon, M. N., Morgan, D., Hatcher, J. M., Hope, C. E., and Diamond, D. M. (2001). "Progressive, age-related behavioral impairments in transgenic mice carrying both mutant amyloid precursor protein and presenilin-1 transgenes". *Brain Res.* 891:42–53.

103. Dewachter, I., Reverse, D., Caluwaerts, N., Ris, L., Kuiperi, C., Van den Haute, C., Spittaels, K., Umans, L., Serneels, L., Thiry, E., Moechars, D., Mercken, M., Godaux, E., and Van Leuven, F. (2002). "Neuronal deficiency of presenilin 1 inhibits amyloid plaque formation and corrects hippocampal long-term potentiation but not a cognitive defect of amyloid precursor protein [V717I] transgenic mice". *J. Neurosci.* 22:3445–3453.

104. Shen, J., Bronson, R. T., Chen, D. F., Xia, W., Selkoe, D. J., and Tonegawa, S. (1997). "Skeletal and CNS defects in presenilin-1-deficient mice". *Cell* 89:629–639.

105. Feng, R., Rampon, C., Tang, Y. P., Shrom, D., Jin, J., Kyin, M., Sopher, B., Miller, M. W., Ware, C. B., Martin, G. M., Kim, S. H., Langdon, R. B., Sisodia, S. S., and Tsien, J. Z. (2001). "Deficient neurogenesis in forebrain-specific presenilin-1 knockout mice is associated with reduced clearance of hippocampal memory traces". *Neuron* 32:911–926.

106. Veinbergs, I., Jung, M. W., Young, S. J., Van Uden, E., Groves, P. M., and Masliah, E. (1998). "Altered long-term potentiation

in the hippocampus of apolipoprotein E-deficient mice". *Neurosci. Lett.* 249:71–74.

107. Krzywkowski, P., Ghribi, O., Gagne, J., Chabot, C., Kar, S., Rochford, J., Massicotte, G., and Poirier, J. (1999). "Cholinergic systems and long-term potentiation in memory-impaired apolipoprotein E-deficient mice". *Neuroscience* 92:1273–1286.

108. Dawson, G. R., Seabrook, G. R., Zheng, H., Smith, D. W., Graham, S., O'Dowd, G., Bowery, B. J., Boyce, S., Trumbauer, M. E., Chen, H. Y., Van der Ploeg, L. H., and Sirinathsinghji, D. J. (1999). "Age-related cognitive deficits, impaired long-term potentiation and reduction in synaptic marker density in mice lacking the beta-amyloid precursor protein". *Neuroscience* 90:1–13.

109. Herreman, A., Hartmann, D., Annaert, W., Saftig, P., Craessaerts, K., Serneels, L., Umans, L., Schrijvers, V., Checler, F., Vanderstichele, H., Baekelandt, V., Dressel, R., Cupers, P., Huylebroeck, D., Zwijsen, A., Van Leuven, F., and De Strooper, B. (1999). "Presenilin 2 deficiency causes a mild pulmonary phenotype and no changes in amyloid precursor protein processing but enhances the embryonic lethal phenotype of presenilin 1 deficiency". *Proc. Natl. Acad. Sci. USA* 96:11872–11877.

110. Huber, G., Marz, W., Martin, J. R., Malherbe, P., Richards, J. G., Sueoka, N., Ohm, T., and Hoffmann, M. M. (2000). "Characterization of transgenic mice expressing apolipoprotein E4(C112R) and apolipoprotein E4(L28P; C112R)". *Neuroscience* 101:211–218.

111. Watson, A. A., Fairlie, D. P., and Craik, D. J. (1998). "Solution structure of methionine-oxidized amyloid beta-peptide (1–40). Does oxidation affect conformational switching?" *Biochemistry* 37:12700–12706.

112. Price, D. L., Sisodia, S. S., and Borchelt, D. R. (1998). "Genetic neurodegenerative diseases: the human illness and transgenic models". *Science* 282:1079–1083.

113. Khachaturian, Z. S., and Radebaugh, T. S. (1996). *Alzheimer's Disease: Cause(s), Diagnosis, Treatment, and Care.* Boca Raton, FL: CRC Press.

114. Oddo, S., Caccamo, A., Shepherd, J. D., Murphy, M. P., Golde, T. E., Kayed, R., Metherate, R., Mattson, M. P., Akbari, Y., and LaFerla, F. M. (2003). "Triple-transgenic model of Alzheimer's disease with plaques and tangles: intracellular Abeta and synaptic dysfunction". *Neuron* 39:409–421.

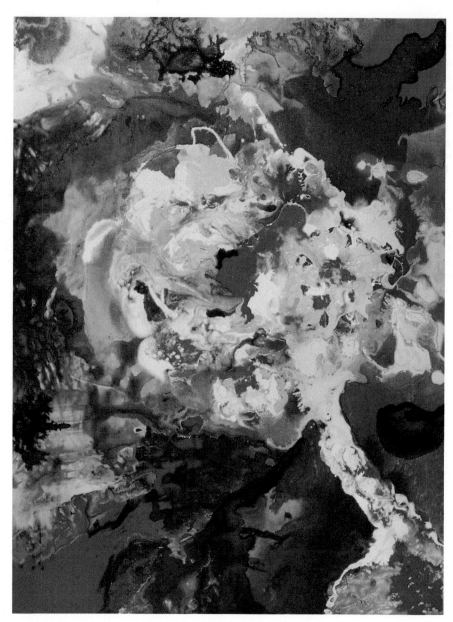

Growth Cone
J. David Sweatt, acrylic on canvas, 2008–2009

Appendix

The Basics of Experimental Design

I. INTRODUCTION

Some people may choose not to read this appendix. For example, those of you who will never: write a research paper; write a grant application; assess the validity of someone else's conclusions; get an advanced degree; or strive to think objectively as you go through life, can skip this part of the book. The rest of us will find this material useful, even if we think of it only as a refresher for things we already know.

In this appendix I am going to formalize and systematize a set of terms related to experimentation, terms that are used consistently throughout this book. Thus, you will be exposed to many terms, both new and already-familiar, in order to establish a vocabulary to use when reading, writing, and talking about experiments. The exposure to any terms that are new to you will, of course, be helpful—that is obvious. However, I encourage you to not gloss over the descriptions of the terms that may already seem familiar to you. Scientific writing, despite all its striving for consistency in terminology, is replete with examples of different scientists using the same term differently. In this chapter I am going to define how I use common terms such as: hypothesis; prediction; experiment; model; etc. In this book we will use these terms in specific ways in order to describe discoveries of how memory works. You have likely used the same terms before, but perhaps slightly differently than how I use them. Appreciating the nuances of how these terms are used in *Mechanisms of Memory* is important.

This appendix will also present a structured way of thinking about how to formulate and test hypotheses. Thus, you will be exposed to both a vocabulary and a conceptual organization to use when thinking about and designing experiments. The vocabulary and the structure for thinking about experimental design are intertwined and intermingled throughout this section. However, they are separable. Even if you choose not to use the term "hypothesis" precisely the same way that I do throughout your career, the *principles* of hypothesis testing and structured reasoning that are presented in this appendix will still serve as a useful foundation for you for the rest of your career. Retain the principles, even if you discard the particulars of the terminology.

Finally, remember that this appendix is woefully incomplete. There is no way that one brief section can describe every variation of every experiment that your clever mind will need to utilize even to get through graduate school. Let the structure that I present be a catalyst for further creative thinking, not a constraint on your creativity. All I ask is that hereafter you are not sloppy with your thinking.

II. INTRODUCTION TO HYPOTHESIS TESTING

To begin with, you need to get familiar with a hierarchy of scientific thought and the terms for various categories within that broad framework (Figure 1). The framework describes levels of scientific thought starting with the broadest, most general, and proceeding through levels of increasing detail to the narrowest and most particular. These categories, in order, are: theories; models; hypotheses; predictions; experiments; and results. I will briefly describe each of these in turn, and then we will proceed to explore hypothesis testing in greater detail.

A. Theories

"That's just a theory" is an oxymoron. Using that phrase is kind of like saying "That's just a fully armed 150 megaton thermonuclear device." A theory is a grand unifying scientific concept, supported by thousands of individual pieces of evidence. "Evolution" is a theory. "General relativity is a theory." "My knockout mouse will be dumb" is not a theory. One theory that this book explores is "Changes in the connectivity between neurons underlies learning and memory."

From considering these examples, it is easy to see that experimental scientists do not deal with theories

on a day-to-day basis. In the modern era, the truly exceptional and fortunate scientist may develop a single meaningful theory over the course of a lifetime of work. A research paper, Ph.D. thesis, or grant application will never test a theory—the amount of evidence required to test a theory is many orders of magnitude larger than that. Nevertheless, a theory is the conceptual starting point for reducing the concept it contains into manageable, testable, pieces.

B. Models

A model deals with one aspect of a theory, a chunk of it, so to speak. Unfortunately, terminology-wise, a model can comprise anything from a very big chunk to a fairly small chunk. Thus, in reality there are gradations within this category. A useful way to think of subdividing the category "models" is to parse it into *unifying models* (which are big) and *working models* (which are manageably sized). The typical research grant application deals with testing specific aspects of one working model, which usually requires five years of full-time effort for 3–5 scientists.

To illustrate the subcategories of models, for the theory of evolution some underlying unifying models would be: the genetic basis of inheritance; natural selection; speciation; epigenetics; etc. These models describe how major aspects of the theory of evolution

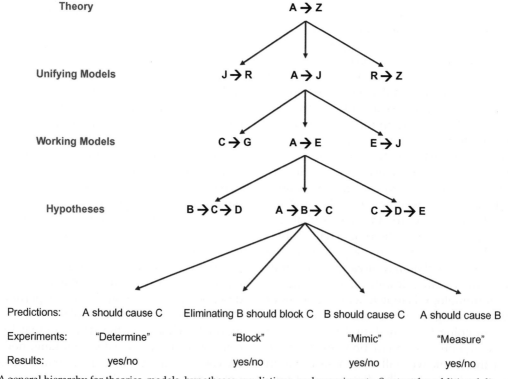

FIGURE 1   A general hierarchy for theories, models, hypotheses, predictions, and experiments. See text for additional discussion.

BOX 1

COMPUTER AND MATHEMATICAL MODELING

How do you proceed if your hypothesis is too complicated to be expressed in a simple A, B, C form such as we have been discussing? Similarly, if your understanding of your experimental system is sufficiently refined and detailed, you may be able to express your hypotheses very precisely as mathematical formulas. Under these circumstances, the ready availability of powerful computers in the modern era allows certain aspects of hypothesis testing to be performed *in silico*. A typical application of this approach in the learning and memory field involves testing very complex, multi-component models of neuronal circuits which incorporate the corresponding biophysical cellular properties of the individual neuronal units that make up the circuit. In many cases realistic circuits, such as those that actually underlie a memory-related behavior, can be modeled.

Roughly speaking, computational approaches package up into one cohesive unit several levels of analysis and experimental design that we have been discussing—this package is referred to as the model. Thus, computational approaches tend to combine the working model, the

hypothesis, prediction, and experiment levels of design, and implement them mathematically so that they can be utilized and analyzed with a computer.

The strengths of the computational modeling approach are many. The model, hypotheses, and predictions are defined very precisely. One can relatively quickly determine whether the various parts of the model are internally consistent, and whether there are any fundamental logical flaws in the model. The parameters that define the underlying assumptions for the model can readily be tweaked and refined. Importantly, modeling of this sort allows one to define the critical nodes in the model that greatly influence its output, which allows predictions of the critical control steps in the overall process. Finally, the strongest variations of modeling *in silico* allow the generation of new predictions that can be tested experimentally in the laboratory (9–12). This particularly strong approach allows for a dynamic from computer to laboratory and *vice versa*, and continuing refinement of the overall model based on biologically realistic parameters.

---

work, mechanistically. Each of these unifying models can comprise thousands of working models to explain various specific aspects or mechanisms of the unifying model. Very roughly speaking, each chapter of this book deals with one or two unifying models relevant to the theory that changes in neuronal connectivity underlie memory. Each chapter subdivision deals with one or a few working models relevant to the unifying model(s) covered in that chapter.

One final comment about "models." Don't confuse the categories for models described in our conceptual hierarchy with the other commonly used variation of the term model: "model system" or "experimental model." These two phrases are also commonly shortened to the single word model (as in: what model do you use?), but used this way the term refers to experimental preparations (the hippocampal slice model), brain region (the cerebellar model), or the species under study (rodent models, the *Aplysia* model, etc.). This is a legitimate, but very different, use of the term model.

C. Hypotheses

For the experimentalist, the hypothesis is the manageable and testable level in the overall hierarchy.

A hypothesis isolates one experimentally-testable aspect of a working model, formalizes it and refines it, and allows predictions to be generated. Testing the predictions allows one to either empirically support or refute (nullify) the hypothesis.

A hypothesis can never be proven correct. A hypothesis is supported by repeatedly testing its predictions, and in the case where the hypothesis reflects the true state of nature, it will bear up under repeated testing and never be nullified. The best a hypothesis can ever do is not be disproven. Not disproven is a long way from proven.

Moreover, as we have already discussed, the entire underpinning of a theory is the experimental testing of hypotheses. Therefore, by extrapolation, it is clear that a theory can never be proven either. This leaves all scientific theories, no matter how well supported, open to the criticism "that's never been proven, it's just a theory." This statement can be used as a hollow, meaningless criticism, perfect for a network sound-bite. The criticism may be completely irrelevant to the discussion at hand, but correct by definition and impossible to refute while maintaining scientific objectivity. This is an example of a case where scientific usage and popular usage of the same term do not mix well.

BOX 2

LEGALITY, ETHICALITY, AND MORALITY

While we will not discuss research ethics in detail in this chapter, in science issues of right and wrong fall broadly into three categories: legality, ethicality, and morality. These three categories fall roughly on a continuum from concrete to abstract (see Figure).

Legal Issues

The extreme left end of the spectrum deals with satisfying the minimal requirements to stay out of jail or not be sued or fined. Slightly more abstract (and certainly more interesting) are issues of copyright, intellectual property, etc., that also are legal issues. This is the realm of your interaction (as a scientist) with commerce and government.

Ethical Issues

The middle of the spectrum deals with your interactions as a scientist with your community and with other scientists. Scientific ethics deals largely with how well you adhere to the scientific community's standards of honesty and truthfulness. As a rule of thumb, most issues of scientific ethics are pretty clear-cut and subject to broad agreement across the scientific community.

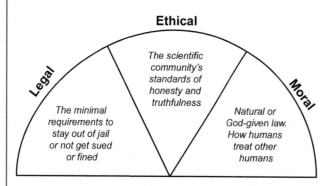

Moral Issues

On the most abstract end of the spectrum is morality. Morality deals with how humans (including scientists) treat other humans. Philosophers and theologians refer to morality as dealing with "natural law" or "God-given law." "Natural law" here does not refer to the laws of nature that scientists study, but rather to fundamental attributes (laws) of human conduct that Nature bestows upon us. Moral issues are issues about which two rational, honest, and clear-thinking individuals may disagree.

It is interesting that a psychological trap for scientists tends to be to dismiss the purely legal or procedural issues because they seem trivial, irrelevant, or uninteresting, because they don't deal with ethics, or because we think we "know better" (e.g., "I don't need to pay attention to this rule against pouring acetic acid down the sink because it's stupid and I know I'm not going to hurt anything."). However, it's very easy to slide over the line from legal violation into ethical violation. If you pour the acetic acid down the sink and then somebody asks you about it, then what? As soon as you tell someone an untruth you have crossed the line from policy violation into unethical behavior.

The best rule to follow is: *if you mess up, 'fess up.* Nobody generally cares if you make an honest or stupid mistake that is a protocol or procedural violation. Where you get into trouble is if you try to ignore the rules that you know (thereby potentially endangering others or the institution), or worse yet trying to cover it up (making you dishonest). Just as in politics, it is the cover-up that gets you in trouble, because that is where you cross the line from honest mistake or technical infraction into scientific misconduct and unethical behavior.

An Abstract Example of a Hypothesis

Let's now generate an abstract example of a hypothesis in order to begin to consider in more detail how we would go about testing this hypothesis. Our made-up theory will be "A causes Z" (see Figure 1). What we are about to do is subdivide this large theory into a series of smaller steps, that can explain in detail all the many causal mechanisms whereby A ultimately leads to Z. In short, we are going to work our way through the entire alphabet from A to Z, dividing it into unifying models, working models, and hypotheses.

Subdividing the theory "A causes Z" into unifying models, we could parse it out into "A causes everything up to J, J causes everything up to T, and T causes everything up to Z." We can then split the first unifying model (A causes J) into two working models: "A causes E, and E causes J." Now we are finally ready to divide one of these two working models into discrete hypotheses: A causes B causes C; C causes D causes E; and so on, up to J. You choose to test the hypothesis that "A causes B causes C" for your research project.

BOX 3

WHAT THE HECK IS A NULL HYPOTHESIS?

In modern experimental design the hypothesis to be tested is assumed to be true: $A \rightarrow B \rightarrow C$ is assumed to be "the true state of nature." Experiments are designed to test predictions of the hypothesis, and if the predictions do not hold up under experimental testing, then the hypothesis is then disproven or nullified. In that case, we then formulate an alternative hypothesis.

In contrast, the classical statistical convention was to assume that the speculated hypothesis was always wrong. The hypothesis was assumed to be nullified if the test results were accurate. This way of thinking gave rise to the term *null hypothesis*—meaning that the hypothesis, as stated, was to be nullified. Null was simply being used as an adjective to describe the presumption that the hypothesis was not true.

Despite the fact that null hypothesis sounds as if it should be the opposite of hypothesis, in fact the two terms mean exactly the same thing. The hypothesis is the hypothesis—the null modifier is supposed to reflect whether your starting assumption is that the hypothesis is correct or incorrect. The hypothesis = $A \rightarrow B \rightarrow C$ = the null hypothesis.

The upshot of all this is that you should just drop the whole null hypothesis jargon. For the most part, nowadays people only throw the phrase into conversation to try to sound impressive or, worse yet, obfuscate. A classically trained intellectual or a rigorous statistician will use the term null hypothesis appropriately—anybody else is likely blowing smoke.

Let's start by rewording the hypothesis into a form that lends itself to discussion and rigorous experimental design. **This is not a trivial consideration.** Many a graduate student, grant writer, and faculty applicant could have saved themselves enormous amounts of grief just by wording their hypothesis simply and in a convenient format from the outset. We will restate our hypothesis "A causes C by activating B."

Phrasing the hypothesis so that it has three components is extremely advantageous. You should always formulate your hypothesis so that it has three components: a trigger (A); an effect (C); and a mechanism (B). Why? This is the definition of a hypothesis! A hypothesis exists in order to allow multiple discrete predictions that can be tested experimentally, in order to support or refute the hypothesis. That is its *raison d'être*. If you can't make multiple discrete, conceptually different, and experimentally testable predictions from your hypothesis it does not serve its intended purpose. Formulate your hypothesis accordingly.

The three components to the hypothesis result in four predictions that one can test. Our example hypothesis is "A causes C by activating B" ($A \rightarrow B \rightarrow C$). This gives us four predictions:

1. A should cause C.
2. Eliminating B should block A from being able to cause C.
3. B should itself be capable of causing C.
4. A should cause B.

Testing each of these four predictions will allow us to support or refute the hypothesis.

How do you test a prediction? You test a prediction with an experiment. The results of each experiment will either support or refute the corresponding prediction, thereby upholding or nullifying the overall hypothesis.

So, in this example, we have worked our way conceptually all the way from theory to experiment, using a unifying scheme that describes the modern experimental approach to science, that is, hypothesis testing (Figure 1). However, as is no doubt painfully evident to you at this point, the language I have used so far is very formalized and stilted, and doesn't lend itself very well to everyday usage. In the next section I will describe a more user-friendly set of terms that help capture the essence of hypothesis testing.

III. THE FOUR BASIC TYPES OF EXPERIMENTS

In general, there are four basic types of experiments that any scientist can perform (1, 2). I refer to them as "block, measure, mimic, and determine" experiments (Figure 2). I have found this categorization a useful mnemonic device throughout my career as a scientist, and I strongly encourage any young scientist who reads this book to incorporate them into their thinking about experimental design. Conveniently, each of the

The Four Basic Types of Experiments

Hypothesis: A → B → C

Experiment	Prediction
Determine	None (A makes C happen)
Block	Blocking B should block A causing C
Mimic	Activating B should cause C
Measure	A makes B happen

FIGURE 2 The four basic types of experiments. See text for discussion.

four basic types of experiments corresponds to testing one of the four types of predictions that are generated by any hypothesis. (This assumes you have had the forethought to phrase your hypothesis correctly.) Do the four types of experiments and you have tested your hypothesis comprehensively.

This framework for thinking about hypothesis testing is very convenient in an everyday context for any working scientist. For example, every time I write or review a research paper, I ask whether the investigation has included all these different types of experiments. Whenever I am writing or reviewing grant applications, where multi-year projects are proposed to comprehensively test a hypothesis, I specifically cross-check myself and others on whether all of these approaches (if technically possible) have been applied to the problem at hand. It is important, because what we do as scientists is test hypotheses, and the testing of any hypothesis is much stronger if a variety of independent lines of evidence are available to support the conclusions reached. "Hypothesis-driven" is the gold standard for grant applications, research reports, and thesis projects. Get the basic paradigm of hypothesis testing squared away in your mind, and you don't have to reinvent the wheel every time you write up or review a piece of scientific work.

What follows is a brief description of each of these four types of experiments. The determine experiment is what sets the stage for even formulating the hypothesis to begin with. For example, you determine that A causes C, and then propose a hypothesis to explain how it happens. One can equally well use the synonym "observe" to describe the originating experimental finding. You have observed that something happens. You will perform additional experiments to understand how it comes about. The determination, or observation, that "A causes C" is what piques your interest initially.

Although, formally speaking, this is the first prediction of a hypothesis, in reality you would already know that "A causes C," in order to have a phenomenon to study. You would have already determined, or observed, that "A causes C" at the outset of your experiments. So, in reality, the "determine" experimental result is already in hand. It is the phenomenon that you are studying.

Determine is also used to describe another experiment that is not really an experiment at all. Used this second way, the determine experiment is to perform a basic characterization of a system or molecule at hand, independent of any experimental manipulation. Examples of this type of pursuit are determining the amino acid sequence of a protein, sequencing a genome, determining the crystal structure of an enzyme or determining the structure of the DNA double helix. Determinations of this sort are not experiments, in that no manipulation of the system is attempted—to do an experiment you tweak the system to see what happens. If you mutate a residue in a protein and see what effect that has on the structure, then you have done an experiment. The basic determination of the structure is not an experiment in and of itself. As mentioned in the last paragraph, basic determinations (or observations) of this sort are what set the stage for subsequent formulation and experimental testing of hypotheses to explain the observation.

Determinations of this sort can be some of the most satisfying laboratory pursuits to undertake, because these are the rare types of studies where definitive data can be obtained. An amino acid sequence is what it is—you get to use unambiguous words like "identical" (versus indistinguishable or similar) and "determined" (versus concluded, inferred, etc.) when describing gene and amino acid sequences. There's slightly more ambiguity in determining protein structures and anatomical structures, but in general this pales in comparison to the ambiguity of a conclusion made on the basis of an experimental manipulation.

The down side of determinations is that, as a practical matter, they can be viewed as boring. It's very difficult to get a grant review study section to recommend approval of a basic anatomical characterization, for example. This is because there is no experimental testing of a hypothesis involved, and in modern biomedical research hypothesis testing is *de rigueur*. However, there is a growing recognition that more sophisticated and detailed basic characterizations are necessary for the next stage of progress in science. It is common nowadays to refer to determination-type approaches as "unbiased," explicitly stating that they are not hypothesis-driven and therefore not susceptible to prejudice based on any predicted result. If it is necessary to propose a determine experiment as part of your project, it is worthwhile to emphasize this philosophically appealing aspect of that approach.

So overall, determine refers to either something that you already know is true, like the observation that "A causes C," or to a basic characterization of a system to identify new and interesting aspects of that system. In either case, the determination sets the stage for subsequent experimentation and hypothesis testing.

Block, measure, and mimic are experiments, and they are all specific types of approaches to test the three remaining predictions of a hypothesis. For the following discussion we will continue to examine testing the hypothesis "A causes C by activating B."

The mimic experiment tests prediction 3 in the list above (see also Figure 2). The mimic experiment tests the prediction that "if B causes C, then if I activate B artificially I should see C happen as a result." The mimic terminology arises from the fact that you are trying to mimic with a drug, etc., an effect that occurs with some other stimulus.

The principal limitation of the mimic experiment is that B may be able to cause C, but in reality A acts independently of B to cause the same effect. B causing C and A causing C may be true, true, and unrelated.

Mimic experiments, in some circumstances, can be very difficult to design and execute. This is because an enormous amount of fundamental understanding of the system under study is necessary, along with the capacity for very subtle manipulation, in order for the experiment to work. For example, suppose I hypothesize that synaptic potentiation underlies learning. Conceptually, the mimic experiment would be to put an electrode in the brain, cause synaptic potentiation, and then the animal would have an altered behavior identical to that caused by a training session. Of course, doing this experiment requires that one knows exactly which synapses to potentiate so that they can selectively achieve the right behavioral output—this is beyond the level of understanding for essentially all mammalian behaviors at this point.

The measure experiment tests the prediction that "A should cause activation of B." This is prediction number 4 in our list above. This is, of course, tested by measuring the activity of B as directly as possible, hence the "measure" terminology. The principal theoretical limitation of the measure experiment is that it is correlative. One can show that A causes activation of B, but that does not demonstrate that activation of B is necessary for C to occur.

The measure experiment has a long and distinguished history in science. Indeed, measure experiments when performed in the context of testing one hypothesis automatically generate an observation that is the basis for a subsequent hypothesis. (The same can be said of the mimic experiment, when the mimicking

agent is an endogenously occurring compound.) This beautiful aspect of hypothesis testing is part of the intellectual engine that has driven science over time to increasingly detailed levels of understanding.

Which brings us to the remaining category, the block experiment; the block experiment tests prediction number 2 in our original list, that "if I eliminate B then A should not be able to cause C." At present, the vast majority of investigations into mechanisms of memory involve this approach, and there are many references to this type of experiment throughout *Mechanisms of Memory*. Specific examples include anatomical lesions, drug infusion studies, and genetic manipulations. The principal theoretical limitation of the block experiment is that it does not distinguish whether activation of B is necessary for C, versus whether the activity of B is necessary for C. For example, suppose that B provides some tonic effect on C that is necessary for it to occur. Inhibiting B will block the production of effect C, when in fact A never has any effect on B. In other words, B is part of the infrastructure necessary for C to happen, but has no place in the causal sequence of events.

In summary, then, the mimic experiment tests sufficiency, the block experiment tests necessity, and the measure experiment tests whether the event does in fact occur. As I have outlined, each type of experiment has its strengths and weaknesses. However, the weakness of each single type of experiment tends to be negated by the strengths of the remaining two. Positive outcomes in testing each of the three experimental predictions for any hypothesis make for clear, strong support of the hypothesis.

IV. AN EXAMPLE OF A HYPOTHESIS AND HOW TO TEST IT

Okay, let's road-test your newfound knowledge of the principles of hypothesis testing, by working through a real-life example. You have made an observation—people get in cars and the cars go places. In considering this phenomenon you have formulated a hypothesis to explain how people make cars go places:

A person makes the car go by pushing the gas pedal.

This is a very reasonable hypothesis. Note that you did not formulate a *theory* of mechanical propulsion, a *unifying model* of automobile operation, or a *working model* of manual control of car function. You also did not formulate an overly ambitious hypothesis that included how people start cars or engage transmissions—these other aspects of the larger working model will be tested using other hypotheses. In formulating your hypothesis you have used a scientific, reductionist approach, and formulated a specific hypothesis testable by experimentation. Your hypothesis proposes to provide a mechanism to explain a manageable-sized piece of a much larger overall phenomenon.

You have also formulated and worded your hypothesis in a way that lends itself to effective and efficient experimental design:

A person (A) makes a car go (C) by pushing the gas pedal (B)

This fits our general algorithm for hypothesis formulation and testing:

$$A \rightarrow B \rightarrow C$$

and therefore you can conveniently formulate the four predictions of this hypothesis. Before we proceed any further, take a moment and mentally work out the four predictions for your hypothesis that *a person makes a car go by pushing the gas pedal.* Write them down, and use them for reference as we next walk through how we will test this hypothesis. Having the predictions in hand should make the experimental design much easier.

What tools will you need in order to test this hypothesis? First, you will need the two components of the initial observation, because they are required to generate the phenomenon you are studying. In this case you will need a car and a person. Given what we are about to do in order to test the hypothesis, you probably would prefer to use someone else's car. Maybe you can also get your annoying little brother to volunteer to be the person. So, in gathering these first two tools, you have in hand both the stimulus (a person), and the output machinery for the phenomenon (a car).

You will also need a way to assess the output, and quantitate the phenomenon under study. Hence, you will need some device to monitor car movement. This will allow you to observe and quantify objectively when the car goes. In our example this can be something as simple as an impartial observer that scores pluses or minuses for car movement. As long as the observer doesn't stand directly in front of the car, this is a pretty safe role to play, so you might ask a favorite family member to do this for you.

The most sophisticated tool you will need for your experiments is an assay system to quantitate "pushing the gas pedal." You have the stimulus (a person) and a way to assess the output (making the car go), but you will need a way to monitor the hypothetical intervening mechanism (pushing the gas pedal). A device such as a digital video camera would suffice. Your annoying little brother always seems to have one of those handy, especially at the wrong times, so you can borrow his. The final tool that you will need is some device to manipulate the system experimentally. I suggest a brick.

Okay, with the five necessary tools in hand, you are ready to proceed to testing your hypothesis experimentally. What experiments are you going to do? The answer is easy—block, mimic, and measure.

What is the block experiment? The block experiment tests the prediction that if I block B from happening, A should no longer be able to cause C. Thus, if you block pushing the gas pedal, a person should no longer be able to make the car go. To perform this experiment, you place the brick underneath the gas pedal, and assess whether a person can still make the car go. If the answer is "no," this prediction of your hypothesis has stood up under experimental testing. In this particular example of the block experiment, you are using the brick as an *antagonist* or *inhibitor* of pushing the pedal. A variation of the block experiment would be to remove the gas pedal—this would be a "lesioning" experiment.

What is the mimic experiment? The mimic experiment tests the prediction that if you artificially activate B, then C will result. Thus, if you artificially mimic pushing the gas pedal, then the car should go. To perform this experiment you place the brick on top of the gas pedal, pushing it down in the absence of a person being in the car, and assess whether the car goes. If the answer is "yes," the hypothesis is further supported.

There is a variation on the mimic experiment called an "occlusion" experiment. If your hypothesis is correct, then adding the normal stimulus (a person) on top of the mimicking agent (the brick on the gas pedal) should result in no additional or greater car movement. Thus, to perform this experiment you put the person in the car, the brick on the gas pedal, and assess whether the car goes any farther or faster with both than with the brick alone. If not, then the hypothesis is supported by this additional result. (This experiment is why you chose your annoying little brother and someone else's car for your experiments.)

In these mimic experiments you are using the brick as an agonist or activator for pushing the pedal. You can also perform a very nice combination-type experiment to confirm the specificity of the brick as an agonist/activator. In this control experiment, as an example, you would block or lesion (remove) the gas pedal exactly as in the block experiment, and demonstrate that placing a brick on top of the pedal (or placing it where the pedal used to be) does not make the car go. This is a control for specificity of your experimental manipulations. An additional type of control experiment for specificity would be to block or lesion a similar component of the car that is not what you hypothesize makes the car go. For example, you might remove the brake pedal, or place a brick under it, as a control for the specificity of your gas pedal manipulation.

Finally, what is the measure experiment? The measure experiment tests the prediction that A actually makes B happen. The first and simplest form of the measure experiment is to confirm that there is actually a gas pedal in the car. In other words, you measure the presence or absence of the gas pedal. By extension, you would also predict that every time a person gets into a car and makes it go, there should be a gas pedal present. You would measure the frequency of occurrence of gas pedals in cars that are going.

However, that simplest form of measure experiment does not fully test the hypothesis, the way it is formulated. Your hypothesis states that a person makes the car go by pushing the gas pedal. Thus, every time you observe a person make the car go there should be a measurable pushing of the gas pedal. Therefore, the fullest implementation of the measure experiment is not just to ascertain if cars have gas pedals, or even to ascertain if people are capable of pushing the gas pedal. Ideally the measure experiment is to ascertain whether a person pushing a gas pedal happens every time the car goes. Gas pedal pushing should be *correlated* with car movement. A makes B happen *every time* A makes C happen. If that is the case, then your hypothesis has stood up to the third experimental test.

Part of why I point this out is that in real life sometimes you may not be able to fully implement the measure experiment. For example, if your pesky little brother will not lend you his digital video camera, you won't be able to document pushing the pedal. You would then be limited to assessing the presence or absence of gas pedals in cars.

On the other hand, having the capacity to fully execute the measure experiment can lead to further refinement of your hypothesis. For example, you might notice while doing the measure experiment that the car's speed of movement seems to correlate with how far the gas pedal is pushed down. You might use this observation to generate a new, more mechanistically detailed hypothesis that you can subsequently test.

As a final note, being able to fully execute the measure experiment also affords you the opportunity to do some nice additional control experiments. For example, you can use the pedal measuring device to confirm that indeed the brick pushes the pedal down when placed on top of it. You can also confirm that the brick blocks the ability of a person to move the gas pedal. These combinations of the measure determination and the block and/or mimic determinations are positive controls for the effectiveness of your experimental manipulations.

In summary, then, let's review how the various experiments you have performed relate to testing specific predictions of your hypothesis, relating them back to the A, B, C format that we have been using.

Hypothesis: $A \rightarrow B \rightarrow C$

Prediction 1: "A should cause C." This was your original observation—people get in a car and make it go.

Prediction 2: "Eliminating B should block A from being able to cause C." This was your block experiment—placing the brick under the pedal, or removing the pedal entirely, blocked a person from being able to make the car go.

Prediction 3: "B should itself be capable of causing C." This was your mimic experiment—placing the brick on top of the gas pedal made the car go.

Prediction 4: "A should cause B." This was your measure experiment—every time a person got in the car and made it go, they pushed the gas pedal.

Given all these results, your hypothesis has been supported by rigorous experimental testing. The entire package of the various types of different experiments makes for a very solid case that the hypothesis is correct; formally speaking that it reflects the true state of nature.

This does not mean that the hypothesis has been proven irrefutably. One can still make up scenarios where all the predictions test out as true, but the hypothesis is incorrect. It is a worthwhile exercise to think up some examples of how this could happen. In doing so, you will realize that it takes some serious mental gymnastics and a proposal of very complex interacting, but not causally related, mechanisms to explain the results but have the hypothesis be incorrect. For this reason, the simple hypothesis, "A causes B causes C," is referred to as the most *parsimonious* explanation for the observed results. A rule of thumb for hypothesis testing (referred to as Ockham's Razor, or the Law of Parsimony), states that in the absence of confounding evidence, always operate on the assumption that the simplest explanation is correct. However, for illustrative purposes, in the next section we will mention a few possible ways that the interpretation of our results might be confounded, sticking with the car example for the sake of convenience.

All the predictions can test true, but the hypothesis can still be wrong in certain circumstances. For example, let's say that you have finished all your experiments with testing your car hypothesis. Then, your smart-aleck little brother puts the car in neutral, gets behind it, and pushes it to make it go. He points out that he has made the car go without pushing the gas pedal. This is an example of an *alternative mechanism*. It doesn't mean that your hypothesis is incorrect, but it does mean that the hypothesized mechanism does not operate in all circumstances. The hypothesized mechanism is not the only mechanism by which A can cause C. Your hypothesis is insufficient, and does not encompass all possible mechanisms. There is nothing wrong with this inadequacy of the hypothesis, but this is an important consideration to keep in mind when using a reductionist experimental approach.

Alternative mechanisms are also particularly relevant for block (or lesion) experiments. This is because the blocking or lesioning may actually recruit the alternative mechanism. For example, if I remove the gas pedal from someone's car as part of my experiment, they may put the car in neutral and push it to the service station down the street. My experimental manipulation has triggered the use of an alternative mechanism to make the car go. This is not the mechanism they would normally use, but it is a mechanism which can compensate for the absence of the normal mechanism. In the real world of experimental biology, this is not a trivial consideration. The compensatory and redundant mechanisms available in complex biological systems may be extensive.

Experimentally, the existence and utilization of the compensatory mechanism would lead me to a *false negative* conclusion about the original hypothesis. The block experiment would not appear to support the prediction of the hypothesis, i.e., the car would still go in the absence of pushing the gas pedal. The compensatory mechanism would cause you to erroneously negate your hypothesis, when it was in fact valid under normal circumstances.

Alternative mechanisms can also confound the results of the mimic experiment. In some cases you might apply an activator of B that causes C, but the activator may actually be acting by stimulating the alternative (not the normal) mechanism. In this circumstance you would make a *false positive* conclusion that the hypothesis was supported, based on the outcome of your mimic experiment result.

A. Some Real-life Examples of Hypothesis Testing

It is extremely useful to practice designing experiments, even if you have no intention in real-life of actually doing those experiments. Formulating and thought-testing hypotheses (along with designing the attendant experiments), is practice in solving complex and interesting puzzles. You can get a lot of practice in the basics of experimental design this way, without ever having to step into a laboratory. Practicing these fundamentals of scientific endeavor will serve you well in setting the stage for a career as a researcher. It should not escape your attention that formulating and thought-testing hypotheses on a large scale, and using experiments that you actually propose to do, is exactly what writing a research grant or fellowship application entails.

In the last section we worked through a simple example of testing a hypothesis, based on thinking about how a person makes a car go. Next, I would like you to think through a real-life hypothesis. That hypothesis is: "Serotonin causes synaptic potentiation by activating adenylyl cyclase."

There are a few pieces of basic information that you need to know to begin to work through this hypothesis. Serotonin is a neurotransmitter and is also known as 5-HT, 5-hydroxy-tryptamine. It can bind to specific receptors on the surface of certain types of neurons, and cause increases in synaptic strength or synaptic potentiation. Adenylyl cyclase is an enzyme present in neuronal membranes that can be activated by serotonin if the appropriate molecular machinery is there. Adenylyl cyclase is the enzyme that makes cyclic AMP, an intracellular second messenger.

I will not walk through the specifics of testing this thought hypothesis—I leave it to you to consider as an exercise. I have, however, provided an "answer sheet," of sorts, for you to refer to. Chapter 3 of this book describes a real-life solution to this problem based on work in the *Aplysia californica* experimental system (3–4). The work that allowed a real-life answer to this problem helped Eric Kandel win a Nobel Prize. Just as an aside, I know from first-hand experience that Eric enjoys working through thought-hypotheses. Put yourself in good company by being the same way.

For illustrative purposes Table 1 gives a brief overview of testing another real-life hypothesis (5–8). This hypothesis is: norepinephrine (NE) activates adenylyl cyclase in neuronal membranes by acting through the beta-adrenergic receptor (βAR). NE is another neurotransmitter, and it can potentially bind to one of several subtypes of receptors in order to activate adenylyl cyclase. For this exercise, you will test the hypothesis that NE acts through the βAR subtype of NE receptor. I will not describe testing this hypothesis in any kind of detail at this point. The idea is that by working through the example in Table 1 on your own, you will begin to generalize the approach to hypothesis testing and experimental design that we have been discussing.

V. SOME ADDITIONAL TERMINOLOGY OF HYPOTHESIS TESTING

In this final section I would like to add a few more terms and concepts to your repertoire. This section principally defines a group of terms that are commonly used in thinking and writing about experimental results. It is important to be familiar with them for this reason. In addition, however, in several instances these definitions draw your attention to some specific

TABLE 1 Testing a Thought Hypothesis

The beta-adrenergic receptor hypothesis: Norepinephrine (NE) acts through beta-adrenergic receptors (βAR) in order to elevate cAMP in neurons

$$NE \rightarrow \beta AR \rightarrow Elevate\ cAMP$$

Observation: Adding NE to neurons causes an increase in cellular cAMP levels.

The block experiment: βAR-selective antagonists block the NE effect on cAMP.

The mimic experiment: βAR-selective agonists (NE is not specific) elevate cAMP.

The measure experiment: Immunoblotting or radioligand binding confirms the presence of βAR. Also, ligand-binding experiments confirm that NE actually binds to the βAR (Note—the measure experiment is *not* simply measuring cAMP; it is measuring the presence of the βAR and the capacity of NE to bind to it.)

Assay system: The means by which βAR or cAMP levels are measured, for example a radioimmunoassay.

The lesion variant of the block experiment: The effect of NE is lost in βAR knockout mice.

The occlusion variant of the mimic experiment: NE gives no additional cAMP when added on top of a maximally effective concentration of βAR agonist.

Refine the hypothesis: The β-2 subtype of βAR is the receptor isoform involved.

Alternative mechanism: Over-expression of alpha-AR subtype receptors compensates for the loss of βAR in the knockout mice.

Control experiments: Forskolin, a direct activator of adenylyl cyclase, still elevates cAMP in the knockout mice or when βAR antagonists are applied. Beta-AR agonists do not elevate cAMP when βAR antagonists are present. These are controls for the selectivity of the experimental manipulations.

---

ways I use these terms in this book—ways that can differ slightly from the way other writers may use them. Highlighting these differences is important to help you avoid being confused if someone else uses the term "hypothesis" in a different way than I do, for example.

In several instances these differences arise from scientists using the same term in two different ways—statistically versus experimentally. Modern biomedical research is experimentally driven, and I have used experimentally-related definitions throughout this chapter. However, the statistically oriented use of the terms is, of course, found frequently in the literature.

A. Hypothesis Versus Prediction

For example, there is another usage for "hypothesis," different from the way I use the term that is valid and common in the scientific literature. This alternative usage arises historically from statistical testing literature. There is a vast body of that literature that deals with the theory of experimental design and hypothesis testing from a statistical analysis perspective. In general, statistical analysis deals with whether a specific set of experimental results (i.e., the *numbers* that are generated

as the output of the experiment) support or refute the anticipated (hypothesized) outcome of the experiment. In statistical terminology, then, the term hypothesis is used in a way that is essentially equivalent to what I call a prediction for an experiment. Statisticians hypothesize a predicted outcome of an experiment, and utilize mathematical algorithms to assess whether the predicted outcome actually occurred.

Thus, using this terminology I might have called the four predictions of our general hypothesis ($A \rightarrow B \rightarrow C$) the four hypotheses resulting from our hypothesis. I could also have called the block experiment the block hypothesis, the mimic experiment the mimic hypothesis, and so on. As I have said, these would all be legitimate usages of the term hypothesis. However, using "hypothesis" in this way, it rapidly becomes very difficult to keep straight what is the overall hypothesis, what is the prediction, and what is the experiment.

The point here is that some authors will use hypothesis synonymously with what I have called a prediction of a hypothesis. Just be mindful of that, and keep straight what level of the hierarchy they are referring to. In this book, I always use the term hypothesis as I have in the earlier parts of this appendix, to refer to a proposed mechanistic explanation for a phenomenon that can be tested with a series of different types of experiments.

B. Accuracy, Precision, and Reproducibility

The evolution of scientific terminology has also given rise to slightly different usages for the term "precision" in the statistics versus the biomedical fields. Since "accuracy versus precision" is one of the classic topics in beginning science classes, even in grade-school, briefly mentioning how these terms are used by experimentalists is useful.

The classic definitions of accuracy versus precision are illustrated by the familiar bulls-eye diagram (Figure 3). In this diagram accuracy is illustrated by the bullet holes being grouped around the center of the bulls-eye of the target, while precision is illustrated by the bullet holes being closely grouped, but away from the center. This is an accurate analogy for statistical testing terminology, for reasons that I won't go into here. However, this is not the way that biomedical researchers use the term precision. What theoretical statisticians call precision we would call reproducibility, meaning that the same result is consistently obtained when repeating an experiment over, and over again. Experimentalists use "precision" to refer to how many decimal places of reliability we have in our assay systems. In the bulls-eye analogy, an experimentalist would equate precision with the size of the bullet holes.

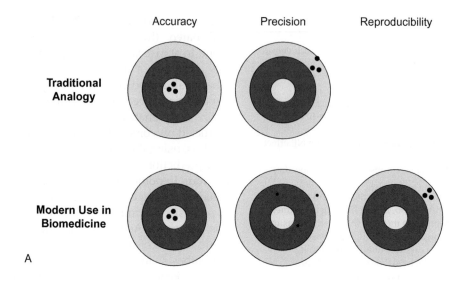

	Group 1 Answers	Group 2 Answers	Group 3 Answers
Subject 1	4	1.000	3.000
Subject 2	4	2.000	3.00
Subject 3	4	7.000	3.000
Subject 4	4	6.000	3.00
	High Accuracy	Low Accuracy	Low Accuracy
	Low Precision	High Precision	High Precision
B	High Reproducibility	Low Reproducibility	High Reproducibility

FIGURE 3 (A) Accuracy, precision, and reproducibility. The traditional bulls-eye analogy of accuracy and precision (upper row) does not correctly capture the more modern usages of accuracy, precision, and reproducibility in experimental biomedicine (bottom row). (B) A mathematical example to illustrate accuracy, precision, and reproducibility.

I will illustrate this with a simple example. I am going to ask you a question, repeat the question four times, and analyze your answers for accuracy, reproducibility, and precision.

The question: "What is 2 + 2?" (the question is repeated four times).

Student One answers: 4, 4, 4, 4. She is highly accurate.

Student Two answers: 3, 3, 3, 3. He is highly reproducible.

Student Three answers: 2.000, 3.000, 1.000, 9.000. He is, if nothing else, highly precise.

Interestingly, you could analyze these data and conclude that Student Three is, on average, more "accurate" than Student Two. That would be an example of lying with statistics. I will leave it as an exercise for you to work out the various combinations of accuracy, reproducibility, and precision.

In summary, then:

$2 + 2 = 4$, accurate
$2 + 2 = 4.000$, precise
$2 + 2$ always $= 4$, reproducible

C. Type I and Type II Errors

The classical literature, especially as related to statistical methodologies, frequently utilizes two terms that you will likely encounter. These terms, Type I error and Type II error, refer to incorrect conclusions that can be made after obtaining inaccurate results in experiments.

A Type I error is a false positive. A Type I error is also sometimes referred to as an alpha error. A Type I error arises when you accept the hypothesis based on an experimental result, when the experimental result

BOX 4

RANDOM ERROR AND SYSTEMATIC ERROR

Random error is one cause of false negative results, also known as a Type II Error. The presence of random error increases the noise in your data, but doesn't alter the arithmetic mean of the grouped data. This is illustrated by the two distributions shown in Panel A, which represent two different groups of samples that were drawn from an identical population. One group of samples (the narrower distribution) has a lower random error for the process used to generate them than the other (the wider distribution). Panel B illustrates bar graphs of data generated with a high degree of random error, leading to a false negative result. The stimulated group, in reality, is larger than the control, but the high random error in the measurement obscures this fact. This is referred to by statisticians as a Type II error.

Frequently, random error arises from uncontrolled variability in the assay system that is used to generate the raw data. For example, if you are measuring cAMP using a radioimmunoassay there will be a certain amount of random error introduced by the multiple pipetting steps involved in preparing and quantitating each sample.

You can reduce random error by performing multiple replicate determinations for each sample, and averaging the replicates to derive a single data point to describe that sample. This allows you to average out the error arising from each single determination, and decreases the overall noise due to the assay system *per se*. Standard statistical tests allow you to use the standard error of the mean (SEM) to describe the overall pooled data if you use multiple replications for determining the value of each single data point. The SEM is a lower value than the standard deviation (SEM = standard deviation divided by the square root of n, the number of data points averaged together), in recognition of the reduced random error associated with the determinations.

Systematic error is one cause of false positive results, also known as a Type I error. Systematic error can also be referred to as *bias*. The presence of systematic error leads to an inaccurate overall conclusion, because you have sampled the control and the experimental groups in an inconsistent fashion for some reason. For example, say you are taking samples from two separate populations (control and experimental) which in reality are not different from each other, but are consistently sampled differently from

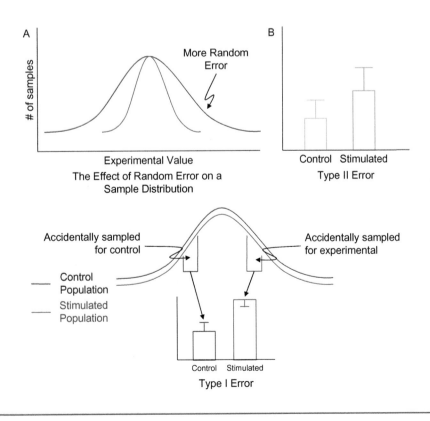

Continued

BOX 4 —cont'd

RANDOM ERROR AND SYSTEMATIC ERROR

each other. As illustrated in Figure B, systematic error can give you results that have an *apparent* difference in arithmetic mean, when in fact the two groups are not different.

Systematic error typically arises in behavioral experiments, for example, when the raw data are generated by direct human observation and scoring of the task that the experimental animals are performing. The experimenter (observer) may unconsciously skew the data by having an anticipated experimental result already in mind, thereby biasing their perception of the behavior of the test subjects. In behavioral experiments where humans are the subjects, even the subject may bias the outcome by altering their behavior in accordance with what they think is supposed to happen.

Human bias of this sort is the rule rather than the exception. The placebo effect, wherein human subjects alter their behavior because they think they have been given a drug or other treatment, is one of the most robust behavioral phenomena ever reported. Given the number of times placebos have been used as controls in human drug testing, the placebo effect is likely the most highly replicated behavioral result ever published.

The ubiquity of human bias means that it needs to be controlled for wherever possible. This is accomplished by "blinding" the experimental observer and/or the subjects to which group is the control and which group is the experimental. The observer should always be blinded in animal behavioral experiments if there is any subjectivity to the behavioral scoring. In experiments with human subjects, a single-blind experiment is one in which the subjects do not know whether they are controls or experimentals. In double-blind experiments neither the human subjects nor the observers know which individuals are controls or experimentals. In the occasional triple-blind experiment, neither the subjects, observers, nor the statisticians analyzing the data know which groups are which. In my laboratory we sometimes perform the quadruple-blind experiment, where nobody knows what's going on. This is also known as "losing the @!&*#^ piece of paper with the secret code."

---

is in fact attributable to chance. Using our example hypothesis of A→B→C, your experimental results in the measure experiment might indicate that B is activated, when in reality it is not. How might this situation arise? When you assay for B in response to A, B might appear to increase because you have a *systematic error* (see Box 4), such that your measurement of B is inaccurate and artificially high.

One sobering consideration is that no matter what, if you set your test of statistical significance at p <0.05, Type I errors will happen to you about 1 out of 20 times. In other words, at p = 0.05, five percent of the time your test will say that you have an effect when in reality you do not. This is pretty scary when you consider how many experiments you might be involved in across your entire career.

Overall, then, how frequently you make a Type I error will depend on the accuracy of your assay system(s), that is, whether they are subject to systematic error, and the stringency of your statistical tests.

A Type II error is a false negative, and this is also referred to as a beta error. A Type II error arises, for example, when your experiments are not detecting a difference when there actually is one. Specifically, for our A→B→C hypothesis, your measure experiment to assess whether A causes B might not detect an increase in B when it fact one was really there. This can arise if there is so much noise in your assay (random error, see Box 4) that you don't detect a difference when there really is one. How frequently this happens will depend on the accuracy and reproducibility of your assay system

VI. SUMMARY

The theme of this chapter has been the basics of hypothesis testing. We covered, in an abstract sense, the four fundamental types of experiments that one has available for testing various predictions of a hypothesis. These basic experimental types are referred to many, many times throughout this book. While we discussed them specifically as pertains to studies of learning and memory and their attendant cellular and molecular mechanisms, mastery of the basic concepts of hypothesis testing is crucial for students, whatever their ultimate field of endeavor. Working through their application in the context of learning and memory will undoubtedly be useful as a mental exercise, helpful beyond the specifics of their application to any one scientific subdiscipline.

BOX 5

HUMAN CLINICAL STUDIES

This appendix, and *Mechanisms of Memory* overall, focuses on studies using non-human subjects, and I will not address the design of clinical therapeutic studies using human patients at all. However, there are some terms widely used in designing clinical and pharmaceutical studies that I feel are useful to introduce at this point. This will provide you with some basic terminology that you can use if you ever need to venture into this literature. More importantly, how are you going to know which Big Pharma and Biotech Start-up stocks to buy if you can't read a stock prospectus and company annual report?

The gold standard of experimental design for human clinical testing is the randomized, double-blind, placebo-controlled study. "Randomized" simply means that individuals in the patient population are randomly assigned to control or experimental groups, therefore avoiding bias in the distribution of test subjects. The term double-blind is covered in Box 4, and "placebo-controlled" means that there is a control group that takes an inactive pill (or injection, etc.) physically indistinguishable from the real drug under study. In many cases the design of clinically based studies is limited by legitimate ethical concerns about the use of human patients. For example, it is almost always inappropriate to take a patient off a known effective therapy in order to assign them to a placebo group.

Preclinical studies are *in vitro* and animal tests that comprise the body of evidence (typically quite large) supporting the idea that the drug will be a reasonably safe and useful treatment for a human disorder. Preclinical studies typically test the safety, efficacy, potency, and pharmacokinetics of the drug under study, in healthy control animals and animal models of the disease of interest.

Phase 0 testing is the first time the drug enters a human. These are simple experiments to get the initial estimates of the human pharmacokinetics (drug half-life, tissue distribution, etc.) and human tolerability of the drug. These studies usually involve single doses and small numbers of healthy human subjects.

Phase I testing usually also involves healthy human subjects, although in some cases where no known treatment exists for a disorder, patients may be used at this stage as well. Phase I testing usually occurs with the subjects staying in a medical clinic in case any significant and unanticipated medical problems arise due to the drug under study. Phase I testing evaluates larger numbers of subjects, and is the initial evaluation of the pharmacologic effects of the drug and a more careful analysis of the pharmacokinetics. The pharmacokinetics of the drug will determine the necessary dosing schedule, etc.

Phase II testing utilizes even larger groups of subjects, and a more comprehensive safety and toxicology assessment of the drug. The numbers of subjects at this stage are large enough that the less-frequent drug side-effects will begin to show up. This principal distinction of Phase II testing, however, is that this is usually the first stage where the effectiveness of the drug for the clinical condition begins to be evaluated. In other words, this is typically the first time the experiment is intended to see if the drug actually leads to a clinical improvement in patients.

Phase III testing involves very large, randomized groups of patients and a comparison of the experimental drug to the best currently available clinical treatment. This is the last phase of testing before the drug is submitted for approval to the Food and Drug Administration (FDA), in the United States at least. If the drug is effective in Phase III testing, this serves as the basis for requesting approval from the FDA to take the drug to market.

Phase IV is what happens after the drug hits the market and begins to be put into whole populations of humans, under relatively uncontrolled circumstances. Phase IV is post-marketing monitoring, to look for the occurrence of rare side-effects and to look at the general tolerability and safety of the drug.

References

1. Sweatt, J. D. (1999). "Toward a molecular explanation for long-term potentiation". *Learn Mem.* 6:399–416.
2. Silva, A. J. (2007). "The science of research: the principles underlying the discovery of cognitive and other biological mechanisms". *J. Physiol. (Paris)* 101:203–213.
3. Byrne, J. H., and Kandel, E. R. (1996). "Presynaptic facilitation revisited: state and time dependence". *J. Neurosci.* 16:425–435.
4. Kandel, E. R. (2004). "Nobel Lecture: The molecular biology of memory storage: a dialog between genes and synapses". *Biosci. Rep.* 24:475–522.
5. Hein, L. (2006). "Adrenoceptors and signal transduction in neurons". *Cell Tissue Res.* 326:541–551.

6. Gibbs, M. E., and Summers, R. J. (2002). "Role of adrenoceptor subtypes in memory consolidation". *Prog. Neurobiol.* 67:345–391.

7. McGaugh, J. L. (2006). "Make mild moments memorable: add a little arousal". *Trends Cogn. Sci.* 10:345–347.

8. Ramos, B. P., and Arnsten, A. F. (2007). "Adrenergic pharmacology and cognition: focus on the prefrontal cortex". *Pharmacol. Ther.* 113(3):523–536.

9. Lorincz, A., and Buzsaki, G. (2000). "Two-phase computational model training long-term memories in the entorhinal-hippocampal region". *Ann. NY Acad. Sci. (Review)* 911:83–111.

10. Smolen, P., Baxter, D. A., and Byrne, J. H. (2006). "A model of the roles of essential kinases in the induction and expression of late long-term potentiation". *Biophys. J.* 90:2760–2775.

11. Medina, J. F., Garcia, K. S., and Mauk, M. D. (2001). "A mechanism for savings in the cerebellum". *J. Neurosci.* 21:4081–4089.

12. Cook, E. P., and Johnston, D. (1997). "Active dendrites reduce location-dependent variability of synaptic input trains". *J. Neurophysiol.* 78:2116–2128.

Index

Printed and bound by CPI Group (UK) Ltd, Croydon, CR0 4YY

03/10/2024

01040316-0011